Documentation for Health Records

**Cheryl Gregg Fahrenholz, RHIA, CCS-P,
and Ruthann Russo, PhD, MPH, RHIT**
Editors

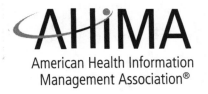

AHIMA
American Health Information
Management Association®

ISBN: 978-1-58426-262-6
AHIMA Product No.: AB100710

AHIMA Staff:
Jessica Block, MA, Assistant Editor
Claire Blondeau, MBA, Managing Editor
June E. Bronnert, RHIA, CCS, CCS-P, Director of Professional Practice Resources
Katie Greenock, MS, Editorial and Production Coordinator
Jason O. Malley, Director, Creative Content Development
Diana M. Warner, MS, RHIA, CHPS, FAHIMA, Manager, Professional Practice Resources
Lou A. Wiedemann, MS, RHIA, CPEHR, FAHIMA, Director of Professional Practice Resources

The websites listed in this book were current and valid as of the date of publication. However, webpage addresses and the information on them may change at any time. The user is encouraged to perform his or her own general web searches to locate any site addresses listed here that are no longer valid.

For more information, including updates, about AHIMA Press publications, visit http://www.ahima.org/publications/updates.aspx.

This book was previously published as *Documentation for Medical Records*, Chicago: AHIMA ©2009.

American Health Information Management Association
233 North Michigan Avenue, 21st Floor
Chicago, Illinois 60601-5809
ahima.org

Brief Contents

Part I	**Clinical Documentation and the Healthcare Delivery System**	**1**

Part II	**Utilization of the Healthcare Record**	**71**

Detail Contents

About the Editors

Cheryl Gregg Fahrenholz, RHIA, CCS-P, is the president of Preferred Healthcare Solutions, LLC and has more than 25 years of experience working with healthcare facilities, providers, and their staff. Her consulting services include revenue cycle performance improvement, documentation and coding audits, operational assessments, charge description master reviews, coding sessions for physician and staff, denial audits, risk and sanction analysis, compliance plan evaluations, electronic health record selection and implementation, expert testimony and defense work, along with interim and retainer professional support and customized project work.

Before establishing her own consulting firm in 1998, Gregg Fahrenholz served as the Director of Documentation, Coding and Reimbursement at the Primary Care Networks of Premier Health Network and as the Manager of Information Management at Miami Valley Hospital. Gregg Fahrenholz holds a B.S. in health information management (HIM) from Bowling Green State University. She is a nationally recognized speaker on the topics of revenue cycle, documentation, coding, and compliance. She has many publications at the national level.

Ruthann Russo, PhD, MPH, RHIT, is the chief executive officer of Cimex Health in Santa Monica, CA. She has worked in the health information management arena since 1980, spending time in a variety of areas including quality assurance, HIM, academics, and consulting. She has founded two successful, award-winning consulting firms and currently is a faculty member teaching complementary and integrative medicine and the director of clinical affiliations and the community connections program for tri-state college of Acupuncture in New York City. She is also managing director with Navigant Consulting's Healthcare Group.

Dr. Russo is the author of nine books and many articles, papers, and presentations on topics spanning the HIM, healthcare, and management disciplines. She has written scripts for and appeared in several video presentations on clinical documentation improvement, reimbursement, and HIM compliance, appeared on radio programs, and participated in several audio conferences for AHIMA and other healthcare organizations. Dr. Russo received her BA from Dickinson College, her JD from American University, her MPH from the Robert Wood Johnson Medical School/University of Medicine & Dentistry of New Jersey, and her PhD from Touro University.

About the Chapter Contributors

Ella L. James, MS, RHIT, CPHQ, is director of corporate health information management and health information security and the privacy officer at Hospital for Special Care in New Britain, Connecticut. James is past president of and twice sat on the board of directors for the Connecticut HIMA and is an AHIMA Community of Practice (CoP) facilitator for long-term care. She chairs the coding committee for the National Association of Long Term Hospitals (NALTH). James has presented programs on HIPAA at the state, regional, and national levels, and has presented educational programs for coders and physicians on long-term acute-care coding for NALTH. She consults on coding and documentation issues for many long-term acute-care hospitals through NALTH. She is the author of *Documentation and Reimbursement for Long-Term Care* and contributing author of the AHIMA publication *Health Information Management Compliance*.

Kathy Munn, RHIA, is the Privacy Officer and Director of Client Records for Mental Health Mental Retardation of Tarrant County in Fort Worth, Texas. She has spent her career in home health, public health, and behavioral health care and continues to consult for long-term care and other community-based services. Munn has spoken on HIM topics for local, regional, and national organizations. She has supported her profession by mentoring many HIM students as an internship instructor and serves as Chair of the HIT Advisory Committee for Tarrant County College.

Susan Rossiter, RHIA, is the operation manager of the HIM Department for 35 university clinics at University of Texas Southwestern Medical Center in Dallas, Texas. Prior to that, she was the Hospital Compliance Officer for Terrell State Hospital and has several years experience in management of HIM departments for acute care, behavioral health and ambulatory care organizations. Rossiter graduated with honors from Texas Woman's University, where she received the Outstanding Senior Student in the State award from the Texas Medical Record Association and the Dallas Outstanding Senior Student award from Texas Woman's University. As chair for the Executive Women in Texas Government, Dallas Affiliate, she supports and promotes women in leadership service to the state of Texas.

Diana M. Warner, MA, RHIA, CHPS, FAHIMA, is a professional practice resources manager with AHIMA. In her role, Warner provides professional expertise on health information management (HIM) practice issues. Her areas of expertise include the management and implementation of electronic health records (EHRs), privacy and confidentiality, and HIM practices in physician practices. She provides her expertise to AHIMA members, the media, and outside organizations through articles publications, and presentations. Warner has more than 20 years of experience in HIM, working in various healthcare settings including physician practice and acute care hospitals. Prior to joining AHIMA in 2009, she was employed as director of HIM at a large academic physician's group, where she participated in the implementation of an EHR. Warner was responsible for the management of the EHR, the paper medical record, and multiple electronic environments. She was also responsible for implementing the organization's privacy and security program.

Margaret J. White, MS, NHA, RHIA, CPHQ, has 30 years experience in the healthcare industry with the last 15 years in long-term care. She is a co-chair of AHIMA's Long-Term Care Practice Council and is co-chair of the Special Interest Council of the Ohio Health Information Management Association. She is on the Ohio Health Information Partnership Advisory Board representing OHIMA and post-acute care and is participating on the adoption and exchange of health information subcommittees. White also serves on the HISPC project steering committee for Ohio as well as being involved in the various working groups representing health information management and post-acute care. Additionally, White is an adjunct faculty member for several HIT programs. White is the assistant licensed nursing home administrator for Columbus Colony Elderly Care of Westerville, Ohio, the only facility in the country "for the deaf, by the deaf."

About the Instructor Manual Contributors

Heather Greene, MBA, RHIA, is a health information technology program coordinator at Bluegrass Community & Technical College in Lexington, KY, where she teaches courses on coding and compliance. She is also a coding and documentation consultant with Kraft Healthcare Consultants. Greene earned her master of business administration from Midway College and her bachelor of science in health information management from Eastern Kentucky University. In addition, Greene is an AHIMA-approved ICD-10 CM/PCS Trainer.

Shanna M. Jones, MPA, RHIA, CCS, currently works as a health information management director at an acute care hospital and rehabilitation center. She is also an adjunct instructor and course author in various HIM/HIT related courses. She has previously worked as a coder and coding coordinator at various hospitals. In a volunteer role, she mentors students from various accredited HIT/HIM programs. She holds a master of public administration degree with a major in Health Services Administration. Her bachelor's degree is from Florida A & M University, and she is also a certified coding specialist.

Karen M. Karban, RHIT, CCS, is the Director of Operations for the HIM Services division of a national technology and HIM consulting firm. Her past activities include development of coding education product lines, numerous audio-conferences on coding topics, serving as an adjunct instructor in Coding and Classification Systems in HIA/HIT programs and development of coding and documentation audit methodologies. She earned her RHIT via the AHIMA Independent Study Program, and is a certified coding specialist and an AHIMA-approved ICD-10-CM/PCS Trainer.

Introduction

Cheryl Gregg Fahrenholz, RHIA, CCS-P

Purpose of Health Record Documentation

The primary focus of a health record is documenting patient care and serving as a mechanism for sharing information about the patient with other healthcare providers. However, the documentation of healthcare is used in a myriad of other areas:

- Serves as the official business record for the provider and facility

- Used for billing and reimbursement

- Used for secondary data sources, such as registries

- Used in research

- Used in evaluation of the quality of care

- Used for internal and external review of quality of care

- Used in the reporting of communicable diseases

- Used for establishing healthcare policy and public health

When we talk about the purpose of the health record, we think about the documentation of care rendered to the patient, communication about the patient among providers, and the health record as the official business and legal record. While clinical documentation is highly important, over the decades, the health record has become the primary source of information for secondary uses such as clinical research, public health reporting, and fraud detection and deterrence. As legislative acts focusing on specific topics were passed, the administrative guidelines often reflected guidelines or requirements for the health record content. See table 1.

TABLE I.1. Selected milestones that shaped healthcare, the health information profession, and the health record

YEAR	MILESTONE
1798	An act was passed for the relief of sick and disabled seamen. This act established a federal network of hospitals for the care of merchant seamen, and was the forerunner of today's US Public Health Service (PHS).
1862	President Lincoln appointed a chemist, Charles M. Wetherill, to serve in the new Department of Agriculture. This was the beginning of the Bureau of Chemistry, forerunner to the Food and Drug Administration (FDA).
1871	The first supervising surgeon (now called surgeon general) was appointed for the Marine Hospital Service, which was organized the prior year.
1887	The federal government opened a one-room laboratory on Staten Island, NY, for research on disease, thereby planting the seed that grew into the National Institutes of Health (NIH).
1902	The Marine Hospital Service was converted into the Public Health and Marine Hospital Service in recognition of its expanding activities in the field of public health. In 1912, the name was shortened to the Public Health Service.
1906	Congress passed the Pure Food and Drugs Act, authorizing the government to monitor the purity of foods and the safety of medicines, now a responsibility of the FDA.
1910	Hospitals began to track every patient it treated long enough to determine whether the treatment was effective. If the treatment was not effective, the hospital would then attempt to determine why, so that similar cases could be treated successfully in the future.
1921	The Bureau of Indian Affairs Health Division was created, the forerunner to the Indian Health Service.
1928	The Association of Record Librarians of North America was created. This organization is now the American Health Information Management Association (AHIMA).
1930	The National Institute (later renamed Institutes) of Health was created out of the Public Health Service's Hygienic Laboratory.
1935	The Social Security Act passed.
1938	The Federal Food, Drug, and Cosmetic Act passed.
1939	The Federal Security Agency was created, bringing together related federal activities in the fields of health, education, and social insurance.
1946	The Communicable Disease Center was established, forerunner of the Centers for Disease Control and Prevention (CDC).
1951	The American College of Physicians (ACP), the American Hospital Association (AHA), the American Medical Association (AMA), and the Canadian Medical Association (CMA) joined with the American College of Surgeons (ACS) to create the Joint Commission on Accreditation of Hospitals (JCAHO, later renamed The Joint Commission), an independent, not-for-profit organization whose primary purpose is to provide voluntary accreditation.
1955	The Salk polio vaccine was licensed. The Indian Health Service was transferred to the Department of Health and Human Services (HHS) from the Department of Interior.
1961	The first White House Conference on Aging was held.
1962	The Migrant Health Act passed, providing support for clinics serving agricultural workers.

YEAR	MILESTONE
1964	The first Surgeon General's Report on Smoking and Health was released.
1965	The Medicare and Medicaid programs were created, making comprehensive healthcare available to millions of Americans.
	The Older Americans Act created the nutritional and social programs administered by HHS' Administration on Aging.
	The Head Start program was created.
1966	Led by the U.S. Public Health Service, the International Smallpox Eradication program was established. The worldwide eradication of smallpox was accomplished in 1977.
	The Community Health Center and Migrant Health Center programs were launched.
1970	The National Health Service Corps was created.
	The Association of Record Librarians became the American Medical Record Association (AMRA), which is now AHIMA.
1971	The National Cancer Act was signed into law.
1977	The Health Care Financing Administration (HCFA) was created to manage Medicare and Medicaid separately from the Social Security Administration.
1980	The federal government began funding to states for foster care and adoption assistance.
1981	Acquired immunodeficiency syndrome (AIDS) was identified in the United States. In 1984, the human immunodeficiency virus (HIV) was identified by PHS and French scientists. In 1985, a blood test to detect HIV was licensed.
1982	Congress mandated the development of a prospective payment system (PPS) to efficiently manage healthcare costs. This system is a per-case reimbursement mechanism in which inpatient admissions are divided into relatively homogeneous categories called diagnosis-related groups (DRGs).
1984	The National Organ Transplantation Act was signed into law.
1989	The Agency for Health Care Policy and Research (now the Agency for Healthcare Research and Quality [AHRQ]) was created.
1990	The Human Genome Project was established.
	The Nutrition Labeling and Education Act was passed, authorizing packaged food labeling.
	The Ryan White Comprehensive AIDS Resource Emergency (CARE) Act began providing support for people with AIDS.
1991	AMRA became AHIMA.
1996	Welfare reform was enacted under the Personal Responsibility and Work Opportunity Reconciliation Act.
	The Health Insurance Portability and Accountability Act (HIPAA) was enacted.
1997	The State Children's Health Insurance Program (SCHIP) was created, enabling states to extend health coverage to more uninsured children.
2000	The human genome sequencing was published.
2001	The Centers for Medicare & Medicaid (CMS) was created, replacing HCFA.
	HHS responds to the nation's first bioterrorism attack—the delivery of anthrax through the mail.

TABLE I.1. (continued)

2002	The Office of Public Health Emergency Preparedness was created to coordinate efforts against bioterrorism and other emergency health threats.
2004	The Office of the National Coordinator for Health Information Technology (ONCHIT, now abbreviated ONC) was created.
2009	The American Recovery and Reinvestment Act (ARRA) of 2009 was passed. This act includes the Health Information Technology for Economic and Clinical Health Act (HITECH Act) of 2009, which includes components that define Medicare and Medicaid incentive payments; introduces meaningful use for certified electronic health records (EHRs); and addresses confidentiality, privacy and security standards.
2010	The Health Care reform bill passed.
2013	International Classification of Diseases, 10th Edition, Clinical Modification/Procedure Coding System (ICD-10-CM/PCS) is implemented in the United States.

Source: HHS n.d.

Evolution of Healthcare Settings Over a Lifetime

Traditionally, the health information profession centered on hospitals, but as patient care expanded to other levels of care, there has been an expanded arena for employment. The evolution of healthcare settings changes during the life span of a patient. As patient care needs shift, healthcare services are provided in different settings. Figure I.1 displays the life span for the patient's continuum of care.

FIGURE I.1. Continuum of care from birth to death

TYPE OF FACILITY/CARE	DESCRIPTION
Birthing center (Excluding hospital maternity facilities and provider offices)	Provides a natural birth experience (labor, delivery, and post-partum care) along with immediate care of newborns
Acute care hospital (Including correctional, Indian Health Services, military, and tribal facilities)	Treatment of brief but severe episode of illness, for conditions that are the result of symptoms, disease, trauma, or recovery from surgery
Provider office (Including correctional, Indian Health Services, military, and tribal facilities)	Primary care, specialty care, and medical home care in an outpatient setting
Retail health clinic	Primary care services provided in a walk-in clinic located within a retail operation
Urgent care	Treatment for non-life threatening illnesses and injuries, typically open seven days a week with hours extending into the evening for unscheduled care requiring immediate attention
Emergency care	Medical–surgical care for injuries or illnesses that could be life threatening or disabling if not treated immediately

TYPE OF FACILITY/CARE	DESCRIPTION
Ambulatory care (freestanding or hospital based, physician offices, group practices, private clinics, community-based clinics, rural health clinics and hospital-based outpatient departments)	Preventive, diagnostic, and therapeutic services provided on a nonresidential basis
Ambulatory surgery center	Surgical and diagnostic medical services provided in a freestanding facility (other than a physician office)
Specialty hospital (long-term care hospitals certified as acute-care hospitals)	Medical care provided to individuals who are clinically complex with multiple acute and chronic conditions requiring an average length of stay greater than 25 days
Behavioral health (dedicated units in acute-care hospitals, psychiatric hospitals, partial hospitalization facilities, intermediate care facilities, residential substance abuse treatment facilities, psychiatric residential treatment center, community-based clinics, physician offices)	Psychiatric and psychological care provided to address mental disorders, developmental disorders, and substance-abuse disorders
End stage renal disease treatment facility	Outpatient treatment facility that provides dialysis treatment, maintenance, and self-care training
Rehabilitative services (dedicated rehabilitation hospitals, community-based facilities, patients' homes, hospital-based outpatient departments)	Therapeutic medical services (speech, physical, and occupational therapy) provided to patients who have been disabled by injuries or illnesses, with the goal of helping patients recover as much function as possible
Health homecare	Medical and/or personal care provided to individuals and families in their place of residence with the goal of promoting, maintaining, or restoring health or minimizing the effects of disabilities and illnesses, including terminal illnesses
Assisted living (residential care, adult living facilities, personal care, board and care, domiciliary care, adult foster care, supported care, retirement residences, custoIdial care)	Facilities that provide assistance with activities of daily living
Skilled nursing facility	Medical, nursing, social and rehabilitative services for persons that require 24-hour nursing care and supervision
Hospice	Palliative and supportive care for terminal conditions where life expectancy is six months or less

Healthcare Statistics Across the Spectrum

The public's increased awareness and involvement in their personal healthcare has resulted in more active communications between patients and their healthcare providers. Whether the communication occurs during a face-to-face service or remotely with the assistance of electronic media, such as e-mail or by phone, the patient is more educated, and many patients come prepared with information that they have read or downloaded from the Internet. Following are recent statistics related to various settings.

Ambulatory care

- Percent of all adults in the United States that have looked for health or medical information on the Internet: 61% (NCHS 2011)

- Percent of adults who had contact with a healthcare professional in the past year: 86% (Pleis, Ward, and Lucas 2010)

- Percent of children who had contact with a healthcare professional in the past year: 91% (Bloom, Cohen, and Freeman 2010)

- Number of physician office visits: 994 million (Hsiao, Cherry, Beatty, and Rechtsteiner 2010)

Emergency department visits (Niska, R., F. Bhuiya, and J. Xu 2010)

- Number of visits: 116.8 million

- Number of injury-related visits: 39.4 million

- Most commonly diagnosed condition: heart disease

- Percent of visits with patient seen in fewer than 15 minutes: 17.8%

- Percent of visits resulting in hospital admission: 12.5%

Hospital inpatient care (Hall, DeFrances, Williams, Golosinskiy, and Schwartzman 2010)

- Number of discharges: 34.4 million

- Discharges per 10,000 population: 1,143.9

- Average length of stay in days: 4.8

- Number of procedures performed: 44.9 million

Importance of Health Information Documentation

The history of health information is closely aligned with the development of medicine, with the earliest medical records traced to the walls of Paleolithic caverns in Spain, about 25,000 BCE. St. Bartholomew's Hospital, London, England, founded in 1123, still has some records of its original patient records. In the 1500s, "The Ordres and Ordinances for the Better Government of the Hospital of Bartholomew the Lesse" addressed the privacy of records as well as the importance of health documentation. Prior to the 20th century, teaching hospitals were keeping records, but it was not until 1905 that physicians began to recognize the value and necessity of appropriate medical records relative to reference for future care and medico legal reasons (Huffman 1976).

Reform movements that began during the late nineteenth century improved the overall quality of medical care in the United States. Specific quality improvement efforts directed at medical school training and hospital care helped improve overall quality. The new, more scientific approach to medicine set the stage for unprecedented advances in biomedicine that were under way at the turn of the twentieth century. Organized efforts among healthcare reformers and private foundations led to the standardization of hospital care, and many private hospitals were established. Care in the new, privately funded hospitals, however, was available only to those who could pay for the services, and underfunded public and charity hospitals continued to serve the poor and indigent.

The development of modern surgical techniques and new pharmaceuticals, as well as the more widespread use of antibiotics after World War II, created an even greater demand for hospital care. As a result, the late 1940s and 1950s saw a hospital-building boom.

Until the late 1980s, hospitals continued to provide most of the diagnostic and therapeutic healthcare services in the United States. Long hospital stays were the norm rather than the exception. Patients usually stayed in the same hospital facility from the time they were admitted for diagnostic testing, through their treatment, until they were well enough to care for themselves at home. Prior to the development of endoscopic and laser surgery, many routine surgical procedures involved long periods of recovery with weeks or even months of professional nursing and follow-up care. Hospitals provided most of that care, and hospitals became places where terminally ill patients went to spend the last days of their lives.

After World War II, employers began offering health insurance coverage to employees and their dependents. This benefited workers and their families because it provided more access to healthcare services and hospital care. However, due to rising costs, many Americans were still unable to pay for healthcare services. As a result, an amendment in 1965 to the Social Security Act established two federal programs, Medicare and Medicaid, to provide health insurance coverage to the aged and poor populations, respectively. With the implementation of Medicare and Medicaid, these federal programs played a pivotal role in the US government becoming the largest payer for healthcare services.

The last decades of the twentieth century brought another wave of revolutionary advances in the biomedical sciences. The development of new pharmaceutical treatments has made it possible for patients with chronic illnesses to stay healthy longer and to postpone or avoid debilitating complications. Developments in surgical technology and anesthesia have shortened surgical recovery times dramatically. Today, many routine surgeries that once meant lengthy hospitalizations now require patients to spend only a few hours or days in the hospital while improving the quality of care provided. Organ transplantations that were innovative just a few years ago have become almost commonplace. Many transplant patients now go home in a matter of days rather than weeks or months after surgery.

Career Opportunities

You have entered the world of health information management and health informatics, and the good news is employment in this area is expected to grow much faster than average. According to the Bureau of Labor Occupational Outlook, 2010-11, job prospects should be very good; technicians with a strong understanding of technology and computer software will be in particularly high demand. Employment of medical records and health information technicians is expected to increase by 20 percent, much faster than the average for all occupations through 2018. In addition, with the increasing use of electronic health records (EHRs), more technicians will be needed to complete the new responsibilities associated with electronic data management. The increasing use of EHRs will continue to broaden and alter the job responsibilities of health information technicians. For example, technicians must be familiar with EHR computer software, maintaining EHR security, and analyzing electronic data to improve healthcare information. Health information technicians use EHR software to maintain data on patient safety, patterns of disease, and disease treatment and outcome. Technicians also may assist with improving EHR software usability and may contribute to the development and maintenance of health information networks (Bureau of Labor Statistics Occupational Outlook 2009).

Salary Information

As documented in the American Health Information Management Association's 2010 Salary Survey, the work force continues to diversify in the setting that health information management (HIM) professionals work. Although the number of settings has increased, the majority (52 percent) of HIM professionals remain in the acute-care hospital setting. See figure I.2 for the diversity of settings for HIM professionals.

Just as in other professions, the base salaries change from year to year. For HIM professionals, that variation is also dependent upon the setting and job level. The average overall salary in 2010 was $59.935 (AHIMA 2010, 4). Figure I.3 displays the average salaries for 2010 by job setting, and figure I.4 illustrates to differences in HIM salaries by the job level.

FIGURE I.2. HIM job settings

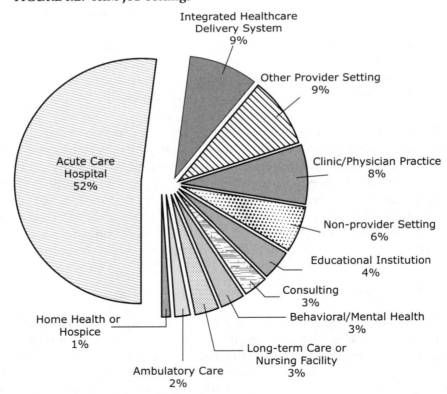

Source: AHIMA 2010, 2.

FIGURE I.3. Average salary by job setting

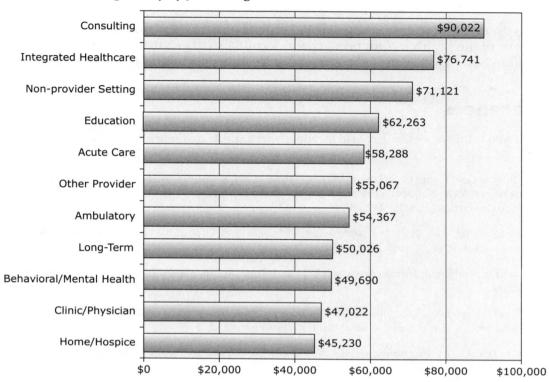

Source: AHIMA 2010, 4.

FIGURE I.4. Average salary by gob level

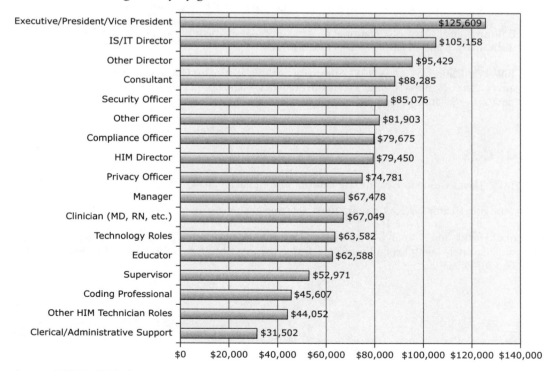

Source: AHIMA 2010, 6.

Summary

This book will address healthcare delivery in the United States, clinical documentation, functions of the health record, primary and secondary data sources, health record documentation best practices, accreditation and regulations, and the continuum of care.

References

AHIMA. 2010 Salary Survey. Chicago: AHIMA. https://ahima.enetrix.com/psitep/%21stmenu_template. main.

Bloom, B., R.A. Cohen, and G. Freeman. 2010. Summary health statistics for U.S. children: National health interview survey, 2009. National Center for Health Statistics. *Vital Health Statistics* 10(247). http://www.cdc .gov/nchs/data/series/sr_10/sr10_247.pdf.

Bureau of Labor Statistics. 2010. *Occupational Outlook Handbook (OOH)*, 2010–11 ed. Washington, DC: US Department of Labor. http://www.bls.gov/oco/.

Department of Health and Human Services (HHS). n.d. Historical highlights. http://www.hhs.gov/about/ hhshist.html.

Hall, M.J., C.J. DeFrances, S.N. Williams, A. Golosinskiy, and A. Schwartzman. 2010. National hospital discharge survey: 2007 summary. *National Health Statistics Reports* (29).

Hsiao, C.J., D.K. Cherry, P.C. Beatty, and E.A. Rechtsteiner. 2010. National ambulatory medical care survey: 2007 Summary. *National Health Statistics Reports* (27).

Huffman, E.K. 1976. *Medical Record Management*. Berwyn, IL: Physicians' Record Co.

National Center for Health Statistics. 2011. NCHS data brief number 66: Use of the Internet for health information: United States, 2009. http://www.cdc.gov/nchs/data/databriefs/db66.htm.

Niska, R., F. Bhuiya, and J. Xu. 2010. National hospital ambulatory medical care survey: 2007 emergency department summary. *National Health Statistics Reports* (26).

Pleis, J.R., B.W. Ward, and J.W. Lucas. 2010. Summary health statistics for U.S. adults: National health interview survey, 2009. National Center for Health Statistics. *Vital Health Statistics* 10(249). http://www.cdc .gov/nchs/data/series/sr_10/sr10_249.pdf.

Resources

Barry, P. 2010. A User's Guide to Health Care Reform. *AARP Bulletin*. 51(4):19–26.

Center for Studying Health System Change. 2003. Tracking health care costs. *Data Bulletin* 25:1–2.

Department of Health and Human Services. 2011. Centers for Medicare and Medicaid National Health Expenditures. National Health Expenditure Data. http://www.cms.hhs.gov/NationalHealthExpendData/01_ Overview.asp#TopOfPage.

PART I

Clinical Documentation and the Healthcare Delivery System

Chapter 1

Healthcare Delivery

Cheryl Gregg Fahrenholz, RHIA, CCS-P

Learning Objectives

- Outline the basic structure of the US healthcare delivery system
- Explain the significance of recent trends in healthcare delivery
- Distinguish between inpatients and outpatients
- Explain the concept of continuum of care
- Present the model of the patient-centered medical home
- Describe healthcare's migration to the electronic health record
- Explain current challenges of the hybrid health record
- Describe the use of personal health records
- Explain the role health information exchange plays in improving healthcare

Key Terms

Accreditation

Acute care

Ambulatory care

American College of Surgeons (ACS)

American Recovery and Reinvestment Act (ARRA)

Behavioral healthcare

Comorbidities

Complications

Continuum of care

Diagnosis-related group (DRG)

Electronic health record (EHR)

Emergency and trauma care

Health Care and Education Reconciliation Act

Health information exchange (HIE)

Health Information Technology for Economic and Clinical Health Act (HITECH)

Health Insurance Portability and Accountability Act (HIPAA)

Healthcare Quality Improvement Act

Home healthcare

Hospice care

Hospitalist

Hybrid health record

Inpatient

Integrated healthcare network

The Joint Commission

Joint Commission on Accreditation of Healthcare Organizations (JCAHO)

Joint Commission on Accreditation of Hospitals (JCAH)

Long-term acute care

Long-term care

Major diagnostic category (MDC)

Medicaid

Medical specialties

Medicare

Medicare severity-diagnosis related groups (MS-DRGs)

Mental Health Parity Act (MHPA)

National Health Information Network (NHIN)

National Quality Forum (NQF)

Office for Civil Rights (OCR)

Office of the National Coordinator for Health Information Technology (ONC)

Omnibus Budget Reconciliation Act (OBRA)

Outpatient

Patient-centered medical home (PCMH)

Patient Protection and Affordable Care Act (PPACA)

Peer Review Act

Personal health record (PHR)

Primary care

Prospective Payment Act

Protected health information (PHI)

Regional health information organization (RHIO)

Rehabilitation care

Secondary care

Skilled nursing care

Subacute care

Surgical specialties

Tax Equity and Fiscal Responsibility Act of 1982 (TEFRA)

Tertiary care

Tethered record

Untethered record

Introduction

In colonial America, many communities opened public hospitals to care for the poor and isolate the sick. Until the twentieth century, most patients received medical care at home from physicians with little formal training. In remote areas of the new settlements, there was often little or no help available for the injured and sick, and the mortality rate among early settlers was very high.

Reform movements that began during the late nineteenth century improved the overall quality of medical care in the United States. Specific quality improvement efforts directed at medical school training and hospital care led to significant improvements. The new, more scientific approach to medicine set the stage for unprecedented advances in biomedicine at the turn of the twentieth century. The thrust for hospital reform guided the formation of the **American College of Surgeons (ACS)** in 1913. The ACS was instrumental in developing the Minimum Standards, a set of hospital standards that were used in 1918 to review the performance of 692 hospitals. Only eighty-nine hospitals fully met the Minimum Standards. As a result, the standards became the foundation of the Hospital Standardization Program, which directed the origin of the current day **accreditation** process (Cassidy 2010, 11).

The number of hospitals and hospital admissions increased dramatically during the early decades of the twentieth century. Organized efforts by healthcare reformers and private foundations led to the standardization of hospital care and the establishment of many private hospitals. Care in these hospitals, however, was available only to those who could pay for the services, and underfunded public and charity hospitals continued to serve the poor and indigent.

The development of modern surgical techniques and new pharmaceuticals, as well as the more widespread use of antibiotics after World War II, created an even greater demand for hospital care. As a result, the late 1940s and 1950s saw a hospital-building boom.

The ACS continued to guide the Hospital Standardization Program until 1952. The American College of Physicians (ACP), the American Medical Association (AMA), the American Hospital Association (AHA), and the Canadian Medical Association (CMA) joined forces in 1951 to create the **Joint Commission on Accreditation of Hospitals** (JCAH) and began performing the accreditation process in 1953, following the Standards for Hospital Accreditation. In 1965, Congress passed the Social Security Amendment, which aligned the accreditation process with the Medicare Conditions of Participation for Hospitals. This meant that hospitals accredited by JCAH automatically met the Medicare compliance requirements and were thus able to participate in Medicare and Medicaid programs. The JCAH began to accredit more nonhospital healthcare settings, and the name was changed in 1987 to the **Joint Commission on Accreditation of Healthcare Organizations (JCAHO)**. The organization is known today simply as **The Joint Commission**. Currently, acute care hospitals, critical access hospitals, long-term care, behavioral health care, ambulatory health care, home care, and laboratory services are accredited. The Joint Commission's mission is "to continuously improve health care for the public, in collaboration with other stakeholders, by evaluating health care organizations and inspiring them to excel in providing safe and effective care of the highest quality and value" (The Joint Commission 2011). See chapter 8 for more information on accreditation.

Until the late 1980s, hospitals continued to provide most of the diagnostic and therapeutic healthcare services in the United States. Long hospital stays were the norm rather than the exception. Patients usually stayed in the same hospital facility from the time they were admitted for diagnostic testing, through their treatment, until they were well enough to care for themselves at home. Prior to the development of endoscopic and laser surgery, many routine surgical procedures involved long periods of recovery with weeks or even months of professional nursing and follow-up care. Hospitals provided most of that care. Hospitals also became places where terminally ill patients spent the last days of their lives.

After World War II, employers began to offer health insurance coverage to employees and their dependents. This benefited workers and their families because it provided more access to healthcare services and hospital care. However, due to rising costs, many Americans were still unable to pay for healthcare services. A 1965 amendment to the Social Security Act established two federal programs, **Medicare** and **Medicaid,** to provide health insurance coverage to the aged and the poor. With the implementation of Medicare and Medicaid, the US government became the largest payer for healthcare services.

During the 1980s and 1990s, significant regulations were enacted to monitor the quality of care provided and the medical necessity of services. Some of those regulations included the **Peer Review Act** of 1982; the **Tax Equity and Fiscal Responsibility Act (TEFRA) of 1982**; the **Prospective Payment Act** of 1982; the **Omnibus Budget Reconciliation**

Acts **(OBRA)** of 1985, 1986, 1989, and 1990; the **Healthcare Quality Improvement Act** of 1986; the **Health Insurance Portability and Accountability (HIPAA) Act** of 1996; and the **Mental Health Parity Act (MHPA)** of 1996 (Cassidy 2010, 17–18).

The last decades of the twentieth century brought another wave of revolutionary advances in the biomedical sciences. The development of new pharmaceutical treatments has made it possible for patients with chronic illnesses to stay healthy longer and to postpone or avoid debilitating complications. Developments in surgical technology and anesthesia have dramatically shortened surgical recovery times. Today, many routine surgeries that once meant lengthy hospitalizations now require patients to spend only a few hours or days in the hospital. Organ transplantations that were innovative just a few years ago have become almost commonplace. Many transplant patients now go home in a matter of days rather than weeks or months after surgery.

Since colonial times, physicians and other healthcare providers have documented the customer services they provide, but increases in costs and in the complexity of healthcare delivery require progressively sophisticated documentation and data collection processes. Documentation of healthcare services and computerization of health record systems have become critical components of the services performed and affect the quality and efficiency of the national healthcare delivery system.

Modern Healthcare Delivery

The US healthcare delivery system is made up of thousands of independent providers and facilities that offer a bewildering array of health-related services. Providers are reimbursed for healthcare services through a complex system of private insurance plans, government-funded programs, and self-payments. The cost of medical–surgical care and pharmaceuticals has grown so much over recent years that many Americans who do not qualify for private or government-sponsored health insurance are unable to find affordable healthcare.

According to the US Census Bureau, the number of Americans with health insurance dropped between 1987 and 2009. (See **TABLE 1.1**.) In 2009, 50.6 million Americans were without health insurance coverage. The percentage of Americans who qualified for employer-based health coverage decreased from 58.5 percent in 2008 to 55.8 percent in 2009. At the same time, the number of people covered by government-sponsored health insurance programs continued to rise, and in 2009 this number was 30.6 percent (DeNavas-Walt, Proctor, and Smith 2011, 71). There is grave concern that the rapid enrollment increase in government-sponsored plans will cause the funds allotted to these plans to be depleted sooner than anticipated. The population is living longer, which contributes to the increase in Medicare enrollment, and legislation has been proposed that would expand the age and condition range for Medicaid eligibility. Healthcare is more expensive than ever, and economists worry about its impact on the nation's economic future.

Healthcare Providers and Facilities

Professional healthcare providers include the following:

- Physicians (doctors of medicine [MDs] or doctors of osteopathic medicine [DOs])
- Nurse practitioners (NPs)

TABLE 1.1. Health insurance coverage: 1987 to 2009[1]

YEAR	NUMBER	PERCENT
2009	50,674	16.7
2008	46,340	15.4
2007	45,657	15.3
2006	46,995	15.8
2005	44,815	15.3
2004	43,498	14.9
2003	43,404	15.1
2002	42,019	14.7
2001	39,760	14.1
2000	38,426	13.7
1999	38,767	14.0
1999	41,014	15.0
1998	42,943	15.8
1997	42,359	15.7
1996	41,093	15.4
1995	40,582	15.4
1994	39,718	15.2
1993	39,713	15.3
1992	38,641	15.0
1991	35,445	14.1
1990	34,719	13.9
1989	33,385	13.6
1988	32,680	13.4
1987	31,026	12.9

[1] Numbers in thousands. People as of March of the following year who are uninsured. For information on confidentiality protection, sampling error, nonsampling error, and definitions, see http://www.census.gov/apsd/techdoc/cps/cpsmar10.pdf.

Source: DeNavas-Walt, Proctor, and Smith 2011, 71.

- Certified nurse midwives (CNMs)

- Clinical nurse specialists (CNSs)

- Physician assistants (PAs)

- Licensed clinical psychologists (LCPs) and clinical social workers (CSWs)

- Physical, respiratory, speech, and occupational therapists (PTs, RTs, STs, OTs)

- Certified registered nurse anesthetists (CRNAs)

- Nurses (registered nurses [RNs] and licensed nurses [LPNs])

- Dentists (DDMs), registered dental assistants (RDAs), and registered dental hygienists (RDHs)

- Medical technologists (MTs) and cytotechnologists (CTs)

- Clinical nutritionists (CCNs) and certified diabetic educators (CDEs)

- Patient-care technicians (PCTs) and certified emergency paramedics (CEPs)

- Podiatrists (DMPs) and chiropractors (doctors of chiropractic [DCs])

- Medical assistants (MAs)

The innumerable public and private facilities in which healthcare services are provided include the following:

- Public and community hospitals operated by local governments

- Teaching hospitals affiliated with university medical schools

- Specialty hospitals dedicated to providing specialized services (for example, cardiology, behavioral health, and rehabilitation care)

- Private hospitals affiliated with religious organizations

- Private hospitals affiliated with for-profit corporations

- Private hospitals operated by nonprofit organizations

- Inpatient psychiatric hospitals, partial hospitalization programs, and psychiatric residential treatment centers

- Integrated healthcare networks (made up of hospitals, postacute care facilities, ambulatory care facilities, skilled nursing facilities, and physician practices operated by the same corporate entity)

- Physicians' offices, group practices, and private medical and school clinics

- Community-based clinics, public health departments, and homeless shelters

- Community mental health centers and intermediate care facilities for the mentally retarded

- Residential substance abuse treatment facilities

- Urgent care clinics

- Retail clinics

- Hospital-based and freestanding ambulatory, diagnostic, and surgical centers

- Hospital-based and freestanding ambulatory rehabilitation centers

- Hospital-based, freestanding, and mobile imaging centers

- Federally qualified health centers (FQHCs)

- Skilled nursing facilities

- Long-term care and assisted-care residential facilities

- Home healthcare and hospice care agencies

- Prisons and correctional institutions
- Facilities providing immediate care for the developmentally disabled

Healthcare Services

Generally, healthcare services are categorized according to the setting in which they are provided and/or the illness toward which they are directed. For example, **acute care** can be defined as the short-term medical and nursing care provided in an inpatient hospital setting to treat the acute phase of a patient's injury or illness. Following are descriptions of other broad categories of healthcare services.

- **Ambulatory care**: The surgical services or preventive, diagnostic, and therapeutic medical services provided on a nonresidential basis in healthcare practitioners' offices, group practices, private clinics, community-based clinics, school-based clinics, urgent care centers, retail clinics, hospital-based outpatient departments, and ambulatory surgery centers

- **Behavioral healthcare**: The psychiatric and/or psychological care provided to address mental disorders, developmental disorders, and substance abuse disorders; it is provided in a variety of settings, including dedicated units in acute care hospitals, psychiatric hospitals, community-based clinics, intermediate care facilities for the mentally retarded, residential treatment facilities, and physicians' offices

- **Emergency and trauma care**: The medical–surgical care provided to individuals whose injuries or illnesses require urgent care to address conditions that could be life threatening or disabling if not treated immediately; it is provided through a network of designated hospitals and emergency transportation systems

- **Home healthcare**: The medical and/or personal care provided to individuals and families in their place of residence with the goal of promoting, maintaining, or restoring health or minimizing the effects of disabilities and illnesses, including terminal illnesses

- **Hospice care**: The medical and/or personal care provided to individuals with life expectancies of six months or less who elect to receive palliative care in place of standard medical treatment for their illnesses; it is provided in patients' homes and in residential treatment facilities

- **Long-term acute care**: The medical care provided to individuals who are clinically complex and have multiple acute and chronic conditions requiring an average length of stay greater than 25 days in long-term care hospitals certified as acute care hospitals

- **Long-term care**: The medical and/or personal care services provided to chronically ill, aged, disabled, or mentally handicapped individuals who reside in dedicated nursing facilities on a permanent basis

- **Rehabilitation care**: The therapeutic medical services (speech, physical, and occupational therapy) it is provided to patients who have been disabled by injuries or illnesses; it is provided in dedicated rehabilitation hospitals, community-based facilities, patients' homes, and hospital-based outpatient departments with the goal of helping patients recover as much function as possible

- **Skilled nursing care**: The professional nursing care and related medical, therapeutic, psychosocial, and personal services provided in a residential setting to individuals recovering from injuries or illnesses or the residual effects of injuries or illnesses after the acute phase of the condition has resolved; it is sometimes called **subacute care**

Trends in Healthcare Delivery

Medical services provided in the United States are often described as the best in the world. Nonetheless, many critics of the US healthcare delivery system consider it too costly and inefficient. The current system is a complex amalgam of payers, providers, and facilities that function more or less independently. There are ongoing concerns related to uneven accessibility, quality, over- and underutilization of services, and cost inflation.

In 2009, more than 16.7 percent of Americans had no health insurance coverage, according to the US Census Bureau (DeNavas-Walt, Proctor, and Smith 2011, 71). Families who do not receive insurance coverage through their employers and do not qualify for Medicaid assistance are finding it difficult or impossible to obtain and pay for medical care. Public healthcare facilities are overcrowded, underfunded, and unable to fully address the needs of their communities. Some economists fear that the high cost of pharmaceuticals will threaten the stability of the Medicare and Medicaid programs. The federal government passed a drug benefit plan intended to give everyone with Medicare, regardless of income, health status, or prescription drug usage, access to prescription drug coverage as of January 2006. The benefit provides access only for the elderly (those older than age 65) and disabled, while many low-income and uninsured people younger than age 65 must rely on community resources to get needed medications. Low-income and uninsured people face many barriers because community resources do not adequately meet growing prescription drug needs, according to a study by the Center for Studying Health System Change (Ginsburg et al. 2006), a nonpartisan policy research organization.

Since the 1960s, the cost of healthcare services has grown at a much faster rate than overall inflation. For example, in 2000, the cost of inpatient hospital services increased by about 6 percent while the overall consumer price index increased by less than 4 percent. In 2010, the cost of inpatient hospital services increased by 8.6 percent over the previous year with a utilization increase of only 0.3 percent, and the overall cost of medical care rose almost7.3 percent. In contrast, overall cost inflation for that period was 1.5 percent (Milliman 2011).

Concerns over the growing cost of healthcare services have brought about significant changes in the healthcare system over the past two decades. The most significant has been the movement of most diagnostic services and noncritical therapeutic services away from the acute care hospital setting. The **diagnosis-related groups (DRGs)** prospective payment system, implemented in the 1980s, started the movement toward outpatient services. This payment system allowed Medicare to group patients based on their diagnosis. Patients within a given DRG were likely to receive equivalent services that utilized the same hospital resources.

On October 1, 2007, **Medicare severity-diagnosis related groups** (MS-DRGs) were implemented. This system, which includes 25 **major diagnostic categories** (MDCs), is the first step toward identifying the proper MS-DRG to a claim. Within each MDC, decision trees help users assign the proper MS-DRG. The identification or absence of **complications** or **comorbidities**, also known as CCs, may determine the final medical or surgical MS-DRG. The final product is a single MS-DRG assigned to each case, which in turn determines the reimbursement due to the hospital.

In response to competition from ambulatory care facilities, many hospitals have enhanced their service offerings in the areas of ambulatory, diagnostic, and surgical services and subacute nursing care. Additionally, many hospitals have merged with other general and specialty hospitals and subacute and ambulatory care providers to form integrated healthcare networks. An **integrated healthcare network** is a group of healthcare organizations that collectively provides a full range of coordinated health-related services. These services range from simple, preventive care to complex surgical care.

Hospital-Based Services

Acute care hospitals reserve inpatient services for the sickest patients and the most invasive medical procedures. Noninvasive diagnostic procedures, same-day surgeries, chemotherapy, and radiation therapy are routinely performed in separate ambulatory care facilities or in the outpatient departments of acute care hospitals. Most convalescent care is provided in dedicated skilled nursing facilities or through home health agencies, but some hospitals have opened dedicated nursing units to care for patients who no longer require acute care services but are too ill to return home. Similarly, most rehabilitation care has transitioned to dedicated rehabilitation hospitals, skilled nursing facilities, freestanding community-based facilities, or hospital-based outpatient departments.

Patients who receive healthcare services in a hospital are categorized as either inpatients or outpatients. An **inpatient** receives healthcare services, room, board, and continuous nursing care in a hospital unit dedicated to providing around-the-clock patient care. An **outpatient** receives healthcare services in a hospital-based clinic or department but is not admitted to a dedicated acute care unit. For example, a patient treated exclusively in the emergency department of a hospital is considered an outpatient rather than an inpatient. However, if that same patient is admitted to an acute care unit of the hospital after receiving emergency services, he is then considered an inpatient for the rest of his hospital stay.

Continuum of Care

Hospital-based services are only one component of the broad spectrum of healthcare services. The healthcare delivery system is extremely complex, and until recently, little effort was made to coordinate the services offered by the hundreds or thousands of independent healthcare practitioners and providers working in any one community. Since the early 1990s, healthcare organizations, accreditation and standards organizations, healthcare-related trade and professional associations, and federal agencies have been attempting to integrate the components of the delivery system. The goals are to improve the quality of medical care provided to Americans and to make healthcare services more affordable and accessible.

The concept of a continuum of care was initially developed during the mid-1990s in response to increasing healthcare costs. Ideally, every patient would receive the appropriate service at the appropriate time from the appropriate practitioner or facility. The **continuum of care** can be defined as the range of healthcare services provided to a patient, from routine ambulatory care to intensive acute care, with an emphasis on communication among caregivers. The services that make up the continuum can be categorized into three levels of care: primary, secondary, and tertiary. The levels of care reflect the cost of the services as well as their intensity. For example, the basic services provided in physicians' offices are generally the least expensive, and the intensive medical services provided in acute care hospitals are generally the most expensive.

Primary Care

Most routine healthcare services are provided at the **primary care** level by physicians working in private offices, group practices, private clinics, or community-based clinics. Primary care physicians usually receive their training in the more general fields of medicine: family practice, pediatrics, and general internal medicine. Many women of reproductive age receive primary care services from physicians specializing in gynecology. Nurse practitioners (nurses who hold advanced clinical degrees) provide direct primary care to patients and have a collaborative arrangement with physicians. Physician assistants provide primary care services to patients under the supervision of physicians.

Primary care physicians also coordinate their patients' hospital care, diagnostic services, specialty care consultations, and psychosocial services. Primary care services include the following:

- Preventive care (such as immunizations)

- Early detection of neoplastic diseases and other serious illnesses through routine screening and laboratory tests (such as mammograms and blood tests)

- Periodic physical examinations (such as well-baby checkups, well-child checkups, and annual checkups for adults)

- Diagnosis and treatment of minor infectious illnesses (such as influenza and other viral infections) and common bacterial and fungal infections (such as strep throat and athlete's foot), which may be diagnosed with a combination of examination and laboratory testing and treated with prescription drugs

- Diagnosis and management services for chronic illnesses (such as asthma, hypertension, congestive heart failure, and diabetes), which are monitored through periodic examinations and laboratory testing and treated with prescription drugs

- Diagnosis and treatment of minor injuries (such as lacerations, sprains, and uncomplicated orthopedic injuries)

A new option for coordinated primary care services comes through the **patient-centered medical home (PCMH)**. This concept was introduced by the American Academy of Pediatrics (AAP) in 1967. In 2002, the AAP expanded the definition of medical home to include accessible, continuous, comprehensive, family-centered, coordinated, compassionate, and culturally effective care and identified specific activities that should be included in the medical home model. In 2005, the American College of Physicians (ACP) developed an advanced medical home model that included evidenced-based medicine, clinical decision support, the chronic care model, medical care plans, enhanced and convenient access to care, quantitative indicators of quality, health information technology, and feedback on performance. (Barr and Ginsburg 2006).

The largest primary care organizations in the United States (American Academy of Family Physicians [AAFP], AAP, ACP, and American Osteopathic Association [AOA]) joined forces in 2007 to publish the *Joint Principles of the Patient-Centered Medical Home*. Supported by the American Medical Association (AMA), the following principles were documented (AAFP et al. 2007):

- Personal physician: Each patient has an ongoing relationship with a personal physician trained to provide first contact, continuous, and comprehensive care.

- Physician-directed medical practice: The personal physician leads a team of individuals at the practice level who collectively take responsibility for the ongoing care of patients.

- Whole person orientation: The personal physician is responsible for providing for all the patient's healthcare needs or appropriately arranging care with other qualified professionals.

- Coordination of care: Care is coordinated and/or integrated, for example across specialists, hospitals, home health agencies, and nursing homes.

- Quality and safety: Quality and safety are ensured by a care planning process, evidence-based medicine, clinical decision-support tools, performance measurement, active participation of patients in decision making, information technology, a voluntary recognition process, quality improvement activities, and other measures.

- Enhanced access: Access to care is expanded to include, for example, open scheduling, extended hours, and new options for communication.

- Payment: Payment must appropriately reflect the added value to patients who have a patient-centered medical home. It should account for the value of work that falls outside of the face-to-face visit, support adoption and use of health information technology for quality improvement, and recognize case-mix differences in the patient population being treated within the practice.

Many accreditation organizations joined the patient-centered medical home initiative. In 2008, then-presidential-candidate Barack Obama wrote, "I support the concept of a patient centered medical home, and as part of my health care plan, I will help providers establish them. As president, I will encourage and provide appropriate payment for providers who implement the medical home model, including physician-directed, interdisciplinary teams, disease management and care coordination programs, quality assurance mechanisms, and health IT systems which collectively will help to improve care for those with chronic conditions" (Obama 2008). By 2009, many states had introduced bills to promote medical homes. In 2009, the Accreditation Association for Ambulatory Health Care (AAAHC) began accrediting medical homes, and the National Committee for Quality Assurance (NCQA) released *Physician Practice Connections–Patient-Centered Medical Home* (PPC-PCMH), which outlined the voluntary standards for physician recognition as medical homes. In January 2011, NCQA released new standards for the PCMH program that focus on more patient-centered care and reinforce federal meaningful-use incentives for primary care practices to adopt health information technology (NCQA 2011).

Secondary Care

Secondary care encompasses the diagnostic and therapeutic services provided by medical specialists working in private offices, specialty group practices, private clinics, community-based clinics, and general and community hospitals. Patients may arrange to consult specialists directly. However, it is more common for primary care physicians to refer patients to specialists for the diagnosis and treatment of complex conditions that require more intensive services than the primary care physician can provide.

Specialty care can be divided into two groups of services: medical and surgical. The **medical specialties** include the following:

- Addiction medicine
- Allergy/immunology
- Cardiology
- Chiropractic medicine
- Critical care medicine
- Dermatology
- Emergency medicine
- Endocrinology
- Family practice
- Gastroenterology
- General practice
- Geriatric medicine
- Hematology
- Hospice and palliative care
- Infectious disease
- Internal medicine
- Nephrology
- Neurology
- Neuropsychiatry
- Oncology

- Optometry
- Osteopathic manipulative medicine
- Pediatric medicine
- Physical medicine and rehabilitation
- Psychiatry
- Pulmonology
- Radiology and nuclear medicine
- Rheumatology
- Sports medicine

The **surgical specialties** include:

- Anesthesiology
- Cardiac electrophysiology
- Cardiac surgery
- Cardiovascular surgery
- Colorectal surgery (formerly proctology)
- General surgery
- Hand surgery
- Interventional pain management
- Interventional radiology
- Maxillofacial surgery
- Neurosurgery
- Obstetrics/gynecology
- Ophthalmology
- Oral surgery (dentists only)
- Orthopedic surgery
- Otorhinolaryngology
- Pathology
- Plastic and reconstructive surgery
- Podiatry
- Surgical oncology
- Thoracic surgery

- Trauma surgery

- Urology

Most medical and surgical specialists provide both office-based and hospital-based care. However, because of the nature of their specialties, some specialists, such as pathologists, radiologists, and anesthesiologists, work predominantly in hospitals and ambulatory surgery settings.

Another provider who performs services only in the hospital is called a **hospitalist.** According to the Society of Hospital Medicine (SHM), a hospitalist is a physician who specializes in the practice of comprehensive medical care to hospitalized patients (SHM 2009). In the traditional patient care model, the primary care physician who treats a patient in her office will also treat the patient in the hospital. The travel time to and from the hospital has led some physicians to use hospitalists to treat their patients at the hospital. When hospitalists first evolved, they were typically internist or family practitioners for adults and pediatric providers for children. They have since extended into medical specialties, including obstetrics hospitalists, neurohospitalists, and surgical hospitalists.

Tertiary Care

Tertiary care is centered on the provision of highly specialized and technologically advanced diagnostic and therapeutic services in inpatient and outpatient hospital settings. Medical specialists working in large, urban hospitals and specialty clinics affiliated with nearby medical schools and universities provide most tertiary care.

Tertiary care services include medical–surgical services such as trauma care; burn care; organ transplantation; and medical–surgical intensive care for neonatal, pediatric, and adult patients. In addition, tertiary care hospitals perform medical research and conduct resident training programs for physicians and other healthcare practitioners.

Clinical Documentation in Healthcare: Moving Toward the Electronic Health Record

Hospitals, like other American businesses, began to apply computer processing to operations and management in the 1960s. Until then, clinical documentation consisted of paper-based methodologies. Computer technology was first applied in financial management, admissions, and billing. By 2000, virtually every clinical laboratory in the United States had implemented computer-based diagnostic systems with automatic reporting capabilities. Many of today's sophisticated diagnostic, medical, and surgical procedures would not be possible without the support of accurate and reliable software systems.

Health information technologies—such as **electronic health records (EHRs)**, computerized ordering of prescriptions and medical tests, clinical decision-support tools, and secure exchange of authorized information—improve quality, reduce medical errors, and prevent deaths. Most healthcare facilities, while implementing the many components of the EHR, operate with patient data and information in paper and electronic formats. Although some documents may be easily integrated into the EHR, many will remain challenging to integrate. According to the American Health Information Management Association (AHIMA), a **hybrid health record** (AHIMA 2010a) "is a system with functional components that include any of the following:

- Both paper and electronic documents *without* a central electronic document management system where all patient information is maintained

- Manual and electronic processes to compile components of the health record

- Multiple repositories (paper or electronic) of information that need to be accessed by the end user to compile the health records for a single episode of care

Some examples of hybrid health record scenarios are:

- Dictation, laboratory, and X-ray results are available electronically, whereas progress notes, ancillary care, provider information, graphic sheets, and doctors' orders are on paper.

- Patient health information may be maintained on various other media types, such as film, video, or an imaging system.

- Patient information may be scanned images that are accessed in a separate part of the system versus being integrated together in a chronological packet of information defined as the legal health record.

- Hospital records are automated, but clinic records are on paper and processed and stored in the clinic, never becoming part of the core EHR."

During the transition to the EHR, the hybrid environment requirements are challenging and costly. Part of the cost is due to the duplicative efforts by staff to manage both paper and electronic documentation, and another part is due to the interface design and integration in a partially EHR system. The potential of error is also greater when compiling and retrieving information in a hybrid environment.

In comparison, the progression of applying electronic information management to health record systems has increased. Many acute care organizations now depend on mixed-media health record systems made up of computer-generated laboratory reports, digital images, transcribed medical–surgical reports, and handwritten orders and progress notes. The cost of electronic clinical documentation systems has been one challenge in the implementation of EHRs. For more details on health record formats, such as hybrid health records and EHRs, see chapter 6.

President Obama's Healthcare Reform

In February 2009, President Obama signed the **American Recovery and Reinvestment Act (ARRA)** into law. Part of ARRA's goal is to encourage healthcare organizations to adopt EHRs through financial incentives. Because of the slowness of adoption, funding barriers, concurrent regulatory compliance timelines, competing technical priorities, strained human resources, and the lack of industry education, many healthcare providers find themselves maintaining a hybrid health record as an alternative to full automation. The **Health Information Technology for Economic and Clinical Health Act (HITECH)** passed as part of ARRA and the **Patient Protection and Affordable Care Act** (PPACA) as amended by the **Health Care and Education Reconciliation Act** of 2010 (referred to collectively as the Affordable Care Act) were landmark legislation (AHIMA 2010).

Section 3001(c)(3) of the Public Health Service Act, as added by the HITECH Act, requires the national coordinator to update and publish the Federal Health IT Strategic Plan through extensive collaboration with the federal government, the private sector, and the public. The result is the **Office of the National Coordinator for Health Information Technology's (ONC)** plan for realizing Congress and the administration's health information technology (IT) agenda: improving the quality, efficiency, safety, and patient-centeredness of healthcare. This proposed plan has six goals with associated objectives (ONC 2011):

1. Achieve adoption and information exchange through meaningful use of health IT

   a. Accelerate adoption of EHRs

   b. Facilitate information exchange to support meaningful use of EHRs

   c. Support health IT adoption and information exchange for public health and populations with unique needs

2. Improve care, improve population health, and reduce health care costs through the use of health IT

   a. Support more sophisticated uses of EHRs and other health IT to improve health system performance

   b. Better manage care, efficiency, and population health through EHR-generated reporting measures

   c. Demonstrate health IT-enabled reform of payment structures, clinical practices, and population health management

   d. Support new approaches to the use of health IT in research, public and population health, and national health security

3. Inspire confidence and trust in health IT

   a. Protect confidentiality, integrity, and availability of health information

   b. Inform individuals of their rights and increase transparency regarding the uses of protected health information

   c. Improve safety and effectiveness of health IT

4. Empower individuals with health IT to improve their health and the health care system

   a. Engage individuals with health IT

   b. Accelerate individual and caregiver access to their electronic health information in a format they can use and reuse

   c. Integrate patient-generated health information and consumer health IT with clinical applications to support patient-centered care

5. Achieve rapid learning and technological advancement

   a. Lead the creation of a learning health system to support quality, research, and public and population health

6. Broaden the capacity of health IT through innovation and research

According to Rode (2010):

> Milestones for PPACA and ARRA-HITECH fall between October 2010 and at least 2016. The HIPAA upgrade is scheduled for completion on January 1, 2012, and the compliance date for the ICD-10 conversion is October 1, 2013. Representatives from the Centers for Medicare and Medicaid Services have reaffirmed the ICD-10 deadline during events, on the CMS Web site, and in education meetings in the spring. Come January 1, 2012, health plans will be free to reject any claim or other HIPAA transaction that is not in the form of an Accredited Standards Committee X12 version 5010 (and NCPCD version D.0 for retail pharmacies). Likewise, on October 1, 2013, claims carrying ICD-9-CM codes may be rejected. New EHR system software or other healthcare technology such as system software that cannot accommodate and comply with the HIPAA and ICD-10 changes will have to be retrofitted, which is an expensive process. Costs can be lowered if the requirements are built into new software.

Successful projects will establish strategic plans that cover all four of these factors. Quality information, documentation processes, and the ability to "collect once and use many" will be components to an organization's strategic plan. For example, both ARRA and PPACA contain numerous provisions on quality and quality measurement reporting. The **National Quality Forum (NQF)**, the authority on most quality measures, recently noted the need to coordinate quality measure components with ICD-10 classifications. Therefore, the healthcare industry and the government are now becoming much more cognizant of these four factors. Healthcare data are becoming as much a factor in an organization's bottom line as financial factors.

More details on regulations, such as ARRA, HITECH, and meaningful use can be found in chapter 8.

Personal Health Records

The Markle Foundation established Connecting for Health, a public-private collaborative intended to coordinate and enhance the visibility of government, provider, and industry efforts to accelerate the adoption of electronically connected health information systems (Connecting for Health 2004a). The 2002 initiative had two phases. Phase 1 included the recommendation to engage the American public in developing **personal health records (PHRs)**. Phase 2 resulted in the following recommendations (Connecting for Health 2004b):

- PHR development should be accelerated.

- PHRs will help increase consumer health awareness, activation, and safety.

- There is no single pathway to a universal PHR.

- A common data set is a vital starting point.

AHIMA defines the PHR as an electronic, universally available, lifelong resource of health information needed by individuals to make health decisions. Individuals own and manage the information in their PHRs, which comes from healthcare providers and the individuals. The PHR is maintained in a secure and private environment, and the individual determines rights of access. The PHR is separate from and does not replace the legal record of any provider.

PHR formats vary, but all are designed to make more information available at the point of care, improve communication between patient and physician, and increase consumer engagement in healthcare. Recognition of the PHR is growing, and the document can play a major role in helping patients (who may also be referred to as consumers) and their caregivers make better health decisions. PHRs are patient-controlled repositories of individual health data. They may contain excerpts from or summaries of physician records generated from clinical encounters, claims data, lab and imaging results, prescription information, and (very important) patient-entered data. PHRs can include functions such as decision support, appointment making, referral requests, medication refills, and bill paying. Patients can contribute their own data to the PHR and can determine what data will be accessible to clinicians and others. To date, most PHRs are not standards based, and few are easy to transport among different EHR products. However, Google and Microsoft, the two largest vendors of web-based PHRs, recently agreed on mechanisms to enable the free exchange of information between their respective PHR systems, and others may follow (US Executive Office of the President 2010). It is important to emphasize that the consumer, not the provider, maintains the PHR and that it does not replace any provider's legal health record. Simply put, the PHR is the consumer's compilation of her health information from all providers. This **untethered** model differs from a **tethered record** (sometimes also called a PHR), which is a subset of information compiled by the provider and offered to the consumer, often through the provider's website. A tethered record functions as a patient view into the provider's electronic record. Some providers offer patients the opportunity to build and maintain their PHRs through the providers' websites. Tethered and untethered models can offer similar benefits—the two-way sharing of health information between patient and provider—but the untethered stresses patient control and the inclusion of information from multiple providers.

Along with being patient controlled, an important feature of PHRs is that they travel with the patient. A patient could schedule a visit with a new physician or a specialist and allow that provider access to his PHR. PHRs can allow patients to become more involved in their own healthcare by enabling them to input their own data, research health issues, and potentially meet and share information with patients who have similar conditions (US Executive Office of the President 2010).

PHRs are gaining in popularity, and not only with patients and physicians. The Office of the National Coordinator for Health Information Technology includes PHRs as part of its strategy for implementing EHRs and the **National Health Information Network (NHIN)**. Vendors have introduced a proliferation of PHR products in recent years. For consumers to embrace PHRs, the healthcare industry must provide education on their proper use—including security and confidentiality—and the technical standards that facilitate the exchange of PHR information.

The future of the PHR is electronic. At this point, however, neither the provider community nor the consumer is ready to rely exclusively on EHRs. Today, people create and maintain their PHRs using common media sources, such as paper, personal computers, the Internet, flash drives, smart cards, mobile phones, vendor-developed software, smartphones, or a combination of these.

In October 2003, AHIMA launched myPHR (http://www.myphr.com), a guide to understanding and managing personal health information for the general public. The site defines a health record, provides instructions on accessing health information and compiling and keeping a PHR, and explains privacy rights. Since its inception, the site has broadened its consumer resources to include healthcare literacy, sample PHRs, and blogs. MyPHR also features the most recent and relevant health information from a variety of industry sources (AHIMA 2010b).

Health Information Exchange

Public- and private-sector stakeholders are focusing efforts on **health information exchange (HIE)** because increasing evidence suggests that health IT can improve healthcare quality and patient safety by reducing errors and unnecessary expenditures. HIE is electronically moving health information among organizations while adhering to national standards. HIE stakeholders include hospitals, clinicians, laboratories, pharmacies, payers, employers, public health departments, quality improvement organizations, and consumers. A 2010 eHealth Initiative survey found that there are currently 73 operational HIE initiatives, up from 57 in 2009 (Warner 2011). Health information organizations that bring these stakeholders together within a geographic area are called **regional health information organizations (RHIOs)**. The RHIO governs HIE among the stakeholders with the purpose of improving healthcare in the region.

One advantage of any HIE is that it provides immediate access to clinical information at the point of patient care. Federal and state laws and regulations and the policies and procedures that govern HIE ensure the security and integrity of electronically accessed health information. HIE may also provide a structure for public health reporting, clinical quality measurements, biomedical surveillance, consumer health informatics research, and the like (AHIMA 2010c).

Many regulations safeguard the confidentiality and integrity of **protected health information (PHI)**, including the Privacy Act of 1974, HIPAA, and HITECH. HITECH expands the current federal protections for the privacy and security of PHI under HIPAA (HHS 2010). It requires all business associates to comply with HIPAA and extends business associate status to HIEs.

Other federal laws and regulations that affect the exchange of health information include the Medicare Conditions of Participation, the federal regulations regarding confidentiality of alcohol and drug abuse patient records, the Family Educational Rights and Privacy Act, the Gramm-Leach-Bliley Act, and the Food, Drug, and Cosmetic Act. If a state has more stringent laws to govern and manage the privacy and security of PHI, those laws preempt the federal laws and regulations. Compliance with all federal and state laws and regulations is particularly important when a single RHIO extends the HIE activities along the borders of two different states (AHIMA 2011).

The ONC's "National Privacy and Security Framework for Electronic Exchange of Individually Identifiable Health Information" outlines principles that, when taken together, constitute good data stewardship and form a foundation of public trust in the collection of, access to, use of, and disclosure of personal information by HIEs. To complement the framework, the **Office for Civil Rights (OCR)** published a series of fact sheets that clarify how the HIPAA privacy rule applies to and can be used to help structure privacy policies behind electronic HIE. ONC's framework and OCR's fact sheets call for the following principles in an HIE (AHIMA 2011):

- Individual Access: HIEs should provide consumers with a "simple and timely means to access and obtain their individually identifiable health information in a readable form and format," according to ONC's framework (HHS, ONC 2008). OCR's guidance further states, "An individual's right to access his or her PHI is a critical aspect of the Privacy Rule, the application of which naturally extends to an electronic environment. The Privacy Rule's specific standards address individuals' requests for access and timely action by the covered entity, including the provision of access, denial of access, and documentation."

- Correction: HIEs should provide patients with "a timely means to dispute the accuracy or integrity of their individually identifiable health information, and to have erroneous information corrected or to have a dispute documented if their requests are denied" (HHS, ONC 2008). OCR notes that the privacy rule provides individuals with the "right to have their protected health information (PHI) amended in a manner fully consistent" with the framework (OCR 2011b).

- Openness and Transparency: Policies, procedures, and technologies that directly affect individuals or their individually identifiable health information should be open and transparent, according to ONC and OCR. Entities that participate in HIE should provide "clear notice of their policies and procedures regarding how an individual's identifiable health information" is protected, used, and disclosed (OCR 2011d).

- Individual Choice: HIEs should provide individuals with "a reasonable opportunity and capability to make informed decisions about the collection, use, and disclosure of their individually identifiable health information" (HHS, ONC 2008). OCR further notes that the framework "emphasizes the opportunity and ability of an individual to make choices with respect to the electronic exchange of their individually identifiable health information" (OCR 2011c).

- Collection, Use, and Disclosure Limitation: "Individually identifiable health information should be collected, used, and/or disclosed only to the extent necessary to accomplish a specified purpose" (HHS, ONC 2008). OCR notes that the framework "emphasized that appropriate limits should be set on the type and amount of information collected, used, and disclosed, and that authorized persons and entities should only collect, use, and disclose information necessary to accomplish a specified purpose" (OCR 2011a).

- Safeguards: "Individually identifiable health information should be protected with reasonable administrative, technical, and physical safeguards (HIPAA security rule) to ensure its confidentiality, integrity, and availability and to prevent unauthorized or inappropriate access, use, or disclosure" (HHS, ONC 2008). OCR notes that the HIPAA privacy rule "supports the Safeguards Principle by requiring covered entities to implement appropriate safeguards to protect the privacy of protected health information (PHI)" (OCR 2011e).

Summary

Healthcare services in the United States are distributed via a complex delivery system made up of numerous clinical professionals, allied health professionals, healthcare administrators, and healthcare provider organizations in a multitude of settings. Many organizations and government agencies manage healthcare reimbursement processes, institute healthcare standards and policies, and conduct healthcare-related research. Although the US healthcare system is considered one of the best in the world, the cost of providing services and the challenge of meeting the needs of every American are a concern today and will likely remain so for some time.

Clinical documentation in today's healthcare environment is migrating from a paper-based health record to an electronic health record. Most healthcare facilities are in the process of implementing electronic health records—a daunting and costly undertaking. These facilities are managing hybrid health records that contain paper-based and electronic health information.

An individual's personal health record is an electronic, universally available, lifelong resource of health information. Personal health records are gaining popularity and are a strategic focus of the National Coordinator for Health Information Technology. The future of the PHR is electronic. However, neither the provider community nor the consumer has completely migrated to a standardized personal health record.

Access to patient information is critical in improving patient care. Stakeholders involved in RHIO projects are pioneers navigating new terrain as they develop regional networks to improve the health of their communities. As this trend evolves and improves, RHIOs may prove to be a valuable stepping stone on the road to a national system in which a customer's medical information is available anywhere, at any time, to authorized users.

References

AHIMA. 2011. HIE Management and Operational Considerations. *Journal of AHIMA* 82 (5): 56–61.

AHIMA. 2010a. Managing the Transition from Paper to EHRs. (Updated November 2010.) Chicago: AHIMA.

AHIMA. 2010b. Role of the Personal Health Record in the EHR. (Updated November 2010.) Chicago: AHIMA.

AHIMA. 2010c. Understanding the HIE Landscape. *Journal of AHIMA* 81 (9): 60–65.

American Academy of Family Physicians (AAFP), American Academy of Pediatrics (AAP), American College of Physicians (ACP), and American Osteopathic Association (AOA). 2007. Joint Principles of the Patient-Centered Medical Home. http://www.acponline.org/advocacy/where_we_stand/medical_home/approve_jp.pdf.

Barr, M., and J. Ginsburg. 2006. *The Advanced Medical Home: A Patient-Centered, Physician-Guided Model of Health Care.* American College of Physicians. http://www.acponline.org/advocacy/where_we_stand/policy/adv_med.pdf.

Cassidy, B. 2010. The US Healthcare Delivery System. In *Health Information Management: Concepts, Principles, and Practice,* 3rd ed., edited by K. LaTour and S. Eichenwald Maki. Chicago: AHIMA.

Connecting for Health. 2004a. Connecting Americans to their Healthcare: Final Report. http://www.markle.org/sites/default/files/CnctAmerHC_fullreport.pdf.

Connecting for Health. 2004b. Achieving Electronic Connectivity in Healthcare: A Preliminary Roadmap from the Nation's Public and Private-Sector Healthcare Leaders. http://www.markle.org/sites/default/files/white_roadmap_072004.pdf.

DeNavas-Walt, C., B. D. Proctor, and J. C. Smith. 2011. Income, Poverty, and Health Insurance Coverage in the United States: 2009. Washington, DC: US Census Bureau.

Ginsburg, P. B., B. C. Strunk, M. I. Banker, and J. P. Cookson. 2006. Tracking Health Care Costs: Spending Growth Remains Stable at High Rate in 2005. Center for Studying Health System Change. http://www.hschange.com/CONTENT/879/.

The Joint Commission. 2011. "The Joint Commission History." http://www.jointcommission.org/about_us/history.aspx.

Milliman. 2011. 2011 Milliman Medical Index. http://publications.milliman.com/periodicals/mmi/pdfs/milliman-medical-index-2011.pdf.

National Committee for Quality Assurance (NCQA). 2011. Physician Practice Connections–Patient-Centered Medical Home (PPC-PCMH). http://www.ncqa.org/tabid/631/Default.aspx.

Obama, B. 2008. Obama Responds to American Academy of Family Physicians. Barack Obama 2012. http://my.barackobama.com/page/community/post/sultanr/gGxkpL.

Office for Civil Rights (OCR). 2011a. Collection, Use, and Disclosure Limitation. http://www.hhs.gov/ocr/privacy/hipaa/understanding/special/healthit/collectionusedisclosure.pdf.

Office for Civil Rights. 2011b. Correction. http://www.hhs.gov/ocr/privacy/hipaa/understanding/special/healthit/correction.pdf.

Office for Civil Rights. 2011c. Individual Choice. http://www.hhs.gov/ocr/privacy/hipaa/understanding/special/healthit/individualchoice.pdf.

Office for Civil Rights. 2011d. Openness and Transparency. http://www.hhs.gov/ocr/privacy/hipaa/understanding/special/healthit/opennesstransparency.pdf.

Office for Civil Rights. 2011e. Safeguards. http://www.hhs.gov/ocr/privacy/hipaa/understanding/special/healthit/safeguards.pdf.

Office of the National Coordinator for Health Information Technology. 2011. The Federal Health IT Strategic Plan. http://healthit.hhs.gov/portal/server.pt/community/federal_health_it_strategic_plan_-_overview/1211.

Rode, D. 2010. Navigating the Perfect Storm: HIM Roles in Steering through Healthcare Reform, ARRA, ICD-10, and HIPAA. *Journal of AHIMA* 81 (6):18–20.

Society of Hospital Medicine (SHM). 2009. Definition of a Hospitalist and Hospital Medicine." Society of Hospital Medicine. http://www.hospitalmedicine.org/AM/Template.cfm?Section=Hospitalist_Definition&Template=/CM/HTMLDisplay.cfm&ContentID=24835.

US Department of Health and Human Services (HHS). 2010. HHS Strengthens Health Information Privacy and Security through New Rules. Press release. http://www.hhs.gov/news/press/2010pres/07/20100708c.html.

US Department of Health and Human Services, Office of the National Coordinator for Health information Technology (HHS, ONC). 2008. National Privacy and Security Framework for Electronic Exchange of Individually Identifiable Health Information. December 15. http://healthit.hhs.gov/portal/server.pt/community/healthit_hhs_gov__privacy___security_framework/1173.

US Executive Office of the President. President's Council of Advisors on Science and Technology. 2010. Report to the President Realizing the Full Potential of Health Information Technology to Improve Healthcare for Americans: The Path Forward. http://library.ahima.org/xpedio/groups/public/documents/government/bok1_048515.pdf#xml=http://library.ahima.org/xpedio/idcplg?IdcService=GET_XML_HIGHLIGHT_INFO&QueryText=%28Personal+Health+record%29%3cand%3e%28xPublishSite%3csubstring%3e%60BoK%60%29&SortField=xPubDate&SortOrder=Desc&dDocName=bok1_048515&HighlightType=PdfHigh.

Warner, D. 2011. HIE Patient Consent Model Options. *Journal of AHIMA* 82 (5):48–49.

Chapter 2

Clinical Documentation and the Health Record

Cheryl Gregg Fahrenholz, RHIA, CCS-P

Learning Objectives

- Discuss the purposes of health records

- Describe the functions of clinical documentation and health records

- List users of health records

- Explain the importance of defining the legal health record

- Review documentation requirements in the health record

- Discuss factors driving healthcare organizations toward the electronic health record

Key Terms

Administrative information

Allied health professional

Certification Commission for Healthcare Information Technology (CCHIT)

Computer-based patient record (CPR)

Covered entities

Critical-access hospital

Derived data

Destruction

Electronic health record (EHR)

Health information management (HIM) professionals

Health Information Exchange Organization (HIO)

Health Insurance Portability and Accountability Act (HIPAA)

Health Level Seven (HL7)

Health record

HITECH Act

Hybrid health record

Legal health record

Longitudinal health record

National Committee on Vital and Health Statistics (NCVHS)

National Council for Prescription Drug Programs (NCPDP)

Nationwide Health Information Network Exchange

Nationwide Health Information Network (NHIN)

Personal health record (PHR)

Picture archiving and communications
    system (PACS)

Protected health information

Release and disclosure

Release of information (ROI)

Retention

Telemedicine

Systematized Nomenclature of Medicine–
    Clinical Terms® (SNOMED CT®)

Source-system data

Working document

Introduction

Regardless of the healthcare setting, healthcare organizations must meet regulatory
and accreditation standards when collecting and storing health information. These
standards require a separate health record for each individual patient and address
minimum documentation requirements to ensure that these records provide for continuity of patient care among providers. The health record serves many purposes, such
as documenting services for quality care, reimbursement, and outcomes management;
protecting legal interests; reporting for public health; and supplying clinical data for
research. It supports the operational management of the healthcare organization as
it is used for training and education and to plan services that support community
health needs.

Each organization must define the parameters of its legal health record according to
its own needs and state laws. Using a paper-based record as the legal health record seems
simplistic when compared to an electronic health record (EHR). The EHR can be accessed
simultaneously by multiple users and can have multiple versions, different views for displaying the same information, and other features that are not present in paper-based
records.

The healthcare industry lags behind other industries in the application of information technology. The same factors that have influenced the development of information
technology in healthcare have also advanced the development of standards for EHR con-
formity and interoperability.

Clinical Documentation and
the Health Record

Every healthcare provider is required to document the clinical services she performs on
behalf of individual patients. Healthcare providers include licensed practitioners such as
physicians, psychologists, clinical social workers, nurses, **allied health professionals**,
and licensed independent practitioners (for example, nurse practitioners, clinical nurse
midwives, and physician's assistants).

Accreditation and regulatory standards require healthcare providers to create and
maintain a separate record for each individual patient treated, regardless of the healthcare setting. Clinical documentation may be stored in a paper-based format, a mixed-
media or hybrid format, or a computer-based electronic format. Regardless of the format,
specific data elements are required.

Accreditation standards, licensing requirements, and federal and state statutes determine the specific health-related information that must be collected for each patient. Standards and regulations specify when the information must be collected and by whom. The content and style of clinical documentation depend on a combination of other factors, including the following:

- The profession and specialty training of the healthcare provider (for example, a physician, surgeon, nurse practitioner, clinical nurse midwife, or respiratory therapist)

- The healthcare setting (for example, a physician's office, ambulatory surgery center, skilled nursing facility, or acute care hospital)

- The type of healthcare service provided (for example, routine screening, cataract surgery, cardiac catheterization, obstetrical delivery, or pulmonary intensive care)

Purpose and Value of Documentation

Federal and state statutes, licensing requirements, and accreditation standards provide minimum guidelines to ensure accurate and complete documentation. Such documentation facilitates effective communication among caregivers to provide continuity of patient care.

The **health record** is the document healthcare providers use to collect and store clinical data for individual patients. In the context of the overall healthcare delivery system, health records serve several important purposes, including the following:

- Ensuring continuity of patient care among providers and along the continuum of care

- Providing a means for evaluating outcomes, quality, and peer review

- Providing documentation to substantiate reimbursement, claim submissions, and medical necessity of care

- Protecting the legal interests of customers, caregivers, and healthcare organizations

- Providing clinical data for biomedical research

- Supporting professional education and training for physicians, nurses, and allied health professionals

- Supporting operational management of healthcare organizations

- Providing health-services data for public health planning and governmental policymaking

Owners of the Health Record

Health records and other documentation related to patient care are the property of the hospital or healthcare provider that created them; however, the information in each record belongs to the individual patient. To ensure their validity and confidentiality, original health records must remain under the facility's physical control except in certain legal situations.

Consumers have a right to control how information in their health records is used. Patients can review, copy, and amend their records when necessary. However, outside healthcare providers, third-party payers, clinical researchers, and others who have a legitimate interest in the contents of health records also need access to health records. To meet the growing demand for healthcare information, hospitals and other healthcare providers must develop processes for fulfilling legitimate requests for health information while protecting the confidentiality of health records and the privacy of patients. Hospitals and providers must ensure that records remain accessible for legitimate purposes for a reasonable period after a healthcare episode is complete.

Until 2002, few federal regulations protected the confidentiality of health information. Federal laws did protect records in a few specialized settings, such as chemical dependency treatment and human immunodeficiency virus (HIV) status. Many states had laws in place to govern the use and disclosure of health information, but the protection of patient privacy and health record security generally was the responsibility of individual healthcare providers. In the hospital setting, **health information management (HIM) professionals** primarily managed the privacy of confidential health information and the security of health records.

The implementation of the **Health Insurance Portability and Accountability Act (HIPAA)** Privacy Rule in 2003 established a consistent set of privacy and security rules. These rules, designed to protect the privacy of patients, also attempted to simplify the sharing of health information for legitimate purposes. For example, before implementation of HIPAA, a healthcare provider who needed access to a health record maintained by another provider usually could not directly request the information. The former provider required the patient's written authorization to release information to the current provider. In many cases, the patient or the patient's legal representative had to facilitate the transfer of medical information to a current healthcare provider. Under federal privacy regulations, the healthcare provider can directly request protected medical information, and a written authorization from the patient is not required when the information is used for treatment purposes. The privacy rule states that **protected health information** used for treatment, payment, or healthcare operations does not require patient authorization to allow providers access, use, or disclosure. However, only the minimum necessary information needed to satisfy the specified purpose can be used or disclosed. The release of information for purposes unrelated to treatment, payment, or healthcare operations still requires the patient's written authorization. In 2006, the Enforcement Rule of HIPAA (codified at 45 CFR Part 160, Subparts C, D, and E) was finalized. This rule assigned civil and criminal penalties for healthcare-related offenses. Although it created several provisions, the most significant was the Administrative Simplification Rules. These rules were intended to increase the efficiency of the healthcare system through standards for use and dissemination of health information.

The Administrative Simplification Rules apply to **covered entities**, which include health plans; healthcare clearinghouses, such as billing services; and healthcare providers that transmit healthcare data in an electronic format that is regulated under HIPAA. In July 2009, the secretary of Health and Human Services (HHS) delegated to the director of the Office for Civil Rights (OCR) the authority to administer and enforce the HIPAA Security Rule (HHS 2011a).

HIPAA established consumers' right to access and amend their own health records. Before the Internet and widespread applications of information technology, most patients were unfamiliar with the contents of their health records. In fact, state regulations and provider policies allowed patients limited access to their records. Today, patients are more aware of the huge wealth of personal information stored in their health records, and they are more concerned about the information's accuracy and the record's security.

Users of the Health Record

The number of organizations and individuals who legitimately need access to confidential patient information has grown as the healthcare delivery system has become more complex. Physicians, psychologists, nurse practitioners, nurses, allied health professionals, and other healthcare providers administer clinical services directly to patients. Staff working in administrative and nonclinical roles support healthcare providers and have a legitimate need to use the health record. During a short hospital stay, dozens of clinicians, ancillary staff, administrative staff, and support staff will access the information in a patient's health record.

The processes that make health record information available to legitimate users are known collectively as **release and disclosure.** *Release of information* **(ROI)** is another term to describe disclosure of patient information. The processes of storing health information and destroying it when it is no longer needed are called **retention** and **destruction**. The development of EHRs has given healthcare organizations the ability to retain and store health information without the physical space restriction of paper-based health records. These processes are subject to specific regulations in many states. Federal regulations and accreditation standards also include specific guidelines on the release and retention of patient-identified health information.

The Institute of Medicine broadly defines the users of health records as "those individuals who enter, verify, correct, analyze, or obtain information from the record, either directly or indirectly through an intermediary" (Dick, Steen, and Detmer 1997, 75). All users influence customer care in some way, but they use the information for various reasons and in different ways. Some users (for example, physicians, nurses, and allied health professionals) consult the health records of specific patients as an integral part of their daily work responsibilities. In contrast, users such as researchers and statisticians never have direct access to the records of individual patients. Instead, they use aggregate (summarized and de-identified) clinical and demographic data derived from health record documentation.

The main users of health records are the clinicians responsible for direct patient care. They are authorized to document and access clinical information for the patients to whom they provide services. Most clinicians are only authorized to access the records of their own patients. Accessing or disclosing health record information without a valid reason is considered a violation of the ethical principles of every healthcare profession and the federal privacy rule. Part of the HIPAA Enforcement Rule of 2006 was determination of the amount of civil money penalties for unauthorized access or disclosure: The civil money penalties for each violation shall not exceed $100 for each violation or $25,000 for identical violations during a calendar year beginning in January (DHHS 2011b). Either of these practices would also violate institutional policies protecting the confidentiality of patient information.

FIGURE 2.1. Representative users of the health record: Individuals*

Patient Care Delivery—Providers

- Physicians
- Residents
- Nurse practitioners
- Dental hygienists
- Dentists
- Dietitians
- Laboratory technologists
- Chaplains
- Nurses
- Pharmacists
- Physical therapists
- Behavioral health providers
- Social workers

Patient Care Delivery—Consumers

- Patients
- Families
- Patients' legal representatives

Providers of Patient Care Management and Support

- Health information management professionals
- Administrators
- Financial managers and accountants
- Quality managers
- Allied health professionals
- Risk managers
- Unit clerks
- Utilization review managers

Patient Care Reimbursement

- Benefit managers
- Insurers (federal, state, and private)

Other

- Accreditors
- Government policy makers and legislators
- Lawyers
- Healthcare researchers and clinical investigators

*This is a representative (not exhaustive) list of users

Interns and students supervised by hospital, clinical, or medical staff access patient-identifiable information for the purpose of training and learning. Coding and billing staff consult patient-identifiable information as the basis for clinical coding and reimbursement. **Figure 2.1** provides a list of representative users of health record information.

Patients (along with their next of kin and/or legal representatives) have the right to access their health records. However, HIM professionals must validate the appropriateness of access. When a patient's next of kin or legal representative requests information belonging to the patient, HIM professionals should be familiar with state and federal laws regarding the right to access and who can authorize the use or disclosure of the information at issue.

According to the Code of Federal Regulations, an individual has a right of access to inspect and obtain a copy of protected health information about the individual in a designated record set for as long as the protected health information is maintained in the designated record set. In some cases, such as with psychotherapy notes, the patient may be denied access to this protected health information (CFR 2011b). Guidelines for charging the patient for obtaining copies of health information are documented in the Privacy Rule as well as in many state regulations.

A number of healthcare-related organizations use information derived from health records. Healthcare providers such as HMOs and physicians' practices use patient-identifiable information, as do third-party payers. Quality improvement organizations and other entities working under contracts with hospitals or with third-party payers such as Medicare often review copies of health record documentation. Many other organizations use aggregate health information in accreditation, research, and policymaking. (See **Figure 2.2** for a more comprehensive list of the institutions that rely on information from health records.)

FIGURE 2.2. Representative users of the health record: Institutions*

Healthcare Delivery (Inpatient and Outpatient)
- Alliances, associations, networks, and systems of providers
- Ambulatory surgery centers
- Donor banks (blood, tissue, organs)
- Health maintenance organizations
- Home care agencies
- Hospices
- Hospitals (general and specialty)
- Nursing homes
- Preferred provider organizations
- Physician offices (large and small group practices, individual practitioners)
- Psychiatric facilities
- Public health departments
- Substance abuse programs

Management and Review of Care
- Medicare peer review organizations
- Quality management companies
- Risk management companies
- Utilization review and utilization management companies

Reimbursement of Care
- Business healthcare coalitions
- Employers
- Insurers (federal, state, and private)

Research
- Disease registries
- Health data organizations
- Healthcare technology developers and manufacturers (equipment and device firms, pharmaceutical firms, and computer hardware and software vendors for patient record systems)
- Research centers

Education
- Allied health professional schools and programs
- Schools of medicine
- Schools of nursing
- Schools of public health

Accreditation
- Accreditation organizations
- Institutional licensure agencies
- Professional licensure agencies

Policy Making
- Federal government agencies
- Local government agencies
- State government agencies

*This is a representative (not exhaustive) list of users.
Source: Dick, Steen, and Detmer 1997, 77.

Definition of the Health Record for Legal Purposes

Until the use of computer technology became widespread in the last part of the twentieth century, the definition of a legal health record seemed relatively straightforward. The contents of the paper-based health record became the provider's legal business record of the services provided.

Defining the legal record becomes complex as organizations transition to EHRs with inherent capabilities that do not exist in paper-based records. For example, an EHR can have multiple versions, display information in multiple ways, and contain features, such as alerts and reminders, that provide clinical decision support. Because these functions and features are not available in a paper-based health record, the healthcare organization must determine which parts of the EHR are included in the legal record and which parts are not.

In a 2011 practice brief, the American Health Information Management Association (AHIMA) recognized the need to define the legal health record and designated record set regardless of the technologies employed or users involved (AHIMA 2011). This practice brief is included as **APPENDIX 2A**. The need to define the legal health record for disclosure purposes is paramount.

There is no one-size-fits-all definition of the legal health record and designated record set. Laws and regulations governing the content vary by practice setting and state. However, following common principles ensures that a health record serves the legal needs of the provider or facility, whether in a paper-based, hybrid (a combination of paper and electronic), or electronic format. Each organization must consider individual state laws, federal regulations, accrediting agency standards, standards of care, and requirements of third-party payers that permit the health record to serve and represent the legal business record. Regardless of the format of the health record, it must represent and fulfill the legal and business needs of the organization.

Legal Health Record

The **legal health record** can be defined as the official business record used for evidentiary purposes created by or for the healthcare organization (AHIMA 2011). The legal health record is the portion of the health record that will be disclosed upon request to parties outside the organization. It does not affect the discoverability of other information held by the organization. The legal health record includes documentation of healthcare services provided to an individual during any aspect of healthcare delivery in any type of healthcare organization as well as the source of the documentation. It contains individually identifiable information stored on any medium and collected and directly used in documenting healthcare or health status. The legal health record serves to (AHIMA 2011):

- Support the decisions made in a patient's care

- Support the revenue sought from third-party payers

- Document the services provided as legal testimony regarding the patient's illness or injury, response to treatment, and caregiver decisions

- Serve as the organization's business and legal record

The documentation that composes the legal health record may physically exist in a combination of paper, electronic, and computer databases. The result is a **hybrid health record**, or one that consists of information created with both paper documents and electronic media.

Organizational policies should require documentation and identification of the source (paper or electronic) of all information contained in the legal health record. A transition plan and policy should define the "legal source of truth," reflecting whether the legal health record is paper, hybrid, or fully electronic. This should include a specific schedule that provides retrospective and prospective dates wherein the user can identify the sources of all information in the record. The location where each portion of a patient's legal health record is located must be clearly indicated.

An **electronic health record (EHR)** system is the portal through which clinicians access patients' health records, order treatments or therapy, and document care delivered to patients. Although healthcare providers may eliminate the paper record when documenting in an electronic system, hard copies (typically paper) are often released for disclosure purposes. The release of information format has shifted somewhat since technical standards for interoperability enable health information exchange between providers and other users of health records.

Different portions of an EHR are usually located in various electronic systems such as laboratory databases, pharmacy information systems, **picture archiving and communications systems (PACS)**, cardiology information systems, results reporting systems, computerized provider order-entry systems, nurse care-planning systems, word-processing systems, and fetal trace monitoring systems, to name a few. Depending on their size and structure, healthcare providers may store structured clinical and administrative data in a database or clinical data repository. In addition, healthcare providers may store unstructured patient clinical data in separate databases or repositories (such as PACS and fetal trace archives) and provide pointers from the clinical portal to these various repositories.

The HIPAA Privacy Rule defines the designated record set as a group of records maintained by or for a covered entity that may include patient medical and billing records; the enrollment, payment, claims, adjudication, and cases or medical management record systems maintained by or for a health plan; or information used in whole or in part to make care-related decisions. It also contains clinical data and individually identifiable data stored on any medium that is collected and directly used in documenting healthcare, health status, and billing operations.

The designated record set is generally broader than the legal health record because it addresses all protected health information. While the legal health record is generally the information used by the patient care team to make decisions about the treatment of a patient, the designated record set contains protected health information along with business information unrelated to patient care.

Under HIPAA, the designated record set is used to clarify the rights of individuals to access, amend, restrict, and acquire an accounting of disclosures. Individuals have the right to inspect and obtain a copy, request amendments, and set restrictions and accountings of medical and billing information used to make decisions about their care (AHIMA 2011).

Defining the Subset of Information That Constitutes the Legal Health Record

The challenge for HIM professionals in defining a legal health record or designated record set is to determine which data elements, electronic-structured documents, images, audio files, and video files become part of the legal EHR. An HIM-driven team of patient care members can use several considerations to guide their identification of a legal health record and designated record set.

- **Step 1**: Determine which legal entities enforce relevant regulations, guidelines, standards, or laws on health records. Although various entities may have defined a legal health record in paper terms, their definitions must become the basis for the organization's legal health record definition.

- **Step 2**: Determine whether the records are created in the regular course of business of the healthcare provider or entity. Source-system or raw data, the data from which interpretations, summaries, and notes are derived, may be designated part of the legal health record, whether or not they are integrated into a single system or maintained as part of the source system. Records from source systems and clinical decision-making systems may be considered part of the legal health record based on the content of the source system's record.

  The determining factor in whether information is to be considered part of the legal health record is how it is used and whether it is reasonably expected to be routinely released as part of a complete health record.

  Some documents are commonly excluded from the legal health record. Documents used for disclosures made for purposes of discovery or e-discovery under court order and working notes used by a provider to complete a final report that were not available to others providing patient care are two examples of such exclusions.

  Several states have laws or regulations that spell out the requirements and conditions under which health information from another healthcare organization or provider must be redisclosed. In the absence of more stringent state law, the HIPAA privacy rule prevails. However, because any medical or billing information that was used to make decisions about the individual is included as part of the designated record set under the HIPAA privacy rule, information must be disclosed or redisclosed if requested by the individual to whom it pertains, regardless of whether the information is external or internal.

- **Step 3**: Ensure that all components of the legal health record are properly retained. Electronic data storage presents many challenges. Create a matrix that defines each document type in the legal health record and determines the medium in which each element will appear. (See **Figure 2.3**.) Such a matrix could include a column indicating the transition date of a particular document from the paper-based to the electronic environment. Guidelines for release of information vary by state.

- **Step 4**: Determine how information may be appropriately released. While it is easy to declare something such as an EKG WAVE file part of the legal health record or designated record set, the organization must consider how it will be reproduced. Will the system have the capability to print or download to a CD? How will the requester access the health information? Components of the legal health record and designated record set must be reproducible in an accessible format.

FIGURE 2.3. Health record matrix

Type of Document	Name of Document	Primary Source*	Primary Source System Start Date	Source of the Health Record/ Designated Record Set	Legal Health Record, Designated Record Set, or Both	Comments
Nursing	ICU nursing assessment	Electronic nursing documentation system	MM/DD/YYYY	Enterprise document management system	Both	Phased implementation
Physician orders	Congestive heart failure order set	Computerized physician order entry system	MM/DD/YYYY	EHR	Both	Downtime paper orders scanned
Emergency department	Emergency department treatment record	Paper	MM/DD/YYYY	Enterprise document system	Both	
Discharge summary	Discharge summary	Transcription system	MM/DD/YYYY	EHR	Both	
Claims	Billing report	Patient financial system	MM/DD/YYYY	Patient financial system	Designated record set	

*Includes scanned images
Source: AHIMA 2011.

- **Step 5**: Determine how to classify external records received by the organization. Some state laws address this classification; however, in the absence of state law, the organization must determine whether external records will be a part of the health record.

  Ultimately, the admissibility of the requested information in court is not the concern of the party producing the information. Compliance with the terms of the subpoena or order is required (AHIMA 2011).

As stated previously, there is no one-size-fits-all definition of the legal health record because laws and regulations governing the content vary by practice setting and by state. Final definition of the legal health record rests with individual healthcare organizations and their legal counsels. When defining the content of the legal health record (whether in a paper-based or electronic format), organizations should consider the items listed in **FIGURE 2.4**.

Additionally, some areas of the EHR do not exist in paper-based health records. During the transition to an EHR, healthcare organizations should review the following list of considerations and determine whether or not these items will be included in the legal health record or designated record set (AHIMA 2011).

- **Annotations/sticky notes:** Additional information that is added as a layer on top of the item. The annotation or sticky note may be suppressed when viewing or printing. These may be considered part of the health record. This documentation may become a permanent part of the record and is maintained in a manner similar to any other information contained within the health record.

FIGURE 2.4. Items to consider when defining legal health record content

- Advance directives
- Alerts, reminders, and pop-ups
- Allergy records
- Anesthesia records
- Care plans
- Consent forms for care, treatment, and research
- Consultation reports
- Continuing care records
- Diagnostic images
- Discharge instructions
- Discharge summaries
- E-mail messages containing patient–provider or provider–provider communications regarding care or treatment of specific patients
- Emergency department records
- Fetal monitoring strips from which interpretations are derived
- Functional status assessments
- Graphic records
- History and physical examination records
- Immunization records
- Instant messages containing patient–provider or provider–provider communications regarding care or treatment of specific patients
- Intake and output records
- Medication administration records
- Medication orders
- Medication profiles
- Minimum data sets (MDS, OASIS, IRF-PAI)
- Nursing assessments
- Operative and procedure reports
- Orders for treatment, including diagnostic tests for laboratory and radiology

- Pathology reports
- Patient education or teaching documents
- Patient identifiers (such as a health record number)
- Patient-submitted documentation
- Photographs (digital and analog) for identification purposes only
- Post-it® notes and annotations containing patient–provider or provider–provider communications regarding care or treatment of specific patients
- Practice guidelines or protocols and clinical pathways that imbed patient data
- Problem lists
- Progress notes and documentation (multidisciplinary, excluding psychotherapy notes)
- Psychology and psychiatric assessments and summaries (excluding psychotherapy notes)
- Records received from another healthcare provider if they were relied on to provide healthcare to the patient (see "Continuing care records," above)
- Research records of tests and treatments
- Respiratory, physical, speech, and/or occupational therapy records
- Results of tests and studies from laboratory and radiology
- Standing orders
- Telephone messages containing patient–provider or provider–provider communications regarding care or treatment of specific patients
- Telephone orders
- Trauma tapes
- Verbal orders
- Wave forms such as ECGs and EMGs, from which interpretations are derived
- Any other information required by the Medicare *Conditions of Participation* (2006), state provider licensure statutes or rules, or any third-party payer as a condition of reimbursement

- **Clinical decision support systems:** A subcategory of clinical information systems that is designed to help healthcare professionals make knowledge-based clinical decisions. Currently there are no generally accepted rules on including decision support such as system-generated notifications, prompts, and alerts as part of the health record. Alerts, reminders, pop-ups, and similar tools are used as aids in the clinical decision-making process. The tools themselves are usually not considered part of the legal health record; however, associated documentation is considered a component. At a minimum, the EHR should include documentation of the clinician's actions in response to decision support. This documentation is evidence of the clinician's decision to follow or disregard decision support. The organization should define the extent of exception documentation required (for example, what no documentation means). When an organization decides to include the decision support trigger as part of the health record, the organization will need to clarify whether all triggers will be part of the record or just the clinical decision support triggers. For example, alerts for patient appointment reminders may not be considered part of the legal health record, but alerts for drug–drug interaction may be.

- **Coding queries:** A routine communication and education tool used to advocate complete and compliant documentation. Retention of the query varies by healthcare organization. First, an organization must determine whether the query will be part of the health record. If the query is not part of the health record, the organization must decide whether to keep the query as part of the business record or only maintain the outcome of the query in a database.

- **Continuing care records:** Records received from another healthcare provider. Historically, these records were generally not considered part of the legal health record unless they were used in the provision of patient care. In the EHR, it may be difficult to determine whether information was viewed or used in delivering healthcare. It may be necessary to define such information as part of the legal health record. Policies should reflect the proper disposition of health records from external sources (such as other healthcare providers) if they are not integrated into the electronic and legal health record.

- **Data/documents:** Documentation of patient care that took place in the ordinary course of business by all healthcare providers.

- **Data from source systems:** Written results of tests. Data from which interpretations, summaries, notes, flowcharts, and so on are derived.

- **Discrete structured data:** Laboratory orders/refills, orders/medication orders/MARs, online charting and documentation, and any detailed charges.

- **Document completion (lockdown):** Organizations must determine when users can no longer create or make changes to electronic documentation. Organizations with several source systems should consider locking down documents at some determined time after a patient encounter. EHR handling of this function may present limitations, which organizations will need to factor into their policies.

- **External records and reports:** Healthcare records created by providers outside of the organization that are received by the organization for patient care. The decision regarding which category external records and reports fall into depends on the applicability of HIPAA privacy rules, state laws or regulations, the source of the request, and the type of request. If external records and reports are used to make decisions about an individual, they become part of the designated record set. If those decisions are care decisions, in most cases those same records and reports will also be included in the provider's legal health record, especially if they are created pursuant to a contract.

- **Personal health records (PHRs):** Copies of PHRs that are created, owned, and managed by the patient and are provided to a healthcare organization (s) may be considered part of the health record if so defined by the organization.

- **Research records:** Organizational policy should differentiate whether research records are part of the health record and specify how these records will be kept.

- **Version control:** Organizations must decide whether all versions or just the final version of a document or ancillary report will be displayed.

- **Diagnostic image data:** CT, MRI, ultrasound, nuclear medicine, and the like.

- **Signal tracing data:** EKG, EEG, fetal monitoring signal tracings, and the like.

- **Audio data:** Heart sounds, voice dictations, annotations, and the like.

- **Video data:** Ultrasound, cardiac catheterization examinations, and the like.

- **Text data:** Radiology reports, transcribed reports, UBS, itemized bills, and the like.

- **Original analog document image data:** Signed patient consent forms, handwritten notes, drawings, and the like.

Patient-identifiable Source Data

Various types of patient-identifiable source data are collected and stored in source systems. Source-system data must be evaluated for inclusion in the legal health record. **Source-system data** are the data from which interpretations, summaries, and notes are derived. Examples of source-system data are radiological film or scans, laboratory values, pathology slides, video and audio recordings, and EKG tracings. They may be designated part of the legal health record whether or not they are integrated into a single system or maintained as part of the source system.

Historically, reports or findings on which clinical decision making is based are part of the legal health record. For example, the written result of a test such as an X-ray, ECG, or other similar procedure are always part of the record, whether these reports are integrated into a single system or part of a source system.

Working notes used by a provider in completing a final report are not considered part of the legal health record unless they are made available to others providing care to a patient. However, documents that are kept in a separate record system, such as notes from a particular specialty that are kept separately but are final products, are always considered part of the record.

The determining factor in whether data are considered part of the legal health record is not the format or location but, rather, how the data are used and whether it is reasonable to expect the data to be routinely released when a request for a complete health record is received.

Equally important, healthcare organizations need to identify information to be excluded from the legal health record or designated record set. Documents that fall outside the legal health record and designated records set can be found in **FIGURE 2.5**.

FIGURE 2.5. Documents that fall outside the legal health record and designated record set

Outside the Designated Record Set	Examples
Health information generated, collected, or maintained for purposes that do not include decision making about the individual	• Data collected and maintained for research • Data collected and maintained for peer review purposes • Data collected and maintained for performance improvement purposes • Appointment and surgery schedules • Birth and death registers • Surgery registers • Diagnostic or operative indexes • Duplicate copies of information that can also be located in the individual's medical or billing record
Psychotherapy notes	The notes of a mental health professional about counseling sessions that are maintained separate and apart from the regular health record
Information compiled in reasonable anticipation of or for use in a civil, criminal, or administrative action or proceeding	Notes taken by a covered entity during a meeting with the covered entity's attorney about a pending lawsuit
CLIA	• Requisitions for laboratory tests • Duplicate lab results when the originals are filed in the individual's paper chart
Employer records	• Pre-employment physicals maintained in human resource files • The results of HIV tests maintained by the infectious disease control nurse on employees who have suffered needle-stick injuries on the job
Business associate records that meet the definition of designated record set but that merely duplicate information maintained by the covered entity	Transcribed operative reports that have been transmitted to the covered entity
Education records	Records generated and maintained by teachers and teachers' aides employed by a school district or patients in acute care hospitals, institutions for the developmentally disabled, and rehabilitation care centers
Source (raw) data interpreted or summarized in the individual's medical or health record	• Pathology slides • Diagnostic films • ECG tracings from which interpretations are derived
Versions	Management of multiple revisions of the same document. By versioning, each iteration of a document is tracked.
Metadata	Data that provides a detailed description about other data. "Information about a particular data set or document that describes how, when, and by whom it was collected, created, accessed, or modified and how it is formatted".
Audits	Results of reviews to identify variations from established baselines or used to track an individual's activity in an electronic system (e.g., view, print, edit).
Pending reports	Reports that have been initiated by a member of the healthcare team but not yet authenticated and may not be available for viewing by staff until completed. An EHR system will keep these documents in a pending or incomplete status.

Administrative Information

Administrative information includes patient-identifiable documentation used for administrative, regulatory, healthcare operations, and payment (financial) purposes. Administrative information should have the same level of confidentiality as the legal health record. Two types of administrative information are created and maintained by healthcare organizations. The first type consists of documentation that is typically part of the health record, such as consents for treatment or surgery and research forms that would be produced in response to a subpoena. The second type of administrative information should not be considered part of the legal health record and would not be produced in response to a court order, subpoena, or request for the health record. Healthcare organizations might more appropriately consider such administrative information **working documents**. Examples of administrative data include (AHIMA 2011):

- Audit trails related to the EHR

- Authorization forms for release of information

- Birth and death certificate worksheets

- Correspondence concerning requests for records

- Databases containing patient information

- Event history and audit trails

- Financial and insurance forms

- Incident or patient safety reports

- Institutional review board lists

- Logs

- Notice of privacy practices acknowledgments (unless the organization chooses to classify them as part of the health record)

- Patient-identifiable data reviewed for quality assurance or utilization management

- Protocols and clinical pathways, practice guidelines, and other knowledge sources that do not imbed patient data

- Work lists and works in progress

Derived data

Derived data consist of factual details aggregated or summarized from a group of health records that provide no means to identify specific patients. These data should have the same level of confidentiality as the legal health record. However, derived data should not be considered part of the legal health record and would not be produced in response to a court order, subpoena, or request for the health record.

The following are examples of derived data:

- Accreditation reports

- Anonymous patient data for research purposes

- Best-practice guidelines created from aggregate patient data

- OASIS reports

- ORYX, Quality Indicator, Quality Measure, or other reports

- Public health reports that do not contain patient-identifiable data

- Statistical reports

- Transmission reports for MDS, OASIS, and IRF-PAI

Emerging Issues

As EHR technology evolves, challenges to the definition of the legal health record are emerging. Organizations must resolve these challenges with their legal counsel and information technology departments. Many items have not historically been included in the legal health record and will entail new storage and retrieval costs if they are defined as part of the record. Following are some examples of documents and data that should be evaluated for inclusion or exclusion in the legal health record:

- Audio files of dictation

- Alerts and reminders (including resolutions/responses)

- Audio files of patient telephone calls

- Nursing shift-to-shift reports (handwritten or audio)

- Patient–physician e-mails

- Telephone consultation audio files

- Videos of office visits

- Videos of procedures

- Videos of telemedicine consultations

Personal Health Records

Organizational policy should address how personal health information provided by the patient will or will not be incorporated into the patient's health record. Copies of **personal health records (PHRs)**, created, owned, and managed by the patient, are considered part of the legal health record when the organization uses them to provide treatment; however, the PHR does not replace the legal health record.

Types of PHRs

Paper-Based

This type of PHR is currently the most common. These PHRs consist of folders or notebooks filled with information from physician practices, hospitals, pharmacies, insurance companies, and ancillary centers, such as laboratories. Lists of emergency contacts, allergies, current medications, and contact information for all physicians are typically included in paper-based EHRs.

Personal Computer-Based

This type of PHR includes typed reports or scanned health information documents stored on a desktop or laptop computer. There may or may not be software to organize the health information. Personal computers are not able to readily exchange health information between healthcare providers and the patient. Unfortunately, PHRs kept on a personal computer are not accessible to healthcare providers when they need them for healthcare treatment purposes. This silo of health information has limited ability to be updated, shared, accessed, and used for treatment decisions.

Web-Based

This type of PHR is obtained through private online accounts accessed via a web browser. Patients log into the account with a unique user name and password. Web-based platforms can include videoconferencing for **telemedicine**, document sharing with providers who have been granted permission, and secure e-mailing. This 24-hour-a-day access offers a wonderful solution for making healthcare treatment decisions using only an Internet connection. Healthcare facilities, employers, and payers may offer this type of PHR to consumers.

Hybrid Desktop/Web-Based

This type of PHR offers the flexibility of uploading health information onto a web server. The patient uses a personal (desktop or laptop) computer to maintain his health information on the web server. Providers can access the information 24 hours a day, primarily in a read-only format. Updating and maintenance are restricted to the personal computer linked to the account.

Portable Devices

Acceptance and use of this type of PHR is growing rapidly. Smart cards, memory devices, and smart phones are among the portable devices used to house PHRs. This allows the patient to easily carry her personal health information wherever she goes. A portable device may also be used in conjunction with all other types of PHRs (AHIMA 2010).

Organizations must address how and when to incorporate PHRs into their legal health records. They must determine when information is used to provide patient-care services; review patient data; or document observations, actions, or instructions. This includes patient owned, managed, and populated tracking records, such as medication records and glucose and insulin records.

Documentation Guidelines

Health records may be called by different names in different healthcare settings, for example:

- Resident records (in long-term care facilities)
- Client records (in behavioral health hospitals and clinics)

- Patient records (in physicians' offices)

- Surgery records (in ambulatory surgery centers)

- Health records (in hospitals)

The style and content of health records depend on the setting in which the healthcare services are provided. Regulatory and accreditation requirements for the various healthcare settings are quite different, as are reimbursement requirements, patient demographics, and services mix.

Documentation requirements for acute care facilities are unique to the setting, and different types of acute care hospitals must comply with different specialty documentation requirements. For example, the documentation for diagnostic and therapeutic services, care of developmental disabilities, and counseling for behavioral conditions are somewhat different from the documentation for acute care medical-surgical services. Other specialty hospitals, such as children's hospitals and women's hospitals, provide services similar to those of general acute care facilities and follow the same general guidelines, although there are specific and unique types of documentation for pediatric care and obstetrics and gynecology specialties. The same is true of **critical-access hospitals**, very small and geographically isolated hospitals that provide a limited range of services.

Long-term acute care hospitals treat patients who require intensive medical services for acute and chronic conditions. Rehabilitation hospitals provide nursing, medical, and rehabilitative services to individuals (such as stroke patients) who require physical, speech, and/or occupational therapy—in addition to medical and nursing services—but are no longer in the acute phase of their illness.

Almost all healthcare settings must comply with federal documentation guidelines established by CMS (2010) for Medicare participants. In addition, most hospitals choose to participate in voluntary accreditation programs, which also publish health record documentation standards.

Regardless of setting, good documentation contains sufficient data and information to identify and support the diagnosis or condition and treatment of the patient. Documentation justifies the care, treatment, and services and promotes continuity of care among providers. Although they vary by setting, high-quality documentation practices are always required.

The transition from paper to hybrid to fully EHRs is a complex process (AHIMA 2011). (See **APPENDIX 2A**.) An attorney should review policies related to legal documentation to ensure adherence to the most current standards and case law. Regardless of the legal health record format, HIM professionals should fully understand the principles of maintaining a legally sound health record and the potential ramifications when the record's legal integrity is questioned. Documentation guidelines that originally applied to paper can translate to electronic documentation; however, additional guidelines will be needed to maintain a legally sound health record. The ultimate goal for managing EHR information is that it is kept in a manner that supports a facility's business and legal processes and eliminates the need to maintain a duplicate paper process.

FIGURE 2.6 lists guidelines that organizations should consider to establish sound documentation principles for health records.

FIGURE 2.6. Health record documentation guidelines

1. Policies should be based on all applicable standards, including accreditation standards, state and local licensure requirements, federal and state regulations, reimbursement requirements, and professional practice standards.

2. The content and format of health records should be uniform.

3. Health record entries should be legible and complete.

4. Individuals documenting the health record should have the authority and right to document as defined by the organization's policies and procedures. The authorship of health record entries should be clearly identified in the documentation.

5. The definition of a legally authenticated entry should be established, and rules should be set for prompt authentication of every entry in the health record by the author responsible for ordering, providing, or evaluating the service furnished.

6. Entries should be made as soon as possible after an event or observation is made at the point of care. An entry should never be made in advance.

7. All entries in the health record should include the complete date and time. Time must be included in all types of narrative notes, even if it may not seem important to the type of entry. Narrative documentation should reflect the actual time the entry was made. Effective January 2007, CMS added the requirement that hospitals must time all entries in health records (CMS 2010).

8. The record should always reflect factual information and be written using specific language and factual statements. Avoid using vague or generalized language.

9. For patient safety reasons, organizational written policies must address the uses of standardized terminology, definitions, abbreviations, acronyms, symbols, and dose designations. Hospitals should publish a list of abbreviations and symbols that are prohibited when documenting in the health record (Joint Commission 2011).

10. Policies should specify the parties responsible for receiving and transcribing verbal or telephone orders of physicians.

11. All entries in the health record, regardless of form or format, must be permanent (paper-based or electronic records). The rules of evidence require that policies and procedures must be in place to prevent alteration, tampering, or loss.

12. Documentation errors should never be obliterated or changed. Instead, documentation errors should be corrected according to the procedure established in the organization's documentation policy and/or medical staff rules.

13. Organizational policies should address how the patient or patient's representative can request corrections and amendments to the record. The amendment should refer back to the information questioned and include date and time. At no time should the documentation in question be removed from the chart or obliterated in any way. The patient has the right to request that a correction be made to his health information, such as with an amendment; however, it is the healthcare organization's discretion as to whether or not the request will be granted" (DHHS 2011a).

14. The qualitative and quantitative analyses of health record documentation should be conducted according to procedures developed and implemented by the hospital's health information management department.

15. Organizational policies should differentiate whether research records are part of the legal health record or if the research center maintains its own records. This should be verified with the institutional review board, since this may influence whether research records are part of the legal health record.

The Future of Clinical Documentation

Healthcare has lagged far behind other fields in the application of information technology to operations and communications. However, the development and implementation of computer-based systems, including EHR systems, is inevitable for all healthcare organizations.

As mentioned in chapter 1, the evolution of computer-based systems in acute care facilities began with the development of automated systems for administrative operations (admissions, billing, and claims processing). In the 1980s and 1990s, automated systems for laboratory and pharmacy services were implemented in most hospitals. Today, hospitals use a wide variety of computer-based technologies to provide clinical services and support administrative functions. Yet, the application of advanced computer technology to health record documentation has been slow. The term *electronic health record* is now preferred over **computer-based patient record (CPR)**, a term that was in use during the 1990s.

HIPAA is driving the universal adoption of EHR systems. Standardized transactions and code sets, when electronically transmitting healthcare information, must comply with HIPAA format and content. Standardized transactions include such items as claims information, encounter information, payment, remittance advice, claim status inquiry and response, and eligibility inquiry and response. Code sets identify specific diagnoses and clinical procedures on claims and encounter forms. The *International Classification of Diseases*, Ninth Revision, Clinical Modification (ICD-9-CM), *Current Procedural Terminology*, Fourth Edition (CPT-4), and Healthcare Common Procedure Coding System (HCPCS) are examples of code sets for procedures and diagnoses.

The **National Committee on Vital and Health Statistics (NCVHS)**, a public policy advisory board made up of representatives from numerous healthcare, trade, and professional organizations, recommended to the US Department of Health and Human Services that standards-developing organizations be encouraged to adopt standards that promote interoperability of EHRs and PHRs. NCVHS recognizes that the interoperability of EHRs provides an opportunity to improve the safety and quality of patient care. Providers will need to use specific terminology, data structure, and transport and security standards to connect healthcare entities. In a 2006 report to the Department of Health and Human Services, NCVHS recommended the minimal functional requirements needed for the initial definition of the **Nationwide Health Information Network (NHIN)** to exchange data (NCVHS 2006).

NHIN efforts play a major role in the future of health information exchange. Through the Office of the National Coordinator for Health Information Technology, the NHIN contains a set of standards, services, and policies that enable secure health information exchange over the Internet. The NHIN provides the framework for the exchange of health information across the country and assists in achieving the goals of the HITECH Act. Some goals of the NHIN are to enable health information to follow the consumer, to make health information available for clinical decision making, and to support appropriate use of healthcare information beyond direct patient care.

The **Nationwide Health Information Network Exchange** demonstrates the ability to exchange health information on a national level. Currently, participants include local-, regional-, and state-level **health information exchange organizations (HIOs)**, integrated delivery systems, and government agencies. By the end of 2011, it is expected that approximately 35 entities, including small provider practices, will securely share live health information as part of this exchange (ONC 2011).

Health Level Seven (HL7) International, a nonprofit organization that develops standards for interoperability of health information technology, was founded in 1987. This global authority has affiliates in more than 30 counties and members in 55 countries. HL7 is the ANSI-accredited standards development organization dedicated to providing a comprehensive framework and related standards for the exchange, integration, sharing, and retrieval of electronic health information that supports clinical practice and the management, delivery, and evaluation of health services (HL7 2011).

EHRs and EHR networks are certified by the **Certification Commission for Healthcare Information Technology (CCHIT)**. The organization was founded in 2004 and began certifying in 2006. The commission "established the first comprehensive, practical definition of what capabilities were needed in these systems" (CCHIT n.d.). The US federal government officially recognizes CCHIT as a certifying body.

The **Systematized Nomenclature of Medicine–Clinical Terms (SNOMED CT)** provides a common language for indexing, storing, retrieving, and aggregating clinical data across specialties and healthcare providers. SNOMED CT is a comprehensive clinical terminology, originally created by the College of American Pathologists and, as of April 2007, owned, maintained, and distributed by the International Health Terminology Standards Development Organisation, a not-for-profit association in Denmark. SNOMED CT has an advanced structure that meets most criteria for a machine-readable terminology, is one of a suite of designated standards for use in US federal government systems for the electronic exchange of clinical health information, and is a required standard in interoperability specifications of the US Healthcare Information Technology Standards Panel (NIH 2011).

The **National Council for Prescription Drug Programs (NCPDP)** creates and promotes data interchange standards for the pharmacy services sector of the healthcare industry. Medicare has mandated e-prescribing for Medicare plans to reduce prescription errors due to illegible handwriting. The NCPDP is an ANSI-accredited standards development organization and the official standard for HIPAA pharmacy claims (NCPDP 2011). The implementation of EHR systems may also support the development of longitudinal health records. A **longitudinal health record** is a health record that includes all of the health-related information generated for an individual during her lifetime. These records have many benefits for consumers. However, maintaining such records for every American will be impossible until every healthcare provider in the country has implemented an EHR system.

Under the current system of mixed-media records, providers keep a separate health record for every patient they treat. As a result, an individual's medical history is documented in hundreds of separate records created over his lifetime. The NHIN would provide the necessary connectivity to link one or more of the customer's EHRs to a single, longitudinal health record, regardless of where the information resides. The NHIN is a critical component to reaching the longitudinal record.

Summary

The quality of the clinical documentation in patients' health records is essential in virtually every aspect of healthcare, including delivery, reimbursement, education, and research. HIM professionals play a vital role by ensuring the availability, completeness, and accuracy of health record documentation. They protect the consumers' right to confidentiality and privacy. To be effective, HIM professionals must understand every aspect of the healthcare environment, including state and federal laws and regulations, accreditation standards and processes, quality improvement practices, and information system technology.

References

AHIMA 2011. Fundamentals of the Legal Health Record and Designated Record Set. *Journal of AHIMA* 82(2): expanded online version.

AHIMA 2010. Role of the Personal Health Record in the EHR (Updated). (Updated November 2010). Chicago: AHIMA.

Centers for Medicare and Medicaid Services (CMS) 2010. Conditions of Participation for Hospitals; Final rule. 42 CFR Part 482. *Federal Register* 71(227): 68672–68695. http://ecfr.gpoaccess.gov/cgi/t/text/text-idx?c=ecfr&sid=dee029e8667b45b65efaf4c6b967bb9c&rgn=div8&view=text&node=42:5.0.1.1.1.3.4.4&idno=42.

Certification Commission for Health Information Technology (CCHIT). n.d. About the Certification Commission for Health Information Technology. http://www.cchit.org/about.

Code of Federal Regulations (CFR). 2011a. Title 45, Volume 1, Part 164, Section 164.501: Definition of a Covered Entity. http://hipaa.ohio.gov/tools/CEDefinition.pdf.

Code of Federal Regulations (CFR). 2011b. Title 45, Volume 1, Part 164, Subpart E, Section 164.524: Access of Individuals to Protected Health Information. http://edocket.access.gpo.gov/cfr_2002/octqtr/45cfr164.524.htm.

Dick, R. S., E. B. Steen, and D. E. Detmer, eds. 1997. *The Computer-Based Patient Record: An Essential Technology for Health Care*, revised ed. Washington, DC: National Academies Press.

Health Level Seven (HL7). 2011. Health Level Seven International. http://www.hl7.org.

The Joint Commission. 2011. *2011 Comprehensive Accreditation Manual for Hospitals: The Official Handbook*. Oakbrook Terrace, IL: Joint Commission.

National Committee on Vital and Health Statistics (NCVHS). 2006. Personal Health Records and Personal Health Record Systems. http://www.ncvhs.hhs.gov/0602nhiirpt.pdf.

National Council for Prescription Drug Programs (NCPDP). 2011. About. http://www.ncpdp.org/about.aspx.

National Institutes of Health (NIH). US National Library of Medicine. 2011. SNOMED Clinical Terms. http://www.nlm.nih.gov/research/umls/Snomed/snomed_main.html.

Office of the National Coordinator for Health Information Technology (ONC). 2011. Health IT. http://healthit.hhs.gov/portal/server.pt/community/healthit_hhs_gov__nhin_exchange/1407.

US Department of Health and Human Services (HHS). 2011a. Health Information Privacy. http://www.hhs.gov/ocr/privacy/index.html.

US Department of Health and Human Services (HHS). 2011b. The HIPAA Enforcement Rule. http://www.hhs.gov/ocr/privacy/hipaa/administrative/enforcementrule/index.html.

Appendix 2A

Fundamentals of the Legal Health Record and Designated Record Set

For years healthcare organizations have struggled to define their legal health records and align them with the designated record set required by the HIPAA Privacy Rule. Questions often arise about the differences between the two sets because both identify information that must be disclosed upon request.

The expanding scope of health records adds to the challenge of defining and compiling these record sets. An individual's record can consist of a facility's record, outpatient diagnostic test results or therapies, pharmacy records, physician records, other care providers' records, and the patient's own PHR. Administrative and financial documents and data may be intermingled with clinical data.

In addition, the type of media on which information is recorded is also expanding. Source records may include diagnostic images, video, voice files, and e-mail. The organization must determine which of these data elements, electronic-structured documents, images, audio files, and video files to include.

The emergence of EHRs is also complicating organizational efforts to define and disclose information. Information in EHRs is often stored in multiple systems, inhibiting the ability to succinctly pull together the record for either the legal health record or the designated record set.

These input systems may include laboratory information, pharmacy information, picture archiving and communications, cardiology information, results reporting, computerized provider order entry, nurse care planning, transcription, document imaging, and fetal trace monitoring systems, as well as a myriad of home grown or individual clinical department systems.

However, the same criteria that organizations used to determine what paper records to retain and include in their legal health records and designated record sets can be applied to electronic records. Questions organizations must ask include:

- What information can be stored long term?

- What is clinically useful long term?

- What is the cost of storage?

- How can the organization effectively and succinctly assemble the EHR for long-term use?

This practice brief compiles and updates guidance from four previously published practice briefs to provide an overview of the purposes of the designated record set and the legal health record and helps organizations identify what information to include in each. It also provides guidelines for disclosing health records from the sets.

AHIMA. 2011. Fundamentals of the Legal Health Record and Designated Record Set. *Journal of AHIMA* 82(2): expanded online version.

Defining the Legal Health Record and Designated Record Set

There is no one-size-fits-all definition for the legal health record and designated record set. The healthcare organization must explicitly define both in a multidisciplinary team approach. Medical staff, for example, should provide guidance to ensure that patient care needs will be met for immediate, long-term, and research uses.

In addition, organizations should consider the capabilities of their electronic systems, both immediate and long term. Additional considerations include ease of access to different components of patient care information and guidance from the organization's legal counsel considering community standards of care, federal regulations, state laws and regulations, standards of accrediting agencies, and the requirements of third-party payers. See boxed section, Other Federal Laws and Regulations.

Other Federal Laws and Regulations

In addition to the HIPAA privacy rule, other federal laws and regulations give individuals the right to access their health information. Organizations must meet these obligations, as well as protect the confidentiality of patient records by ensuring that they are released to or accessed by authorized individuals only.

The Privacy Act of 1974, like the HIPAA Privacy Rule, gives individuals the right to access and request amendments to their records. The act defines a record as "any item, collection, or grouping of information about an individual that is maintained by an agency, including, but not limited to, his education, financial transactions, medical history, and criminal or employment history and that contains his name, or the identifying number, symbol, or other identifying particular assigned to the individual, such as a finger or voice print or a photograph."[1]

The Medicare Conditions of Participation for state long-term care facilities state that the resident or his or her legal representative has the right to access "all records pertaining to himself or herself," including current clinical records.[2] In addition to clinical records, the term "records" includes all records pertaining to the resident, such as trust-fund ledgers pertinent to the resident and contracts between the resident and the facility.[3]

The Confidentiality of Alcohol and Drug Abuse Patient Records regulation allows federally subsidized alcohol and drug abuse programs to give patients access to their own records, including the opportunity to inspect and copy any records that the program maintains about the patient. The regulation defines records as "any information, whether recorded or not, relating to a patient received or acquired by a federally assisted alcohol or drug program."[4]

The Occupational Safety and Health Administration requires employers to document certain employee injuries, including medical care provided in relation to those injuries. Employees and their designated representatives generally have access to such injury reports and related health records.[5]

(Continued)

The HIPAA privacy rule clearly indicates that its intent is not to preempt other federal laws and regulations. Therefore, if an individual's rights of access are greater under another federal law, the individual should be afforded the greater access.

State Laws

Many states have laws or regulations that give individuals the right to their health information. Some state laws may define health information more broadly than the privacy rule. Some states may not limit access and amendment to personal health information in a designated record set. When state laws or regulations afford individuals greater rights of access, the covered entity must adhere to state law.

Notes

1. Privacy Act of 1974. 5 USC, Section 552A. Available online at www.justice.gov/opcl/privstat.htm.
2. Centers for Medicare and Medicaid Services. "Part 483-Requirements for States and Long Term Care Facilities." Title 42-Public Health. Chapter IV. Available online at www.access.gpo.gov/nara/cfr/waisidx_01/42cfr483_01.html.
3. Centers for Medicare and Medicaid Services. "State Operations Manual: Appendix PP-Guidance to Surveyors for Long Term Care Facilities." Revised December 2, 2009. Available online at http://cms.gov/manuals/Downloads/som107ap_pp_guidelines_ltcf.pdf.
4. "Confidentiality of Alcohol and Drug Abuse Patient Records." 42 CFR, Part 2. Available online at http://ecfr.gpoaccess.gov/cgi/t/text/text-idx?c=ecfr&rgn=div5&view=text&node=42:1.0.1.1.2&idno=42.l.
5. Occupational Safety and Health Administration, Department of Labor. "Recording and Reporting Occupational Injuries and Illnesses." 29 CFR, Chapter 17, Part 1904.35, Section 657. 2002. Available online at www.osha.gov/pls/oshaweb/owastand.display_standard_group?p_toc_level=1&p_part_number=1904.

Organizations should follow the following common principles when defining their legal health record and designated record set.

Legal Health Record Definition and Role

The legal health record serves to identify what information constitutes the official business record of an organization for evidentiary purposes. The legal health record is a subset of the entire patient database. The elements that constitute an organization's legal health record vary depending on how the organization defines it.

The legal health record is the documentation of healthcare services provided to an individual during any aspect of healthcare delivery in any type of healthcare organization. An organization's legal health record definition must explicitly identify the sources, medium, and location of the individually identifiable data that it includes (i.e., the data collected and directly used in documenting healthcare or health status). The documentation that composes the legal health record may physically exist in separate and multiple paper-based or electronic systems.

The legal health record serves to

- Support the decisions made in a patient's care

- Support the revenue sought from third-party payers

- Document the services provided as legal testimony regarding the patient's illness or injury, response to treatment, and caregiver decisions

- Serve as the organization's business and legal record

The legal health record is typically used when responding to formal requests for information for evidentiary purposes. It does not affect the discoverability of other information held by the organization.

When defining the legal health record, healthcare organizations should consider:

- The available functions in the EHR system that may generate relevant information. For example, does the EHR have clinical decision support, digital image import, or patient portals? Will information sent to or by the patient through the portal be inserted into the record and considered part of the legal record?

- The storage capacity and cost for the required retention period of the health record. For example, what is the cost and storage capacity for WAVE files, transcribed records, and scanned documents or images?

- The data's importance for long-term use. For example, organizations should define how to differentiate between different types of raw data. Some source documentation for test results, whether digital or paper, generally is considered useful only for short-term use (for example, EEG tracings).

- Whether the EHR system is able to provide both readable electronic and paper copies of all components of the legal health record.

Designated Record Set Definition and Role

The HIPAA Privacy Rule defines the designated record set as a group of records maintained by or for a covered entity that may include patient medical and billing records; the enrollment, payment, claims, adjudication, and cases or medical management record systems maintained by or for a health plan; or information used in whole or in part to make care-related decisions.

The designated record set also contains individually identifiable data stored on any medium and collected and directly used in documenting healthcare or health status. It includes clinical data such as WAVE files, images (for example, X-rays), and billing information.

The designated record set is generally broader than the legal health record because it addresses all protected health information. While the legal health record is generally the information used by the patient care team to make decisions about the treatment of a patient, the designated record set contains protected health information along with business information unrelated to patient care.

Organizations must define the types of documentation that comprise the designated record set and identify where the records physically exist, such as in separate and multiple paper-based or electronic systems.

Under HIPAA, the designated record set is used to clarify the rights of individuals to access, amend, restrict, and acquire an accounting of disclosures. Individuals have the right to inspect and obtain a copy, request amendments, and set restrictions and accountings of medical and billing information used to make decisions about their care.

Guidance for Defining Record Sets

The challenge for HIM professionals in defining the legal health record or designated record set is to determine which data elements, electronic-structured documents, images, audio files, and video files to include. The primary consideration in defining the legal health record and designated record set must always be the needs for immediate and long-term patient care. An HIM committee comprised primarily of patient care team members can guide this process. Members of this committee should decide what information is clinically meaningful.

1. Identify Relevant Regulations, Standards, and Laws

Based on the committee's clinical direction, the first step in defining the legal health record and designated record set is to determine what legal entities enforce relevant regulations, guidelines, standards, or laws on health records. Although these entities may have defined a legal record in paper terms (for example, requiring a medication sheet rather than an electronic medication administration record), their definitions must become the basis for the organization's legal health record definition.

2. Determine Records Created in the Course of Business

The second step is to determine whether the records are created in the provider or entity's ordinary course of business. Source-system or raw data are the data from which interpretations, summaries, and notes are derived. They may be designated part of the legal health record, whether or not they are integrated into a single system or maintained as part of the source system.

Records from source systems may be considered part of the legal health record based on the content of the source system's record. Historically, reports or findings upon which clinical decision making is based are parts of the legal health record. For example, the written result of a test such as an X-ray, an ECG, or other similar procedure is always part of the record, whether these reports are integrated into a single system or are part of a source system.

Working notes used by a provider to complete a final report are not considered part of the health record unless they are made available to others providing patient care. However, documents that are kept in a separate system (such as notes from a particular area of specialty that are kept separately but are treatment records) are always considered part of the health record.

The determining factor in whether information is to be considered part of the legal health record is not where it resides or the format it takes, but rather how it is used and whether it may be reasonably expected to be routinely released when a request for a complete health record is received.

Uses of the information for business and legal purposes are usually, but not always, drawn from the legal health record. The most notable exceptions are those disclosures made for purposes of discovery or e-discovery in which any information requested under the court order must be provided.

Several states have laws or regulations that spell out the requirements and conditions under which health information from another healthcare organization or provider must be redisclosed. In the absence of more stringent state law, the HIPAA privacy rule prevails. However, because any medical or billing information that was used to make decisions about the individual is included as part of the designated record set under the HIPAA privacy rule, information must be disclosed or redisclosed if requested by the individual to whom it pertains, regardless of whether the information is external or internal.

3. Address Retention Requirements

The third step in determining the legal health record is ensuring that components are retained appropriately. Storing EHR components in disparate systems can cause problems. HIM professionals must identify and collaborate with IT professionals and system owners to define retention policies and practices. Without adequate retention of the EHR, compiling the complete record for release could be impossible.

A tool such as a matrix is critical for tracking the paper and electronic portions of the health record. As records are transitioned from paper to electronic, dates should be documented to provide a guide for staff when retrieving the patient's health information. (A sample matrix is provided in **APPENDIX 2A.1,** Health Record Matrix.)

4. Consider How Data Would Be Produced

The fourth step in defining the legal health record and designated record set is to determine how information may be appropriately released. While it is easy to declare something such as an EKG WAVE file part of the legal health record or designated record set, the organization must consider how it will be reproduced.

Questions to ask include if the source system can print or download to a CD, how it will be accessed by the requester, and if it will be in an understandable format. Components of the legal health record and designated record set must be reproducible in an accessible format. See **APPENDIX 2A.2** for a comparison of the legal health record versus the designated record set.

5. Classify External Records

The fifth step is determining how to classify external records received by the organization. Some state laws address how to classify external records; however, in the absence of state law, the organization must determine if external records will be a part of the health record.

There is a school of thought that these external records cannot and should not become part of the legal health record because of the inability to attest to how they were originally created. To include them as part of the legal health record may result in implied liability for any inaccuracies the external records contain.

The opposing view is that if the external records were relied upon to make care decisions they should be included as part of the legal record. In addition, the College of American Pathologists requires that the laboratory director be involved with the decision on what lab results should be included in the EHR.

However, including external records as part of the designated record set and making them available in all appropriate disclosures, including disclosures in response to a subpoena, may accomplish the same purpose. The organization's legal counsel should be consulted prior to determining policy regarding the inclusion of external records as part of the legal health record.

Ultimately, the admissibility of the requested information in court is not the concern of the party producing the information. Compliance with the terms of the subpoena or order is required.

Additional Elements and Functions to Consider

As technology continues to evolve, other features will need to be evaluated and reflected in the legal health record and designated record set policies. Consideration needs to be given to documents that are not yet complete or are in interim/pending status. Functions such as clinical decision support triggers and annotations need to be considered as well. **APPENDIX 2A.3** lists the features and functions that should be evaluated when creating the policy for the organization's designated record set and legal health record.

Equally as important, organizations need to identify information that is not in the legal health record or designated record set. Data such as audit trails, metadata, and psychotherapy notes are not included in the definitions for these record sets. See **APPENDIX 2A.4** for a sample list of items outside the legal health record and designated record set.

Recommendations for Clarifying Disclosure

Healthcare organizations can take the following basic steps to help clear up confusion around the legal health record and the designated record set and the disclosure of information from both:

- Develop and maintain an inventory of documents and data that comprise the legal health record. Consider whether other types of information that are not document based are part of the legal health record (for example, e-mail, electronic fetal monitoring strips, diagnostic images, digital photography, and video).

- Develop a detailed inventory of items that compose the designated record. Declare the official legal health record and designated record set in organizational policy.

- Consider a single repository for legal retention requirements.

- Consider the use of records management software that supports the records declaration process and records life cycle management, particularly for messaging records (such as e-mail or instant messages that are considered part of the legal health record or designated record set).

- Collaborate with clinicians to develop procedures for identifying external information that has been used in patient care. Once identified as such, provisions should be made for including this in the patient's record, whether paper or electronic. Within the record, consideration should be given to filing or indexing the external information under a separate tab or section of the electronic or paper record developed for this purpose. Review state statutes that may require inclusion of external information.

- Promptly return to the patient (if feasible) or dispose of (in accordance with the organization's destruction procedures) any health information that is not used or not solicited.

- Consider developing policies and procedures that confine the ability to request health information from external sources and to place such information in the patient's record to specified staff or personnel.

- Develop written policies and procedures as well as staff training for clinical users that address the use of external information. Train HIM staff on procedures related to redisclosure of health information.

- Identify the records the organization believes individuals have the right to access and amend under state and federal laws and regulations

- Apply HIPAA's pre emption standards where individuals' rights to access and amend are not the same under other federal or state laws and regulations

There may be times when an individual has a legitimate need to access source data that are not considered part of the legal health record or designated record set. The organization's legal counsel should advise whenever there is uncertainty. **APPENDIX 2A.5** contains policy definitions that can be included in organizational policy. **APPENDIX 2A.6** offers a sample template for the legal health record, and **APPENDIX 2A.6** features a sample template for a designated record set policy.

References

AHIMA. 2010. Guidance for clinical documentation improvement programs. *Journal of AHIMA* 81 (5): expanded Web version. AHIMA Body of Knowledge. http://www.ahima.org.

Centers for Medicare and Medicaid Services, Department of Health and Human Services. Title 42-Public Health. Chapter IV, Subchapter G-Standards and Certification. Part 482-Conditions of Participation for Hospitals, Subpart C-Basic Hospital Functions. Section 482.24-Condition of Participation: Medical Record Services. http://cfr.vlex.com/vid/482-condition-participation-record-19811382#ixzz13345288z.

Department of Health and Human Services. 2002. "Standards for Privacy of Individually Identifiable Health Information; Final Rule." 45 CFR Parts 160 and 164. *Federal Register* 67, no. 157 (Aug. 14). http://aspe.hhs.gov/admnsimp/final/pvcguide1.htm.

Joint Commission. The Joint Commission Standards. http://www.jointcommission.org/Standards.

NCHICA Designated Record Sets Work Group and Privacy and Confidentiality Focus Group. 2002. Guidance for Identifying Designated Record Sets under HIPAA. August 16. http://www.nchica.org/HIPAA Resources/Samples/DesRecSets.pdf.

Servais, Cheryl E. 2008. *The Legal Health Record*. Chicago: AHIMA.

Warner, Diana. 2010. Evaluating alerts and triggers: determining whether alerts and triggers are part of the legal health record. *Journal of AHIMA* 81 (3): 40-41. AHIMA Body of Knowledge.http://www.ahima.org.

Appendix 2A.1

Health Record Matrix

The matrix below is a tool organizations can use to help identify and track the paper and electronic portions of the health record during an EHR implementation and ongoing maintenance. HIM professionals can customize this matrix to their organization's needs and add specific items that should be considered when implementing an EHR. It is up to each individual organization to determine what health information is considered part of their legal health record and their designated record set.

Type of Document	Name of Document	Primary Source*	Primary Source System Start Date	Source of the Legal Health Record/ Designated Record Set	Legal Health Record, Designated Record Set, or Both	Comments
Nursing	ICU nursing assessment	Electronic nursing documentation system	MM/DD/YYYY	Enterprise document management system	Both	Phased implementation
Physician orders	Congestive heart failure order set	Computerized physician order entry system	MM/DD/YYYY	EHR	Both	Downtime paper orders scanned
Emergency department	Emergency department treatment record	Paper	MM/DD/YYYY	Enterprise document system	Both	
Discharge summary	Discharge summary	Transcription system	MM/DD/YYYY	EHR	Both	
Claims	Billing report	Patient financial system	MM/DD/YYYY	Patient financial system	Designated record set	

*Includes scanned images.

Appendix 2A.2

Comparison of the Designated Record Set versus the Legal Health Record

This side-by-side comparison of the designated record set and the legal health record demonstrates the differences between the two sets of information, as well as their purposes.

	Designated Record Set	Legal Health Record
Definition	A group of records maintained by or for a covered entity that is the medical and billing records about individuals; enrollment, payment, claims adjudication, and case or medical management record systems maintained by or for a health plan; information used in whole or in part by or for the HIPAA-covered entity to make decisions about individuals.	The business record generated at or for a healthcare organization. It is the record that would be released upon receipt of a request. The legal health record is the officially declared record of healthcare services provided to an individual delivered by a provider.
Purpose	Used to clarify the access and amendment standards in the HIPAA privacy rule, which provide that individuals generally have the right to inspect and obtain a copy of protected health information in the designated record set.	The official business record of healthcare services delivered by the entity for regulatory and disclosure purposes.
Content	Defined in organizational policy and required by the HIPAA privacy rule. The content of the designated record set includes medical and billing records of covered providers; enrollment, payment, claims, and case information of a health plan; and information used in whole or in part by or for the covered entity to make decisions about individuals.	Defined in organizational policy and can include individually identifiable data in any medium collected and directly used in documenting healthcare services or health status. It excludes administrative, derived, and aggregate data.
Uses	Supports individual HIPAA right of access and amendment.	Provides a record of health status as well as documentation of care for reimbursement, quality management, research, and public health purposes; facilitates business decision making and education of healthcare practitioners as well as the legal needs of the healthcare organization.

Categorizing record types can assist in understanding the similarities and differences and help organizations develop policies for each. Some record types are found in both the designated record set and the legal health record, while others are specific to the designated record set. The following table provides examples of different types of records and shows the similarities and differences between the two sets of information.

Sorting Record Types

Some record types belong in both the designated record set and the legal health record. Some belong in the designated record set only. Categorizing record types helps organizations set policies for each record set.

Clinical Record	Source Clinical Data	External Records and Reports
• History and physical • Orders • Progress notes • Lab reports (including contract lab) • Progress notes • Vital signs • Assessments • Consults • Clinical reports • Authorizations and consents • Designated record set and legal health record	• X-rays • Images • Fetal strips • Videos • Pathology slides • Designated record set and legal health record	• External records referenced for patient care: other providers' records, records provided upon transfer • Patient-generated records • Personal health records • Designated record set and legal health record*

*There are two points of view on whether external records referenced for patient care are part of the legal health record. One view is that they should be if they were relied upon to make care decisions. The other view is that although they are part of the designated record set and are available for patient care and disclosures, they should not be because of the organization's inability to attest to how the external records were originally created. Organizations should consult with their counsels to weigh the risks and benefits of either approach.

Committee Reports (of patient-specific care decisions)	Administrative and Financial	Secondary/Administrative and Statistical
• Ethics committee or tumor board, if deciding on a course of treatment for an individual patient Note: Documentation of findings could be reported in the patient's health record. Other legal privileges may apply to these records. • Designated record set only	• Super bills/encounter forms • Remittance advice • Case management records • Designated record set only	• Tumor registries data • QI/QM reports and abstracts • Statistical data • Committee minutes (not patient-specific treatment related) • Neither

Appendix 2A.3

Considerations for the Legal Health Record and Designated Record Set

The move toward EHRs is complicating organizational efforts to define and disclose information. Many of the items within the EHR have not historically been included in the legal health record and the designated record set. Examples of documents and data that should be evaluated for inclusion or exclusion include, but are not limited to:

- **Administrative data/documents:** Patient-identifiable data used for administrative, regulatory, healthcare operations, and payment (financial) purposes.[1]

- **Annotations/"sticky notes":** Additional information that is added as a layer on top of the note. The annotation or sticky note may be suppressed when viewing or printing. These may be considered part of the health record. This documentation may become a permanent part of the record and is maintained in a manner similar to any other information contained within the health record.

- **Clinical decision support systems:** A subcategory of clinical information systems that is designed to help healthcare professionals make knowledge-based clinical decisions.[2] Currently there are no generally accepted rules on including decision support such as system-generated notifications, prompts, and alerts as part of the health record.[3] Alerts, reminders, pop-ups, and similar tools are used as aids in the clinical decision-making process. The tools themselves are usually not considered part of the legal health record; however, associated documentation is considered a component.[4] At a minimum the EHR should include documentation of the clinician's actions in response to decision support. This documentation is evidence of the clinician's decision to follow or disregard decision support. The organization should define the extent of exception documentation required (e.g., what no documentation means).[5] When an organization decides to include the decision support trigger as part of the health record, the organization will need to determine if all triggers will be part of the record or just the clinical decision support triggers. For example, alerts for patient appointment reminders may not be considered part of the legal health record, but alerts for drug–drug interaction may be.[6]

- **Coding queries:** A routine communication and education tool used to advocate complete and compliant documentation. Retention of the query varies by healthcare organization. First, an organization must determine if the query will be part of the health record. If the query is not part of the health record, then the organization must decide if the query is kept as part of the business record or only the outcome of the query is maintained in a database.[7]

- **Continuing care records:** Records received from another healthcare provider. Historically, these records were generally not considered part of the legal health record unless they were used in the provision of patient care. In the EHR it may be difficult to determine if information was viewed or used in delivering healthcare. It may be necessary to define such information as part of the legal health record. Policies should reflect the proper disposition of health records from external sources (e.g., other healthcare providers) if they are not integrated into the electronic and legal health record.[8]

- **Data/documents:** Documentation of patient care that took place in the ordinary course of business by all healthcare providers.[9]

- **Data from source systems:** Written results of tests. Data from which interpretations, summaries, notes, flowcharts, etc. are derived.[10]

- **Discrete structured data:** Laboratory orders/refills, orders/medication orders/MARs, online charting and documentation, and any detailed charges.[11]

- **Document completion (lockdown):** Organizations must determine when users can no longer create or make changes to electronic documentation. Organizations with several source systems should consider locking down documents at some determined time after a patient encounter. There may be limitations regarding how the EHR handles this function, which organizations will need to factor into their policies.[12]

- **External records and reports:** Healthcare records that are created by providers outside of the organization that are received by the organization for patient care. The decision regarding which category external records and reports fall into depends on the applicability of HIPAA Privacy Rules, state law or regulation, source of the request, and type of request. If external records and reports are used to make decisions about an individual, they become part of the designated record set. If those decisions are care decisions, in most cases those same records and reports will also be included in the provider's legal health record, especially if they are created pursuant to a contract.[13]

- **Personal health records (PHRs):** Copies of PHRs that are created, owned, and managed by the patient and are provided to a healthcare organization(s) may be considered part of the health record if so defined by the organization.[14]

- **Research records:** Organizational policy should differentiate whether research records are part of the health record and how these records will be kept.[15]

- **Version control.** Organizations must decide whether all versions of a document or ancillary report will be displayed or just the final version.[16]

- **Diagnostic image data:** CT, MRI, ultrasound, nuclear medicine, etc.[17]

- **Signal tracing data:** EKG, EEG, fetal monitoring signal tracings, etc.[18]

- **Audio data:** Heart sounds, voice dictations, annotations, etc.[19]

- **Video data:** Ultrasound, cardiac catheterization examinations, etc.[20]

- **Text data:** Radiology reports, transcribed reports, UBS, itemized bills, etc.[21]

- **Original analog document/document image data:** Signed patient consent forms, handwritten notes, drawings, etc.[22]

Appendix 2A.3 Notes

1. AHIMA EHR Practice Council. 2007. "Developing a Legal Health Record Policy: Appendix A." *Journal of AHIMA* 78, no. 9 (Oct.): Web extra. AHIMA Body of Knowledge. www.ahima.org.

2. AHIMA. 2009. *Pocket Glossary of Health Information Management and Technology.* Chicago: AHIMA.

3. AHIMA EHR Practice Council. 2007. "Developing a Legal Health Record Policy." *Journal of AHIMA* 78, no. 9 (Oct.): 93–97. AHIMA Body of Knowledge. www.ahima.org.

4. AHIMA e-HIM Work Group on the Legal Health Record. 2005. "Update: Guidelines for Defining the Legal Health Record for Disclosure Purposes." *Journal of AHIMA* 76, no. 8 (Sept.): 64A–G. AHIMA Body of Knowledge. www.ahima.org.

5. AHIMA EHR Practice Council. "Developing a Legal Health Record Policy."

6. Warner, Diana. 2010. "Evaluating Alerts and Triggers: Determining Whether Alerts and Triggers Are Part of the Legal Health Record." *Journal of AHIMA* 81, no. 3 (Mar.): 40–41. AHIMA Body of Knowledge. www.ahima.org.

7. AHIMA. 2010. "Guidance for Clinical Documentation Improvement Programs." *Journal of AHIMA* 81, no. 5 (May): expanded Web version. AHIMA Body of Knowledge. www.ahima.org.

8. AHIMA e-HIM Work Group on the Legal Health Record. "Update: Guidelines for Defining the Legal Health Record for Disclosure Purposes."

9. AHIMA EHR Practice Council. "Developing a Legal Health Record Policy: Appendix A."

10. Ibid.

11. Ibid.

12. AHIMA EHR Practice Council. "Developing a Legal Health Record Policy."

13. Dougherty, Michelle, and Lydia Washington. 2008. "Defining and Disclosing the Designated Record Set and the Legal Health Record." *Journal of AHIMA* 79, no. 4 (Apr.): 65–68. AHIMA Body of Knowledge. www.ahima.org.

14. AHIMA EHR Practice Council. "Developing a Legal Health Record Policy: Appendix A."

15. Ibid.

16. AHIMA EHR Practice Council. "Developing a Legal Health Record Policy."

17. AHIMA EHR Practice Council. "Developing a Legal Health Record Policy: Appendix A."

18. Ibid.

19. Ibid.

20. Ibid.

21. Ibid.

22. Ibid.

Appendix 2A.4

Documents that Fall Outside the Designated Record Set and Legal Health Record

In its definition of the designated record set the privacy rule does not specifically address source data such as pathology slides, diagnostic films, and tracings. However, narrative throughout the preamble suggests that providing interpretations from source data would generally be acceptable in the designated record set. In most cases, individuals cannot interpret source data, so such data are meaningless. On the other hand, the interpretations of source data provide individuals with information needed to make informed decisions about their healthcare.

There may be times, however, when an individual has a legitimate need to access source data. When such a need arises, the covered entity will want to provide the individual with greater rights of access, allowing the individual access to or copies of the source data when possible.

The following table provides examples of those documents that are not included in the designated record set.

Outside the Designated Record Set	Examples
Health information generated, collected, or maintained for purposes that do not include decision making about the individual	• Data collected and maintained for research • Data collected and maintained for peer review purposes • Data collected and maintained for performance improvement purposes • Appointment and surgery schedules • Birth and death registers • Surgery registers • Diagnostic or operative indexes • Duplicate copies of information that can also be located in the individual's medical or billing record
Psychotherapy notes	The notes of a mental health professional about counseling sessions that are maintained separate and apart from the regular health record
Information compiled in reasonable anticipation of or for use in a civil, criminal, or administrative action or proceeding	Notes taken by a covered entity during a meeting with the covered entity's attorney about a pending lawsuit
CLIA	• Requisitions for laboratory tests • Duplicate lab results when the originals are filed in the individual's paper chart
Employer records	• Pre employment physicals maintained in human resource files • The results of HIV tests maintained by the infectious disease control nurse on employees who have suffered needle-stick injuries on the job

(continued)

Business associate records that meet the definition of designated record set but that merely duplicate information maintained by the covered entity	Transcribed operative reports that have been transmitted to the covered entity
Education records	Records generated and maintained by teachers and teachers' aides employed by a school district or patients in acute care hospitals, institutions for the developmentally disabled, and rehabilitation care centers
Source (raw) data interpreted or summarized in the individual's medical or health record	• Pathology slides • Diagnostic films • ECG tracings from which interpretations are derived
Versions	Management of multiple revisions of the same document. By versioning, each iteration of a document is tracked.
Metadata	Data that provide a detailed description about other data. "Information about a particular data set or document that describes how, when, and by whom it was collected, created, accessed, or modified and how it is formatted."[1]
Audits	Results of reviews to identify variations from established baselines or used to track an individual's activity in an electronic system (e.g., view, print, edit).
Pending reports	Reports that have been initiated by a member of the healthcare team but not yet authenticated and may not be available for viewing by staff until completed. An EHR system will keep these documents in a pending or incomplete status.

Administrative and Derived Data

There are many types of patient-identifiable data elements that are pulled from the patient's healthcare record that are not included in the legal health record or designated record set definitions. Administrative data and derived data and documents are two examples of patient-identifiable data that are used in the healthcare organization.

Administrative data are patient-identifiable data used for administrative, regulatory, healthcare operation, and payment (financial) purposes. Examples of administrative data include:

- Audit trails related to the EHR
- Authorization forms for release of information
- Birth and death certificate worksheets
- Correspondence concerning requests for records
- Databases containing patient information
- Event history and audit trails
- Financial and insurance forms

- Incident or patient safety reports

- Institutional review board lists

- Logs

- Notice of privacy practices acknowledgments (unless the organization chooses to classify them as part of the health record)

- Patient-identifiable data reviewed for quality assurance or utilization management

- Protocols and clinical pathways, practice guidelines, and other knowledge sources that do not imbed patient data

- Work lists and works-in-progress

Derived or administrative data are derived from the primary healthcare record and contain selected data elements to aid in the provision, support, evaluation, or advancement of patient care. Derived data and documents should be provided the same level of confidentiality as the legal health record. However, derived data should not be considered part of the health record and would not be produced in response to a court order, subpoena, or request for the health record.

Derived data consist of information aggregated or summarized from patient records so that there are no means to identify patients. Examples of derived data are

- Accreditation reports

- Anonymous patient data for research purposes

- Best-practice guidelines created from aggregate patient data

- OASIS reports

- ORYX, Quality Indicator, Quality Measure, or other reports

- Public health reports that do not contain patient-identifiable data

- Statistical reports

- Transmission reports for MDS, OASIS, and IRF PAI

Appendix 2A.4 Note

1. Sedona Conference. "The Sedona Guidelines: Best Practice Guidelines and Commentary for Managing Information & Records in the Electronic Age." September 2005. Available online at www.thesedonaconference.org/content/miscFiles/TSG9_05.pdf.

Appendix 2A.5

Policy Definitions

Definitions

The following definitions may be helpful for organizations when creating the legal health record and designated record set policies. Any key terms the organization identifies should also be included in the organization's final policy.

Business record: "A recording/record made or received in conjunction with a business purpose and preserved as evidence or because the information has value. Because this information is created, received, and maintained as evidence and information by an organization or person, in pursuance of legal obligation or in the transaction of business, it must consistently deliver a full and accurate record with no gaps or additions."[1]

Data: Basic facts about people, processes, measurements, and conditions represented in dates, numerical statistics, images, and symbols. An unprocessed collection or representation of raw facts, concepts, or instructions in a manner suitable for communication, interpretation, or processing by humans or automatic means.[2]

Data element: A combination of one or more data entities that forms a unit or piece of information, such as a patient identifier, diagnosis, or treatment.[3]

Electronic health record: Medical information compiled in a data-gathering format for retention and transferral of protected information via a secured, encrypted communication line. The information can be readily stored on an acceptable storage medium such as compact disc.[4]

Evidence: Information that a fact finder may use to decide an issue. Information that makes a fact or issue before court or other hearing more or less probable.[5]

Legal health record: AHIMA defines the legal health record as "generated at or for a healthcare organization as its business record and is the record that would be released upon request. It does not affect the discoverability of other information held by the organization. The custodian of the legal health record is the health information manager in collaboration with information technology personnel. HIM professionals oversee the operational functions related to collecting, protecting, and archiving the legal health record, while information technology staff manage the technical infrastructure of the electronic health record."[6]

The legal health record is a formally defined legal business record for a healthcare organization. It includes documentation of healthcare services provided to an individual in any aspect of healthcare delivery by a healthcare organization.[7,8] The health record is individually identifiable data in any medium, collected and directly used in documenting healthcare or health status. The term also includes records of care in any health-related setting used by healthcare professionals while providing patient care services, reviewing patient data, or documenting observations, actions, or instructions.[9]

Original document: An authentic writing as opposed to a copy.[10]

Regular course of business: Doing business in accordance with the normal practice of business and custom, as opposed to doing it differently because an organization may be or is being sued.[11]

Source systems: The systems in which data were originally created.

- **Primary source system:** An information system that is part of the overall clinical information system in which documentation is most commonly first entered or generated.

- **Source of legal health record:** The permanent storage system where the documentation for the legal health record is held.

Appendix 2A.5 Notes

1. AHIMA e-HIM Work Group on e-Discovery. "New Electronic Discovery Civil Rule." *Journal of AHIMA* 77, no. 8 (Sept. 2006): 68A–H.

2. AHIMA e-HIM Work Group on the Legal Health Record. 2005. "Update: Guidelines for Defining the Legal Health Record for Disclosure Purposes." *Journal of AHIMA* 76, no. 8 (Sept.): 64A–G.

3. Ibid.

4. Ibid.

5. Ibid.

6. Ibid.

7. Amatayakul, Margaret, et al. "Definition of the Health Record for Legal Purposes." *Journal of AHIMA* 72, no. 9 (Oct. 2001): 88A–H.

8. AHIMA e-HIM Work Group on the Legal Health Record. "Update: Guidelines for Defining the Legal Health Record for Disclosure Purposes."

9. Ibid.

10. Ibid.

11. Ibid.

Appendix 2A.6

Legal Health Record Sample Template

Policy Name: The Health Record for Legal and Business Purposes

Effective Date:

Departments Affected: HIM, Information Systems, Legal Services, *[any additional departments affected]*

Purpose: This policy identifies the health record of *[organization]* for business and legal purposes and to ensure that the integrity of the health record is maintained so that it can support business and legal needs.

Scope: This policy applies to all uses and disclosures of the health record for administrative, business, or evidentiary purposes. It encompasses records that may be kept in a variety of media, including, but not limited to, electronic, paper, digital images, video, and audio. It excludes those health records not normally made and kept in the regular course of the business of *[organization]*.

Note: The determining factor in whether a document is considered part of the legal health record is not where the information resides or its format, but rather how the information is used and whether it is reasonable to expect the information to be routinely released when a request for a complete health record is received. The legal health record excludes health records that are not official business records of a healthcare provider. Organizations should seek legal counsel when deciding what constitutes the organization's legal health record.

Policy: It is the policy of *[organization]* to create and maintain health records that, in addition to their primary intended purpose of clinical and patient care use, will also serve the business and legal needs of *[organization]*.

It is the policy of *[organization]* to maintain health records that will not be compromised and will support the business and legal needs of *[organization]*.

Routine disclosures will only include information needed to fulfill the intent of the request. It excludes information determined to not be included in the legal health record.

Responsibilities

It is the responsibility of the Health Information Management Director, working in conjunction with the Information Services Department (IS) and the Legal Department *[or other appropriate departments]*, to

- Maintain a matrix or other document that tracks the source, location, and media of each component of the health record. *[Reference an addendum or other source where the health record information is found.]*

- Identify any content that may be used in decision making and care of the patient that may be external to the organization (outside records and reports, PHRs, e-mail, etc.) that is not included as part of the legal record because it was not made or kept in the regular course of business.

- Develop, coordinate, and administer a plan that manages all information content, regardless of location or form, that comprises the legal health record of *[organization]*.

- Develop, coordinate, and administer the process of disclosure of health information.

- Develop and administer a health record retention schedule that complies with applicable regulatory and business requirements.

- Ensure appropriate access to information systems containing components of the health record

- Execute the archiving and retention schedule pursuant to the established retention schedule

- *[Other responsibilities]*

[Additional responsibilities for other individuals or departments]

Appendix 2A.7

Sample Designated Record Set Template

Policy Name: Designated Record Set Policy

Effective Date:

Departments Affected: HIM, Information Systems, Legal Services, *[any additional departments affected]*

Purpose: The purpose of this policy is to establish guidelines for the definition and content of the *[organization]* designated record set in accordance with the Health Insurance Portability and Assurance Act (HIPAA) of 1996.

Scope: This policy applies to all uses and disclosures of the health record. It encompasses records that may be kept in a variety of media including, but not limited to, electronic, paper, digital images, video, and audio. It excludes those health records not normally made and kept in the regular course of the business of *[organization]*.

Note: The determining factor in whether a document is considered part of the designated record set is not where the information resides or its format, but rather how the information is used and whether it is reasonable to expect the information to be routinely released when a request from the individual to inspect, copy, or request an amendment. The designated record set excludes health records that are not official business records of a healthcare provider. Organizations should seek legal counsel when deciding what constitutes the organization's designated record set.

Policy: To define the specific information or records that patients may access and amend under the HIPAA and state privacy laws. The standards provide that individuals have the right to inspect and obtain a copy and request amendment of medical information used to make decisions about their care and billing information.

Definitions:

Designated Record Set: A group of records maintained by or for *[organization]* that includes the health records and billing records about individuals that are used in whole or part by or for *[organization]* to make decisions about individuals. The term "record" is defined as any item, collection, or grouping of information that includes protected health information and is maintained, collected, used, or disseminated by or for *[organization]*.

Includes:

- Legal health record (refer to your organization's legal health record policy)

- Patient-specific claim information such as encounter forms, claims submitted, account balances, payment agreements, ABN letters, notice of noncoverage letters, etc.

- Outside facility or provider records used in whole or in part by [*organization*] to make decisions about individuals

- Patient-submitted documentation and referral letters

- Other patient-specific information such as consents and authorizations

Excludes:

- Administrative data, which is patient identifiable and used for administrative, regulatory, or other healthcare operations, such as event history/audit trails, data used for quality assurance or utilization management, data prepared in anticipation of legal action, etc.

- Derived data stored in aggregate or summarized that is not patient identifiable, such as data used for accreditation reports, research data, statistical reports, best practice guidelines, etc.

- Psychotherapy notes maintained separate from the rest of the patient's health record

- Patient information created as part of a research study to which the patient has temporarily waived right to access

- Records that have been destroyed because they exceeded their required retention period or were rendered unusable due to fire, flood, or other circumstances

- Information that is subject to a legal privilege, such as peer review or attorney/client privilege

Excluded from designated record set but may be disclosed with appropriate authorization:

- Source data such as radiology films, videos, photographs, slides, EKG strips, fetal monitor strips, etc., when available.

Responsibilities

It is the responsibility of the Health Information Management Director, working in conjunction with the Information Services Department and the Legal Department *[or other appropriate departments]*, to

- Maintain a matrix or other document that tracks the source, location, and media of each component of the health record *[reference an addendum or other source where the health record information is found]*

- Identify any content that may be used in decision making and care of the patient that may be external to the organization (outside records and reports, PHRs, e-mail, etc.) that is not included as part of the legal record because it was not made or kept in the regular course of business

- Develop, coordinate, and administer a plan that manages all information content, regardless of location or form, that comprises the legal health record of *[organization]*

- Develop, coordinate, and administer the process of inspecting, copying, and amending health information

- Develop and administer a health record retention schedule that complies with applicable regulatory and business requirements

- Ensure appropriate access to information systems containing components of the health record

- Execute the archiving and retention schedule pursuant to the established retention schedule

- *[Other responsibilities]*

[Additional responsibilities for other individuals or departments]

PART II

Utilization of the Healthcare Record

Chapter 3

Principal and Ancillary Functions of the Healthcare Record

Cheryl Gregg Fahrenholz, RHIA, CCS-P

Learning Objectives

- Identify and explain the principal functions of a health record

- Define the terms *information* and *data* and distinguish between them

- Identify the ancillary functions of the health record; explain the special roles health records play in accreditation, licensure and certification, biomedical research, clinical education, credentialing and privileging, legal proceedings, and reporting of morbidity and mortality rates

- Discuss the right to access, release and disclosure, and retention and destruction of health records; list the most common secondary indexes, registries, and databases maintained by hospitals and explain the content and purpose of each

Key Terms

Accountable care organization (ACO)

Accreditation

Accreditation organization

Advanced decision support

Allied health professional

Biomedical research

Case management

Case-mix analysis

Centers for Disease Control and Prevention (CDC)

Centers for Medicare and Medicaid Services (CMS)

Certificate of destruction

Certification

Clinical practice guidelines

Clinical privilege

Confidentiality

Continuous quality improvement (CQI)

Core measure

Corporate negligence

Court order

Credentialing

Data

Demographic data

Diagnostic code

e-discovery

Electronic health record (EHR)

Face sheet

Federal Rules of Civil Procedure (FRCP)

Financial data

Health Insurance Portability and Accountability Act (HIPAA)

Health Level Seven (HL7)

Health record

Healthcare Integrity and Protection Data Bank (HIPDB)

ICD-10-CM and ICD-10-PCS

Incident

Incident report

Information

Informed consent

Liability

Licensure

Loss prevention

Loss reduction

Master patient index (MPI)

Medical necessity

Medical staff bylaws

Morbidity

Mortality

National Practitioner Data Bank (NPDB)

National Vital Statistics System (NVSS)

Notifiable diseases

Patient-centered medical home (PCMH)

Performance improvement (PI)

Population-based statistics

Privacy

Privileged communication

Procedural code

Protected health information (PHI)

Quality improvement organization (QIO)

Quality indicator

Redisclosure

Reimbursement

Risk management (RM)

Risk prevention

Statute of limitations

Subpoena

Subpoena duces tecum

Systematized Nomenclature of Medicine–Clinical Terms® (SNOMED CT®)

Third-party payer

Transcriptionist

Unique identifier

Utilization management (UM)

Utilization review (UR)

World Health Organization (WHO)

Introduction

The health records created and maintained by hospitals contain large amounts of clinical documentation stored as data and information. That documentation must be readily accessible for legitimate healthcare functions and yet protected from unauthorized access, damage, and loss.

The terms *data* and *information* are often used interchangeably, but the two terms have distinctly different meanings when they are used in reference to health records. **Data** represent objective descriptions of processes, procedures, people, and other observable things and activities. Data are collected in the form of dates, numbers, symbols, images, illustrations, texts, lists, charts, and equations. The analysis of data for a specific purpose results in **information**. Data represent facts; information conveys meaning. In other words, data themselves have no meaning until they are considered in the context of a specific purpose or function.

For example, a chart showing a series of columns with times, dates, initials, numbers, and symbols would have little meaning outside the context of patient care. Put in context, the numbers and symbols would represent observations of the vital signs of a specific patient, and the times, dates, and initials would constitute authentication of the health record documentation of those observations. The data would have even more specific meaning if it were considered in the context of the patient's age and medical condition.

Before the widespread use of computer technology in healthcare, all the information in healthcare records was collected and stored in paper format. Each record was a compilation of handwritten progress notes and orders, paper forms, photographs, graphic tracings, and typewritten reports. Many of the typewritten reports of medical findings and operative procedures were originally dictated by physicians or surgeons and converted into written format by medical **transcriptionists** (specially trained typists who understand medical terminology). The paper record was organized in a paper folder called a chart. When an episode of care was complete, the paper record was removed from the patient-care unit and stored in a large file room. After a predetermined amount of time, the record might be moved to a more remote storage facility or converted to a film image (called microfiche) that consumed much less space in storage. Eventually, the paper records were destroyed.

Many healthcare organizations, including hospitals, continue to use paper-based health record systems. Most combine handwritten documentation with computer print-outs and documents generated in other media, such as digital or video images and e-mail communications.

Hospitals and other large healthcare organizations are accelerating their adoption of new information technologies. Although the costs of implementing an electronic health record are high, healthcare facilities cannot afford to be left behind and risk hindering reimbursements. This accelerated movement toward **electronic health record (EHR)** systems has occurred since the implementation of the **Health Insurance Portability and Accountability Act (HIPAA)** in 1996. Similarly, the future adoption of the new diagnostic and procedural coding system **(ICD-10-CM and ICD-10-PCS)** and the standardized definitions from the **Systematized Nomenclature of Medicine–Clinical Terms® (SNOMED CT®)** have spurred the inevitable transition from paper and mixed media to EHR systems. Health information technology (IT) adoption moves forward as the first deadlines for stage 1 meaningful use approach, which means more and more physicians are making technology investments. **Health Level Seven (HL7)** began working on a functional model for EHRs in 2003. (HL7 is a standards development organization that addresses issues at the applications [or seventh] level of healthcare system interconnections.) When HL7 and industry stakeholders adopted the functional model, it provided momentum to develop new technology to support the interoperability of the EHR. The HL7 standards are a critical tool for evaluating the function of an organization's EHR.

The focus on pay for performance and outcomes, both clinically and financially, served as a catalyst to the adoption of new technology. **Accountable care organizations (ACOs)** and **patient-centered medical homes (PCMHs)** are prime examples. Both initiatives require a high level of connectivity across not only a health system but also the patient's continuum of care. This cannot be easily achieved in a paper-based environment. The complexity of the components, such as care plans, real-time updates to patient care, evidence-based decision support, and centralized financial management, requires data to be free-flowing, secure from unauthorized users, and accessible to authorized users. Any silos of healthcare data by a single provider will negate the effectiveness of the EHR. Trust and connectivity must be achieved and maintained for a successful program.

The bidirectional exchange of data between individual providers and healthcare systems requires a collaborative approach and full participation of all players involved in the clinical workflow (AHIMA 2011b). Health information management (HIM) professionals play a vital role in evaluating the effectiveness of the EHR by analyzing workflow and daily needs for copies or information from the patient's record. The management of health information requires HIM professionals to possess solid knowledge of data sets and terminology. To reach consensus on what data elements should be collected and how they should be defined while keeping an eye to the HL7 functional model, HIM professionals must work with those who set standards. HIM professionals with this skill set will secure their role in the management of quality data (Giannangelo and Hyde 2010).

Principal Functions of the Health Record

Regardless of its storage format, the functions of the health record remain the same. The **health record** serves as the principal repository for clinical documentation relevant to the care and treatment of a specific patient. The principal functions are related to specific healthcare encounters between providers and patients. The ancillary functions are related to the environment in which healthcare services are provided.

Administrative Information and Demographic Data

For elective hospital admissions, the patient or the admitting physician's office staff often provide administrative information and demographic data before the patient comes to the hospital. Alternatively, the patient may provide the information to the hospital's registration staff on the day of admission or through a secure page of the organization's website prior to admission. In the case of an unplanned admission, the patient or the patient's representative provides administrative information.

Admitting and Registration Information

The patient access or registration staff collects personal details about the patient and information about the patient's health insurance coverage at the time of admission. Nearly all hospitals use a computer-based registration system linked to a database called the **master patient index (MPI)**. When patients are readmitted, patient access or registration staff check the patient's personal information against the data in the database to ensure that it is current and correct. The patient's administrative information is then recorded on an identification sheet or screen in the EHR, which is often called a **face sheet**. In paper-based record systems, a printout of the face sheet is used as the front page of the patient's record. It identifies the patient and contains demographics, original date of admission, insurance coverage or payment source, referral information, hospital stay dates, physician information, and discharge information. It also contains the names of the responsible party, emergency contacts, additional contacts, and the patient's diagnosis.

In an electronic format, data collected from the face sheet may be captured on several screens but displayed in a logical manner to those who need it. For instance, clinical staff caring for the patient should be able to quickly identify the patient by name, health record number, and account number and locate emergency contacts for the patient, whereas the billing office needs the patient's name, account number, and insurance information. While EHR systems may display information differently, all the information gathered for the health record is available online and displayed in a logical manner to those who need it (James 2009).

Demographic Data

The term *demographics* refers to the study of statistical data about human populations. In the context of healthcare, **demographic data** includes basic factual details about the individual patient. The demographic data collected from the patient include the following:

- Last, first, and middle names
- Address
- Telephone number(s), including work and mobile phone numbers
- E-mail address
- Gender
- Date of birth
- Place of birth
- Race or ethnic origin
- Marital status
- Name and address of next of kin
- Social Security number (optional)

The main purpose of collecting demographic data is to confirm the patient's identity. Hospitals and other healthcare-related organizations use the demographic data collected from patients as the basis of statistical records, research, and resource planning.

In past years, Social Security numbers were often used to help positively identify patients because they are a **unique identifier**, that is, a number that represents one and only one individual. Hospitals assign unique identifiers to individual health records to make sure information in the records is easily retrievable and not misplaced or lost. With the increase in identity theft, the trend is to reduce, if not eliminate, the use of Social Security numbers as a form of unique identification. Examples of variations of a full Social Security number are the use of only the last four digits or restricting the display and transmission of the full or partial number (FTC 2008). For employee system access, another unique identifier should be used to validate the user's identification (AHIMA 2010b).

Financial Data

Details about the patient's occupation, employer, and insurance coverage are collected at the time of treatment. Healthcare providers use these data to complete claims forms that will be submitted to third-party payers. **Financial data** include the following:

- Patient's name
- Name of the insured party and his or her relationship to the patient, if the patient is a dependent of the insured party
- Insured party's member identification number
- Insured party's date of birth

- Name of the insurance company and the group policy number

- Employer's name and address

Clinical Data

Basic clinical data, such as type of surgery or reason for the visit, are collected and recorded during the intake process. From this, the treating or admitting physician can provide the patient's preliminary diagnosis and the reason the patient is seeking treatment.

Accurate clinical data collection is important because it becomes the basis of care plans and helps determine medical necessity.

Patient-Care Delivery

The health record combines information about the patient's illness with documentation of the services provided. Clinical observations of the patient, results of physical examinations and diagnostic tests, details of medical–surgical procedures, and descriptions of therapeutic outcomes are all compiled in one record. This record is accessible to all of the clinical professionals and **allied health professionals** who provide services to the patient.

The health record serves as a documentation tool that constitutes a permanent account of services the patient received. Communication between the patient's caregivers is very important, and the health record ensures the continuity of customer services. Information recorded in the patient's health record helps physicians make informed decisions about the patient's current condition and treatment requirements. The health record assists with patient assessment and care planning. Nursing assessments document the level of nursing assistance and personal care the patient needs. To facilitate continuity of customer care, the health record also serves as the basis for discharge planning. Discharge planning is meant to ensure that the patient will receive appropriate follow-up care.

Information documented in the health record forms the basis for evaluations of potential threats to the welfare of individual customers or the healthcare organization. Using the health record as a risk assessment tool helps manage the risk of the organization.

Because EHRs are based on sophisticated information-processing technology, they offer clinical functions that conventional paper-based records cannot, such as the following:

- The EHR performs as an **advanced decision support** instrument. Advanced decision support makes the latest clinical guidelines and research findings available to physicians at a click.

- Medication errors can be easily detected in the EHR, so it can be considered a medical error prevention tool. Drug interaction and dosage warnings are issued automatically when conflicting medication orders are entered into the record. Other reminders for clinicians can also be issued automatically.

- Testing is completed only as necessary, since test results from multiple physical locations can be viewed in the EHR. Healthcare costs are reduced as duplicate tests are avoided, and results are available electronically.

- Discharge planning is enhanced. EHR systems can be linked to clinic schedules so that patients can make follow-up appointments before they leave the hospital. EHRs can automatically provide patient-specific aftercare or discharge instructions.

Patient-Care Management and Support

Patient-care management encompasses the activities related to the management of services provided directly to patients. Many of these activities require an analysis of health records to determine an organization's financial health and the relevance of its services or to develop clinical guidelines.

To determine Medicare reimbursement, a hospital will analyze its case mix. **Case-mix analysis** is a method of grouping patients according to a predefined set of characteristics.

Health record information provides the basis for case management. **Case management** is the ongoing review of clinical care conducted during the patient's hospital stay. The purpose of case management is to ensure the necessity and quality of the services provided to the patient.

Clinicians use health record information to develop clinical pathways and other **clinical practice guidelines**, which help clinicians make knowledge- and experience-based decisions on medical treatment. These guidelines make it easier to coordinate multidisciplinary care and services.

The healthcare organization must allocate the necessary resources for patient care. An analysis of health record information helps determine appropriate staffing, plan new service lines, and forecast future demand for services or equipment acquisitions.

Quality Management and Performance Improvement

Accreditation organizations and licensing bodies expect hospitals and other healthcare organizations to strive for the highest possible quality in customer care. These organizations have written standards that healthcare organizations must meet to be accredited. **Third-party payers** review the quality of care their members receive. Most payers have written administrative manuals (either paper based or electronic) that document the expectations a healthcare organization must meet to become a participating healthcare organization with the payer.

Quality Management

The Joint Commission (2011) uses the Quality Report to differentiate healthcare organizations that achieve safety and quality goals. The Joint Commission's **Quality Indicators** are measurements for comparing hospitals on a state and a national level. The Quality Indicators include the following (Joint Commission 2011):

- National Patient Safety Goals: Healthcare organizations are required to abide by these goals when relevant services are provided. Performance is assessed as meeting the goal, not meeting the goal, or the goal's being not applicable for the healthcare organization.

- National Quality Improvement Goals: These goals are chosen by The Joint Commission and reflect treatments that affect thousands of patients every year. The Quality Report tracks outcomes for ORYX core measure sets, such as heart attack, heart failure, pregnancy, pneumonia, children's asthma, and the Surgical Care Improvement Project (SCIP) for infection prevention, cardiac, and venous thromboembolism. Currently, hospitals that submit these data are required to report on four of the six measure sets. Pediatric, psychiatric, and small rural hospitals are not required to submit core measure data due to their size or patient population. Performance is measured against a target range or value.

The designations are above, similar to, below, not applicable for the healthcare organization, or not displayed.

The Medicare program first established a system of quality review in 1982. Today, local **quality improvement organizations (QIOs)** work under contract with the **Centers for Medicare and Medicaid Services (CMS)**, the federal agency that administers the Medicare and Medicaid programs. QIO contracts set targets related to CMS's federal targets at the state level based on a focused set of publicly reported quality measures. The mission of a QIO program is to improve the effectiveness, efficiency, economy, and quality of services delivered to Medicare beneficiaries. For example, special projects in the hospital setting focus on acute myocardial infarction, heart failure, pneumonia, and surgical care. All of these projects are intended to improve patient outcomes.

Based on this statutory charge and CMS's program experience, CMS identifies the core functions of the QIO program as follows (CMS 2011):

- Improving quality of care for beneficiaries

- Protecting the integrity of the Medicare Trust Fund by ensuring that Medicare pays only for services and goods that are reasonable and necessary and that are provided in the most appropriate setting

- Protecting beneficiaries by expeditiously addressing individual complaints, such as beneficiary complaints, provider-based notice appeals violations of the Emergency Medical Treatment and Labor Act (EMTALA), and other related responsibilities as articulated in QIO-related law

Healthcare organizations submit patient information collected from health records to the QIOs, which then review the appropriateness of delivered care. In August 2008, work began on the QIO Program's Ninth Statement of Work (SOW), which extended through July 31, 2011. The Ninth SOW has six main sections. Three of them are required of all 53 QIO contractors, while completion of the other three will be conducted among the QIOs subnationally (CMS 2011).

For all QIOs:

1. Beneficiary Protection

2. Patient Safety

3. Core Prevention

Subnational tasks for some QIOs:

4. Chronic Kidney Disease Project

5. Care Transitions Project

6. Prevention: Efforts to Reduce Health Disparities among Diabetes Patients

The SOW has specific tasks for providers in settings such as nursing homes, home health, hospitals, critical-access hospitals/rural prospective payment system hospitals, and physicians' practices. Managed care organizations and other third-party payers review information on services provided to their beneficiaries. The appropriateness and quality of care provided to customers is the focus.

Another element of quality management in the healthcare setting is medical staff credentialing. Credentialing is the process of obtaining, verifying, and assessing a practitioner's qualifications to provide care or services in or for a healthcare organization (Joint Commission 2011). Credentialing standards guide the process.

Performance Improvement

Healthcare organizations systematically review processes and outcomes to ensure the quality of their services. Many hospitals employ quality management professionals who work directly with clinical and ancillary staff to identify patient-care issues and improve processes. Historically, quality assurance efforts were concentrated on the identification of mistakes and substandard individual performance. In contrast, present-day **performance improvement (PI)** efforts emphasize the importance of identifying the shortcomings of processes and systems rather than those of individuals.

Hospitals use different PI models, and the models tend to go in and out of fashion rather quickly. PI processes driven by patient-care information are the most effective. Currently, most healthcare organizations use some form of **continuous quality improvement (CQI)**, also known as total quality management (TQM). The CQI philosophy emphasizes the critical importance of three factors:

1. Knowing and meeting customer expectations

2. Reducing variation within processes

3. Relying on data to build knowledge for process improvement

CQI entails a continuous cycle of planning, measuring, and monitoring performance and making periodic knowledge-based improvements. Quality managers use a number of tools to monitor performance and identify areas for improvement. Many hospitals use a model originally developed by the Hospital Corporation of America (Eichenwald and Oachs 2010). See **FIGURE 3.1** for this model: FOCUS-PDCA.

Like other CQI models, FOCUS-PDCA applies the plan–do–check–act process, which is basically a cycle of trial, measurement, and learning. During the planning phase, the PI team analyzes the process to be improved. They identify the process, how it currently works, who is involved, and other performance factors. Then they propose a change to address the identified problem. Team members develop a system for measuring the outcomes of the proposed change to determine whether it brings about an improvement. In the doing phase, the proposed improvement is implemented for a trial period, and data are collected. The checking phase involves analyzing those data. If the change resulted in a measurable improvement, the cycle moves on to the action step. The change is either adjusted based on the knowledge gained or implemented. If the proposed change had no observable effect, the team develops another solution and repeats the entire PDCA cycle until they find a solution that works.

Utilization Management

The process of **utilization management (UM)** focuses on how healthcare organizations use their resources. Hospital UM programs ensure that each customer receives the appropriate level of services and that the services are performed in an efficient and cost-effective way. UM review is based on health record information. State and federal government regulations require hospitals to conduct UM reviews. Most commercial health insurance

FIGURE 3.1. FOCUS-PDCA model

The FOCUS phase helps to narrow the team's attention to a discrete opportunity for improvement		
F	Find	Find a process that needs improvement. Define the process and its customers. Decide who will benefit from the improvement. Understand how the process fits within the hospital's system and priorities.
O	Organize	Select a team that is knowledgeable about the process. Determine team size, identify potential members who represent various levels in the organization, select members, and prepare to document their progress.
C	Clarify	Clarify the current knowledge of the process. Define the process as it is and as it should be. The team reviews current knowledge and then must understand the process to be able to analyze it and differentiate the way it actually works and the way it is meant to work.
U	Understand	Understand the causes of variation. The team will measure the process and learn the causes of variation. They will then formulate a plan for data collection, collect the data, and use the information to establish specific, measurable, and controllable variations.
S	Select	Select the potential process improvement. Determine the action that needs to be taken to improve the process (must be supported by documented evidence.)
The PDCA phase allows the team to pursue that opportunity and review its outcome.		
P	Plan	Plan the improvement/data collection. Plan the change by studying the process, deciding what could improve it, and identifying data to help.
D	Do	Do the improvement/data collection/data analysis. Execute the plan on a small scale or by simulation.
C	Check	Check the data for process improvement. Observe the results of the change. Document the results of the change. Modify the change, if necessary and possible.
A	Act	Act to hold the gain/continue improvement. Implement the change if it is working. If it fails, abandon the plan and repeat the cycle.

Source: HCA n.d.

plans conduct their own UM reviews for inpatient and outpatient services to ensure that high-quality care is performed in the most appropriate setting by the most appropriate provider. Evidence-based guidelines are often used for this purpose.

Utilization review (UR) is a formal process conducted to determine the medical necessity of the services provided to, or planned for, an individual patient. Determinations of **medical necessity** are based on whether the services can be expected to have a reasonably beneficial effect on the patient's physical needs and quality of life.

The Medicare Conditions of Participation for Hospitals specifically require acute-care facilities to perform URs for Medicare and Medicaid patients to determine the medical necessity of hospital admissions, lengths of stay, and professional services, including drugs and biological substances. This process uses preestablished, objective screening criteria based on the severity of the patient's illness and the intensity of the services needed to effectively treat the illness. Hospitals may conduct UR at several points before, during, and after the patient's stay to determine whether the patient's condition and need for services necessitates inpatient treatment. In most cases, the Medicare regulations permit hospitals to conduct UR for a sample of patients rather than for every Medicare or Medicaid patient.

UR conducted by commercial health insurance plans may include a pre-authorization process that occurs before a service is performed. Concurrent reviews may be conducted to ensure that evidence-based care guidelines are being followed and the patient's transition of care needs are being fulfilled. Review may also be conducted after the treatment has occurred.

Risk Management

Health record information is used in risk management activities. The main purpose of **risk management (RM)** is prevention of situations that might put hospital patients, caregivers, or visitors in danger. RM includes investigating reported incidents, reviewing liability claims, and working with the hospital's legal counsel. Hospitals employ professional risk managers, who may manage the hospital's safety programs and disaster planning, depending on the size and complexity of the organization. Additional information regarding risk management can be found later in this chapter.

Billing and Reimbursement

According to Homan (2011, 37):

> Healthcare **reimbursement** is based on the documentation contained in the health record. By referring to the records of individual patients, coding specialists identify the patients' diagnoses as well as the therapeutic procedures they underwent and the services they received. Using this information, coding specialists assign appropriate **diagnostic** and **procedural codes.** The coded information is then used to generate a patient bill and/or a claim for reimbursement to a third-party payer, such as a commercial health insurance company or government-sponsored health program such as Medicare.
>
> Some third-party payers require billers to submit copies of portions of the health record along with the claims. The health record documentation substantiates the need for services and the fact that such services were provided.

A traditional principle among health information managers—"if it wasn't documented, it didn't happen"—reflects the importance of complete, timely, and accurate clinical documentation. The quality of the information in health records is especially critical because of the complexity of patient care and the potentially serious consequences incorrect or incomplete information can have for patients and caregivers. Less obvious is the effect poor quality documentation can have on the facility's ability to claim appropriate reimbursement from patients and third-party payers. This, in turn, can damage the organization's short-term and long-term financial stability, affect its continued ability to provide high-quality patient care with the most cost-effective means, and hinder its ability to use technological advances.

Documentation must accurately reflect the healthcare services rendered to the patient. According to Bowman (2008):

> Claims should be submitted only when appropriate documentation supporting them is present in the health record and available for audit and review. Processes for ensuring that health record documentation is adequate and appropriate to support the coded diagnoses and procedures need to be in place.

See **FIGURE 3.2** for a list of questions to challenge and improve documentation for reimbursement purposes and to help ensure compliance with federal regulations.

Ancillary Functions of the Health Record

The ancillary functions of the health record are not associated with specific patients and specific healthcare encounters, but with the environment in which patient care is provided. Accreditation, certification, and licensure processes are linked to the operation of health-

FIGURE 3.2. Questions to ask when evaluating documentation

- Is the chief complaint and/or reason for the patient encounter or hospitalization documented?
- Do the initial orders for patient care reflect the level of care to be provided?
- Is there an appropriate history and physical examination?
- Are all services that were provided documented?
- Does documentation clearly explain why support services, procedures, and supplies were provided?
- Is assessment of the patient's condition included in the documentation?
- Does documentation include information on the patient's progress and treatment outcome?
- Is there a documented treatment plan?
- Does the plan for care include, as appropriate, treatments and medications (including frequency and dosage), any referrals and consultations, patient and family education, and follow-up instructions?
- Are changes to the treatment plan, including rationale, documented?
- Is there documentation of the medical rationale for services rendered?
- Does documentation support standards for medical necessity?
- Are abnormal test results addressed in the physician documentation? If abnormal test results are returned after discharge, are they documented in an addendum, along with the action taken?
- Are relevant health risk factors identified?
- Does documentation support intensity of patient evaluation and/or treatment, including thought processes and complexity of decision making?
- Are significant changes in the patient's condition and action taken documented?
- Is the status of unresolved problems documented?
- Is planned follow-up care documented?
- Is the hospital discharge status, including transfers to another hospital or to postacute care, clearly documented? Are any plans for home health services clearly documented?
- Does documentation support the level of care provided?
- Does documentation meet the criteria for the evaluation and management code billed?
- Does the documentation for the patient encounter include an assessment, clinical impression, or diagnosis?
- Are all diagnoses and procedures documented as specifically as possible?
- Are all complications and comorbidities documented?
- Do clinical reports include all elements required by regulatory and accreditation agencies?
- Are health record entries appropriately dated and authenticated?
- Is the documentation legible?
- Is surgery done in the emergency department documented in the final progress note?
- Are symptoms used when etiologic factors are known?
- Is there a summation of the visit or hospitalization in the final progress note?
- Is the source identified for patients admitted with pathologic factors?
- Are indications for transfusions clearly documented?
- Are all cancer sites identified as primary or secondary? If there is metastasis, has the site it has spread to been documented?
- Do all diagnoses on the final progress note agree with those on the discharge summary?
- Are surgical procedures that were omitted from the final progress note on the operative record?
- Do pathology reports have findings that do not appear in the health record?
- Do medication sheets often show administration of medication without an associated diagnosis clearly documented in the health record?
- Do diagnoses on the outpatient referral form relate to the ordered test or service?
- Do physicians write "rule out" of certain conditions as the reason for the visit?

Source: Adapted from Bowman 2008, 39.

care organizations and require health record information. State and federal regulations include a number of specific operational and informational reporting requirements. Biomedical research and clinical education use information in the health record, which is another example of an ancillary function.

Health record data are the basis of morbidity and mortality (vital statistics) reports and healthcare-related indexes, registries, and databases. (**Morbidity** refers to illness, and **mortality** refers to death.) Many of the statistical data collected in hospital reports, indexes, registries, and databases are submitted to state, federal, and international agencies. These agencies are responsible for policymaking on healthcare delivery, services, research, and education. For example, the **World Health Organization (WHO)**, a component of the United Nations, uses record-based statistics to track the incidence of disease worldwide and to plan public health initiatives accordingly.

Accreditation, Licensure, and Certification

Hospitals and other healthcare organizations are subject to a number of practice standards, which are intended to ensure the safety of patients and the quality of medical care. The accreditation, licensure, and demanding certification processes that hospitals undergo are based on these standards. **Accreditation** is the process of granting formal approval to a healthcare organization. Approval is based on whether the organization meets a set of voluntary standards developed by the accrediting organization. The Joint Commission (2011) publishes operational standards for several types of healthcare organizations. The purpose of accreditation is to confirm the quality of the services provided. After an organization receives initial accreditation by The Joint Commission, periodic surveys further assess whether the facility continues to meet the standards. Accreditation benefits hospitals and other healthcare organizations. For example, after a hospital receives accreditation by The Joint Commission, Medicare automatically allows the hospital to participate in the Medicare and Medicaid programs for reimbursement purposes. Accredited hospitals also have a competitive advantage over nonaccredited hospitals in their geographic area because The Joint Commission's stamp of approval lets the consumer know he is receiving care from an organization that has met higher standards.

Licensure is the state's act of granting a healthcare organization or individual practitioner the right to provide healthcare services of a defined scope in a limited geographic area. State governments establish licensure requirements, which vary from state to state. However, it is illegal in all fifty states to operate healthcare facilities and practice medicine without a license. Unlike accreditation, which is a voluntary process, licensure is mandatory. To practice in a particular state, an individual physician, dentist, or nurse must obtain a license in that state.

Certification is the process of granting an organization the right to provide healthcare services to a specific group of individuals. For example, healthcare organizations must meet certain federal regulations to receive Medicare funding. These regulations are published in the Medicare Conditions of Participation (Shaw et al. 2010, 334).

Many individual healthcare practitioners undergo voluntary certification. Clinical and ancillary professional certifications are based on requirements established by specialized professional organizations. For example, a physician specializing in dermatology would seek certification from the American Academy of Dermatologists, while HIM administrators and technicians are certified through the American Health Information Management Association (AHIMA).The requirements usually include a certain level of education, and most involve passing certification examinations. In addition, most certified professionals are required to meet continuing education requirements to maintain their credentials.

Biomedical Research

Biomedical research is the process of systematically investigating subjects related to the functioning of the human body. It often leads to a greater understanding of disease processes and the development of new or improved treatments and medical technologies. For example, research conducted over the past thirty years has led to the development of new drugs that control several debilitating mental illnesses, including clinical depression and schizophrenia. Similarly, the development of endoscopic, laser, and computer-assisted technology has revolutionized the way many surgical procedures are performed.

The goal of scientific research is to prove or disprove theoretical explanations of observable phenomena. To be valid, research results must be reproducible in subsequent studies conducted by different research teams. The general purpose of biomedical research is to develop or improve treatment interventions. Such developments are the cumulative result of multiple studies conducted over many years.

Biomedical research is usually conducted at large, urban hospitals affiliated with universities and medical schools. Funding comes from different sources, including the federal government, pharmaceutical and medical equipment manufacturers, and charitable foundations. Many acute-care facilities are not involved in long-term research projects, although they often participate in clinical trials.

Biomedical research studies explore the safety and effectiveness of drugs, diagnostic procedures, therapeutic procedures, and disease prevention approaches. A large portion of biomedical research is conducted on the microscopic level or with nonhuman subjects. However, many studies involve human subjects or clinical cases gleaned from health records.

Studies that involve human subjects must meet federal and international ethical guidelines intended to protect the welfare of human subjects. Internationally, the Declaration of Helsinki represents the ethical principles approved by the World Medical Association to be followed in biomedical studies involving biological specimens or clinical data that come from an identifiable human source (Watzlaf 2010, 562).

In the United States, the Department of Health and Human Services (HHS) Code of Regulations (45 CFR 46) contains three provisions to protect human subjects involved with biomedical research.

1. Institutional Assurances of Compliance—A documented commitment from a healthcare organization to comply with HHS regulations for the protection of human subjects.

2. Institutional Review Board (IRB) Review and Approval—A committee established to protect the rights and welfare of human research subjects.

3. Informed Consent—A thoughtful and respectful explanation of information so that a potential participant may decide whether or not to be included in the research. It should contain the three fundamentals: information, comprehension, and voluntariness.

The Office of Human Research Protection (OHRP) is the federal agency that provides leadership and oversight on the protection of human subjects participating in research supported by HHS. Participating healthcare organizations must agree to comply with the human subject protection regulations found in the Code of Federal Regulations (Watzlaf 2010, 563–69).

Federal regulations require that researchers provide human subjects with specific information before biomedical studies are initiated. The information is meant to make it possible for the subjects to give their **informed consent** to participation. (See **APPENDIX 3A**.) This information must include at least the following (45 CFR 46.116 2011):

- A statement that the study involves research, a description of the purpose of the research, the expected duration of the subject's participation, a description of the procedures to be followed, and identification of any experimental procedures involved.

- A description of any reasonably foreseeable risks or discomforts. The description must be accurate and reasonable, and participants must be informed of previously reported adverse events.

- A description of the possible benefits to the subject or others who may reasonably benefit from the research.

- A disclosure of any alternative procedures or courses of treatment, if any, that might benefit the subject. When appropriate, a statement that supportive care with no additional disease-specific treatment is an alternative.

- A statement that describes the level of **confidentiality** that will be applied to any records that identify the subject. That statement should include full disclosure and description of approved agencies—such as the Food and Drug Administration (FDA)—that may have access to the records.

- An explanation of the compensation or medical treatment available to address possible injuries during the study if the study involves more than minimal risk for the subject. Research-related injury may include physical, psychological, social, financial, or other injuries.

- An explanation of where the subject may find information if she is injured during the study and a contact who will answer questions about the research or the subject's rights.

- A statement explaining that participation is voluntary, that refusal to participate will involve no penalties or loss of benefits, and that the subject may discontinue participation at any time

The Joint Commission Rights and Responsibilities of the Individual (Joint Commission 2011, RI.01.03.05) manual states, "The hospital protects the patient and respects his or her rights during research, investigation, and clinical trials." These specific standards relate to research and clinical trials conducted in hospitals. They are similar to the federal regulations on human research. To meet the accreditation standards, the following eight elements of performance must be accomplished:

1. The hospital reviews all research protocols and weighs the risks and benefits to the patient participating in the research.

2. To help the patient determine whether or not to participate in research, investigation, or clinical trials, the hospital provides the patient with all of the following information:

- An explanation of the purpose of the research

- The expected duration of the patient's participation

- A clear description of the procedures to be followed

- A statement of the potential benefits, risks, discomforts, and side effects

- Alternative care, treatment, and services available to the patient that might prove advantageous to the patient

3. The hospital informs the patient that refusing to participate in research, investigation, or clinical trials, or discontinuing participation at any time will not jeopardize the patient's access to care, treatment, and services unrelated to the research.

4. The hospital documents the following in the research consent form: That the patient received information to help determine whether or not to participate in the research, investigation, or clinical trials.

5. The hospital documents the following in the research consent form: That the patient was informed that refusing to participate in research, investigation, or clinical trials, or discontinuing participation at any time will not jeopardize her access to care, treatment, and services unrelated to the research.

6. The hospital documents the following in the research consent form: The name of the person who provided the information and the date the form was signed.

7. The research consent form describes the patient's right to privacy, confidentiality, and safety.

8. The hospital keeps all information given to subjects in the health record or research file along with the consent forms.

The Health Insurance Portability and Accountability Act (HIPAA) contains the Standards for Privacy of Individually Identifiable Health Information, known as the Privacy Rule. This rule was effective on April 14, 2001, with a compliance date of April 14, 2003. It defines the means by which human research participants are informed of how their personal medical information will be used or disclosed. It also outlines their rights to access the information. Further, it protects the privacy of individually identifiable information while ensuring that researchers have access to the medical information they need to conduct their research. Investigators are permitted to use and disclose protected health information (PHI) for research with individual authorization or without individual authorization under limited circumstances (Horton 2011, 590). Patient information considered protected is listed in **FIGURE 3.3**.

Clinical Education

Health records are used as educational tools by medical schools, dental schools, nursing schools, and allied health training programs. The case studies derived from health record information provide real-world experience for students. Case studies are useful for academic and in-service training for all of the health professions, including HIM.

FIGURE 3.3. Examples of protected health information

The privacy rule allows covered entities to de-identify data by removing the following 18 elements that may be used to identify the individual or the individual's relatives, employers, or household members.

1. Names

2. All geographic subdivisions smaller than a state, including street address, city, county, precinct, zip code, except for the initial three digits of a zip code if, according to the current publicly available data from the Bureau of the Census:

   a. The geographic unit formed by combining all zip codes with the same three initial digits contains more than 20,000 people

   b. The initial three digits of a zip code for all such geographic units containing 20,000 or fewer people are changed to 000

3. All elements of dates (except year) for dates directly related to an individual, including birth date, admission date, discharge date, date of death; and all ages over 89 and all elements of dates (including year) indicative of such age, except that such ages and elements may be aggregated into a single category of age 90 or older

4. Telephone numbers

5. Facsimile numbers

6. E-mail addresses

7. Social Security numbers

8. Medical record numbers

9. Health plan beneficiary numbers

10. Account numbers

11. Certificate/license numbers

12. Vehicle identifiers and serial numbers, including license plate numbers

13. Device identifiers and serial numbers

14. Web universal resource locators (URLs)

15. Internet protocol (IP) address numbers

16. Biometric identifiers, including fingerprints and voiceprints

17. Full-face photographic images and any comparable images

18. Any other unique identifying number, characteristic, or code, unless permitted by the privacy rule for re-identification

Source: Horton 2011, 591.

Medical Staff Appointments and Privileges

Physicians directly perform or manage the medical-surgical care provided to patients in an acute care setting. Except in teaching hospitals, some of the physicians who provide medical or surgical services in hospitals are independent practitioners rather than employees or agents of the hospital. However, hospitals assume accountability for the quality of all medical treatment provided in their facilities. For example, say a physician who is not qualified to perform orthopedic surgery treats a patient with a broken leg in the emergency department of a hospital. If the physician injures the patient by providing substandard care, the physician and hospital are jointly liable for the patient's injury. This case represents an example of **corporate negligence**, a legal doctrine that was established by a 1965 court case.

In *Darling v. Charleston Community Hospital* (1965), the court ruled specifically that hospital governing boards have a duty to institute a means to evaluate and counsel medical staff who personally perform services on a patient that results in harm due to unreasonable risk (Pozgar 2012). The court's ruling established the hospital's obligation to appoint only highly qualified practitioners to the medical staff. Owing to that obligation, hospitals may be held liable when a member of the medical staff fails to meet established standards of patient care.

Most states have statutes that regulate the medical staff appointment processes. In addition, accreditation programs generally require hospitals to confirm the qualifications of practitioners before clinicians are given the right to practice in the facilities.

Hospital governing boards (sometimes called boards of directors or trustees) are legally responsible for the overall operation of a hospital. Every hospital's governing board has a duty to establish medical staff policies to ensure that unqualified practitioners do not provide medical services in the facility. These policies establish a hospital's medical staff qualification criteria and process.

Physicians and other clinical practitioners who wish to practice in a hospital must first become members of that hospital's medical staff. Although the governing board considers the recommendations of medical staff leaders in making medical staff appointments, the ultimate responsibility for such decisions rests with the board.

The governing board generally relies on the hospital's medical staff leaders to manage independent clinical practitioners by implementing medical staff bylaws. **Medical staff bylaws** describe the rights and responsibilities of individual members and the means by which medical staff leaders govern the conduct of members.

Credentialing Process

Before making medical staff appointments and reappointments, hospitals evaluate the qualifications of physicians, surgeons, podiatrists, dentists, clinical psychologists, nurse practitioners, and other practitioners through a systematic process called credentialing. **Credentialing** involves the review and validation of an individual practitioner's qualifications to practice medicine. (See **Figure 3.4**.)

Initial credentialing reviews typically include the following types of information:

- Verifications of the applicant's undergraduate, medical, and postdoctoral education

- Verifications of the applicant's residency and fellowship training and continuing medical education

- Past and current medical staff appointments at other facilities

- Past and current work history with practice locations

- Current state licenses to practice medicine

- Current specialty board certifications

- Additional certifications, such as Basic Life Support (BLS), Advanced Cardiac Life Support (ACLS), Advanced Life Support in OB (ALSO), Pediatric Advanced Life Support (PALS), Advanced Trauma Life Support (ATLS), Neonatal Advanced Life Support (NALS), or Cardiopulmonary Resuscitation (CPR)

- Current Drug Enforcement Administration registration

- Documentation of professional liability insurance

- References and recommendations from the applicant's professional peers

- Information on the applicant's health status

- Past and current liability status

As part of every medical staff appointment process, hospitals and other healthcare organizations are required by federal law to send inquiries to two national databases: the

FIGURE 3.4. Credentialing and privileging processes

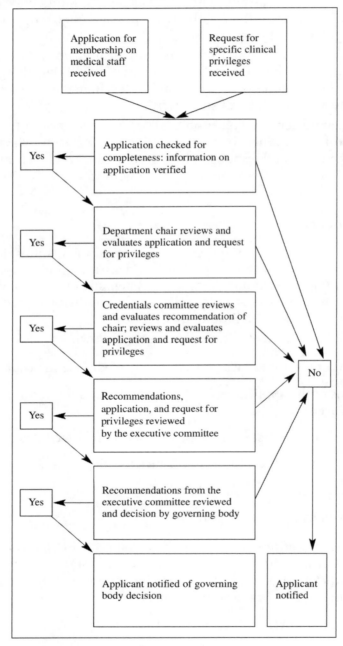

Source: Adapted from Zeman 2010, 543.

National Practitioner Data Bank (NPDB) and the **Healthcare Integrity and Protection Data Bank (HIPDB)**. The NPDB collects information on medical malpractice settlements, clinical privilege actions, and medical society actions taken against licensed healthcare providers in the United States. The HIPDB collects information on legal actions taken against licensed healthcare providers, including civil judgments and criminal convictions. Both banks are located at "the Data Bank" under the HHS and can be found online at http://www.npdb-hipdb.hrsa.gov/index.jsp.

The hospital's medical staff executive committee reviews a practitioner's application after verifying credentials and determining that the practitioner meets established qualification criteria. The committee subsequently submits its recommendation to the governing board for final action.

Privileging Process

With the board's approval, the hospital grants the practitioner medical staff privileges. These **clinical privileges** authorize the practitioner to provide patient services in the hospital, but only those specific services that fall within her area of medical expertise. For example, a cardiovascular surgeon's clinical privileges would allow her to perform cardiac bypass surgery but not cataract surgery. Criteria for granting clinical privileges must be documented in the medical staff bylaws. According to The Joint Commission (MS.06.01.07), medical staff privileges are granted for a period not to exceed two years (Joint Commission 2011).

Reappointments include a review of the practitioner's current qualifications and require new queries to the NPDB and HIPDB. Hospitals consider how often the practitioner used his privileges during the preceding period to determine whether the practitioner is still proficient in the clinical services for which he is seeking privileges. Outcome data for the practitioner's patients and peer review information help determine whether his privileges will continue.

Reappointment decisions consider whether the practitioner fulfilled his administrative responsibilities as specified in the hospital's medical staff bylaws. For example, the bylaws may require members to attend a specific percentage of medical staff meetings or participate on medical staff committees.

Medical staff reappointments review the practitioner's health record delinquency status. Practitioners with consistently high delinquency rates may lose their medical staff privileges.

Risk Management and Incident Reporting

Although hospitals and caregivers make every effort to ensure the safety of patients, visitors, and staff, unforeseen events can occur. Whether accidents or mistakes, some of these unforeseen events result in serious and sometimes fatal injuries.

Hospitals devise systems for responding to such events and taking steps to prevent similar problems in the future. Several terms are used to describe unforeseen events that lead to injuries and other losses, including *incidents, adverse events, potentially compensable events*, and *adverse occurrences*. The Joint Commission (2011) uses the term *sentinel event* and requests that the most serious be reported to them and to government agencies as required by federal or state law. Hospitals develop internal reporting processes to help identify risks within the organization. Internal and external reporting procedures are part of every hospital's risk management program.

Risk management (RM) is the process of overseeing the hospital's internal medical, legal, and administrative operations with the goal of minimizing the hospital's exposure to liability. In this context, *risk* is a formal insurance term referring to situations that may lead to liability claims. **Liability** is the legal responsibility to compensate individuals for injuries and losses sustained as the result of negligence.

Successful RM programs include three components: loss prevention, loss reduction, and risk prevention.

1. **Loss prevention** includes developing and revising facility-wide and department-specific policies and procedures, including education of all staff.

2. **Loss reduction** encompasses techniques used to manage events or claims that have already taken place. This component includes investigating and reviewing claims, working with defense counsel, and assisting with depositions, to name a few.

3. **Risk prevention** includes developing early warning and reporting programs, providing training on safety and adverse occurrences, creating databases to track events, and performing similar activities.

Health records constitute the hospital's legal record of the services provided to individual patients from the time they are admitted until they are discharged. Health record documentation must be objective and based on actual observations rather than on opinions and conjecture.

Like other events and outcomes during the patient's stay in the hospital, adverse events must be completely and accurately described in the patient's health record. However, it is extremely important that the health record documentation of adverse events remains entirely objective, with no comments from caregivers that suggest blame or speculate on causation.

Hospital internal RM policies usually define the circumstances that constitute a reportable **incident** (an event that is considered inconsistent with accepted standards of care) and address the steps to be taken in response. Most hospitals require the preparation of incident reports. Some facilities use the terms *occurrence* and *occurrence report* in this context.

An **incident report** describes the occurrence (time, date, and location); identifies the individual(s) involved (patients, visitors, and/or staff); and documents the current condition of the individual(s) affected. The report should include witness statements and should be completed as soon as possible after the incident to ensure accuracy and thoroughness.

Incident reports are prepared for RM, performance improvement, and staff education purposes but not for direct patient care. The report contains subjective information from witnesses and individuals involved in the incident. For these reasons, incident reports must never be included or mentioned in a patient's legal health record. Instead, incident reports should be stored in separate, secure databases or files in the facility's RM or performance improvement department. In anticipation of future court action, incident reports should be marked as confidential and addressed to the hospital's attorney. Incident reports should not be copied, and the original should not be disseminated internally or externally to anyone other than the individuals designated by the hospital's RM policies (McWay 2010, 262–64). Incident reports are not disseminated because of the risk of copies being filed in another file, which would make them discoverable. When kept as discussed, incident reports are generally not discoverable.

Health Records as Legal Documents

The health record is generally considered a business record, and as such, its contents are admissible as evidence in legal proceedings. Patients who have been treated for injuries related to automobile accidents or violent crimes often become involved in private liability lawsuits or criminal court cases. Patients suffering from employment-related injuries or illnesses may file workers' compensation claims. Sometimes patients or their families who believe they have been harmed by medical mistakes file malpractice lawsuits against physicians, hospitals, and other healthcare providers. Information documented in the health record plays a critical part in the decisions eventually handed down by judges and juries. Because many court cases do not go to trial until years after the original events, the written documentation in health records may be the only reliable information available. For this reason, the importance of complete and accurate health records cannot be overemphasized.

For healthcare information to be considered admissible in court, it must represent the health record of one of the persons involved in the legal proceedings. In other words, the contents of the record must be relevant to the issue being decided. Patient authorization or notification is not required for disclosures related to legal proceedings when the proper subpoena or court order is presented.

Legal Proceedings

The contents of health records constitute the healthcare organization's legal business record. For a health record to be admissible as evidence, four basic principles must be met.

1. The record must be documented in the normal course of business.

2. The record must be kept in the regular course of business.

3. The record must be created at or near the time the events occurred.

4. The record must be created by a person within the business with knowledge of the acts, events, conditions, and observations described in the record.

Generally, statements made outside the court by a party in a lawsuit are considered hearsay and not admissible as evidence. Documentation in the health record is technically hearsay; however, Federal Rules of Evidence (803[6]) and the Uniform Business and Public Records Act adopted by most states allow exception to the hearsay rule for records maintained in the regular course of business, including health records. All records must be identified and authenticated prior to determining their admissibility in court (AHIMA e-HIM Work Group on Maintaining the Legal EHR 2005). (See **APPENDIX 3B**.)

These conditions apply to paper-based health records and EHRs as long as the records are shown to be accurate and trustworthy. To be considered trustworthy, records must be secured in a manner that protects them from tampering. The health record is admissible because it passes the business rule of evidence and is not considered hearsay in a court of law. (See **APPENDIX 3B** for additional guidelines.)

Personal injury lawsuits and other legal proceedings are often conducted long after the original events take place. Eyewitness testimony is often contradictory; written evidence is more reliable. The patient's health record usually provides reliable evidence to substantiate the care and treatment the patient received. Incomplete or illegible documentation can lead to judgments against the facility and caregivers.

Subpoenas and Court Orders

When the court has determined that a health record is relevant to a particular case, the judge will issue a subpoena or a court order to the owner of the record. A **subpoena** is a direct command that requires an individual or a representative of an organization to appear in court or present an object to the court. The common elements in a valid subpoena are the following (McWay 2010, 54):

1. Name of the court where the lawsuit is brought

2. Names of parties to the lawsuit

3. Docket number of the case

4. Date, time, and place of requested appearance

5. Specific documents to be produced if a subpoena duce tecum is involved

6. Name and telephone number of the attorney who requested the subpoena

7. Signature, stamp, or seal of the official empowered to issue the subpoena

8. Witness fees, where provided by law

In the healthcare context, a **subpoena duces tecum** directs a hospital's representative (usually the director of HIM) to submit a specific health record or other business record to the court that holds jurisdiction over the pending proceedings. With the advice of legal counsel, an HIM director may decide that it is inappropriate for the hospital to release a subpoenaed record. In such cases, a **court order** must be issued in place of a subpoena when the disclosure of the material would otherwise be prohibited by state or federal statutes or regulations (McWay 2010, 54).

The method used to respond to subpoenas and court orders depends on the regulations of the state in which the court is located. Some states allow hospitals to make certified copies of the health records in question and mail the copies to the clerk of the court or to another designated individual. In other states, a representative of the hospital must deliver the original records in person and then testify to their authenticity.

e-Discovery

This section was adapted from Kimberly Baldwin-Stried Reich's article "Developing a Litigation Response Plan," originally published in the October 2007 issue of the *Journal of American Health Information Management Association.*

The e-discovery amendments to the **Federal Rules of Civil Procedure (FRCP)** (updated in 2010) and the Uniform Rules Relating to the Discovery of Electronically Stored Information (approved in August 2007 at the National Conference of Commissioners on Uniform State Laws) have created responsibilities for legal counsel and HIM professionals. Organizations must know how they will respond to e-discovery requests for information. The process by which electronic information is produced in response to threatened or impending litigation is changing, and those closely involved with the process must be knowledgeable on the requirements for producing information.

The Advisory Committee on the Rules of Civil Procedure amended the FRCP to specifically address **e-discovery**, or the discovery and production of electronically stored information. Congress established the legal rules that dictate allowable methods for discovery, at the federal court level. The FRCP, state legislative efforts regarding e-discovery and the Uniform Rules Related to the Discovery of Electronically Stored Information (2007) define the e-discovery process for all healthcare organizations. Legal counsels throughout the country are educated about e-discovery, information systems, and records management in an effort to protect organizations and their information. As a result, discussion of HIM operations has moved to the boardroom, and HIM professionals help shape and design their organizations' e-discovery processes.

In general terms, *discovery* is the formal pretrial legal process the parties in a lawsuit use to obtain information. Discovery helps ensure that neither party is subjected to surprises at trial. The scope of information that can be obtained through discovery is not limited to what will be used at trial. Federal courts and most state courts allow a party to discover any information relevant to the claim. Parties often disagree about what information must be exchanged and what is considered privileged. These disputes are resolved through court rulings on discovery motions.

Historically, discovery was the production of relevant information or paper documents. This information is generally produced after an individual or organization has been served with a subpoena or subpoena duces tecum. Other common discovery devices include depositions, interrogatories, requests for admissions, document production requests, and requests for inspection of records. The legal process for the discovery of electronically stored information (ESI) varies significantly from the discovery process that legal HIM professionals know today. Federal Rules of Civil Procedure sections 16, 26, and 34 compel parties and their counsel to enter into early discussion of key issues about discovery of ESI. As a result, it is incumbent upon legal counsel and HIM and IT professionals to evaluate how their roles and responsibilities will change with regard to the production and discovery of ESI.

The basic principles regarding preservation of relevant ESI are essentially the same as those governing the preservation of relevant paper-based business records. That is, at the moment when litigation is reasonably anticipated (known, threatened, or pending), the normal disposition and processing of information in either format should be suspended. The duty to preserve relevant ESI also supersedes an organization's record retention and management policies that would normally result in the destruction of ESI.

Judges now have a heightened sensitivity to the preservation of ESI and its loss, known as spoliation. In *Pension Committee of the University of Montreal Pension Plan v. Banc of America Securities*, a new opinion written by Judge Shira A. Scheindlin provided the criteria a court should review in evaluating ESI preservation. During discovery in the case, settled in January 2010, Judge Scheindlin determined that the plaintiffs were negligent in preserving and collecting ESI, which led to the spoliation of relevant evidence. The court imposed sanctions on the plaintiffs. The judge identified the factors that would establish negligent conduct supporting the imposition of sanctions:

- Failure to obtain records from employees who had some involvement with the issues at stake in the litigation but were not key players

- Failure to assess the accuracy and validity of search terms used to search ESI

- Failure of counsel to supervise the preservation and production of ESI

In addition, Judge Scheindlin found that some of the plaintiffs were grossly negligent in satisfying their e-discovery obligations. Specifically, they failed to: issue a written litigation hold; identify all key players and ensure that their records were preserved; preserve e-mail; collect information from former employees' files while within parties' control, custody, or possession; and preserve backup tapes when they were the sole source of relevant information or relate to key players. As a result of this gross negligence, the court charged the jury with the discovery abuses and informed the jurors that they should presume that any missing evidence would have been adverse to the grossly negligent plaintiffs (DeLoss 2010).

Once litigation can be reasonably anticipated, an organization should establish a legal (litigation) hold and take reasonable measures to identify and preserve all information relevant to the claim. A court may or may not issue a legal hold (also known as a preservation order). An organization's key determination in establishing a legal hold is whether litigation is "reasonably anticipated." For example, once an individual or organization is served with a complaint, subpoena, or subpoena duces tecum or receives notice of a government investigation, litigation can be reasonably anticipated. A legal hold should then be immediately established, and reasonable measures should be taken to identify and preserve relevant information. The duty to preserve could arise well before an individual or organization is served with any of these documents or notices. Determining when the legal hold should be established is not a rote decision. When faced with potential litigation, the facts of each situation must be carefully weighed.

Morbidity and Mortality Reporting

In the United States, official vital statistics are maintained under the **National Vital Statistics System (NVSS)**, a federal agency that operates within the **Centers for Disease Control and Prevention (CDC)**. The CDC is a group of federal agencies that oversee health promotion, disease control, and disease prevention activities in the United States. Vital statistics include data on the number of births and deaths that occur during a calendar year. Hospitals and other healthcare providers report the births and deaths in their facilities to designated state authorities. Most states have their own reporting requirements for vital statistics. State authorities report the required statistics to the NVSS. State and federal agencies collect and report other types of morbidity and mortality data submitted by healthcare providers. The source of all these data is the health record.

To ensure consistency in data collection, the NVSS provides standard forms and procedures. Data collection forms are revised about every ten years. Standard forms include the US Standard Certificate of Live Birth (**Figure 3.5**), the US Standard Certificate of Death (**Figure 3.6**), and the US Standard Report of Induced Termination of Pregnancy (1988) (**Figure 3.7**). The US Standard Report for Fetal Deaths is very similar to the certificate of live birth (CDC 2003).

Individual states maintain public health databases to manage data on the incidence of communicable diseases. The CDC maintains a database that contains similar data. The WHO's international health regulations require incidence reporting from participating nations so that the organization can track potential worldwide epidemics. The WHO is the United Nations' agency that oversees global health initiatives. The SARS epidemic that spread from China to Europe, Canada, and the United States in 2003 and the H1N1 pandemic that spread throughout the world in 2009 are examples of how quickly communicable diseases can be carried from continent to continent via international transportation systems.

FIGURE 3.5. Sample US Standard Certificate of Live Birth

U.S. STANDARD CERTIFICATE OF LIVE BIRTH

LOCAL FILE NO.   BIRTH NUMBER:

C H I L D

1. CHILD'S NAME (First, Middle, Last, Suffix)	2. TIME OF BIRTH (24 hr)	3. SEX	4. DATE OF BIRTH (Mo/Day/Yr)

5. FACILITY NAME (If not institution, give street and number)	6. CITY, TOWN, OR LOCATION OF BIRTH	7. COUNTY OF BIRTH

M O T H E R

8a. MOTHER'S CURRENT LEGAL NAME (First, Middle, Last, Suffix)	8b. DATE OF BIRTH (Mo/Day/Yr)

8c. MOTHER'S NAME PRIOR TO FIRST MARRIAGE (First, Middle, Last, Suffix)	8d. BIRTHPLACE (State, Territory, or Foreign Country)

9a. RESIDENCE OF MOTHER-STATE	9b. COUNTY	9c. CITY, TOWN, OR LOCATION

9d. STREET AND NUMBER	9e. APT. NO.	9f. ZIP CODE	9g. INSIDE CITY LIMITS? □ Yes □ No

F A T H E R

10a. FATHER'S CURRENT LEGAL NAME (First, Middle, Last, Suffix)	10b. DATE OF BIRTH (Mo/Day/Yr)	10c. BIRTHPLACE (State, Territory, or Foreign Country)

C E R T I F I E R

11. CERTIFIER'S NAME: _____ TITLE: □ MD □ DO □ HOSPITAL ADMIN. □ CNM/CM □ OTHER MIDWIFE □ OTHER (Specify)_____	12. DATE CERTIFIED _____ / _____ / _____ MM DD YYYY	13. DATE FILED BY REGISTRAR _____ / _____ / _____ MM DD YYYY

INFORMATION FOR ADMINISTRATIVE USE

M O T H E R

14. MOTHER'S MAILING ADDRESS: 9 Same as residence, or: State:	City, Town, or Location:
Street & Number:	Apartment No.: Zip Code:

15. MOTHER MARRIED? (At birth, conception, or any time between) □ Yes □ No IF NO, HAS PATERNITY ACKNOWLEDGEMENT BEEN SIGNED IN THE HOSPITAL? □ Yes □ No	16. SOCIAL SECURITY NUMBER REQUESTED FOR CHILD? □ Yes □ No	17. FACILITY ID. (NPI)

18. MOTHER'S SOCIAL SECURITY NUMBER:	19. FATHER'S SOCIAL SECURITY NUMBER:

INFORMATION FOR MEDICAL AND HEALTH PURPOSES ONLY

M O T H E R

20. MOTHER'S EDUCATION (Check the box that best describes the highest degree or level of school completed at the time of delivery)	21. MOTHER OF HISPANIC ORIGIN? (Check the box that best describes whether the mother is Spanish/Hispanic/Latina. Check the "No" box if mother is not Spanish/Hispanic/Latina)	22. MOTHER'S RACE (Check one or more races to indicate what the mother considers herself to be)
□ 8th grade or less □ 9th - 12th grade, no diploma □ High school graduate or GED completed □ Some college credit but no degree □ Associate degree (e.g., AA, AS) □ Bachelor's degree (e.g., BA, AB, BS) □ Master's degree (e.g., MA, MS, MEng, MEd, MSW, MBA) □ Doctorate (e.g., PhD, EdD) or Professional degree (e.g., MD, DDS, DVM, LLB, JD)	□ No, not Spanish/Hispanic/Latina □ Yes, Mexican, Mexican American, Chicana □ Yes, Puerto Rican □ Yes, Cuban □ Yes, other Spanish/Hispanic/Latina (Specify)_____	□ White □ Black or African American □ American Indian or Alaska Native (Name of the enrolled or principal tribe)_____ □ Asian Indian □ Chinese □ Filipino □ Japanese □ Korean □ Vietnamese □ Other Asian (Specify)_____ □ Native Hawaiian □ Guamanian or Chamorro □ Samoan □ Other Pacific Islander (Specify)_____ □ Other (Specify)_____

F A T H E R

23. FATHER'S EDUCATION (Check the box that best describes the highest degree or level of school completed at the time of delivery)	24. FATHER OF HISPANIC ORIGIN? (Check the box that best describes whether the father is Spanish/Hispanic/Latino. Check the "No" box if father is not Spanish/Hispanic/Latino)	25. FATHER'S RACE (Check one or more races to indicate what the father considers himself to be)
□ 8th grade or less □ 9th - 12th grade, no diploma □ High school graduate or GED completed □ Some college credit but no degree □ Associate degree (e.g., AA, AS) □ Bachelor's degree (e.g., BA, AB, BS) □ Master's degree (e.g., MA, MS, MEng, MEd, MSW, MBA) □ Doctorate (e.g., PhD, EdD) or Professional degree (e.g., MD, DDS, DVM, LLB, JD)	□ No, not Spanish/Hispanic/Latino □ Yes, Mexican, Mexican American, Chicano □ Yes, Puerto Rican □ Yes, Cuban □ Yes, other Spanish/Hispanic/Latino (Specify)_____	□ White □ Black or African American □ American Indian or Alaska Native (Name of the enrolled or principal tribe)_____ □ Asian Indian □ Chinese □ Filipino □ Japanese □ Korean □ Vietnamese □ Other Asian (Specify)_____ □ Native Hawaiian □ Guamanian or Chamorro □ Samoan □ Other Pacific Islander (Specify)_____ □ Other (Specify)_____

Mother's Name   Mother's Medical Record No.

26. PLACE WHERE BIRTH OCCURRED (Check one) □ Hospital □ Freestanding birthing center □ Home Birth: Planned to deliver at home? 9 Yes 9 No □ Clinic/Doctor's office □ Other (Specify)_____	27. ATTENDANT'S NAME, TITLE, AND NPI NAME: _____ NPI:_____ TITLE: □ MD □ DO □ CNM/CM □ OTHER MIDWIFE □ OTHER (Specify)_____	28. MOTHER TRANSFERRED FOR MATERNAL MEDICAL OR FETAL INDICATIONS FOR DELIVERY? □ Yes □ No IF YES, ENTER NAME OF FACILITY MOTHER TRANSFERRED FROM: _____

REV. 11/2003

FIGURE 3.5. (continued)

MOTHER	29a. DATE OF FIRST PRENATAL CARE VISIT ___/___/___ ☐ No Prenatal Care M M D D YYYY	29b. DATE OF LAST PRENATAL CARE VISIT ___/___/___ M M D D YYYY	30. TOTAL NUMBER OF PRENATAL VISITS FOR THIS PREGNANCY _____ (If none, enter ʌ0".)

31. MOTHER'S HEIGHT _____ (feet/inches)	32. MOTHER'S PREPREGNANCY WEIGHT _____ (pounds)	33. MOTHER'S WEIGHT AT DELIVERY _____ (pounds)	34. DID MOTHER GET WIC FOOD FOR HERSELF DURING THIS PREGNANCY? ☐ Yes ☐ No

35. NUMBER OF PREVIOUS LIVE BIRTHS (Do not include this child)	36. NUMBER OF OTHER PREGNANCY OUTCOMES (spontaneous or induced losses or ectopic pregnancies)	37. CIGARETTE SMOKING BEFORE AND DURING PREGNANCY	38. PRINCIPAL SOURCE OF PAYMENT FOR THIS DELIVERY

37. CIGARETTE SMOKING BEFORE AND DURING PREGNANCY
For each time period, enter either the number of cigarettes or the number of packs of cigarettes smoked. IF NONE, ENTER ʌ0".

35a. Now Living Number _____ ☐ None	35b. Now Dead Number _____ ☐ None	36a. Other Outcomes Number _____ ☐ None

Average number of cigarettes or packs of cigarettes smoked per day.

	# of cigarettes		# of packs
Three Months Before Pregnancy	_____	OR	_____
First Three Months of Pregnancy	_____	OR	_____
Second Three Months of Pregnancy	_____	OR	_____
Third Trimester of Pregnancy	_____	OR	_____

38. PRINCIPAL SOURCE OF PAYMENT FOR THIS DELIVERY
☐ Private Insurance
☐ Medicaid
☐ Self-pay
☐ Other
(Specify) _____

35c. DATE OF LAST LIVE BIRTH ___/___ MM YYYY	36b. DATE OF LAST OTHER PREGNANCY OUTCOME ___/___ MM YYYY	39. DATE LAST NORMAL MENSES BEGAN ___/___/___ M M D D YYYY	40. MOTHER'S MEDICAL RECORD NUMBER

MEDICAL AND HEALTH INFORMATION

41. RISK FACTORS IN THIS PREGNANCY (Check all that apply)

Diabetes
☐ Prepregnancy (Diagnosis prior to this pregnancy)
☐ Gestational (Diagnosis in this pregnancy)

Hypertension
☐ Prepregnancy (Chronic)
☐ Gestational (PIH, preeclampsia)
☐ Eclampsia

☐ Previous preterm birth

☐ Other previous poor pregnancy outcome (Includes perinatal death, small-for-gestational age/intrauterine growth restricted birth)

☐ Pregnancy resulted from infertility treatment-If yes, check all that apply:
 ☐ Fertility-enhancing drugs, Artificial insemination or Intrauterine insemination
 ☐ Assisted reproductive technology (e.g., in vitro fertilization (IVF), gamete intrafallopian transfer (GIFT))

☐ Mother had a previous cesarean delivery
 if yes, how many _____

☐ None of the above

42. INFECTIONS PRESENT AND/OR TREATED DURING THIS PREGNANCY (Check all that apply)

☐ Gonorrhea
☐ Syphilis
☐ Chlamydia
☐ Hepatitis B
☐ Hepatitis C
☐ None of the above

43. OBSTETRIC PROCEDURES (Check all that apply)

☐ Cervical cerclage
☐ Tocolysis

External cephalic version:
☐ Successful
☐ Failed

☐ None of the above

44. ONSET OF LABOR (Check all that apply)

☐ Premature Rupture of the Membranes (prolonged, ∃12 hrs.)
☐ Precipitous Labor (<3 hrs.)
☐ Prolonged Labor (∃ 20 hrs.)
☐ None of the above

45. CHARACTERISTICS OF LABOR AND DELIVERY (Check all that apply)

☐ Induction of labor
☐ Augmentation of labor
☐ Non-vertex presentation
☐ Steroids (glucocorticoids) for fetal lung maturation received by the mother prior to delivery
☐ Antibiotics received by the mother during labor
☐ Clinical chorioamnionitis diagnosed during labor or maternal temperature ≥38°C (100.4°F)
☐ Moderate/heavy meconium staining of the amniotic fluid
☐ Fetal intolerance of labor such that one or more of the following actions was taken: in-utero resuscitative measures, further fetal assessment, or operative delivery
☐ Epidural or spinal anesthesia during labor
☐ None of the above

46. METHOD OF DELIVERY

A. Was delivery with forceps attempted but unsuccessful?
 ☐ Yes ☐ No

B. Was delivery with vacuum extraction attempted but unsuccessful?
 ☐ Yes ☐ No

C. Fetal presentation at birth
 ☐ Cephalic
 ☐ Breech
 ☐ Other

D. Final route and method of delivery (Check one)
 ☐ Vaginal/Spontaneous
 ☐ Vaginal/Forceps
 ☐ Vaginal/Vacuum
 ☐ Cesarean
 If cesarean, was a trial of labor attempted?
 ☐ Yes
 ☐ No

47. MATERNAL MORBIDITY (Check all that apply) (Complications associated with labor and delivery)
☐ Maternal transfusion
☐ Third or fourth degree perineal laceration
☐ Ruptured uterus
☐ Unplanned hysterectomy
☐ Admission to intensive care unit
☐ Unplanned operating room procedure following delivery
☐ None of the above

NEWBORN INFORMATION

NEWBORN

48. NEWBORN MEDICAL RECORD NUMBER

49. BIRTHWEIGHT (grams preferred, specify unit)
_____ 9 grams   9 lb/oz

50. OBSTETRIC ESTIMATE OF GESTATION:
_____ (completed weeks)

51. APGAR SCORE:
Score at 5 minutes:_____
If 5 minute score is less than 6,
Score at 10 minutes: _____

52. PLURALITY - Single, Twin, Triplet, etc.
(Specify)_____

53. IF NOT SINGLE BIRTH - Born First, Second, Third, etc. (Specify) _____

54. ABNORMAL CONDITIONS OF THE NEWBORN (Check all that apply)

☐ Assisted ventilation required immediately following delivery
☐ Assisted ventilation required for more than six hours
☐ NICU admission
☐ Newborn given surfactant replacement therapy
☐ Antibiotics received by the newborn for suspected neonatal sepsis
☐ Seizure or serious neurologic dysfunction
☐ Significant birth injury (skeletal fracture(s), peripheral nerve injury, and/or soft tissue/solid organ hemorrhage which requires intervention)
9 None of the above

55. CONGENITAL ANOMALIES OF THE NEWBORN (Check all that apply)

☐ Anencephaly
☐ Meningomyelocele/Spina bifida
☐ Cyanotic congenital heart disease
☐ Congenital diaphragmatic hernia
☐ Omphalocele
☐ Gastroschisis
☐ Limb reduction defect (excluding congenital amputation and dwarfing syndromes)
☐ Cleft Lip with or without Cleft Palate
☐ Cleft Palate alone
☐ Down Syndrome
 ☐ Karyotype confirmed
 ☐ Karyotype pending
☐ Suspected chromosomal disorder
 ☐ Karyotype confirmed
 ☐ Karyotype pending
☐ Hypospadias
☐ None of the anomalies listed above

Mother's Name
Mother's Medical Record No. _____

56. WAS INFANT TRANSFERRED WITHIN 24 HOURS OF DELIVERY? 9 Yes 9 No IF YES, NAME OF FACILITY INFANT TRANSFERRED TO:_____	57. IS INFANT LIVING AT TIME OF REPORT? ☐ Yes ☐ No ☐ Infant transferred, status unknown	58. IS THE INFANT BEING BREASTFED AT DISCHARGE? ☐ Yes ☐ No

Source: CDC 2011.

FIGURE 3.6. Sample US Standard Certificate of Death

U.S. STANDARD CERTIFICATE OF DEATH

LOCAL FILE NO.   STATE FILE NO.

1. DECEDENT'S LEGAL NAME (Include AKA's if any) (First, Middle, Last)	2. SEX	3. SOCIAL SECURITY NUMBER

4a. AGE-Last Birthday (Years)	4b. UNDER 1 YEAR — Months / Days	4c. UNDER 1 DAY — Hours / Minutes	5. DATE OF BIRTH (Mo/Day/Yr)	6. BIRTHPLACE (City and State or Foreign Country)

7a. RESIDENCE-STATE	7b. COUNTY	7c. CITY OR TOWN

7d. STREET AND NUMBER	7e. APT. NO.	7f. ZIP CODE	7g. INSIDE CITY LIMITS? ☐ Yes ☐ No

8. EVER IN US ARMED FORCES? ☐ Yes ☐ No	9. MARITAL STATUS AT TIME OF DEATH ☐ Married ☐ Married, but separated ☐ Widowed ☐ Divorced ☐ Never Married ☐ Unknown	10. SURVIVING SPOUSE'S NAME (If wife, give name prior to first marriage)

11. FATHER'S NAME (First, Middle, Last)	12. MOTHER'S NAME PRIOR TO FIRST MARRIAGE (First, Middle, Last)

13a. INFORMANT'S NAME	13b. RELATIONSHIP TO DECEDENT	13c. MAILING ADDRESS (Street and Number, City, State, Zip Code)

14. PLACE OF DEATH (Check only one: see instructions)

IF DEATH OCCURRED IN A HOSPITAL:
☐ Inpatient ☐ Emergency Room/Outpatient ☐ Dead on Arrival

IF DEATH OCCURRED SOMEWHERE OTHER THAN A HOSPITAL:
☐ Hospice facility ☐ Nursing home/Long term care facility ☐ Decedent's home ☐ Other (Specify):

15. FACILITY NAME (If not institution, give street & number)	16. CITY OR TOWN , STATE, AND ZIP CODE	17. COUNTY OF DEATH

18. METHOD OF DISPOSITION: ☐ Burial ☐ Cremation ☐ Donation ☐ Entombment ☐ Removal from State ☐ Other (Specify):	19. PLACE OF DISPOSITION (Name of cemetery, crematory, other place)

20. LOCATION-CITY, TOWN, AND STATE	21. NAME AND COMPLETE ADDRESS OF FUNERAL FACILITY

22. SIGNATURE OF FUNERAL SERVICE LICENSEE OR OTHER AGENT	23. LICENSE NUMBER (Of Licensee)

NAME OF DECEDENT — For use by physician or institution
To Be Completed/ Verified By: FUNERAL DIRECTOR:

ITEMS 24-28 MUST BE COMPLETED BY PERSON WHO PRONOUNCES OR CERTIFIES DEATH

24. DATE PRONOUNCED DEAD (Mo/Day/Yr)	25. TIME PRONOUNCED DEAD

26. SIGNATURE OF PERSON PRONOUNCING DEATH (Only when applicable)	27. LICENSE NUMBER	28. DATE SIGNED (Mo/Day/Yr)

29. ACTUAL OR PRESUMED DATE OF DEATH (Mo/Day/Yr) (Spell Month)	30. ACTUAL OR PRESUMED TIME OF DEATH	31. WAS MEDICAL EXAMINER OR CORONER CONTACTED? ☐ Yes ☐ No

CAUSE OF DEATH (See instructions and examples)

32. PART I. Enter the chain of events--diseases, injuries, or complications--that directly caused the death. DO NOT enter terminal events such as cardiac arrest, respiratory arrest, or ventricular fibrillation without showing the etiology. DO NOT ABBREVIATE. Enter only one cause on a line. Add additional lines if necessary.

Approximate interval: Onset to death

IMMEDIATE CAUSE (Final disease or condition ———> resulting in death)
a._____ Due to (or as a consequence of): _____

Sequentially list conditions, if any, leading to the cause listed on line a. Enter the **UNDERLYING CAUSE**
b._____ Due to (or as a consequence of): _____

(disease or injury that initiated the events resulting in death) **LAST**
c._____ Due to (or as a consequence of): _____

d._____

PART II. Enter other significant conditions contributing to death but not resulting in the underlying cause given in PART I

33. WAS AN AUTOPSY PERFORMED? ☐ Yes ☐ No
34. WERE AUTOPSY FINDINGS AVAILABLE TO COMPLETE THE CAUSE OF DEATH? ☐ Yes ☐ No

35. DID TOBACCO USE CONTRIBUTE TO DEATH? ☐ Yes ☐ Probably ☐ No ☐ Unknown	36. IF FEMALE: ☐ Not pregnant within past year ☐ Pregnant at time of death ☐ Not pregnant, but pregnant within 42 days of death ☐ Not pregnant, but pregnant 43 days to 1 year before death ☐ Unknown if pregnant within the past year	37. MANNER OF DEATH ☐ Natural ☐ Homicide ☐ Accident ☐ Pending Investigation ☐ Suicide ☐ Could not be determined

38. DATE OF INJURY (Mo/Day/Yr) (Spell Month)	39. TIME OF INJURY	40. PLACE OF INJURY (e.g., Decedent's home; construction site; restaurant; wooded area)	41. INJURY AT WORK? ☐ Yes ☐ No

42. LOCATION OF INJURY: State: City or Town: Street & Number: Apartment No.:   Zip Code:

43. DESCRIBE HOW INJURY OCCURRED:	44. IF TRANSPORTATION INJURY, SPECIFY: ☐ Driver/Operator ☐ Passenger ☐ Pedestrian ☐ Other (Specify)

45. CERTIFIER (Check only one):
☐ Certifying physician-To the best of my knowledge, death occurred due to the cause(s) and manner stated.
☐ Pronouncing & Certifying physician-To the best of my knowledge, death occurred at the time, date, and place, and due to the cause(s) and manner stated.
☐ Medical Examiner/Coroner-On the basis of examination, and/or investigation, in my opinion, death occurred at the time, date, and place, and due to the cause(s) and manner stated.

Signature of certifier:_____

46. NAME, ADDRESS, AND ZIP CODE OF PERSON COMPLETING CAUSE OF DEATH (Item 32)

47. TITLE OF CERTIFIER	48. LICENSE NUMBER	49. DATE CERTIFIED (Mo/Day/Yr)	50. **FOR REGISTRAR ONLY**- DATE FILED (Mo/Day/Yr)

To Be Completed By: MEDICAL CERTIFIER

51. DECEDENT'S EDUCATION-Check the box that best describes the highest degree or level of school completed at the time of death. ☐ 8th grade or less ☐ 9th - 12th grade; no diploma ☐ High school graduate or GED completed ☐ Some college credit, but no degree ☐ Associate degree (e.g., AA, AS) ☐ Bachelor's degree (e.g., BA, AB, BS) ☐ Master's degree (e.g., MA, MS, MEng, MEd, MSW, MBA) ☐ Doctorate (e.g., PhD, EdD) or Professional degree (e.g., MD, DDS, DVM, LLB, JD)	52. DECEDENT OF HISPANIC ORIGIN? Check the box that best describes whether the decedent is Spanish/Hispanic/Latino. Check the "No" box if decedent is not Spanish/Hispanic/Latino. ☐ No, not Spanish/Hispanic/Latino ☐ Yes, Mexican, Mexican American, Chicano ☐ Yes, Puerto Rican ☐ Yes, Cuban ☐ Yes, other Spanish/Hispanic/Latino (Specify) _____	53. DECEDENT'S RACE (Check one or more races to indicate what the decedent considered himself or herself to be) ☐ White ☐ Black or African American ☐ American Indian or Alaska Native (Name of the enrolled or principal tribe) _____ ☐ Asian Indian ☐ Chinese ☐ Filipino ☐ Japanese ☐ Korean ☐ Vietnamese ☐ Other Asian (Specify)_____ ☐ Native Hawaiian ☐ Guamanian or Chamorro ☐ Samoan ☐ Other Pacific Islander (Specify)_____ ☐ Other (Specify)_____

54. DECEDENT'S USUAL OCCUPATION (Indicate type of work done during most of working life. DO NOT USE RETIRED).

55. KIND OF BUSINESS/INDUSTRY

To Be Completed By: FUNERAL DIRECTOR

REV. 11/2003

Source: CDC 2011.

FIGURE 3.7. Sample US Standard Report of Induced Termination of Pregnancy

TYPE/PRINT IN PERMANENT BLACK INK FOR INSTRUCTIONS SEE HANDBOOK

U.S. STANDARD
REPORT OF INDUCED TERMINATION OF PREGNANCY

STATE FILE NUMBER

1. FACILITY NAME (if not clinic or hospital, give address)	2. CITY, TOWN, OR LOCATION OF PREGNANCY TERMINATION	3. COUNTY OF PREGNANCY TERMINATION
Merrywood Clinic	Louisville	Jefferson

4. PATIENT'S IDENTIFICATION	5. AGE LAST BIRTHDAY	6. MARRIED?	7. DATE OF PREGNANCY TERMINATION (Month, Day, Year)
25466	23	☐ YES ☒ NO	November 20, 1997

8a. RESIDENCE-STATE	8b. COUNTY	8c. CITY, TOWN, OR LOCATION	8d. INSIDE CITY LIMITS? (Yes or No)	8e. ZIP CODE
Ohio	Hamilton	Cincinnati	☒ YES ☐ NO	45202

9. OF HISPANIC ORIGIN? (Specify No or Yes – If yes, specify Cuban, Mexican, Puerto Rican, etc.) ☐ No ☒ Yes Specify: Puerto Rican

10. RACE
☐ American Indian
☐ Black
☒ White
☐ Other (Specify) _____

11. EDUCATION (Specify only highest grade completed)
Elementary/Secondary (0-12)	College (1-4 or 5+)
12	

12. DATE LAST NORMAL MENSES BEGAN (Month, Day, Year)	13. CLINICAL ESTIMATE OF GESTATION (Weeks)	14. PREVIOUS PREGNANCIES (Complete each section)			
		LIVE BIRTHS		OTHER TERMINATIONS	
		14a. Now Living	14b. Now Dead	14c. Spontaneous	14d. Induced (Do not include this termination)
September 5, 1997	10 weeks	Number _____ ☒ None	Number _____ ☒ None	Number _____ ☒ None	Number _____ ☒ None

15. TYPE OF TERMINATION PROCEDURE (Check only one)

☒ Suction Curettage

☐ Medical (Nonsurgical), Specify Medication(s) _____

☐ Dilation and Evacuation (D&E)

☐ Intra-Uterine Instillation (Saline or Prostaglandin)

☐ Sharp Curettage (D&C)

☐ Hysterotomy/Hysterectomy

☐ Other (Specify) _____

16. NAME OF ATTENDING PHYSICIAN (Type/Print)	17. NAME OF PERSON COMPLETING REPORT (Type/Print)
Edmund Matthew Stone, M.D.	Julia Lynn Koval

7-0795

U.S. DEPARTMENT OF HEALTH AND HUMAN SERVICES — CENTERS FOR DISEASE CONTROL AND PREVENTION — NATIONAL CENTER FOR HEALTH STATISTICS — 1997 REVISION

Source: CDC 1997, 15.

A number of communicable illnesses must be reported to the CDC, as shown in **FIGURE 3.8**. National data on these diseases (classified as **notifiable diseases**) are reported weekly. Case-specific information is included in the CDC's reports. The CDC investigates cases where the cause of an illness or the source of an epidemic cannot be determined at the local level.

Hospitals calculate population-based health statistics at the local level. **Population-based statistics** represent estimates of the incidence of a disease as a percentage of the total population that could have been affected. For example, the crude birth rate for a community can be calculated by dividing the number of live births in the community during a specified time period by the estimated population of that community during the same time.

Morbidity statistics are calculated as incidence rates (the number of people who contracted the same disease during a specific time period compared to the number of people who could have contracted the disease). Incidence rates usually include race, gender, and

FIGURE 3.8. Infectious diseases that require notification

- Anthrax
- Arboviral neuroinvasive and non-neuroinvasive diseases
  - California serogroup virus disease
  - Eastern equine encephalitis virus disease
  - Powassan virus disease
  - St. Louis encephalitis virus disease
  - West Nile virus disease
  - Western equine encephalitis virus disease
- Babesiosis
- Botulism
  - Botulism, foodborne
  - Botulism, infant
  - Botulism, other (wound and unspecified)
- Brucellosis
- Chancroid
- *Chlamydia trachomatis* infection
- Cholera
- Coccidioidomycosis
- Cryptosporidiosis
- Cyclosporiasis
- Dengue
  - Dengue fever
  - Dengue hemorrhagic fever
  - Dengue shock syndrome
- Diphtheria
- Ehrlichiosis/anaplasmosis
  - *Ehrlichia chaffeensis*
  - *Ehrlichia ewingii*
  - *Anaplasma phagocytophilum*
  - Undetermined
- Giardiasis
- Gonorrhea
- *Haemophilus influenzae*, invasive disease
- Hansen disease (leprosy)
- Hantavirus pulmonary syndrome
- Hemolytic uremic syndrome, post-diarrheal
- Hepatitis
  - Hepatitis A, acute
  - Hepatitis B, acute

- Hepatitis B, chronic
- Hepatitis B, perinatal infection
- Hepatitis C, acute
- Hepatitis C, past or present
- HIV infection*
  - HIV infection, adult/adolescent (age ≥ 13 years)
  - HIV infection, child (age ≥ 18 months and < 13 years)
  - HIV infection, pediatric (age < 18 months)
- Influenza-associated pediatric mortality
- Legionellosis
- Listeriosis
- Lyme disease
- Malaria
- Measles
- Meningococcal disease
- Mumps
- Novel influenza A virus infections
- Pertussis
- Plague
- Poliomyelitis, paralytic
- Poliovirus infection, nonparalytic
- Psittacosis
- Q Fever
  - Acute
  - Chronic
- Rabies
  - Rabies, animal
  - Rabies, human
- Rubella
- Rubella, congenital syndrome
- Salmonellosis
- Severe acute respiratory syndrome-associated coronavirus (SARS-CoV) disease
- Shiga toxin-producing *Escherichia coli* (STEC)
- Shigellosis
- Smallpox
- Spotted fever rickettsiosis
- Streptococcal toxic-shock syndrome
- *Streptococcus pneumoniae*, invasive disease
- Syphilis

FIGURE 3.8. (continued)

o Primary	• Vancomycin-intermediate *Staphylococcus aureus* (VISA)
o Secondary	• Vancomycin-resistant *Staphylococcus aureus* (VRSA)
o Latent	• Varicella (morbidity)
o Early latent	• Varicella (deaths only)
o Late latent	• Vibriosis
o Latent, unknown duration	• Viral hemorrhagic fevers, due to
o Neurosyphilis	o Ebola virus
o Late, non-neurological	o Marburg virus
o Stillbirth	o Arenavirus
o Congenital	o Crimean-Congo hemorrhagic fever virus
• Tetanus	o Lassa virus
• Toxic-shock syndrome (other than streptococcal)	o Lujo virus
• Trichinellosis (trichinosis)	o New world arenaviruses (Gunarito, Machupo, Junin, and Sabia viruses)
• Tuberculosis	• Yellow fever
• Tularemia	
• Typhoid fever	

*AIDS has been reclassified as HIV stage III

Source: CDC 2011.

age data so that the rates among different populations can be compared. Examples of commonly computed mortality statistics include the following:

- Crude death rate

- Neonatal mortality rate

- Postneonatal mortality rate

- Infant mortality rate

- Crude mortality rate

- Cause-specific mortality rate

- Maternal mortality rate

Management of the Healthcare Delivery System

CMS collects data from reimbursement claims in a national database. This database is the basis for decisions related to the effectiveness of healthcare delivery systems and reimbursement systems. Federal and state governments use the data reported by hospitals and other healthcare organizations to develop public health policies.

Professional and trade organizations, such as the American Medical Association, the American College of Surgeons, and the American Hospital Association, use information reported from health records to develop professional practice standards. Their support for public actions on healthcare policy issues is based on clinical information derived from health records.

Form and Content of Health Records

State laws and regulations establish legal requirements related to the form and content of health records for facilities located within the covered geopolitical area. Health record regulations are usually developed by the state administrative agency responsible for licensing healthcare organizations. Some state regulations have minimal standards for maintaining clinical records. Others require that clinical records be complete and accurate. In a few states, health record regulations interpret the specific categories of information that hospitals must collect. In addition, some state regulations integrate the health record requirements of the Medicare Conditions of Participation or pertinent accreditation standards.

Public health regulations in many states require hospitals to routinely report specific confidential, health-related information collected directly from health records. Most public health regulations require the reporting of vital statistics data such as births and deaths. Many states require the collection and reporting of information about the public's health, safety, and welfare. The required reporting of communicable diseases and injuries that resulted from a violent crime would fit in this category. In addition, many states require that hospitals and other healthcare providers report cases of suspected child or adult abuse or neglect to the appropriate legal authorities.

Failure to comply with state health record or public health regulations may result in a penalty such as forfeiture of a hospital's operating license, fines, and criminal sanctions.

The Consumer's Right to Health Record Access

Many states have statutes that address the patient's right to view, copy, and/or correct her health record. The Medicare Conditions of Participation for Hospitals establish the individual's right to access her health information. As noted in chapter 2, the HIPAA privacy act describes the situations in which patient access is available. Hospital policies should encompass state regulations, the HIPAA privacy act, and the Conditions of Participation to ensure that all applicable state and federal requirements address the patient's right to access her record.

Release and Disclosure of Confidential Health Information

Before the HIPAA (2003) privacy standard was implemented, there were no federal statutes or regulations to specifically protect the confidentiality of health records. The privacy rights of patients and the confidentiality of health records were addressed in a patchwork of state and federal regulations, professional practice standards, and individual facility policies.

When the Medicare program was established in the late 1960s, the Conditions of Participation required the confidentiality of health records for Medicare beneficiaries. In the 1970s, federal legislation was implemented to ensure the privacy of patients in some types of treatment programs operated or supported by the federal government. The drug and alcohol treatment legislation passed in 1970 and amended in 2000 established strict confidentiality requirements for substance-abuse treatment records, but only for records maintained by facilities that receive federal funding. Similarly, the provisions of the Privacy Act of 1974 apply only to facilities operated by the federal government.

In contrast, the HIPAA privacy standard established consistent rules that apply to virtually every healthcare facility, healthcare professional, healthcare information clearinghouse, and health plan in the United States. The standard supersedes state regulations that permit less stringent privacy practices.

Although the federal privacy standard has preempted some state health record regulations, many are still relevant. The federal regulations constitute a minimum standard for protecting confidential records. Some states have no additional laws, while others require that specific patient authorization language be obtained prior to release. One state (Minnesota Department of Health 2008) has developed its own universal consent form. When state regulations require stricter privacy practices, hospitals and other healthcare organizations must follow these regulations in addition to the federal privacy standard. Healthcare organizations must comply with the public health reporting regulations and licensure and certification requirements in their geopolitical area (AHIMA 2008).

Many states base the confidentiality rights of patients on the concept of **privileged communication**. According to this concept, medical practitioners, like lawyers and other professionals, are not allowed to disclose the confidential information they learn in their capacity as professional service providers. There are very few exceptions to this basic rule for medical practitioners.

The HIPAA privacy standard does not require healthcare organizations to obtain the patient's formal consent to use health information for treatment, reimbursement, operational, and reporting purposes. However, some state regulations may still require hospitals and other healthcare providers to obtain written consent from the patient or the patient's legal representative before sharing the patient's confidential health information with external healthcare providers and third-party payers.

Even in the absence of state and federal requirements, many hospitals choose to document the patient's consent for routine uses and disclosures of confidential information. Patients are usually asked to sign general consents during the admissions process. (See **Figure 3.9** for Minnesota's Universal Consent Form.) Consents relevant to confidential information are treated as separate documents rather than as elements of the general consent to treatment, which is obtained at admission (Hjort and Hughes 2002).

State regulations governing the release and disclosure of confidential health information take a variety of approaches. Implicitly or explicitly, however, they all grant patients or their legal representatives two basic rights: the right to limit access to their records under certain circumstances and the right to waive their confidentiality rights when they choose. State regulations can be found online at the URLs listed in **Table 3.1**. For states not shown, search the state's official website or the AHIMA Component State Association website.

In general, healthcare facilities and practitioners are required to obtain the patient's explicit written permission before disclosing information for any purpose not related to treatment, reimbursement, operations, or public health reporting. Federal and state regulations, accreditation standards, and professional practice guidelines dictate the specific form and content of such consents and authorizations.

Redisclosure of Confidential Health Information

Health records sometimes include clinical data originally collected by other healthcare providers. For example, surgeons often supply copies of preadmission laboratory test results for patients scheduled to undergo elective surgery in the hospital. Such documents become a permanent part of the patient's acute-care record only when used during the patient's course of treatment in the hospital.

The process of disclosing health record documentation originally created by a different provider is called **redisclosure**. Federal and state regulations provide specific rediscolsure guidelines. When in doubt, follow the same release and disclosure guidelines for other types of health record information (AHIMA 2009).

FIGURE 3.9. Minnesota's Uniform Consent Form

Instructions for Minnesota Standard Consent Form to Release Health Information

Important: Please read all instructions and information before completing and signing the form.

An incomplete form may not be accepted. Please follow the directions carefully. If you have any questions about the release of your health information or this form, please contact the organization you will list in section 3.

This standard form was developed by the Minnesota Department of Health as required by the Minnesota Health Records Act of 2007. If completed properly, this form must be accepted by the health care organization(s), specific health care facility(ies), or specific professional(s) identified in section 3.

A fee may be charged for the release of the health information.

The following are instructions for each section. Please type or print as clearly and completely as possible.

1| Include your full and complete name. If you have a suffix after your last name (Sr., Jr., III), please provide it in the "last name" blank with your last name. If you used a previous name(s), please include that information. If you know your medical record or patient identification number, please include that information. All these items are used to identify your health information and to make certain that only your information is sent.

2| If there are questions about how this form was filled out, this section gives the organization that will provide the health information permission to speak to the person listed in this section. **Completing this section is optional.**

3| In this section, state who is sending your health information. **Please be as specific as possible.** If you want to limit what is sent, you can name a specific facility, for example Main Street Clinic. Or name a specific professional, for example chiropractor John Jones. Please use the specific lines. Providing location information may help make your request more clear. Please print "All my health care providers" in this section if you want health information from all of your health care providers to be released.

4| Indicate where you would like the requested health information sent. It is best to provide a complete mailing address as not everyone will fax health information. A place has been provided to indicate a deadline for providing the health information. **Providing a date is optional.**

5| Indicate what health information you want sent. If you want to limit the health information that is sent to a particular date(s) or year(s), indicate that on the line provided.

For your protection, it is recommended that you initial instead of check the requested categories of health information. This helps prevent others from changing your form. EXAMPLE: _jh_ All health information

If you select **all health information**, this will include any information about you related to mental health evaluation and treatment, concerns about drug and/or alcohol use, HIV/AIDS testing and treatment, sexually transmitted diseases and genetic information.

Important: There are certain types of health information that require special consent by law.

Chemical dependency program information comes from a program or provider that specifically assesses and treats alcohol or drug addictions and receives federal funding. This type of health information is different from notes about a conversation with your physician or therapist about alcohol or drug use. To have this type of health information sent, mark or initial on the line at the bottom of page 1.

Psychotherapy notes are kept by your psychiatrist, psychologist or other mental health professional in a separate filing system in their office and not with your other health information. **For the release of psychotherapy notes, you must complete a separate form noting only that category. You must also name the professional who will release the psychotherapy notes in section 3.**

6| Health information includes both written and oral information. If you do not want to give permission for persons in section 3 to talk with persons in section 4 about your health information, you need to indicate that in this section.

7| Please indicate the reason for releasing the health information. If you indicate marketing, please contact the organization in section 4 to determine if payment or compensation is involved. If payment or compensation to the organization is involved, indicate the amount.

8| This consent will expire one year from the date of your signature, unless you indicate an earlier date or event. Examples of an event are: "60 days after I leave the hospital," or "once the health information is sent."

9| Please sign and date this form. If you are a legally authorized representative of the patient, please sign, date and indicate your relationship to the patient. You may be asked to provide documents showing that you are the patient or the patient's legally authorized representative.

 This form was approved by the Commissioner of the Minnesota Department of Health on January 30, 2008.   JAN2008

105

FIGURE 3.9. (continued)

Minnesota Standard Consent Form to Release Health Information

PAGE 1 OF 2

1 | Patient information

First name_____ Middle name _____ Last name _____

Patient date of birth ___ / ___ / _____ Previous name(s) _____
  MM   DD   YYYY

Home address _____

City_____ State_____ Zip code _____

Daytime phone _____ E-mail address (optional)_____

Medical Record/patient ID number (optional)_____

2 | Contact for information about how this form was filled out (optional) :

I give permission for the organization(s) listed in section 3 permission to talk to

First name_____ Last name_____ about how this form was completed,

this person can be reached at: Daytime phone _____ E-mail address (optional)_____

3 | I am requesting health information be released from at least one of the following:

Organization(s) name _____

Specific health care facility or location(s) _____

Specific health care professional's name(s) _____

4 | I am requesting that health information be sent to:

Organization(s) name _____

And/or person: First name _____ Last name_____

Mailing address _____

City_____ State_____ Zip code_____

Phone (optional) _____ Fax (optional) _____

Information needed by (date) ___ / ___ / _____ (optional)
           MM   DD   YYYY

5 | Information to be released

IMPORTANT: indicate only the information that you are authorizing to be released.

☐ Specific dates/years of treatment _____

☐ All health information *(see description in instructions for what is included)*

OR to only release specific portions of your health information, indicate the categories to be released:

☐ History/Physical   ☐ Mental health   ☐ HIV/AIDS testing

☐ Laboratory report   ☐ Discharge summary   ☐ Radiology report

☐ Emergency room report   ☐ Progress notes   ☐ Radiology image(s)

☐ Surgical report   ☐ Care plan   ☐ Photographs, video, digital or other images

☐ Medications   ☐ Immunizations   ☐ Billing records

☐ Other information or instructions _____

The following information requires special consent by law. Even if you indicate **all health information**, you must specifically request the following information in order for it to be released:

☐ Chemical dependency program *(see definition in instructions)*

☐ Psychotherapy notes *(this consent cannot be combined with any other; see instructions)*

This form was approved by the Commissioner of the Minnesota Department of Health on January 30, 2008.

JAN2008

FIGURE 3.9. (continued)

Minnesota Standard Consent Form to Release Health Information

Patient's name _____   PAGE 2 OF 2

6 | **Health information includes written and oral information**

By indicating any of the categories in section 5, you are giving permission for written information to be released **and** for a person in section 3 to talk to a person in section 4 about your health information.

If you do not want to give your permission for a person in section 3 to talk to a person in section 4 about your health information, indicate that here (check mark or initials) _____

7 | **Reason(s) for releasing information**

- ☐ Patient's request
- ☐ Review patient's current care
- ☐ Treatment/continued care
- ☐ Payment
- ☐ Insurance application
- ☐ Legal
- ☐ Appeal denial of Social Security Disability income or benefits
- ☐ Marketing purposes   (payment or compensation involved?   ☐ NO   ☐ YES, amount _____)
- ☐ Other (please explain) _____

8 | I understand that by signing this form, I am requesting that the health information specified in Section 5 be sent to the third party named in section 4 above.

I may stop this consent at any time by writing to the organization(s), facility(ies) and/or professional(s) named in section 3. If the organization, facility or professional named in section 3 has already released health information based on my consent, my request to stop will not work for that health information.

I understand that when the health information specified in section 5 is sent to the third party named in section 4 above, the information could be re-disclosed by the third party that receives it and may no longer be protected by federal or state privacy laws.

I understand that if the organization named in section 4 is a health care provider they will not condition treatment, payment, enrollment or eligibility for benefits on whether I sign the consent form.

If I choose not to sign this form and the organization named in section 4 is an insurance company, my failure to sign will not impact my treatment; I may not be able to get new or different insurance; and/or I may not be able to get insurance payment for my care.

This consent will end one year from the date the form is signed unless I indicate an earlier date or event here:

Date ___ / ___ / _____ Or specific event _____
      MM   DD   YYYY

9 | **Patient's signature** _____ Date ___/___/_____
                                                                                    MM DD YYYY

Or legally authorized representative's signature_____ Date ___/___/_____
                                                                                    MM DD YYYY

Representative's relationship to patient (parent, guardian, etc.)_____

[Print Form]

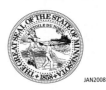

This form was approved by the Commissioner of the Minnesota Department of Health on January 30, 2008.   JAN2008

Source: Minnesota Department of Health 2008.

TABLE 3.1. State regulations for release of information

DOCUMENT TITLE BY STATE	YEAR PUBLISHED	URL	COST	FORMAT
Arkansas Legal Manual for Health Information Management	2006	http://www.arhima.org/	Paper: $175—member, $275—nonmember; CD: $125—member, $250—nonmember; plus shipping and handling	Paper or CD-ROM
Confidentiality and Security–Protecting and Releasing Health Information in California	2003	www.CaliforniaHIA.org	$65—member, $75—nonmember	Paper
A HIPAA Compendium–Patient Privacy and Security in California	2002	www.CaliforniaHIA.org	$40—member, $45—non-member	Paper
The California Patient Privacy Manual	2004	www.calhealth.org	$175—member, $375—nonmember; plus tax and shipping	Paper
Colorado Consent Manual: Guidelines for Consent to Care and Release of Health Information	2008	www.cha.com	$695—member, $995—nonmember	CD-ROM
A Medico-Legal Guide to Healthcare Records in Florida	1987	http://www.fhima.org/	$305 for CD-ROM and notebook set	CD-ROM
Georgia GHIMA 2006 Legal Handbook	2006	http://www.ghima.org/	$150—member, $200—nonmember; plus tax, shipping/handling	CD-ROM
Managing Health Information in Illinois (MHII), A Reference Guide to Health Information and the Law in Illinois	1986	http://www.ilhima.org/	Varies by membership and format	Electronic (PDF file downloadable via password) and paper
Indiana Health Information Management Association (IHIMA) Release of Information Guide	2008	http://www.ihima.org/	Price under revision	CD-ROM
Iowa Guide to Medical Record Laws	2003	http://www.ahima.org/directory/iowa.asp	$125—member, $200—nonmember; plus shipping	CD-ROM and paper
Kentucky Legal Reference for Health Information Management	Not noted	http://www.khima.org/	$225 plus $15 shipping/handling for a paper version plus a CD-ROM	CD-ROM and paper
Louisiana Health Information Law	1999	http://www.hpm.cc/	$149 plus shipping and handling	Paper
Healthcare Practitioner's Guide to Medical and Legal Information (Maine)	Not noted	http://www.mehima.org/	$50 for manual or $5 for each chapter.	CD-ROM
Medico-Legal Guide to Health Record Information (Massachusetts)	1963	http://www.mahima.org/	$179—member, $199—nonmember for a paper version plus a CD-ROM	CD-ROM and paper
Legal Reference Manual for Health Information Management in Minnesota	1990	www.mnhima.org	$175—member, $225—nonmember; plus tax	CD-ROM

TABLE 3.1. (continued)

DOCUMENT TITLE BY STATE	YEAR PUBLISHED	URL	COST	FORMAT
Legal Manual for the Management of Health Information in Missouri	2006	http://www.mohima.org/	CD-ROM: $100—member, $150—nonmember; Paper: $135—member, $150—nonmember	CD-ROM and paper
MHA (Association of Montana Heath Care Providers) Health Care Consent Manual	Not noted	http://www.mtha.org/	Varies by membership and format	CD-ROM and paper
Guide for Privacy, Retention and Disclosure of Health Information (New Hampshire)	2006	http://www.nhima.org/	One free to each NHIMA member; $150 plus tax and shipping/handling—nonmember	CD-ROM
Medico-Legal Manual (New York)	Not noted	http://www.nyhima.org/	$125—member, $200—nonmember, $85—student; plus shipping/handling	CD-ROM and paper
North Carolina Health Information Management Association Legal Reference Manual	1985	http://www.nchima.org/	$125—CD-ROM; $150—paper; prices include shipping and handling	CD-ROM and paper
North Dakota Health Information Management Association Legislative Manual	Not noted	http://www.ahima.org/directory/north_dakota.asp	Information not available	Paper
Oklahoma Health Information and the Law	2005	http://www.okhima.org/	$75—member, $125—nonmember; plus $10 shipping and handling	CD-ROM
South Carolina Health Information Management Association (SCHIMA) Legal Manual	2007	http://www.schima.org/	$155—member, $205—nonmember	CD-ROM
South Dakota Healthcare Information Legal Manual	2006	http://www.sdhima.org/	$60—member, $80—nonmember	Paper
Tennessee Health Information Management Association Legal Handbook 2006	1977	www.thima.org & www.thima.org/whats.new/LEGALHANDBOOKORDERFORM.doc (legal manual order form)	$250—member, $300—nonmember CD-ROM or paper; add shipping and tax	CD-ROM and paper
Washington State Health Information Association Legislative Manual	1961	http://www.wshima.org/files/Legislative_Manual_Order_Form_2007.pdf	Varies according to quantity ordered	CD-ROM
Legal Resource Manual for Patient Health Care Information (Wisconsin)	1994	http://www.whima.org/services/services4.html	Varies according to format	CD-ROM and paper

Source: AHIMA 2008.

Retention of Health Records

Hospitals and other healthcare facilities develop health record retention policies to ensure that health records comply with all applicable state and federal regulations and accreditation standards and meet future patient-care needs. Establishing and following consistent record retention and destruction policies helps control the cost of record storage space, equipment, and labor.

Most states have established regulations that address how long health records and other healthcare-related documents must be maintained before they can be destroyed. Although the Medicare Conditions of Participation for Hospitals stipulate a five-year minimum, many states require longer retention periods. Some states base their retention guidelines on the type of services represented in the record. A few state laws specify how long health records must be retained in their original form before they may be converted to a different storage media. In many states, retention guidelines require facilities to retain the records of infants and children longer than the records of adults.

In states that do not stipulate a retention period, the healthcare providers must preserve and retain all components of the legal health record, whether paper-based or electronic, for the period established by the state's statute of limitations (Reynolds and Bowman 2010). Consideration must be made when EHRs are maintained in disparate systems (AHIMA 2011a). A **statute of limitations** is a law that dictates the maximum period of time that may elapse between an event (for example, an injury or a crime) and any consequent legal action. In most states, the statute of limitations requires legal action in less than ten years. Therefore, in the absence of other state retention guidelines, hospitals and other healthcare providers may decide to maintain health records for a minimum of ten years (Reynolds and Bowman 2010). Similarly, AHIMA recommends that health records be maintained for a minimum period of ten years. It recommends permanent retention for several other types of patient-care records. See **TABLE 3.2** for information on the retention standards recommended by AHIMA.

Although the Medicare Conditions of Participation for Hospitals and various accreditation standards provide some guidance, every hospital should establish its own retention policies to reflect its unique regulatory climate. As a matter of law, retention policies must comply with the applicable local, state, and federal regulations. However, hospitals use health records for purposes other than patient care (for example, medical staff credentialing and performance improvement activities). Hospital retention policies should also take into account the advice of the facility's malpractice insurance carrier and legal counsel.

In addition to patient-care records, hospitals and other healthcare organizations maintain huge amounts of administrative information. The board of directors, executive staff, legal counsel, and medical staff should work together to develop retention guide-

TABLE 3.2. AHIMA's recommended retention standards

HEALTH INFORMATION	RECOMMENDED RETENTION PERIOD
Diagnostic images (such as X-ray film)	5 years
Disease index	10 years
Fetal heart monitor records	10 years after the infant reaches the age of majority
Master patient/person index	Permanently
Operative index	10 years
Patient health/medical records (adults)	10 years after the most recent encounter
Patient health/medical records (minors)	Age of majority plus statute of limitations
Physician index	10 years
Register of births	Permanently
Register of deaths	Permanently
Register of surgical procedures	Permanently

Source: Servais 2008, 350.

lines for all of the facility's records. State and federal regulations on taxation and business reporting must be considered when drafting information-retention policies.

Destruction of Health Records

Because of cost and space limitations, permanently storing paper and microfilm-based health record documents is not an option for most hospitals. The question of how to dispose of original records in a way that protects their confidentiality usually comes up in one of four situations.

1. The retention period for a set of paper-based or micrographic records has elapsed, and the healthcare organization needs to free up storage space for current records.

2. The healthcare organization routinely transfers paper-based records onto microfiche or optical disks for long-term storage and needs to dispose of the original paper documents.

3. The healthcare organization is in the process of implementing an EHR system and needs to dispose of paper records that are scanned and loaded onto the new system.

4. The healthcare organization is being sold or is closing permanently and needs to arrange for the disposition of its health records.

The destruction of patient-identifiable clinical documentation should be carried out in accordance with relevant federal and state regulations and organizational policy, such as e-discovery. Health records related to open investigations, audits, or court cases should not be destroyed for any reason. In an entirely EHR world, selective destruction is possible in which some types of documentation can be retained while others can be destroyed. If this is the organizational choice, the policy for record retention and destruction of EHRs should outline the protocol for selective destruction. Once the statute of limitations has expired on an episode of care, the documentation can be destroyed. In the electronic record, not all documents have the same need for retention. For example, is it really necessary to keep all the nursing graphic documentation after the statute of limitations has expired? Perhaps the progress notes of attending physicians would be retained, but notes of medical students and first-year interns would not. A facility could decide to retain the discharge summary, operative report(s), pathology report(s), and diagnostic data but nothing else. Once decisions are made according to the protocol, electronic files can be destroyed according to facility data security policy (AHIMA 2010a).

Some states require hospitals and other providers to complete certain preparatory activities, such as creating health record abstracts or notifying patients so that they have enough time to request copies, before they destroy health records. Some states establish specific requirements for the method of destruction.

According to AHIMA practice standards, acceptable destruction methods include the following (Hughes 2002):

- **Paper documents**: burning, shredding, pulping, or pulverizing

- **Micrographic film**: recycling or pulverizing

- **CD or optical disks**: shredding or pulverizing

- **Electronic documents**: magnetic degaussing (demagnetizing)

- **Magnetic tapes**: magnetic degaussing (demagnetizing) or zeroization process (writing repeated sequences of ones and zeros over the information)

Some facilities engage record destruction services to process obsolete health records. In such cases, the facility's contract with the vendor must fulfill the requirements of the HIPAA privacy standard.

When workstations, laptops, and servers use hard drives to store patient health information, simply deleting the files or folders containing this information does not necessarily erase the data.

1. To ensure that any patient's health information has been removed, utility software that overwrites the entire disk drive must be used. Total data destruction does not occur until the backup tapes have been overwritten. Magnetic neutralization will leave the domain in random patterns with no preference to orientation, rendering previous data unrecoverable.

2. If the computer is being redeployed internally or disposed of owing to obsolescence, the aforementioned utility must be run against the computer's hard drive, after which the hard drive may be reformatted and a standard software image loaded on the reformatted drive.

3. If the computer is being disposed of owing to damage and it is not possible to run the utility to overwrite the data, then the hard drive must be removed from the computer and physically destroyed. Alternatively, the drive can be erased using a magnetic bulk eraser. This requirement applies to PC workstations, laptops, and servers.

Federal guidelines for data disposal and sanitization can be found in the National Institute of Standards and Technology's Special Publication 800–88, *Guidelines for Media Sanitization* (AHIMA 2010a).

Appropriate documentation of health record destruction must be maintained permanently no matter how the process is carried out. This documentation usually takes the form of a **certificate of destruction**, which should include the following details (Reynolds and Bowman 2010, 225):

- Date of destruction

- Method of destruction (shredding, burning, or other means)

- Description of the disposed record series of numbers or items

- Inclusive dates covered

- A statement that the records were destroyed in the normal course of business

- The signatures of the individuals supervising and witnessing the destruction

Maintaining such documentation in a permanent file provides the facility with legal protection in any future liability actions (McWay 2010, 165). (See **Figure 3.10** for an example of a certificate of record destruction.)

State and federal record retention requirements continue to apply to health records maintained by facilities that have been sold or closed permanently. Before a sale or closure, the organization should develop plans for ensuring that the health

FIGURE 3.10. **Example of a certificate of record destruction**

Anytown General Hospital

**CERTIFICATE OF HEALTH
RECORD DESTRUCTION**

PATIENT LABEL

The information described below was destroyed in the normal course of business pursuant to a proper retention schedule and destruction policies and procedures.

Date of destruction: _____

Description of records or record series disposed of:_____

_____

_____

Inclusive dates covered: _____

Method of destruction: _____

☐ Burning   ☐ Shredding   ☐ Pulping

☐ Demagnetizing   ☐ Overwriting   ☐ Pulverizing

☐ Other: _____

Records Destroyed By: _____
                                    Signature   Date

Witness Signature:_____
                                    Signature   Date

Department Manager: _____
                                    Signature   Date

CERTIFICATE OF HEALTH RECORD DESTRUCTION
0943217 (08/2003)

records of former patients will be stored appropriately and made available for legitimate access over the required retention period. (An AHIMA practice brief provides specific guidance on handling patient information after a facility closure [Rhodes and Brandt 2003].)

Summary

The primary functions of the health record can be grouped into four categories: patient-care delivery, patient-care management, patient-care support, and billing and reimbursement. In examining these functions, this chapter focused on the concept that data represent facts but information conveys meaning. Primary users of the health record include nurses, physicians, allied health professionals, administrative personnel, patients, and their family members or legal representatives.

The ancillary functions of the acute care health record are related to the care environment. Ancillary functions include accreditation, licensure, and certification; biomedical research; clinical education; and morbidity and mortality reporting.

The principal functions of the health record use primary, patient-identifiable information. Most ancillary functions use secondary, de-identified health record information, usually in an aggregate form that protects the confidentiality of patient records.

References

AHIMA. 2011a. Fundamentals of the Legal Health Record and Designated Record Set. *Journal of AHIMA* 82(2): expanded online version.

AHIMA. 2011b. *Regulations Governing Research* (Updated). Chicago: AHIMA.

AHIMA. 2010a. *EHRs as the Business and Legal Records of Healthcare Organizations* (Updated). Appendix A: Issues in Electronic Health Record Management. Chicago: AHIMA.

AHIMA. 2010b. *Information Security—An Overview* (Updated). Chicago: AHIMA.

AHIMA. 2009. Redisclosure of Patient Health Information (Updated). *Journal of AHIMA* 80(2):51–54.

AHIMA. 2008. *Release of Information Workgroup on a Resource Guide On Release of Information For Continuity of Care*. Chicago: AHIMA.

AHIMA e-HIM Work Group on Maintaining the Legal EHR. 2005. Update: Maintaining a Legally Sound Health Record—Paper and Electronic. *Journal of American Health Information Management Association* 76(10):64A–L.

Baldwin-Stried Reich, K. 2007. Developing a Litigation Response Plan. *Journal of American Health Information Management Association* 78(9):76–78, 86.

Bowman, S. 2008. Policies and Procedures. In *Health Information Management Compliance: Guidelines for Preventing Fraud and Abuse*, 4th ed., edited by S. Bowman. Chicago: AHIMA.

Centers for Disease Control and Prevention (CDC). 2011. *Nationally Notifiable Infectious Diseases, United States, 2011*. http://www.cdc.gov/osels/ph_surveillance/nndss/phs/infdis2011.htm.

Centers for Disease Control and Prevention (CDC). 2003. *2003 Revisions of the U.S. Standard Certificates of Live Birth and Death and the Fetal Death*. Hyattsville, MD: National Center for Health Statistics. http://www.cdc.gov/nchs/nvss/vital_certificate_revisions.htm.

Centers for Disease Control and Prevention (CDC). 1997. *Handbook on the Reporting of Induced Termination of Pregnancy*. Hyattsville, MD: National Center for Health Statistics. http://www.cdc.gov/nchs/data/misc/hb_itop.pdf.

Centers for Medicare and Medicaid Services (CMS). 2011. Quality Improvement Organizations. https://www.cms.gov/QualityImprovementOrgs.

Code of Federal Regulations (45 CFR 46). 2011. Title of Public Welfare, Department of Health and Human Services. Part 46 Protection of Human Subjects. §46.116 General requirements for informed consent. http://ohsr.od.nih.gov/guidelines/45cfr46.html#46.116.

DeLoss, G. 2010. E-Discovery from the Judicial Perspective. *Journal of AHIMA* 81(7):48–49.

Eichenwald Maki, S., and P. Oachs. 2010. Work Design and Performance Improvement. In *Health Information Management: Concepts, Principles, and Practice*, 3rd ed., edited by K. LaTour and S. Eichenwald Maki. Chicago: AHIMA.

Federal Trade Commission (FTC). 2008. *Security in Numbers: SSNs and Identity Theft*. http://www.ftc.gov/os/2008/12/P075414ssnreport.pdf.

Giannangelo, K., and L. Hyde. 2010. Retooling Quality Measures for ICD-10. *Journal of AHIMA* 81(6):56–57.

Health Insurance Portability and Accountability Act (HIPAA) of 1996. Public Law 104-191. http://www.gpoaccess.gov/cfr/index.html.

Hospital Corporation of America (HCA). n.d. http://hcahealthcare.com/home/index.dot.

Hjort, B., and G. Hughes. 2002. Practice Brief: Consent for Uses and Disclosures of Information. *Journal of American Health Information Management Association* 73(10).

Homan, C. 2011. Purpose and Function of the Health Record. In *Health Information Management Technology*, 3rd ed., edited by M. Johns. Chicago: AHIMA.

Horton, L. 2011. Healthcare Statistics. In *Health Information Management Technology*, 3rd ed., edited by M. Johns, 590–91. Chicago: AHIMA.

Hughes, G. 2002. Practice Brief: Destruction of Patient Health Information. *Journal of American Health Information Management Association* 73(10).

James, E. 2009. *Documentation and Reimbursement for Long-term Care*, 2nd ed. Chicago: AHIMA.

The Joint Commission. 2011. *2011 Comprehensive Accreditation Manual for Hospitals; The Official Handbook*. Oakbrook Terrace, IL: The Joint Commission.

McWay, D. 2010. *Legal Aspects of Health Information Management*, 3rd ed. Clifton Park, NY: Delmar Learning.

Minnesota Department of Health. 2008. Minnesota Standard Consent Form to Release Health Information. http://www.health.state.mn.us/divs/hpsc/dap/consent.pdf.

National Conference of Commissioners on Uniform State Laws. 2007. *Uniform Rules Relating to the Discovery of Electronically Stored Information*. http://www.law.upenn.edu/bll/archives/ulc/udoera/2007_final.htm.

Pozgar, G. D. 2012. Medical Staff. In *Legal Aspects of Health Care Administration*. 11th ed. Sudbury, MA: Jones & Bartlett Learning.

Reynolds, R., and E. Bowman. 2010. Paper-Based and Hybrid Health Records. In *Health Information Management: Concepts, Principles, and Practice*, 3rd ed., edited by K. LaTour and S. Eichenwald Maki. Chicago: AHIMA.

Rhodes, H., and M. Brandt. 2003. Practice Brief: Protecting Patient Information After a Facility Closure.

Journal of American Health Information Management Association 74(10):64A–C.

Servais, C. 2008. *The Legal Health Record.* Chicago: AHIMA.

Shaw, P., C. Elliot, P. Isaacson, and E. Murphy. 2010. *Quality and Performance Improvement in Healthcare: A Tool for Programmed Learning,* 4th ed. Chicago: AHIMA.

Voigt, C., and S. Torzewski. Direct Results: An HIE Tests Simple Information Exchange Using the Direct Project. *Journal of AHIMA* 82(5):38–41.

Watzlaf, V. 2010. Biomedical and Research Support. In *Health Information Management: Concepts, Principles, and Practice,* 3rd ed., edited by K. LaTour and S. Eichenwald Maki, 561–98. Chicago: AHIMA.

Zeman, V. 2010. Clinical Quality Management. In *Health Information Management: Concepts, Principles, and Practice,* 3rd ed., edited by K. LaTour and S. Eichenwald Maki. Chicago: AHIMA.

Appendix 3A

Sample Informed Consent Document

Revised 6/2/08

SAMPLE INFORMED CONSENT DOCUMENT

Please note that some of the language contained in this sample consent document may not be appropriate for the type of study that you are conducting. If you would like assistance on how to modify the document for your study, please contact the IRB Office.

ONLY INCLUDE THIS HEADER ON ALL CONSENT PAGES IF YOU ARE SUBMITTING A PAPER APPLICATION. IF YOU ARE SUBMITTING AN ELECTRONIC SUBMISSION THROUGH OSIRIS (CURRENTLY REQUIRED FOR ALL NEW PROTOCOLS), PLEASE USE THE WATERMARK THAT IS AVAILABLE THROUGH THE SYSTEM.

(Division, Department, School, or Center Letterhead)   University of Pittsburgh
Institutional Review Board
Approval Date:
Renewal Date:
IRB Number:

CONSENT TO ACT AS A PARTICIPANT IN A RESEARCH STUDY

TITLE: Phase III Evaluation of Iometinol-300 as a Contrast Medium for CT Scans

PRINCIPAL INVESTIGATOR: Cynthia Curie, M.D.
Professor of Radiology
University of Pittsburgh
Room B-319, UPMC Presbyterian
Telephone: 412-647-xxxx

CO-INVESTIGATORS: Ray Rembrant, M.D.
Associate Professor of Radiology
University of Pittsburgh
Room B-325, UPMC Presbyterian
Telephone: 412-647-xxxx

SOURCE OF SUPPORT: January Laboratories, Inc.
Department of Radiology, UPMC

Why is this research being done?

You are being asked to participate in a research study in which we will test whether an "investigational" drug, called Iometinol-300, can further improve the pictures taken during CT scans, compared to drugs used currently. We will also test the safety of this "investigational drug". Computerized tomography (CT scan) is a method to take pictures of internal organs using X-rays. To increase the quality of these pictures, a drug ("X-ray dye") is often given by injection into a vein prior to the CT scan. Iometinol-300 is an "investigational" X-ray dye. This drug is considered "investigational" because it has not received approval from the Food and Drug Administration for general use.

Page 1 of 10   Participant's Initials_____

Revised 6/2/08

In this research study, we will compare the CT scan pictures taken with the study drug, Iometinol-300, to those taken with the standard drug currently used in the radiology department. We will also evaluate if the study drug causes any changes to your body or blood.

Who is being asked to take part in this research study?

You are being invited to take part in this research study because you have already been scheduled for a CT scan of your head using the standard drug. The results of the CT scan using the standard drug will be compared to the results of an extra, research CT scan using the study drug to show us which of the two drugs was better for your particular case.

People invited to participate in this study must be between 18-60 years of age and, if female, cannot be pregnant. The study is being performed on a total of 60 individuals in three different medical centers in the United States. At this medical center, 20 individuals will participate.

What procedures will be performed for research purposes?

If you decide to take part in this research study, you will undergo the following procedures that are not part of your standard medical care:

Screening Procedures:

Procedures to determine if you are eligible to take part in a research study are called "screening procedures". For this research study, the screening procedures include:

1. For women who could possibly be pregnant, a small sample (about 1 teaspoonful) of blood will be taken from a vein in your arm for a pregnancy test. Pregnant women, or women who are currently breast-feeding an infant, will not be allowed to take part in this study.

Experimental Procedures:

If you qualify to take part in this research study, you will undergo the experimental procedures listed below. These procedures will take place in the radiology department.

1. Prior to the injection of the study drug and the extra, research CT scan, we will measure your blood pressure, temperature, and heart rate. In addition, we will obtain a blood sample (about 1 teaspoonful) from a vein in your arm for safety tests. This will require about 30 minutes of your time.

2. The study drug will be injected by vein followed by the extra, research CT scan.

Page 2 of 10   Participant's Initials_____

Revised 6/2/08

<u>Monitoring/Follow-up Procedures:</u>

Procedures performed to evaluate the effectiveness and safety of the experimental procedures are called "monitoring " or "follow-up" procedures. For this research study, the monitoring/follow-up procedures include:

1. One hour after the injection of the study drug, we will again measure your blood pressure, temperature, and heart rate. Thus, the study drug injection, research CT scan, and repeat safety measures will require about 1 hour of your time.

   You are free to leave the radiology department after these measures, but you will need to return 3 hours later for additional safety tests.

2. Four hours after the injection of the study drug, we will once again measure your blood pressure, temperature, and heart rate. These repeat safety measures will require about 15 minutes of your time.

   You are free to go home after these measures, but you will need to return the next day for final safety tests.

3. At about 24 hours (1 day) following injection of the study drug, we will measure your blood pressure, temperature, and heart rate. We will also obtain another sample (about 1 teaspoonful) of blood from your vein for follow-up safety tests. These procedures will require about 30 minutes of your time and will be performed in the radiology department.

4. The investigators will compare your scheduled CT scan using the standard drug to the research CT scan using the study drug.

What are the possible risks, side effects, and discomforts of this research study?

The possible risks of this research study may be due to the study drug, the blood tests, and/or the radiation exposure from the extra CT scan.

<u>Risks of the Study Drug:</u>

Previous human research studies using the study drug have shown that the nature and number of adverse events associated with its use are similar to those which occur with the standard drugs used for CT scans.

   Infrequent adverse events (occur in 1–10%, or 1–10 out of 100 people): Itching, hives, nausea, and vomiting may be expected in 1-2% of the individuals who receive the study drug. These adverse events are usually mild in severity.

Page 3 of 10   Participant's Initials_____

Revised 6/2/08

Rare adverse events (occur in less than 1% , or less than 1 out of 100 people): In about 1 out of every 10,000 injections (0.01%), more severe reactions (e.g., shortness of breath, chest pain, seizure) may occur. In some cases these reactions can be life-threatening.

As with any experimental procedure, there may be adverse events or side effects that are currently unknown and certain of these unknown risks could be permanent, severe, or life threatening.

A physician and emergency drugs and equipment will be readily available should you experience any adverse reactions from administration of the study drug.

Because participation in this study may harm a pregnancy, you and any person with whom you have sex must use an approved form of birth control. If you become pregnant or father a child while you are in this study, you must tell your doctor at once. Also, women must not breast feed while in this study. If you are a woman and you are able to become pregnant, you will have a *(insert the appropriate measurement: blood or urine)* test to make sure that you are not pregnant before you are permitted to undergo the experimental procedures. If you have questions, you are encouraged to speak with either the study doctor or your personal physician. **(Note: Additional examples of acceptable reproductive risk language appear on the IRB web site in a document entitled "Guidance for Reproductive Risk Language for Consents Revised February 22, 2008."**

Risks of the Blood Tests:

Bruising, soreness, or rarely, infection may occur as a result of the needle sticks to obtain blood from your vein.

Risks of Radiation Exposure:

Participation in this research study will involve exposure to radiation from the extra, research CT scan. The amount of radiation exposure that you will receive from this extra CT scan is about 1 rem (a unit of radiation exposure) to your head, with minimum exposure of other areas of your body. For comparison, radiation workers are permitted, by federal regulation, a maximum radiation exposure of 50 rems per year to any single body organ. There is no minimum amount of radiation exposure that is recognized as being totally free of the risk of causing genetic mutations (abnormal cells) or cancer. However, the risk associated with the amount of radiation exposure that you will receive from taking part in this study is felt to be low and comparable to everyday risks.

What are possible benefits from taking part in this study?

You will likely receive no direct benefit from taking part in this research study. Should the study drug be better than the standard drug, it is possible that you may receive some benefit from the higher quality CT scan. However, such a benefit cannot be guaranteed.

Page 4 of 10   Participant's Initials_____

Revised 6/2/08

What treatments or procedures are available if I decide not to take part in this research study?

If you decide not to take part in this research study, you will have only the routine CT scan for which you were scheduled, using the standard drug.

If I agree to take part in this research study, will I be told of any new risks that may be found during the course of the study?

You will be promptly notified if, during the conduct of this research study, any new information develops which may cause you to change your mind about continuing to participate.

Will my insurance provider or I be charged for the costs of any procedures performed as part of this research study?

Neither you, nor your insurance provider, will be charged for the costs of any of the procedures performed for the purpose of this research study (i.e., the Screening Procedures, Experimental Procedures, or Monitoring/Follow-up Procedures described above). You will be charged, in the standard manner, for any procedures performed for your routine medical care (e.g., the CT scan for which you were already scheduled).

(NOTE—IF THE RESEARCH SUBJECTS OR THEIR HEALTH INSURANCE PROVIDER WILL BE RESPONSIBLE FOR ANY COSTS ASSOCIATED WITH THE RESEARCH, PLEASE INCLUDE THE FOLLOWING STATEMENTS):

If you participate in this research study, the cost of the experimental (device or drug, as applicable) and/or the costs of certain procedures performed for the purpose of the research study may be billed to your health insurance provider. You will be notified, in advance of undergoing the research procedures should your health insurance provider refuse to cover certain or all of these research costs and if any of these uncovered research costs will be billed directly to you. In this situation, you will be provided with a price estimate for the uncovered research costs that will be billed to you. If you decide to continue your participation in this research study, you will be required to meet with a hospital financial counselor to arrange for your advance payment of these uncovered research costs. If you do not have health care insurance, you will be provided with a price estimate for the research costs that will be billed to you. If, you decide to continue your participation in this research study, you will be required to meet with a hospital financial counselor to arrange for your advance payment of these research costs.

Will I be paid if I take part in this research study?

You will be paid a total of $150 if you complete all parts of this study. If, for whatever reason, you complete part but not all of the study, the terms of this payment will be as follows: 1) $20 for completing the initial temperature, blood pressure, and heart rate measurements and blood sample (if applicable); 2) an additional $50 for completing the extra, research CT scan using the new drug; 3) an additional $20 for completing the repeat measurements at 1 hour after injection of the study drug; 4) an additional $20 for completing the repeat measurements at 4 hours after injection of the study drug; and 5) an additional $40 for completing the repeat measurements and blood sample at 24 hours after injection of the study drug.

Page 5 of 10   Participant's Initials_____

Revised 6/2/08

In addition, any parking fees related to your participation in this study will be paid for by the study.

Who will pay if I am injured as a result of taking part in this study?

For research that is NOT commercially sponsored but is conducted at Pitt or UPMC facilities utilize the following language:

If you believe that the research procedures have resulted in an injury to you, immediately contact the Principal Investigator who is listed on the first page of this form. Emergency medical treatment for injuries solely and directly related to your participation in this research study will be provided to you by the hospitals of UPMC. Your insurance provider may be billed for the costs of this emergency treatment, but none of those costs will be charged directly to you. If your research-related injury requires medical care beyond this emergency treatment, you will be responsible for the costs of this follow-up care. At this time, there is no plan for any additional financial compensation.

For research that IS commercially sponsored and the protocol is provided by the sponsor, please see Chapter 8 of the IRB Reference Manual for instructions.

Who will know about my participation in this research study?

Any information about you obtained from this research will be kept as confidential (private) as possible. All records related to your involvement in this research study will be stored in a locked file cabinet. Your identity on these records will be indicated by a case number rather than by your name, and the information linking these case numbers with your identity will be kept separate from the research records. You will not be identified by name in any publication of the research results unless you sign a separate consent form giving your permission (release).

Will this research study involve the use or disclosure of my identifiable medical information?

This research study will involve the recording of current and/or future identifiable medical information from your hospital and/or other (e.g., physician office) records. The information that will be recorded will be limited to information concerning the purpose of the CT scan that you were scheduled to undergo for your medical care, the results of this CT scan, and any adverse events that may have been associated with the approved X-ray dye used in this CT scan. This information will be compared to the research CT scan performed using the study drug for the purpose of evaluating the safety and effectiveness of the study drug.

This research study will result in identifiable information that will be placed into your medical records held at UPMC Presbyterian. The nature of the identifiable information resulting from your participation in this research study that will be recorded in your medical record includes the results of the additional CT scan performed for research purposes and information related to any adverse events you may suffer following the injection of the study drug.

Page 6 of 10   Participant's Initials_____

Revised 6/2/08

Who will have access to identifiable information related to my participation in this research study?

In addition to the investigators listed on the first page of this authorization (consent) form and their research staff, the following individuals will or may have access to identifiable information (which may include your identifiable medical information) related to your participation in this research study:

Authorized representatives of the University of Pittsburgh Research Conduct and Compliance Office may review your identifiable research information (which may include your identifiable medical information) for the purpose of monitoring the appropriate conduct of this research study.

In unusual cases, the investigators may be required to release identifiable information (which may include your identifiable medical information) related to your participation in this research study in response to an order from a court of law. If the investigators learn that you or someone with whom you are involved is in serious danger or potential harm, they will need to inform, as required by Pennsylvania law, the appropriate agencies.

Authorized representatives of the sponsor of this research study, January Laboratories, Inc., will review and/or obtain identifiable information (which may include your identifiable medical information) related to your participation in this research study for the purpose of monitoring the accuracy and completeness of the research data and for performing required scientific analyses of the research data. Authorized representatives of the study sponsor may also be present during your participation in CT procedures performed as part of this research study. While the study sponsor understands the importance of maintaining the confidentiality of your identifiable research and medical information, the UPMC and University of Pittsburgh cannot guarantee the confidentiality of this information after it has been obtained by the study sponsor. The investigators involved in the conduct of this research study may receive funding from the sponsor to perform the research procedures and to provide the sponsor with identifiable research and medical information related to your participation in the study.

Authorized representatives of the U.S. Food and Drug Administration may review and/or obtain identifiable information (which may include your identifiable medical information) related to your participation in this research study for the purpose of monitoring the accuracy of the research data. While the U.S. Food and Drug Administration understands the importance of maintaining the confidentiality of your identifiable research and medical information, the University of Pittsburgh and UPMC cannot guarantee the confidentiality of this information after it has been obtained by the U.S. Food and Drug Administration.

Authorized representatives of the UPMC hospitals or other affiliated health care providers may have access to identifiable information (which may include your identifiable medical information) related to your participation in this research study for the purpose of (1) fulfilling orders, made by the investigators, for hospital and health care services (e.g., laboratory tests, diagnostic procedures) associated with research study participation; (2) addressing correct payment for tests and procedures ordered by the investigators; and/or (3) for internal hospital operations (i.e. quality assurance).

Page 7 of 10   Participant's Initials_____

Revised 6/2/08

For how long will the investigators be permitted to use and disclose identifiable information related to my participation in this research study?

The investigators may continue to use and disclose, for the purposes described above, identifiable information (which may include your identifiable medical information) related to your participation in this research study for a minimum of seven years after final reporting or publication of a project.

May I have access to my medical information that results from my participation in this research study?

In accordance with the UPMC Notices of Privacy Practices document that you have been provided, you are permitted access to information (including information resulting from your participation in this research study) contained within your medical records filed with your health care provider.

Is my participation in this research study voluntary?

Your participation in this research study, to include the use and disclosure of your identifiable information for the purposes described above, is completely voluntary. (Note, however, that if you do not provide your consent for the use and disclosure of your identifiable information for the purposes described above, you will not be allowed to participate in the research study.) Whether or not you provide your consent for participation in this research study will have no effect on your current or future relationship with the University of Pittsburgh. Whether or not you provide your consent for participation in this research study will have no effect on your current or future medical care at a UPMC hospital or affiliated health care provider or your current or future relationship with a health care insurance provider.

Your doctor is involved as an investigator in this research study. As both your doctor and a research investigator, s/he is interested both in your medical care and the conduct of this research study. Before agreeing to participate in this research study, or at any time during your study participation, you may discuss your care with another doctor who is not associated with this research study. You are not under any obligation to participate in any research study offered by your doctor.

May I withdraw, at a future date, my consent for participation in this research study?

You may withdraw, at any time, your consent for participation in this research study, to include the use and disclosure of your identifiable information for the purposes described above. (Note, however, that if you withdraw your consent for the use and disclosure of your identifiable medical record information for the purposes described above, you will also be withdrawn, in general, from further participation in this research study.) Any identifiable research or medical information recorded for, or resulting from, your participation in this research study prior to the date that you formally withdrew your consent may continue to be used and disclosed by the investigators for the purposes described above.

To formally withdraw your consent for participation in this research study you should provide a written and dated notice of this decision to the principal investigator of this research study at the address listed on the first page of this form.

Page 8 of 10   Participant's Initials_____

Revised 6/2/08

Your decision to withdraw your consent for participation in this research study will have no effect on your current or future relationship with the University of Pittsburgh. Your decision to withdraw your consent for participation in this research study will have no effect on your current or future medical care at a UPMC hospital or affiliated health care provider or your current or future relationship with a health care insurance provider.

If you decide to withdraw from study participation after you have received the study drug, you should participate in described monitoring follow-up procedures directed at evaluating the safety of the study drug.

If I agree to take part in this research study, can I be removed from the study without my consent?

It is possible that you may be removed from the research study by the researchers if, for example, your pregnancy test proves to be positive. If you are withdrawn from participation in this research study, you will continue to undergo the CT scan for which you were scheduled using the currently approved X-ray dye.

****

VOLUNTARY CONSENT

The above information has been explained to me and all of my current questions have been answered. I understand that I am encouraged to ask questions about any aspect of this research study during the course of this study, and that such future questions will be answered by a qualified individual or by the investigator(s) listed on the first page of this consent document at the telephone number(s) given. I understand that I may always request that my questions, concerns or complaints be addressed by a listed investigator.

I understand that I may contact the Human Subjects Protection Advocate of the IRB Office, University of Pittsburgh (1-866-212-xxxx) to discuss problems, concerns, and questions; obtain information; offer input; or discuss situations that have occurred during my participation.

By signing this form, I agree to participate in this research study. A copy of this consent form will be given to me.

_____   _____   _____

Participant's Signature   Printed Name of Participant   Date

Participant's Initials_____

Revised 6/2/08

CERTIFICATION of INFORMED CONSENT

"I certify that I have explained the nature and purpose of this research study to the above-named individual(s), and I have discussed the potential benefits and possible risks of study participation. Any questions the individual(s) have about this study have been answered, and we will always be available to address future questions as they arise."

_____   _____
Printed Name of Person Obtaining Consent   Role in Research Study

_____   _____
Signature of Person Obtaining Consent   Date

IF THE RESEARCH STUDY INVOLVES CHILDREN OR DECISIONALLY IMPAIRED SUBJECTS, PLEASE SEE CHAPTER 6.0 FOR THE APPROPRIATE LANGUAGE/SIGNATURE SPACES.

Page 10 of 10   Participant's Initials_____

Maintaining a Legally Sound Health Record—Paper and Electronic

The health record is the legal business record for a healthcare organization. As such, it must be maintained in a manner that follows applicable regulations, accreditation standards, professional practice standards, and legal standards. The standards may vary based on practice setting, state statutes, and applicable case law. An attorney should review policies related to legal documentation issues to ensure adherence to the most current standards and case law.

HIM professionals should fully understand the principles of maintaining a legally sound health record and the potential ramifications when the record's legal integrity is questioned. This practice brief will review the legal documentation guidelines for entries in and maintenance of the health record—both paper and electronic. Many of the guidelines that originally applied to paper-based health records translate to documentation in electronic health records (EHRs). In addition, new guidelines and functionalities have emerged specific to maintaining legally sound EHRs. It is of the utmost importance to maintain EHRs in a manner that will support a facility's business and legal processes, otherwise duplicate paper processes will need to be maintained.

AHIMA convened an e-HIM work group to reevaluate and update the 2002 practice brief "Maintaining a Legally Sound Health Record" to address the transition many organizations face in the migration from paper to hybrid to fully electronic health records. Issues unique to EHRs are addressed specifically if they are different or require expansion. Many organizations use a hybrid record (which includes both paper and electronic documentation), scanning paper documents into an electronic document management system. Even though a scanned document ends up in an electronic state, the documentation principles for paper-based records still apply. If there are unique issues for scanned records, they are specified in this brief.

Authentication for Legal Admissibility

Generally, statements made outside the court by a party in a lawsuit are considered hearsay and not admissible as evidence. Documentation in the health record is technically hearsay; however, Federal Rules of Evidence (803[6]) and the Uniform Business and Public Records Act adopted by most states allow exception to the hearsay rule for records maintained in the regular course of business, including health records. All records must be identified and authenticated prior to admissibility in court.

Four basic principles must be met for the health record to be authenticated or deemed admissible as evidence. The record must have been:

- Documented in the normal course of business (following normal routines)

- Kept in the regular course of business

AHIMA e-HIM Work Group on Maintaining the Legal EHR. 2005. Maintaining a Legally Sound Health Record—Paper and Electronic. *Journal of AHIMA* 76(10):64A–L.

- Made at or near the time of the matter recorded

- Made by a person within the business with knowledge of the acts, events, conditions, opinions, or diagnoses appearing in it

EHRs are admissible if the system that produced them is shown to be accurate and trustworthy. The Comprehensive Guide to Electronic Health Records outlines the following facts to support accuracy and trustworthiness:

- Type of computer used and its acceptance as standard and efficient equipment

- The record's method of operation

- The method and circumstances of preparation of the record, including:

  o The sources of information on which it is based

  o The procedures for entering information into and retrieving information from the computer

  o The controls and checks used as well as the tests made to ensure the accuracy and reliability of the record

  o The information has not been altered[1]

As EHRs become more commonplace, the federal courts are beginning to differentiate the standards to be applied to authenticate EHRs, based on the type of information stored. For example, when a computer record contains the assertions of a person, such as a progress note or dictated report, the record must fit within the hearsay exception to be admissible. These records are referred to as computer stored.

In contrast, computer-generated records contain the output of computer programs, untouched by human hands. Examples may include decision-support alerts and machine-generated test results. The admissibility issue here is not whether the information in the record is hearsay, but whether the computer program that generated the record was reliable and functioning properly (a question of authenticity). In most cases, the reliability of a computer program can be established by showing that users of the program actually do rely on it on a regular basis, such as in the ordinary course of business.

Testifying About Admissibility

Typically, the health record custodian is called upon to authenticate records by providing testimony about the process or system that produced the records. An organization's record-keeping program should consist of policies, procedures, and methods that support the creation and maintenance of reliable, accurate records. If so, the records will be admissible into evidence.

Electronic and imaged health records. Case law and the Federal Rules of Evidence provide support to allow the output of an EHR system to be admissible in court. The rule states "if data are stored in a computer or similar device, any printout or other output readable by sight, shown to reflect the data accurately, is an 'original.'"[2] As a result, an accurate printout of computer data satisfies the best evidence rule, which ordinarily requires the production of an original to prove the content of a writing, recording, or photograph. Organizations that maintain EHRs should clearly define those systems that contain the legal EHR or portions of the EHR. Each of these systems should be configured and maintained, ensuring that entries originated in a manner consistent with HIM principles and their business rules, content, and output meet all standards of admissibility.

An important component of this effort is to establish methods to authenticate the electronic data stored in the EHR, namely to verify that data have not been altered or improperly modified consistent with Federal Rules of Evidence. HIPAA security implementation standards require organizations to authenticate protected electronic health information as a means of ensuring data integrity, including data at rest and transmitted data. Cryptographic applications commonly used to authenticate include message authentication codes and digital signatures.

Authorship

Authorship is the origination of recorded information. This is an action attributed to a specific individual or entity, acting at a particular time. Authors are responsible for the completeness and accuracy of their entries in the health record.

AHIMA recommends that anyone documenting in the health record (regardless of media) have the authority and right to document as defined by the organization's policies and procedures. Individuals must be trained and competent in the fundamental documentation practices of the organization and legal documentation standards. Organizations should define the level of record documentation expected of their practitioners based on the practitioners' licensure, certification, and professional experience.

Authentication of Entries

Authentication shows authorship and assigns responsibility for an act, event, condition, opinion, or diagnosis. Health Level Seven (HL7) has defined a legally authenticated document or entry as "a status in which a document or entry has been signed manually or electronically by the individual who is legally responsible for that document or entry."[3] Each organization should establish a definition of a legally authenticated entry and establish rules to promptly authenticate every entry in the health record by the author responsible for ordering, providing, or evaluating the service furnished.

Many states have regulations or rules of evidence that speak to specific characteristics required for authenticating entries. Before adopting any authentication method other than written signature, the organization should consult state statutes and regulations regarding authentication of entries. The medical staff bylaws (where applicable) or organizational policies should also approve computer authentication and authentication of scanned entries and specify the rules for use. Organizations automating health records in a state that does not expressly permit the use of computer keys to authenticate should seek permission from the applicable state agency.

Types of Signatures

For paper-based records, acceptable methods to identify the author generally include written signature, rubber stamp signature, or initials combined with a signature legend on the same document. Acceptable methods of identifying the author in EHRs generally include electronic or digital signatures or computer key. Acceptable methods for authenticating a scanned document may follow paper or electronic guidelines.

Signatures are the usual method to authenticate entries in a paper-based record. The Centers for Medicare and Medicaid Services (CMS) Interpretive Guidelines for Hospitals 482.24(c)(1) require name and discipline at a minimum. A healthcare organization can choose a more stringent standard requiring the author's full name with title or credential to assist in proper identification of the writer. Healthcare organization policies should define the acceptable format for signatures in the health record.

A **counter signature** requires a professional to review and, if appropriate, approve action taken by another practitioner. Countersignatures should be used as required by state licensing or certification statutes related to professional scope of practice. The entries of individuals who are required to practice under the direct supervision of another professional should be countersigned by the individual who has authority to evaluate the entry. Once countersigned, the entry is legally adopted by the supervising professional as his or her own entry. For example, licensed nurses who do not have the authority to supervise should not countersign an entry for a graduate nurse who is not yet licensed. Practitioners who are asked to countersign should do so carefully. The CMS Interpretive Guidelines for Hospitals (482.24[c][1][I]) require that medical staff rules and regulations identify the types of documents or entries nonphysicians may complete that require a countersignature by a supervisor or attending medical staff member.

Rubber stamp signatures are acceptable if allowed by state, federal, and reimbursement regulations. From a reimbursement perspective, some fiscal intermediaries have local policies prohibiting the use of rubber stamp signatures in the health record even though federal regulation allows their use. Healthcare organization policies should state if rubber stamp signatures are acceptable and define the circumstances for their use after review of state regulations and payer policies.

When rubber stamp signatures are used, a list of signatures should be maintained to cross reference each signature to an individual author. The individual whose signature the stamp represents should sign a statement that he or she is the only one who has the stamp and uses it. There can be no delegation to another individual for use of the stamp. Sanctions should be established for unauthorized or inappropriate use of signature stamps.

Initials can be used to authenticate entries such as flow sheets, medication records, or treatment records. They should not be used for such entries as narrative notes or assessments. Initials should never be used for entries where a signature is required by law. Authentication of entries by only initials should be avoided because of the difficulty in positively identifying the author of an entry based on initials alone and distinguishing that individual from others having the same initials.

If a healthcare organization chooses to use initials in any part of the record for authentication of an entry, there should be corresponding full identification of the initials on the same form or on a signature legend. A signature legend may be used to identify the author and full signature when initials are used to authenticate entries. Each author who initials an entry must have a corresponding full signature on record. For EHRs, apply recommendations for computer key signatures.

Fax signatures. The acceptance of fax documents and signatures is dependent on state, federal, and reimbursement regulations. Unless specifically prohibited by state regulations or healthcare organization policy, fax signatures are acceptable. The Federal Rules of Evidence and the Uniform Rules of Evidence allow for reproduced records used during the course of business to be admissible as evidence unless there is a genuine question about their authenticity or circumstances dictate that the originals be admissible rather than the reproductions. Some states have adopted the Uniform Photographic Copies of Business and Public Records Act, which allows for the admissibility of a reproduced business record without the original. The Uniform Business Records as Evidence Act also addresses the admissibility of reproductions. When a fax document or signature is included in the health record, the document with the original signature should be retrievable from the original source.

Electronic signatures are acceptable if allowed by state, federal, and reimbursement regulations. In 2000 the US government passed the Electronic Signatures in Global National Commerce Act, which gives electronic signatures the same legality as handwritten signatures for interstate commerce. State regulations and payer policies must be reviewed to ensure acceptability of electronic signatures when developing healthcare organization policies. ASTM and HL7 have standards for electronic signatures.

Electronic signature software binds a signature or other mark to a specific electronic document. It requires user authentication such as a unique code, biometric, or password that verifies the identity of the signer in the system. If electronic signatures are used in the EHR, the software program or technology should provide message integrity—assurance that the message sent or entry made by a user is the same as the one received or maintained by the system. If electronic signatures are used in the EHR, the software program or technology should also provide for nonrepudiation—assurance that the entry or message came from a particular user. It will be difficult for a party to deny the content of an entry or having created it.

A **digital signature** provides a digital guarantee that information has not been modified, as if it were protected by a tamper-proof seal that is broken if the content were altered.[4]

A **computer key** or other code is an acceptable method to authenticate entries in an EHR if allowed by state, federal, and reimbursement regulations. When computer codes are used, a list of codes should be maintained that links each code to an individual author. Authorized users should sign a statement ensuring that they alone will use the computer key. Sanctions should be established for unauthorized or inappropriate use of a computer key.

Digital ink or digitized signatures differ from electronic signatures in that they use handwritten signatures on a pen pad. The actual written signature is converted into an electronic image. Digitized signatures are acceptable if allowed by state, federal, and reimbursement regulations. State regulations and payer policies must be reviewed to ensure acceptability of digitized signature when developing healthcare organization policies.

Specific Authentication Issues

There are a number of unique authentication scenarios and issues that organizations must address.

Auto-authentication. The author of each entry should take specific action to verify that the entry is his or her entry or that he or she is responsible for the entry and that the entry is accurate. Computer technology has provided opportunities to improve the speed and accuracy of the authentication process. However, authentication standards still require that the author attest to the accuracy of the entry. As a result, any auto-authentication technique that does not require that the author review the entry is likely to fall short of federal and state authentication requirements and place the organization at legal risk.

Failure to disapprove an entry within a specific time period is not an acceptable method of authentication. A method should be in place to ensure that authors authenticate dictated documents after they are transcribed. Auto-authentication methods where the dictator is deemed to have authenticated a transcribed document if no corrections are requested within a specified period of time are not recommended.

Authenticating documents with multiple sections or completed by multiple individuals. Some documentation tools, particularly assessments, are set up to be completed by multiple staff members at different times. As with any entry, there must be a mechanism to determine who completed information on the document. At a minimum, there should be a signature area at the end of the document for staff to sign and date. Staff who have completed sections of the assessment should either indicate the sections they completed at the signature line or initial the sections they completed.

Some EHR documentation tools, particularly assessments, are also intended to be completed by multiple staff members at different times. Here too there must be a mechanism to determine who completed information in the document.

Documenting care provided by a colleague. Individuals providing care are responsible for documenting that care. Documentation must reflect who performed the action. Patient care carried out by another provider, as well as clinical information supplied by another person to the writer of the entry, should be clearly attributed to the source.

Some EHR systems provide the capability to indicate differences between the person who enters information and the author of a document. In either case, documentation must reflect who performed the action. If documentation of care is entered for another provider, at a minimum the document should contain the identification of the person who entered the information along with the date the entry was made and authentication by the actual provider of care with the corresponding date of authentication.

Documentation Principles

Regardless of the format, text entries, canned phrases, or templates should follow fundamental principles for the quality of the entry. Content should be specific, objective, and complete.

Use **specific** language and avoid vague or generalized language. Do not speculate. The record should always reflect factual information (what is known versus what is thought or presumed), and it should be written using factual statements. Examples of generalizations and vague words include "patient doing well," "appears to be," "confused," "anxious," "status quo," "stable," and "as usual." If an author must speculate (that is, diagnosis is undetermined), the documentation should clearly identify speculation versus factual information.

Chart **objective** facts and avoid using personal opinions. By documenting what can be seen, heard, touched, and smelled, entries will be specific and objective. Describe signs and symptoms, use quotation marks when quoting the patient, and document the patient's response to care.

Document the **complete** facts and pertinent information related to an event, course of treatment, patient condition, response to care, and deviation from standard treatment (including the reason for it). Make sure the entry is complete and contains all significant information. If the original entry is incomplete, follow guidelines for making a late entry, addendum, or clarification.

Other Documentation Issues

Organizational policies must address the use of approved abbreviations in the health record. A second emerging documentation issue is the cut-and-paste functionality in EHRs. Organizations must consider whether they will allow cutting and pasting and how they will handle cut-and-paste content from one entry to another.

Use of abbreviations. Every healthcare organization should have a goal to limit or eliminate the use of abbreviations in medical record documentation as part of its patient safety efforts. Healthcare organizations should set a standard for acceptable abbreviations to be used in the health record and develop an organization-specific abbreviation list. Only those abbreviations approved by the organization should be used in the health record. When there is more than one meaning for an approved abbreviation, chose one meaning or identify the context in which the abbreviation is to be used. Every organization should have a list of abbreviations, acronyms, and symbols that should not be used.

EHRs. Abbreviations should be eliminated as information is formatted for the EHR. Electronic order sets, document templates for point-and-click or direct charting, voice recognition, or transcribed documents can be formatted or programmed to eliminate abbreviations.

Cut, copy, and paste functionality is not generally regarded as legitimately available in the paper record. Analogous functions in paper records include photocopying a note, cropping it, and pasting or gluing it into the record. The primary issue with the cut, copy, and paste functionality in the EHR is one of authorship—who is the author and what is the date of origination for a copied entry?

Cutting and pasting saves time; however, it also poses several risks:

- Cutting and pasting the note to the wrong encounter or the wrong patient record

- Lack of identification of the original author and date

- The acceptability of cutting and pasting the original author's note without his or her knowledge or permission

Organizations should develop policy and procedures related to cutting, copying, and pasting documentation in their EHR systems. By following these guidelines and training clinical staff, providers can allow cutting and pasting within certain boundaries.

- In general, the original source author and date must be evidenced in copied information. If users are allowed to copy forward from a previous entry by another person, an attribution statement referring to the original document, date, and author should be attached or incorporated where applicable.

- Cutting, copying, and pasting must not be perceived as "OK unless proven otherwise" but instead should be considered "not OK until proven otherwise."

- Each potential function must be evaluated for policy or procedure acceptance or rejection by a practice.

- In some settings, copy and paste may be acceptable for legal record purposes but not for others (clinical trials data, quality assurance data, pay-for-performance data).

- In the hybrid environment, audit tracking of copy and paste may not be available because it involves different systems.

- In some contexts, it is never legitimate, including settings where the actual function takes personal health information outside the security environment.

- Some systems have an intermediate step allowing information to be brought forward but require another validation step.

- As a mitigation step, boilerplate text or libraries may be devised to describe common or routine information as agreed upon by the organizational standards.

Linking Each Patient to a Record

Every page in the health record or computerized record screen must identify patients by name and health record number. Patient name and number must be on both sides of every page as well as on every form and computerized printout. Paper and computer-generated forms with multiple pages must have the patient name and number on all pages.

EHRs. Each data field in the health record must be linked to the patient's name and health record number. Patient name and number must be on every page of printed, viewed, or otherwise transmitted information. The system in use must have a means of authenticating information reported from other systems.

Referencing another patient in the paper record. If it is necessary to refer to another patient to describe an event, the patient's name should not be used—the record number should be referenced in its place.

Timeliness and Chronology of Entries

Timeliness of an entry is critical to the admissibility of a health record in court as required by the Uniform Rules of Evidence. Entries should be made as soon as possible after an event or observation is made. An entry shall never be made in advance. If it is necessary to summarize events that occurred over a period of time (such as a shift), the notation shall indicate the actual time the entry was made with the narrative documentation identifying the time events occurred, if time is pertinent to the situation.

Timeliness of an entry presumes that the medium to which the entry is made is accessible. The principle of availability has been recognized as also consistent with timeliness, with the understanding that an entry would be made as soon as the record or system is available.

EHRs. Facilities must define what constitutes the legal health record in their organizational policies. Procedures must be in place to define timeliness for each component of the EHR system where there are no real-time automated links between subsystems.

Chronology

The record must reflect the continuous chronology of the patient's healthcare. Tools should be provided for caregivers to view episode-based information. The chronology must be readily apparent in any given view. It is recommended that organizations have a facility-wide standard view. EHR systems should have the capability of producing an output that chronicles the individual's encounter.

Date and Time

Every entry in the health record must include a complete date (including month, day, and year) and a time. Time must be included in all types of narrative notes even if it may not seem important to the type of entry.

Charting time as a block (for example, 7 a.m.–3 p.m.) is not advised, especially for narrative notes. Narrative documentation should reflect the actual time the entry was made. For certain types of flow sheets, such as a treatment record, recording time as a block could be acceptable. For example, a treatment that can be delivered any time during a shift could have a block of time identified on the treatment record with staff signing that they delivered the treatment during that shift. For assessment forms where multiple individuals are completing sections, the date and time of completion should be indicated as well as who has completed each section. (Time is not required on standardized data sets such as the MDS and OASIS.)

EHR systems must have the ability to date- and time-stamp each entry as the entry is made. Every entry in the health record must have a system-generated date and time based on current date and time. Date and time stamps must be associated with the signature at the time the documentation is finalized. For businesses operating across time zones, the time zone must be included in the date and time stamp. The date and time of entry must be accessible by the reviewer. Systems must have the ability for the documenter to enter date and time of occurrence for late entries.

Imaged records. The same standards for paper records apply to imaged records. Additionally, all scanned documents must be date- and time-stamped with the date scanned.

Legibility and Display

All entries to the record should be legible. If an entry cannot be read, the author should rewrite the entry on the next available line; define what the entry is for, referring back to the original documentation; and legibly rewrite the entry. For example: "Clarified entry of [date]" and rewrite entry, date, and sign. The rewritten entry must be the same as the original. All entries to the record should be made in black ink to facilitate legible photocopying of records. Entries should not be made in pencil.

Labels should be procured from a specific vendor to ensure adhesiveness and should not be placed over documentation. Organizations should review written documents as detailed in the practice brief "Ensuring Legibility of Patient Records."[5]

EHRs. Graphic user interface display options should accommodate ergonomic needs of all users (for example, visual acuity). Critical results should not rely on color due to consideration for color-blind users. Asterisks or labels can be used as additional visual cues. Screen resolution should be adjustable for individual user preference. Imaged documents incorporated in the system should require a minimal number of clicks and keystrokes to open. Devices such as bar codes should be part of an organization's quality check protocol. If data are used in multiple organizational systems, legibility should be a shared quality check between applications. Free-text entries should be spellchecked to ensure the legibility requirement of ability to understand.

Imaged records. All entries to be scanned into the record should be made in black ink to facilitate legible reproduction of records. Entries should not be made in pencil. Paper records as well as corresponding microfilm should be retained for the period defined by facility policy.

Legibility of all records, including scanned records, should be included in an organization's quality control processes.

Computer screens must be of sufficient size and resolution to display information appropriate for the intended use and intended users. Displays must support viewing information in its entirety without scrolling. PACS images, especially scanned documents, require close attention to display support of required legibility.

Corrections, Errors, Amendments, and Other Documentation Problems

There will be times when documentation problems or mistakes occur, and changes or clarifications will be necessary. Proper procedures must be followed in handling these situations. ASTM and HL7 have standards that apply to error correction.

Error Correction Process

When an error is made in a health record entry, proper error correction procedures must be followed:

- Draw a line through the entry. Make sure that the inaccurate information is still legible.

- Write "error" by the incorrect entry and state the reason for the error in the margin or above the note if room.

- Sign and date the entry.

- Document the correct information. If the error is in a narrative note, it may be necessary to enter the correct information on the next available line, documenting the current date and time and referring back to the incorrect entry.

Do not obliterate or otherwise alter the original entry by blacking out with marker, using whiteout, or writing over an entry.

EHRs. Correcting an error in an electronic or computerized health record system should follow the same basic principles. The system must have the ability to track corrections or changes to the entry once the entry has been entered or authenticated. When correcting or making a change to an entry in a computerized health record system, the original entry should be viewable, the current date and time should be entered, the person making the change should be identified, and the reason should be noted. In situations where a hard copy is printed from the EHR, the hard copy must also be corrected.

Every entry should be date-, time-, and author-stamped by the system. A symbol that indicates a new or additional entry that has resulted in an additional version should be viewable. It must be clear to the user that there are additional versions of the data being viewed. A preferred method is to apply a strikethrough for the error with commentary and date-, time-, and author-stamp or equivalent functionality to retain original versions linked to the corrected version.

Hybrid records. Organizational policy must define how errors are corrected in imaged documents while preserving in a readable form the original document or image. The practice brief "Electronic Document Management as a Component of the Electronic Health Record" provides guidelines for retraction, resequencing, and reassignment:

- **Retraction** involves removing a document for standard view, removing it from one record, and posting it to another within the electronic document management system. In the record from which the document was removed, the document would not be considered part of the designated record set or visible to anyone. Someone should be designated by the organization to view or print the retracted documents. An annotation should be viewable to the clinical staff so that the retracted document can be consulted if needed.

- **Resequencing** involves moving a document from one place to another within the same episode of care. No annotation of this action is necessary.

- **Reassignment** (synonymous with misfiles) involves moving the document from one episode of care to a different episode of care within the same patient record. As with retractions, someone in the organization should be designated to view or print the reassigned document. An annotation should be viewable to the clinical staff so that the reassigned document can be consulted if needed.[6]

Late Entry

When a pertinent entry was missed or not written in a timely manner, a late entry should be used to record the information in the health record.

- Identify the new entry as "late entry."

- Enter the current date and time. Do not try to give the appearance that the entry was made on a previous date or time.

- Identify or refer to the date and incident for which the late entry is written.

- If the late entry is used to document an omission, validate the source of additional information as much as possible (for example, where you obtained the information to write the late entry).

- When using late entries, document as soon as possible. There is no time limit to writing a late entry; however, the more time that passes, the less reliable the entry becomes.

Amendments

An addendum is another type of late entry that is used to provide additional information in conjunction with a previous entry. With this type of correction, a previous note has been made and the addendum provides additional information to address a specific situation or incident. When making an addendum:

- Document the current date and time.

- Write "addendum" and state the reason for the addendum referring back to the original entry.

- Identify any sources of information used to support the addendum.

- When writing an addendum, complete it as soon after the original note as possible.

- In an electronic system it is recommended that organizations have a link to the original entry or a symbol by the original entry to indicate the amendment. ASTM and HL7 have standards related to amendments.

Healthcare organizations should have policies to address how a patient or his or her representative can enter amendments into the record. The HIPAA privacy rule requires specific procedures and time frames be followed for processing an amendment. A separate entry (progress note, form, typed letter) can be used for patient amendment documentation. The amendment should refer back to the information questioned, date, and time. The amendment should document the information believed to be inaccurate and the information the patient or legal representative believes to be correct. The entry in question should be flagged to indicate a related amendment or correction (in both a paper and electronic system). At no time should the documentation in question be removed from the chart or obliterated in any way. The patient cannot require that the records be removed or deleted.

Version Management

An organization must address management of document versions. Once documentation has been made available for patient care, it must be retained and managed regardless of whether the document was authenticated (if authentication applies). Organizations must decide whether all versions of a document will be displayed or just the final, who has access to the various versions of a document, and how the availability of versions will be flagged in the health record.

It is acceptable for a draft of a dictated and transcribed note or report to be changed before authentication unless there is a reason to believe the changes are suspect and would not reflect actual events or actions. Facility policy should define the acceptable period of time allowed for a document to remain in draft form before the author reviews and approves it (for example, 24 to 72 hours). Once a document is no longer considered a draft or has been authenticated, any changes or alterations should be made following the procedures for a late entry or amendment. The original document must be maintained along with the new revised document.

Chart Content

Organizations must define the content of their legal health records based on regulations and standards of practice. This step is critical in determining the information disclosed upon request that documents clinical encounters and the documentation that must be retained and protected for required periods of time. The practice brief "Update: Guidelines for Defining the Legal Health Record for Disclosure Purposes" provides information on determining the health record content.[7] The following topics address unique content issues.

Decision Support

Decision support, including system-generated notifications, prompts, and alerts, should be evidence-based, validated, and accepted by the organization. The patient health record should include documentation of the clinician's actions in response to decision support. This documentation is evidence of the clinician's decision to follow or disregard decision support. The organization should define the extent of exception documentation required (for example, what no documentation means).

Notification and Communication with Patients or Family

If notification of the patient's physician or family is required or a discussion with the patient's family occurs regarding care of the patient, all such communications (including attempts at notification) should be documented. Include the time and method of all communications or attempts. The entry should include any orders received or responses, the implementation of such orders, and the patient's response. Messages left on answering machines should be limited to a request to return the call and are not considered a valid form of notification. An organization should determine whether copies of letters to patients are retained as part of the legal patient record, if they should be disclosed to others, and their retention period.

Informed Consent

Informed consent entries include explanation of the risks and benefits of a treatment or procedure, alternatives to the treatment or procedure, and evidence that the patient or appropriate legal surrogate understands and consents to undergo the treatment or procedure. This type of information should be carefully documented. Laws, regulations, and organization policy define the format of informed consent (for example, it must it be a distinct form or a documented discussion).

EHRs. With electronic consent, the patient views the consent and electronically signs it. An organization should verify that the electronic signature or authentication protocol meets all legal and regulatory requirements. The informed consent shall contain enough information for the patient to clearly choose various options of care and treatment during the episode of care. The informed consent should not allow for any "striking out" or deleting, but rather a document that provides for standard inclusions or exclusions.

Imaged records. With regard to imaging, regulations, laws, or organization policies should define whether the original paper form or the patient's original ink signature should be retained, the retention period, and the retrieval expectation. Policy should define if the legal medical record and a legal signature include a scanned image of the document or signature. Storage and retention should be consistent with the organization's policy for all other contents of the legal patient record.

Managing Data from Other Facilities or the Patient

Clinical information received from other facilities or from the patient should be evaluated by the clinician. The organization's policy should define whether the data in its entirety or just the data abstracted and transferred by the clinician is incorporated into the patient's health record. The source of the clinical data should be documented.

EHRs. If medical images are received from outside healthcare organizations or the patient, the images may be uploaded into the core clinical system. Retain attribution detail of source organization, author, and date.

Hybrid records. Organizations should define the procedure for the transfer of clinical information received on CD or DVD into the hybrid record. Options may include print to paper then image or upload into EHR or interface with the hybrid record. It must be determined whether laws, regulations, or organization policy require retention of the original media or a photocopy.

Customized Clinical Views

If the EHR system can provide customized clinical views, the organization should determine who is authorized to create and maintain the customized views. When clinical data are pulled into a customized view and used for clinical decision making, the logic or programming should be retained and made retrievable by the organization. The organization is encouraged to retain the methods and logic of customized clinical views; however, the system logic is not considered part of the legal health record.

Templates, Boilerplates, Canned Text

Care must be taken that these methods support clinical care and accurate documentation and are not used simply to expedite the process. Creation and periodic review of these tools should be based on clinically appropriate, standards-based protocols for common or routine information. Documentation by this method should require an active choice in response to the interaction between the patient and provider. When a clinician reviews and authenticates, the author is indicating he or she reviewed and completed the documentation and accepted the accuracy as his or her own.

Flow Sheets

Organization policy should establish form design and documentation standards, including frequency of documentation. All entries are date, time, and author stamped. The policy should define the frequency and standard time frame for documentation of clinical observations and assessments. On paper, if initials identify author only, a full signature should be elsewhere on the form for easy reference.

EHRs. Organization policy should outline the frequency of data entry or capture and standard intervals for display of information (for example, exact time, every five seconds, every 10 minutes, every 30 minutes, every hour). Policy should define the frequency of data captured directly from clinical monitoring systems, machine to machine (for example, continuous, every five seconds, every 15 minutes). All data are date and time stamped with the author noted. The standard frequency for view or print of archived flow sheet data should be defined. The system should provide views of archived data by date, time, author, or data field.

Output Format

Organization policy should determine whether the record must be complete before output is generated and who has the authority to generate output from the EHR. The EHR system must have the capability of providing a chronological record of the patient's encounter. When the EHR output is generated for disclosure, the organization must define the standardized forms, formats, and order based on user needs (for example, different views, formats, and order for lawyers, insurance companies, patients, or healthcare providers). Organizations must also decide what versions of documents will be provided.

The organization should define a standard technology for output according to the information system capability, privacy and security standards, and user need and capability to use the format chosen.

Printing Guidelines

The organization must define the standard form and format of the paper health record and identify who can reproduce paper documents for internal or external disclosure. The organization must also define the scope and reasons for printing paper internally. Printing can be a legal challenge if clinicians print from the EHR and then document on the printouts rather than in the system. Strict control of printing policies should be in place.

EHRs. Organizations must decide if they will reproduce the EHR in paper format. If printing from the EHR system is allowed, organization policies should define who has the authority to print and under what circumstances. Printing should be tracked in the audit trail, and information on user and location should be available if needed. Policies should also define the form and format of documents that print from the EHR. For example, is it a screen print of the clinician view or a form that mimics the traditional paper record forms? What interval of time is printed as a standard—by encounter, date ranges, any point in time, or at discharge?

Organizations must decide which version is printed—only the most current version of a document or other versions as well. If other versions are printed, determine under what circumstances previous archived versions are printed. Organizations must decide whether to print the traditional final lab results report versus all the preliminary results and whether lab result trends are printed. When separate covered entities share a clinical data repository and use shared information for clinical decision making, the organization should define what information from the repository can be printed. An organization should also determine if preliminary, unauthenticated reports can be printed and under what circumstances.

Permanency

All entries in the health record, regardless of form or format, must be permanent (manual or computerized records). The Rules of Evidence require that policies and procedures be in place to prevent alteration, tampering, or loss. The organization must consider the issue of permanency of records in its records management policies. In a paper system, permanency is affected by life span of the actual paper or microfilm that health information is recorded on. Retention policies and schedules developed by the organization determine the permanency of the information.

EHRs. The organization must consider the issue of permanency of records in its electronic records management policies. In an electronic system, permanency is affected by the digital nature of data, which may be more readily subject to change or technology obsolescence than is information recorded on paper. This includes changes to the actual data itself or changes that occur over time in data formats and storage devices. Use of standard file formats and clinical nomenclatures may facilitate data conversion as technology changes and are a major consideration for permanency. Procedures to protect against data degradation and loss of integrity during system conversions must be addressed.

Other Permanency Issues

Ink color. For hard-copy paper records, blue or black ink is preferred to ensure readability when records are copied. The ink should be permanent (no erasable or water-soluble ink should be used). Never use a pencil to document in the health record. Black ink is preferred for records that will be imaged.

Printer. When documentation is printed from a computer for entry in the health record or retention as the permanent record, the print must be permanent. For example, a laser printer should be used rather than an ink-jet printer, because the latter ink is water soluble.

Fax copies. When fax records are maintained in the health record, assurance must be made that the record will maintain its integrity over time. For example, if thermal paper is used, a copy must be made for filing in the health record because the print on thermal paper fades over time. (See section on fax signatures for admissibility as evidence.)

Photocopies. The health record should contain original documents whenever possible. There are times when it is acceptable to have copies of records and signatures, particularly when records are sent from another provider.

Carbon copy paper. If there is a question about the permanency of the paper (for example, NCR or carbon paper), a photocopy should be made. Policy should indicate when items are copied and how the original is disposed. At times, carbon copies of documents may be used on a temporary basis and the original will replace the carbon.

Use of labels. Labels and label paper (adhesive-backed paper) are used for a variety of reasons, including patient demographics, transcription of dictated progress notes, printing of physician orders for telephone orders, medication, or treatment records. When labels are used in the record, a number of issues or concerns must be considered and addressed before implementation. Organization policies and practices should address how and where labels will be placed. Information may not be obscured by the label, and the adhesiveness of the label must be adequate for the retention period of the document.

Retention

Organizations must establish retention schedules for the content of the legal health record that comply with federal and state regulations and the needs for patient care, research, and administrative purposes (such as legal and compliance).

EHRs. Electronic storage media, such as magnetic and optical formats, must meet the organization's retention schedule and include retention of all types of data, including discrete data, text, audio, video, and images. Policies should address backup procedures to ensure retention and protect against data loss.

Organizations should also address retention of data and information that is associated with the EHR but which may not be strictly part of the EHR—items such as audit trails, alerts and reminders, and metadata associated with structured as well as unstructured data. This may be important in certifying the integrity of the information for risk management and legal purposes.

Retention policies should comply with accreditation standards and federal and state law and regulations. Information life cycle management should be built into EHR systems in the development phase. If an EHR crosses multiple disparate information systems, retention policies must be applied to each component. EHR systems must include a function or feature that allows for litigation holds that exempt specific records from the retention policy due to legal, compliance, or other business needs.

Imaged records. With imaged documents, an organization needs to decide how long to retain the paper after scanning. Considerations include provisions for quality assurance in the scanning process, the organization's definition of its legal record (paper, electronic, or both), and the frequency and timing of backups of the scanned images.

Other considerations in retention of paper may include state regulations, requirements of the organization's malpractice risk carrier, and in the case of organizations that conduct research, FDA regulations. When paper is retained after scanning, there must be an established cataloging and indexing method so that it can be retrieved. Schedules or guidelines for conversion of document images from magnetic to optical storage should be addressed.

Depending on the organization's need for longevity of scanned images, it may also wish to consider converting scanned images to microfilm for longer retention periods. Occupational health records, for example, must be retained for 30 years.

Storage

An organization must store health records in a way that prevents loss, destruction, or unauthorized use. Traditional methods for storing paper records include open-space shelving for active files and off-site box storage for archived records.

EHRs. Organizations must ensure that EHR systems provide basic database storage standards, including appropriate security measures. Major considerations include how to store information in order to convey it to an external user in an acceptable medium and the volume of records to be stored (for example, what types must be included).

Obsolescence of Technology

Stored records must be accessible for the length of the retention period regardless of the technology used. When records are stored as microfilm and microfiche, an organization must retain hardware to access or reproduce the records for the length of the retention period.

EHRs. Organizations require a plan to access or reproduce EHR data. As technology changes, consideration must include backwards compatibility or some type of access to previous systems from the new or upgraded system.

Purging and Destruction

Records should be purged and destroyed in a consistent manner based on an established retention schedule, plan, and procedure. Destruction is acceptable unless there is a concern that certain records or documents were selected for destruction. When this happens, behavior is considered suspect, and it can appear that information that was harmful to the organization was destroyed. Plans should include method of destruction (for example, shredding, burning) and should consider security of the destruction process.

EHRs. The organization should have a plan for destruction of storage media, including hard drives and portable media such as diskettes and USB drives. Consideration should be given to determining if an EHR system can indicate records to be purged based on the organization's policy. The organization should have a policy that defines purging versus archiving and how the system will support the policy.

Data Integrity: Access, Audit Trail, and Security

Integrity is defined as the accuracy, consistency, and reliability of information content, processes, and systems. Information integrity is the dependability or trustworthiness of information, which is an important concept in a legal proceeding. Integrity of the health record is maintained through access, network security, audit trail, security, and disaster recovery processes.

To protect the integrity of the paper legal health record, organizations should define the policy and procedures regarding the content and reconciliation processes to ensure accuracy and completeness of the health record.

EHRs. To protect the integrity of the electronic legal health record, policies and procedures must be in place:

- Regarding the reconciliation of electronic processes (such as process for checking individual data elements, reports, files)

- To assess potential data corruption, data mismatches, and extraneous data

- Regarding managing different iterations of documents (version control), with clear indication of when each version is viewable by caregivers for use in making clinical decisions

- To define when the record is complete and permanently filed (locking the record with view-only access), including temporary locking of high-risk charts by certain users

- Regarding downtime processes and ability to capture data following downtime through direct entry or scanning

Performance criteria and functionality should define and minimize the intrinsic risks by appropriate design, deployment, development, and detection of the EHR. Performance criteria and functionality should also define and minimize the extrinsic risks by appropriate test conversion planning, testing and data validation, and minimization of system downtime.

Access Control

Access control is the process that determines who is authorized to access patient information in the health record. Controlling access is an important aspect of maintaining the legal integrity of the health record. In the paper world this is controlled through physical security safeguards, chart tracking, and outguide systems.

EHRs. Access control and validation procedures must be in place to validate a person's access to the system based on role or function. Access should be terminated automatically after a predetermined period of inactivity. Organizations must also define access to information for emergency situations (break-the-glass access). Policies must address facility access controls to meet the HIPAA security rule.

Audit Trail

An audit trail is a business record of all transactions and activities, including access, associated with the medical record. Elements of an audit trail may include date, time, nature of the transaction or activity, and the individual or automated system linked to the transaction or activity. Transactions may include additions or edits to the medical record. Activities may include access to view or read, filing, and data mining. Audit trail functionality is important to support the legal integrity of the record. The purpose of an audit trail is to create a system control to establish accountability for transactions and activities as well as compliance with facility policies, procedures, and protocols related to medical record access and maintenance.

For the paper medical record, an audit trail may include a sign-out sheet, a manual or electronic chart tracking system (such as flagging devices or software), or a log book.

EHRs. Audit trails are critical legal functionality for EHR systems because they record key information on data creation, access, and revision. An audit trail may be one of the following types of business records:

- Electronic file of transactions and activities (data creation, access, revision, along with date and time)

- Hard-copy report of transactions and activities

- Batch file processing report

- Information system data transmission or interface report

- Exception report of unauthorized access attempts

Special Considerations for an EHR Audit Trail

Teaching environment—academic medical centers. The high turnover of students, interns, and residents in an academic facility or a specific clinical department may necessitate the need to maintain a large file of unique EHR access codes or requirements. Timely activation and deactivation of identification and authentication tools may affect the reliability of audit trail data and must be addressed by organization policies to prevent negative impact on legal integrity of the record.

Health systems—mergers, acquisitions, and divestitures. Physicians and other clinicians who provide direct patient care at multiple locations or facility management and staff who work at other institutions may have more than one EHR access code or level of access when facilities merge or acquire other patient care sites with similar EHR software.

EHR Audit Trail Performance Criteria and Functionalities

- Make sure audit trail functionality is turned on in EHR applications.

- Include date and time stamps on all transactions.

- Do not allow back-door access by a staff member (such as the system administrator) to make alterations in the EHR without an audit trail record. If back-door access is possible, have the software vendor fix the problem to ensure that the EHR retains integrity in a legal proceeding.

Network Security

Electronic network security protects EHR data from unauthorized internal or remote access or illegitimate internal or remote transactions. The purpose of an electronic network security protocol is to preserve the integrity of EHR data and to protect patient privacy, consistent with facility and regulatory requirement, as well as accreditation standards. Electronic network security protocols must address the following access mechanisms:

- Remote access through a virtual private network

- Remote access through a local area network

- Remote access through a wireless network

- Remote access through a workstation

- Internal access through a workstation

Disaster Recovery and Business Continuity

An important aspect of maintaining a legally sound health record is securing the record to prevent loss, tampering, or unauthorized use. Rules of evidence require an organization to have policies and procedures in place to protect against alterations, tampering, and loss. Systems and procedures should also be in place to prevent loss (such as tracking and sign-out procedures), establish secure record storage areas or systems, and limit access to only authorized users.

Organizations should develop and implement controls to safeguard data and information, including the clinical record, against loss, destruction, and tampering. Organizations should:

- Develop and implement policies when removal of records is permitted

- Protect data and information against unauthorized intrusion, corruption, or damage

- Prevent falsification of data and information

- Develop and implement guidelines to prevent the destruction of records

- Develop and implement guidelines for destroying copies of records

- Protect records in a manner that minimizes the possibility of damage from fire and water

EHRs. Establish (and implement as needed) policies and procedures for responding to an emergency such as a fire, vandalism, system failure, or a natural disaster that damages systems containing electronic protected health information. Organizations must address and develop the following to adequately prepare for a disaster and prevent loss or destruction of information:

- Data backup plan

- Disaster recovery plan

- Emergency mode operation plan

- Testing and revision procedures

- Applications and data criticality analysis

Business Continuity

Disaster recovery planning includes information and plans on how operations are to continue in the event of a disaster. If a department, business unit, or system is unavailable, a plan must be in place to continue operations. To develop a plan, consider the following:

- List all departments that are directly or indirectly affected by extended system downtime

- List all daily procedures that must be followed to maintain acceptable levels of operations

- List actions (manual procedures) completed during downtimes for each department

- Expand the process to plan for the system if it were unavailable for an extended period of time

- Outline specific steps to integrate backlogged data maintained during the downtime

- List additional procedures to be followed after recovery activities are complete

Conclusion

Maintaining a legally sound health record covers a vast territory from the content of the health record and how entries are recorded to the functionality in the system to access, audit trails, and security. While the electronic age brings new variables to an old and complex problem, the foundation remains the same: health records must be maintained in a manner that follows applicable regulations, accreditation standards, professional practice standards, and legal standards. HIM professionals play a critical role in the transition from paper to electronic records and must partner with clinical, legal, and information technology to adequately address the legal business issues for the health record.

References

AHIMA. 1998. *Health Information Management Practice Standards: Tools for Assessing Your Organization.* Chicago: AHIMA.

AHIMA. 2003. E-mail as a Provider-Patient Electronic Communication Medium and Its Impact on the Electronic Health Record. FORE Library: HIM Body of Knowledge. http://www.ahima.org.

AHIMA. 2003. Implementing Electronic Signatures. FORE Library: HIM Body of Knowledge. http://www.ahima.org.

AHIMA. 2004. The strategic importance of electronic health records management. *Journal of AHIMA* 75. (9) : 80A–B.

Amatayakul, Margret. 2005. Access controls: striking the right balance. *Journal of AHIMA* 76(1): 56–57.

Anderson, Ellen Miller. 2004. Online clinical documentation in the electronic legal medical record. 2004 IFHRO Congress and AHIMA Convention Proceedings. FORE Library: HIM Body of Knowledge. http://www.ahima.org.

ASTM. 2000. *Annual Book of ASTM Standards.* Volume 14.01, Healthcare Informatics, Section 8, Signature Attributes. West Conshohocken, PA: ASTM.

Centers for Medicare and Medicaid Services. 2011. Interpretive guidelines for hospitals. http://www .cms.gov/manuals/1Downloads/som107ap_a_hospitals.pdf.

Dougherty, Michelle. 2002. Maintaining a legally sound health record. *Journal of AHIMA* 73(8): 64A–G.

Fox, Leslie, and Walter Imbiorski. 1994. *The Record That Defends Its Friends,* 6th ed. Chicago: Care Communications.

Center for Medicare and Medicaid Services (CMS). 2003. Health Insurance Reform: Security Standards; Final Rule. 45 CFR Parts 160, 162, and 164. *Federal Register* 68(34). http://www.cms.hhs.gov/hipaa/hipaa2/regulations/security/03-3877.pdf.

Health Level Seven. 1997. Sections 9.4.5-9.4.11, 9.5.5–9.5.10.

Hirsh, Harold L. 1978. Will your medical records get you into trouble?" *Legal Aspects of Medical Practice* 6 (9): 46–51.

Huffman, Edna K. 1994. *Health Information Management,* 10th ed. Berwyn, IL: Physicians' Record Co.

Joint Commission on Accreditation of Healthcare Organizations. 2005. *Comprehensive Accreditation Manual for Hospitals,* Update 3. Oakbrook Terrace, IL: Joint Commission.

Murer, Cherilyn G., Michael A. Murer, and Lyndean Lenhoff Brick. 2000. *The Complete Legal Guide to Healthcare Records Management.* Washington, DC: Healthcare Financial Management Association.

National Institute of Standards and Technology. 2004. Security Considerations in Information System Development Life Cycle. http://csrc.nist.gov/publications/nistpubs.

Quinsey, Carol Ann. 2004. A HIPAA security overview. *Journal of AHIMA* 75 (4): 56A–C.

Roach, William H. Jr., and the Aspen Health Law and Compliance Center. 1998. *Medical Records and the Law,* 3rd ed. Chicago: Aspen Publishers.

Rollins, Gina. 2005. The prompt, the alert, and the legal record: documenting clinical decision support systems. *Journal of AHIMA* 76 (2): 24–28.

Scott, Ronald W. 1994. *Legal Aspects of Documenting Patient Care.* Annville, PA: Aspen Publishers.

Center for Medicare and Medicaid Services (CMS). 2000. Standards for Privacy of Individually Identifiable Health Information; Final Rule. 45 CFR Parts 160 and 164. *Federal Register* 65(250). http://www.hhs.gov/ocr/hipaa/finalreg.html.

Waller, Adele, and Oscar Alcantara. 1998. Ownership of health information in the information age. *Journal of AHIMA* 69 (3): 28–38.

Chapter 4

Documentation for Statistical Reporting and Public Health

Cheryl Gregg Fahrenholz, RHIA, CCS-P

Learning Objectives

- Study how statistics are used in healthcare

- Distinguish between primary and secondary data

- Compare and contrast patient-identifiable data with aggregate data

- Relate how health record data are used for research and statistics

- Define healthcare databases in terms of purpose and content

- Explain the use of health record data in clinical trials

- Identify the role of health record documentation in public health reporting

- Define vital statistics

- Trace the flow of information in reporting vital statistics

- Identify data quality issues to yield statistical information for administrative and clinical decisions

- Describe the role and content of a master patient index

- Recognize secondary data sources

- Identify facility-specific indexes

- List routine healthcare databases

- Identify data elements in standardized clinical data sets

Key Terms

Agency for Healthcare Research and Quality (AHRQ)

Aggregate data

American National Standards Institute (ANSI)

Census

Centers for Disease Control and Prevention (CDC)

Clinical trial

Consolidated Health Informatics (CHI)

Initiatives

Data dictionary

Data sets

Database

Department of Health and Human Services (HHS)

Disease index

Enterprise master patient index (EMPI)

Facility-specific index

Facility-specific registry

Food and Drug Administration (FDA)

Health services research

Healthcare information standards

Incidence

Index

Master patient index (MPI)

National Alliance for Health Information Technology (NAHIT)

National Center for Health Statistics (NCHS)

National Committee on Vital and Health Statistics (NCVHS)

National Practitioner Data Bank (NPDB)

Office of the National Coordinator for Health Information Technology (ONC)

Operation index

Patient-specific/identifiable data

Physician index

Population-based registry

Prevalence

Primary data

Primary data source

Protocol

Public health

Registry

Research

Secondary data

Secondary data source

Vital statistics

Introduction

The primary purpose of healthcare documentation is to chronicle patients' health over time. Although this benefits consumers by ensuring the continuity of their care, the information compiled from healthcare documentation can also reveal trends and contribute to improving healthcare for consumers of all ages. Health record documentation is the source data for statistical reports that guide decisions in local facilities. These decisions can influence the health of a state and even a nation. This chapter provides information on facility-specific, state, and national indexes, registries, and **databases**.

Research and Statistics

Data contained in the health record are required for **research**, statistical reporting, cancer registries, trauma registries, burn registries, disease registries, implant registries, and birth certificate registration, to name a few public health uses. Documentation from disease-specific registries may be utilized with incentive payment systems that are based on the quality of care provided to patients. Documentation needed for research ranges from identification of candidate health records for projects to actual review of selected records and abstract preparation or collection of data from them for physicians or clinical researchers.

Providing research assistance to clinicians and medical staff committees is a health infomation management (HIM) department function. Aggregate statistical data are also useful for clinical and administrative decision support. **Indexes** are used to sort data to assist with the study of certain data elements. HIM departments also collect and calculate various statistics about the operations of the healthcare facilities and clinical practices they serve. Many of these statistics are provided electronically; however, the HIM department provides quality control to ensure the accuracy of calculations and statistical reports.

An HIM professional may be called upon to provide information for a clinical trial. A **clinical trial** is an investigation of the safety and effectiveness of new treatments and tests. The trial proceeds according to a **protocol**, which is the list of rules and procedures to be followed. The **Food and Drug Administration (FDA)** Modernization Act of 1997 mandated the development of a clinical trials database, which enables patients and practitioners to determine which clinical trials are available and applicable. The National Library of Medicine has developed the database, called Clinical Trials, for use by both consumers and practitioners. Information in the database includes the following (Bowman 2010, 502–504):

- Study identification number
- Study sponsor
- Brief title
- Brief summary
- Location of trial
- Recruitment status
- Contact information
- Eligibility criteria
- Study type
- Study design
- Study phase
- Condition
- Intervention
- Data provider
- Date last modified

Public Health Reporting

The health of populations in geopolitical locations is the domain of **public health**. One of the duties of public health agencies is surveillance of the health status of the population within their jurisdictions.

Centers for Disease Control and Prevention WONDER Database

The **Centers for Disease Control and Prevention (CDC)** WONDER database is an integrated information and communication system for public health. Its purposes are twofold (CDC 2010):

1. To promote information-driven decision making by placing timely, useful facts in the hands of public health practitioners and researchers

2. To provide the general public with access to specific and detailed information from the CDC

CDC WONDER furthers the CDC's mission of health promotion and disease prevention by expediting and simplifying access to public health information for state and local health departments, the US Public Health Service, and the academic public health community. The database is valuable in public health research, decision making, priority setting, program evaluation, and resource allocation. It also offers an online database query function that allows users to select specific data sets within a variety of specific diseases to compile ad hoc reports for the analysis of public health data (CDC 2010).

Collection and calculation of various healthcare statistics also depend on the health record. Statistics, including ratios and percentages (for example, percentage of occupancy, death and autopsy rates; hospital **census** reports) are needed to describe the operation of a healthcare facility. Integrated computer information systems generate many of these types of statistics automatically. However, data entry and other errors often produce inaccurate findings, so the HIM department is typically responsible for verifying the accuracy of such statistics.

National Center for Health Statistics

The **National Center for Health Statistics (NCHS)** compiles statistical information to guide actions and policies to improve health. NCHS (2011) uses health statistics to

- Document the health status of the population and of important subgroups

- Identify disparities in health status and use of healthcare by race or ethnicity, socioeconomic status, region, and other population characteristics

- Describe people's experiences with the healthcare system

- Monitor trends in health status and healthcare delivery

- Identify health problems

- Support biomedical and health services research

- Provide information for making changes in public policies and programs

- Evaluate the impact of health policies and programs

NCHS collaborates with the health community and uses a variety of approaches to obtain information. Data are collected from birth and death records, health records, and interview surveys, and through direct physical exams and laboratory testing. NCHS monitors the national public health infrastructure and provides information to identify and address critical health problems (NCHS 2011).

Health record documentation is required to develop the databases used by public health departments to provide information on the **incidence** and **prevalence** of diseases, possible high-risk populations, survival statistics, and trends over time. Data may be collected using interviews, physical examinations of individuals, or review of health records, among other methods. An HIM manager may have input in these databases through information from health records (Bowman 2010, 500).

Department of Health and Human Services Data Council

The **Department of Health and Human Services (HHS)** established its Data Council to coordinate and integrate its data collection and analysis activities. HHS has taken steps to address key data needs, promote a coordinated organization-wide strategy on data issues, and strengthen collaboration with private-sector entities, state and local governments, and other partners (HHS 2009). The Data Council also supports HHS-wide implementation of the Health Insurance Portability and Accountability Act (HIPAA) Administrative Simplification, an initiative to adopt national standards for electronic healthcare transactions.

The Data Council assists in decision making, analysis, and dissemination of information within HHS as well as to public- and private-sector entities with common data interests. In addition, HHS is a national leader in health and human services information policy, including national data standards, privacy policy, and national health information infrastructure issues (HHS 2009).

The National Health Care Survey

The National Health Care Survey is one of the major national public health surveys. It relies on data from patients' health records and includes information on several practice areas. (See **TABLE 4.1**.)

TABLE 4.1. Databases included in the national health care survey

DATABASE	TYPE OF SETTING	CONTENT	DATA SOURCE	METHOD OF DATA COLLECTION
National Ambulatory Medical Care Survey	Office-based physician practice	Data on the patient and the visit	State discharge databases Office-based physician records	Abstract
National Nursing Home Survey	Nursing home	Data on the facility, current and discharged residents	Administrator Nurse caregiver	Interview
National Hospital Ambulatory Medical Care Survey	Hospital emergency departments and outpatient clinics	Data on the patient, the visit, and the method of payment	Emergency department and outpatient clinic records	Abstract
National Home and Hospice Care Survey	Home health and hospice	Facility data and patient data	Administrator Caregiver	Interview
National Electronic Disease Surveillance System (NEDSS)	Public health departments	Possible bioterrorism incidents	Local and state public health departments	Electronic surveillance

Source: Bowman 2010, 339.

Vital Statistics

Vital statistics include data on births, deaths, fetal deaths, marriages, and divorce. Responsibility for the collection of vital statistics rests with the states, which serve as the official repository for birth and death certificates and share information with the NCHS. From the vital statistics collected, states and the national government develop a variety of databases (Bowman 2010, 502). For example, one national database links birth certificates and death certificates for infants who die before reaching age one. Such information is useful in analyzing patterns of infant deaths.

The **National Committee on Vital and Health Statistics (NCVHS)**, formed in 1949, helps connect the interests of the US government, the health industry, and research and public health entities and helps connect to those working on health information policy in other countries (Kanaan 2000). The mission of the NCVHS is to advise the federal government on the information needs underlying health policy. It designs and coordinates improvements in national and international vital and health statistics.

Facility-Specific Indexes

Healthcare facilities establish **facility-specific indexes** to meet their individual, specific needs for customer care or other reporting requirements. These indexes make it possible to retrieve health records in a variety of ways, including by disease, physician, or operation. Prior to computerization, these indexes were kept on cards. Today, most are compiled from databases routinely developed by the facility or with the assistance of electronic health records (EHRs) at facilities that use such technology.

Master Patient Index

The **master patient index (MPI)** is a database of patients within a facility or associated group of facilities (enterprise). The MPI, whether in paper or electronic format, may be considered the most important resource in a healthcare facility because it tracks patient activity across every type of care setting. The MPI identifies all patients who have been treated in a facility or enterprise and lists the health records or identification numbers associated with the names. An index can be maintained manually or as part of a computerized system. Retention of entries depends on the MPI's use. Typically, entries for healthcare facilities are retained permanently, while those for insurers, registries, or others may have different retention periods.

Data Elements

Data elements included in the MPI should

- Accurately match patients being registered for care with their MPI records
- Minimize duplicate records within a facility and across all care settings
- Facilitate merging MPIs to create enterprise MPIs
- Facilitate access to longitudinal health records

Complying with these guidelines will speed access to patient information, resulting in significant benefits for customers and healthcare providers. To achieve this, AHIMA (2010) recommends that MPIs include the core data elements listed in appendix 4A.1. The need to identify patients across departments within a facility has lead to the development of the **enterprise master patient index (EMPI)**. The EMPI consolidates information from registration, scheduling, financial, and clinical software systems. EMPIs may also assist organizations in maintaining HIPAA patient identification and tracking requirements, as listed in **APPENDIX 4A.1**.

See **APPENDIX 4A** for AHIMA's practice brief on building an enterprise master person index.

Physician Index

The **physician index** categorizes patients by primary physician. It guides the retrieval of cases treated by a particular physician. This index is created simply by sorting patients by physician. Information required in a physician index includes the physician's name or code, health record number, diagnosis, operations, disposition of the patients the physician treated, dates of admission and discharge, and gender and age of patients (Cerrato and Roberts 2011, 452–53).

For example, a facility could retrieve all of Dr. Anderson's patients with melanoma and compare their treatment with Dr. Bradford's patients with the same diagnosis. The quantity and quality of care by a physician is considered in credentialing and assignment of privileges.

Disease and Operation Indexes

Disease and **operation indexes** allow the retrieval of patient information by diagnosis or surgical procedure. The index is arranged by diagnostic or procedure codes, facilitating the study of patients with the same or similar conditions or treatment. This sorting guides the locating of health records to conduct quality improvement and research studies or to monitor quality of care. The index is also useful for retrieving records for research studies. The following data elements from the health record are essential for this index (Cerrato and Roberts 2011, 451–52):

- Principal diagnosis and relevant secondary diagnoses with codes
- Associated procedures and codes
- Patient's health record number
- Patient's gender, age, and race
- Attending physician's code or name
- The hospital service
- The end result of hospitalization
- Dates of encounter (including admission and discharge for inpatients)

Most facilities today have an automated index with predetermined data elements captured from the health records, which makes standard and special reports available

FIGURE 4.1. Registries maintained by healthcare facilities

Standard registries	Specialty registries
• Admissions	• Trauma
• Discharges	• Disease-specific (for example, cancer, AIDS, diabetes)
• Operating/surgical	• Birth defects
• Births	• Implants
• Deaths	• Transplants
• Physician	• Immunizations
	• Burn

from the information system. Frequently, the responsibility for entering the index data is assigned to the HIM department.

Registries

A **registry** is a chronological listing of patients with a common characteristic. Registries commonly maintained by healthcare facilities are listed in **FIGURE 4.1**. Creation and maintenance of these registries is often a responsibility of the HIM department.

Registries contain more extensive information than indexes. These reports are typically generated from a facility's existing database. Registries are also used for patient follow-up and aggregate studies.

Registry maintenance consists of the following activities:

- **Case definition**: Describing the patients that are to be included

- **Case finding**: Identifying patients to be included

- **Case abstracting**: Extracting the information to be included from health records

The **Agency for Healthcare Research and Quality (AHRQ)**, an agency within HHS, aims to improve the quality, safety, efficiency, and effectiveness of healthcare for all Americans. One of its functions is to support **health services research**. In 2010, AHRQ and CMS published a handbook to help providers set up registries. The handbook included recommendations for design and data source access and suggestions on ways to encourage participation in registries.

Healthcare Databases

Individual health records are a rich source of data about an individual patient. However, it is not easy to see trends in a population of patients by looking at individual records. To reveal patterns, data must be extracted from individual records and entered into databases. These data may be used in a **facility-specific** or **population-based registry** for research and improvement in customer care. In addition, they may be reported to the state and become part of state and federal databases used to inform health policy and improve healthcare. When a healthcare facility utilizes an EHR, data may be accessed simultaneously by multiple users for a variety of purposes, including databases (Bowman 2010, 480–81).

An HIM professional can perform various tasks in managing secondary records and databases, including setting up databases. This involves determining the content of the database and ensuring compliance with the laws, regulations, and accreditation standards that affect its content and use. All data elements included in the database or registry must be defined in a **data dictionary**. The HIM professional may oversee the completeness and accuracy of the data abstracted for inclusion in the database or registry (Bowman 2010, 481).

National Practitioner Data Bank (NPDB)

As mandated by the Health Care Quality Improvement Act of 1986 and codified at 45 CFR Part 60, the National Practitioner Data Bank (NPDB) provides a database of medical malpractice payments, adverse licensure actions, and certain professional review actions (such as denial of medical staff privileges) taken by healthcare entities such as hospitals against physicians, dentists, other healthcare providers, private accrediting organizations, and peer review organizations. Congress amended this law with the Omnibus Budget Reconciliation Act of 1990, Public Law 101-508, to include "any negative action or finding by such authority, organization, or entity regarding the practitioner or entity." This expansion of mandated reporting implementation is the responsibility of the Bureau of Health Professions, Health Resources and Services Administration, US HHS (NPDB 2011). There are monetary penalties for failure to report.

Since the law requires healthcare facilities to query the NPDB for privileging, credentialing, and recredentialing purposes, the NPDB provides data specific to an individual healthcare practitioner for these purposes. This is particularly helpful to healthcare facilities when a healthcare practitioner has lost his license to practice in one state and moves to another state to practice. Previously the healthcare facility would have been unaware of the action against the healthcare practitioner from the other state. Practitioner-specific information that may be found in the NPDB report includes information about the practitioner, the reporting entity, and the judgment or settlement (Bowman 2010, 498–99).

The NPDB also includes a public-use data file that does not include healthcare practitioner–specific information. These data are used for statistical analysis and come from Medical Malpractice Payment Reports, Adverse Action Reports, and Medicare and Medicaid exclusion actions. The public-use data files are sorted by individual provider type, organizations, federal agencies, state agencies, and health plans. Within each report type, the statistical analysis is further calculated with unique findings specific to each state (NPDB 2011).

Data Quality Issues

Indexes, registries, and databases are only helpful when the data they contain are accurate. Decisions concerning new treatment methods, healthcare policy, and physician credentialing and privileging are based on these databases. Incorrect data will likely result in serious errors in decision making (Bowman 2010, 508). Considerations for protecting the quality of data in indexes, registries, and databases are summarized in **TABLE 4.2**.

TABLE 4.2. Strategies to protect the quality of data in indexes, registries, and databases

DATA QUALITY ELEMENT	DESCRIPTION	METHOD TO ENSURE QUALITY
Validity	Accuracy of data	Incorporate edits
Reliability	Consistency of data	Have more than one person abstract data for the same case
Completeness	Avoidance of missing data	Look at a variety of sources; don't allow blanks
Timelines	Up-to-date data	Set targets for abstract completion

Source: Adapted from Bowman 2006, 421–23.

Primary and Secondary Data Sources

Data are categorized as either **primary** or **aggregate data**. The health record consists entirely of **patient-specific/identifiable data** or primary data. Aggregate data (also referred to as **secondary data**) includes compiled information on groups of people or patients that does not identify any particular patient.

The health record is considered a **primary data source** because it contains patient-specific data and information about a patient that has been documented by the professionals who provided care or services to that patient. Data taken from the health record and entered into registries and databases are considered a secondary data source (Bowman 2010, 481–82).

Secondary data sources provide information that is not readily available from individual health records. Data taken from health records and entered into disease-oriented databases can help researchers determine the effectiveness of alternative treatment methods and monitor outcomes. They can also quickly demonstrate survival rates at different stages of diseases. Types of secondary data sources are listed in **TABLE 4.3**.

A healthcare facility will have internal and external users of secondary data sources. External users include the CDC, NCHS, and NCVHS. Some diseases must be reported to the state department of health. See chapter 3 and figure 3.9 for additional information. Another external user is the federal government, which collects data from the states on vital events such as births and deaths (Bowman 2010, 482–83).

Standardized Clinical Data Sets

Data and information pertaining to individuals who use healthcare services are collected in virtually every setting where healthcare is delivered. These data elements usually describe specific characteristics of individual patients. In healthcare settings, data are stored in the individual's paper or electronic health record. The data elements in the health record are combined, analyzed, and interpreted by the patient's physician and other clinicians.

The original data sets developed to support uniform data collection are inadequate for an electronic environment, and many public and private organizations have been actively engaged in the process of developing **healthcare information standards** to support EHR development and information exchange. The **Consolidated Health Informatics (CHI) initiatives** and the efforts of the **Office of the National Coordinator of Health**

TABLE 4.3. Types of secondary data sources

FACILITY-SPECIFIC INDEXES	HEALTHCARE DATABASES
Master Patient Index (MPI) and **Enterprise Master Person Index** Alphabetic file	Disease registries (specific diagnoses)
Disease and **Operation Indexes** (arranged by code number)	Cancer registries (trends in cancer incidence)
Physician's Index (cases of a physician)	Trauma registries (injuries caused by external physical force)
	Birth defects registries (newborns with defects)
National, State, and County Public Health Databases	Diabetes registries (patient follow-up)
National Healthcare Survey	Implant registries (device tracking by **FDA**)
National Hospital Discharge Survey	Transplant registries (donor organs and recipients)
National Employer Health Insurance Survey	Immunization registries (required childhood immunizations)
National Health Provider Inventory	HIV/AIDS registries
National Ambulatory Medical Care Survey	Cardiac registries
National Nursing Home Survey	Burn registries (monitor outcomes)
National Hospital Ambulatory Medical Care Survey	**National and Administrative Databases**
National Home and Hospice Care Survey	Medicare Provider Analysis and Review File (MEDPAR)—acute care and skilled nursing facility claims data
	National Practitioner Database (NPDB) —medical malpractice payments and sanctions by boards of medical examiners
	Healthcare Integrity and Protection Data Bank (fraud and abuse information)
Other Databases	
Health Services Research Databases—**Agency for Healthcare Research and Quality (AHRQ)** (efficiency and effectiveness of healthcare delivery system)	
Healthcare Cost and Utilization Project (HCUP) • Nationwide Inpatient Sample (NIS) • State Inpatient Database (SID) • State Ambulatory Surgery Database (SASD) • Kids' Inpatient Database (KID)	
National Library of Medicine • MEDLINE • Unified Medical Language System (UMLS) • National Emergency Department Sample (NEDS) • State emergency Department Database (SEDD)	

Information Technology (ONC) are federal initiatives that speak to the importance of healthcare information standards. NCVHS put forward a vision for a national health information infrastructure in its 2001 report *Information for Health* (NCVHS 2001), which was followed in 2002 by its vision for 21st-century health statistics (NCVHS 2002). In 2009, the NCVHS convened its four subcommittees (population health, standards, quality, and privacy/confidentiality/security) to develop a conceptual paper, titled Toward Enhanced Information Capacities for Health. From each subcommittee's perspective, the following healthcare information capacity issues were presented (NCVHS 2010):

- Accessibility and availability of information

- Standards for interoperability, usability, quality, safety, and efficiency

- Privacy, confidentiality, and security

Continued efforts from subcommittees will focus on three areas (NCVHS 2010):

1. Emerging health data needs from person-centered health and health systems with an emphasis on coordinating the continuity of care across a continuum of services

2. Developing recommendations regarding governance and a framework for the identification and appropriate management of sensitive data

3. Seeking to ensure a comprehensive framework and road map for health information standards that support the national health information technology strategic framework

The idea of data standardization became widely accepted during the 1960s. Under the leadership of NCHS and NCVHS, in collaboration with other organizations, data sets were developed for a variety of healthcare settings, first of which were acute care, long-term care, and ambulatory care. Standardizing data elements and definitions makes it possible to compare the data collected at different facilities. With the increased use of computers to retrieve, house, analyze, and disseminate data, the demand for information came from internal and external users. External users, such as third-party payers, government agencies, and accreditation organizations, intensified the use of health information and created demands for standards that promote interoperable electronic interchange of data and information (Giannangelo 2011, 197–98).

Healthcare **data sets** have two purposes:

1. To identify data elements that should be collected for each patient

2. To provide uniform definitions for common terms

Characteristics of several healthcare data sets are detailed in **TABLE 4.4**.

The main trend in collecting secondary data seems to be the increased use of automated data entry. Registries and databases commonly use data already available in electronic form rather than manually abstract all data. The use of EHRs will make separate databases for various diseases and conditions unnecessary. The patient health record itself will be a database that can be queried for information currently obtained from specialized registries.

Coordination efforts are a necessity due to the increased number of organizations developing standards. The **American National Standards Institute (ANSI)** is one example of a standards development organization (SDO). ANSI coordinates the development of voluntary standards in many industries, including healthcare. Most SDOs in the United States are members of ANSI. The Healthcare Information Technology Standards Panel (HITSP), administered by ANSI, is a partnership between the private and public sectors to harmonize and integrate standards that will meet clinical and business needs for sharing information among organizations and systems (HITSP 2009). **TABLE 4.5** lists organizations that are actively involved in developing standards for health-related information management.

TABLE 4.4. Characteristics of data sets

DATA SETS	CHARACTERISTICS
Uniform Hospital Discharge Data Set (UHDDS)	**Patient-specific** data items on every inpatient
	Collected by all short-term general hospitals in the United States
	Incorporated into federal regulations (Medicare and Medicaid)
Uniform Ambulatory Care Data Set (UACDS)	Used in every facility for outpatient care
	Includes optional data items
	Voluntary
Minimum Data Set for Long-Term Care Resident Assessment **Protocols**	Residential facilities, nursing home residents
	Federally mandated
	Collected on admission and at designated reassessment points
	Uses structured lists
	Used for patient assessment
Outcomes Assessment Information Set (OASIS)	Home health industry
	Gathered for Medicare beneficiaries
	Measures patient outcomes
	Assesses quality of care
	Basis for reimbursement
Data Elements for Emergency Department Systems (DEEDS)	Emergency and trauma care
	Hospital-based emergency departments
	Reduces incompatibilities in emergency department records
	Incorporates national standards for electronic data interchange (EDI)
Essential Medical Data Set (EMDS)	Complement to DEEDS
	Part of NHIN
	Used for emergency encounters
	Past medical history
Health Plan Employer Data and Information Set (HEDIS)	Compares performance of managed care plans
	Sponsored by NCQA
	Administrative, claims, health record review data
	Used to develop physician profiles
	Population-based data collection tool
ORYX	Performance measurement
	Promotes a comprehensive, continuous, data-driven Joint Commission accreditation process
National Health Information Network (NHIN)	Allows electronic exchange among healthcare facilities
	Increases patient safety, reduces medical errors, and increases efficiency and effectiveness
	Contains costs

TABLE 4.5. Standards development organizations

Private or government organizations involved in the development of healthcare informatics standards at a national or international level.

RESOURCE	DESCRIPTION	SOURCE
AIIM	AIIM is an ANSI (American National Standards Institute) accredited standards development organization. AIIM also holds the secretariat for the ISO (International Organization for Standardization) committee focused on information management compliance issues. TC171.	http://www.aiim.org
Accredited Standards Committee (ASC) X12	ASC X12 is a designated committee under the Designated Standard Maintenance Organization (DSMO), which develops uniform standards for cross-industry exchange of business transactions through electronic data interchange (EDI) standards. ASC X12 is an ANSI-accredited standards development organization.	http://www.x12.org
American Dental Association (ADA)	The ADA is an ANSI-accredited standards developing organization that develops dental standards that promote safe and effective oral healthcare.	http://www.ada.org/275.aspx
ASTM International	Formerly the American Society for Testing and Materials, ASTM International is an ANSI-accredited standards development organization that develops standards for healthcare data security, standard record content, and protocols for exchange of laboratory data.	http://www.astm.org
European Committee for Standardization (CEN)	CEN contributes to the objectives of the European Union and European Economic Area with voluntary technical standards that promote free trade, the safety of workers and consumers, interoperability of networks, environmental protection, exploitation of research and development programs, and public procurement.	http://www.cenorm.be/cenorm/index.htm
Clinical and Laboratory Standards Institute (CLSI)	A global, nonprofit, standards development organization that promotes the development and use of voluntary consensus standards and guidelines within the healthcare community, Its core business is the development of globally applicable voluntary consensus documents for healthcare testing.	http://www.clsi.org
Clinical Data Interchange Standards Consortium (CDISC)	CDISC is an open, multidisciplinary, nonprofit organization, that has established worldwide industry standards to support the electronic acquisition, exchange, submission, and archiving of clinical trials data and metadata for medical and biopharmaceutical product development.	http://www.cdisc.org/
Designated Standard Maintenance Organization (DSMO)	The DSMO was established in the final HIPAA rule and is charged with maintaining the standards for electronic transactions and developing or modifying an adopted standard.	http://www.hipaa-dsmo.org
Health Industry Business Communications Council (HIBCC)	HIBCC is an industry-sponsored and industry-supported nonprofit organization. As an ANSI-accredited organization, its primary function is to facilitate electronic communications by developing standards for information exchange among healthcare trading partners.	http://www.hibcc.org/
Health Level 7 (HL 7)	An ANSI-accredited standards development organization that develops messaging, data content, and document standards to support the exchange of clinical information.	http://www.hl7.org

TABLE 4.5. (continued)

RESOURCE	DESCRIPTION	SOURCE
Institute of Electrical and Electronic Engineers (IEEE)	A national organization that develops standards for hospital system interface transactions, including links between critical care bedside instruments and clinical information systems.	http://www.ieee.org
International Organization for Standardization (ISO)	ISO is a nongovernmental organization and network of national standards institutes from 157 countries.	http://www.iso.org/iso/en/ISOOnline.frontpage
National Council for Prescription Drug Programs (NCPDP)	A designated committee under the DSMO that specializes in developing standards for exchanging prescription and payment information.	http://www.ncpdp.org
National Information Standards Organization (NISO)	An ANSI-accredited, nonprofit association that identifies, develops, maintains, and publishes technical standards to manage information. NISO standards address areas of retrieval, repurposing, storage, metadata, and preservation.	http://www.niso.org
National Uniform Billing Committee (NUBC)	A designated committee under the DSMO that is responsible for identifying data elements and designing the CMS-1500.	http://www.nubc.org
National Uniform Claim Committee (NUCC)	The national group that replaced the Uniform Claim Form Task Force in 1995 and developed a standard data set to be used in the transmission of noninstitutional provider claims to and from third-party payers.	http://www.nucc.org

Source: Appendix A Data Standards Resource 2007.

Summary

Health record information is valuable to individual patients for continuity of care and documenting evidence of episodes of care. The information is also valuable in an aggregate form to report incidence of disease and effectiveness of care. Statistical reporting of healthcare trends in a variety of indexes, registries, and databases is another common function of HIM services. The HIM professional is responsible for developing, maintaining, and ensuring the accuracy of this aggregate data; transmitting required reports to local, state, and national agencies; and providing statistics to the local facility that guide administrative and clinical decisions.

The HIM professional must understand the importance of healthcare data sets and standards. This role will evolve as healthcare informatics standards and interoperability of these standards are enhanced. This knowledge will be critical to the successful capturing, monitoring, analyzing, and disseminating of health data.

References

Agency for Healthcare Research and Quality (AHRQ). 2010. *Registries for Evaluating Patient Outcomes: A User's Guide*. Rockville, MD: AHRQ.

AHIMA. 2010. *Fundamentals for Building a Master Patient Index/Enterprise Master Patient Index* (Updated). Appendix A: Recommended Core Data Elements for EMPIs. Chicago: AHIMA.

Bowman, E. 2006. Secondary Data Sources. Chapter 9 in *Health Information Management Technology: An Applied Approach,* 2nd ed. Edited by Merida Johns. Chicago: AHIMA.

Bowman, E. 2010. Secondary Records and Healthcare Databases. In *Health Information Management: Concepts, Principles, and Practice,* 3rd ed., edited by K. M. LaTour and S. Eichenwald Maki. Chicago: AHIMA.

Centers for Disease Control and Prevention (CDC). 2010. *CDC WONDER Database.* http://wonder.cdc.gov.

Cerrato, L., and J. Roberts. 2011. Health Information Technology Functions. In *Health Information Management Technology: An Applied Approach,* 3rd ed., edited by M. Johns. Chicago: AHIMA.

Giannangelo, K. 2011. Healthcare Data Sets and Standards. In *Health Information Management Technology: An Applied Approach,* 3rd ed., edited by M. Johns. Chicago: AHIMA.

Health Information Technology Standards Panel. 2009. http://www.hitsp.org.

Johnson, D. L., and C. M. Spielman. 2010. Data and Information Management. In *Health Information Management: Concepts, Principles, and Practice,* 3rd ed., edited by K. M. LaTour and S. Eichenwald Maki. Chicago: AHIMA.

Kanaan, S. B. 2000. *The National Committee on Vital and Health Statistics, 1949–1999: A History.* http://www.ncvhs.hhs.gov/50history.htm.

National Center for Health Statistics. 2011. About NCHS. http://www.cdc.gov/nchs/about.htm.

National Committee on Vital and Health Statistics (NCVHS). 2010. *Toward Enhanced Information Capacities for Health.* http://www.ncvhs.hhs.gov/100526concept.pdf.

National Committee on Vital and Health Statistics (NCVHS). 2002. *Shaping a Health Statistics Vision for the 21st Century.* http://ncvhs.hhs.gov/21st%20final%20report.pdf.

National Committee on Vital and Health Statistics (NCVHS). 2001. *Information for Health: A Strategy for Building the National Health Information Infrastructure.* http://www.ncvhs.hhs.gov/nhiilayo.pdf.

National Plan and Provider Enumeration System (NPPES). 2011. NPI Registry. https://nppes.cms.hhs.gov/NPPES/NPIRegistryHome.do.

National Practitioner Data Bank (NPDB). 2011. The Data Bank. http://www.npdb-hipdb.hrsa.gov.

US Department of Health and Human Services (HHS). 2009. Office of the Assistant Secretary for Planning and Evaluation: The HHS Data Council. http://aspe.hhs.gov/datacncl.

Appendix 4A

Fundamentals for Building a Master Patient Index/Enterprise Master Patient Index

A master patient index (MPI) is an index of known patients within a single organization whose visits are linked together by a single identifier, typically the medical record number. MPI management activities typically pertain to a software application that identifies, coordinates, and lists database information.

Electronic MPIs have been used in healthcare since the 1980s, replacing the past process of manually completing index cards. Interest in electronic MPIs has markedly increased because of the consolidation of healthcare organizations and the implementation of electronic health records (EHRs). Industry efforts such as health information exchange (HIE) and the Nationwide Health Information Network (NHIN) also have provided a spotlight on a new term, *enterprise MPI (EMPI)*, which combines MPIs of two or more organizations.

As the healthcare industry moves to a fully integrated, longitudinal EHR, the MPI and EMPI become vital databases. The information within an MPI is a key component in the accuracy of patient information, such as identification of allergies, medication lists, and prior visits.

This practice brief identifies fundamental components of building accurate MPIs and EMPIs and best practices for maintaining them. For the purpose of this practice brief, the term "MPI" encompasses both organizational- and enterprise-level activities of an electronically generated MPI.

Effect of EHRs

The healthcare industry is on a fast-moving train to implement EHRs. Accurate patient identification and its ability to affect all areas of the healthcare enterprise become the foundation for success. Accurate MPI databases will allow organizations and HIEs to improve patient care, reduce risks, improve operational efficiencies, support information exchange, and enhance the national health infrastructure.

Although MPIs traditionally may have been maintained on index cards, many organizations automated this labor-intensive paper index in the beginning stages of EHR development. The MPI is used during the registration application to ensure a patient is represented accurately and logically once in the database and ensures the same set of demographic and registration data are available throughout the organization.

With the adoption of EHRs, patients with more than one identifier will have isolated packets of information, such as treatment plans, allergies, and important historical medical care documentation, in the system. These isolated pieces of information create

AHIMA. 2010. Practice brief: Fundamentals for building a master patient index/enterprise master patient index. *Journal of AHIMA*.

an actual loss of information because providers may not have a complete health record in front of them when making clinical care decisions.

Organizational-level MPI applications generally are categorized as vendor neutral or "best of breed" or a core vendor solution. The first classification implies that the patient information contained in the MPI can be integrated readily with any other EHR vendor application. Vendor-neutral applications can assist in patient identification across multiple EHR modules, such as laboratory, pharmacy, registration, and billing. A core vendor solution generally is sold as an inherent or add-on module specific to a particular EHR system and may not readily integrate multiple disparate EHR systems across a large healthcare system.

Industry Effect

The American Recovery and Reinvestment Act of 2009 strengthened industry efforts regarding MPI applications. A key component to meeting stage 1 meaningful use criteria and, therefore, incentive payments is an organization's ability to exchange information for the purpose of care coordination. Such coordination requires tremendous efforts at the organizational and HIE levels to ensure care providers have access to the right information, for the right patient, at the right time.

Other industry initiatives include ongoing efforts of the NHIN and Connecting for Health's Common Framework. The NHIN is essentially a set of standards and policies that enables the secure transmission of health information over the Internet within an HIE environment. The NHIN will provide the foundation for health IT standards across organizations and communities and across the nation. This foundation will allow health information to follow patients as they move throughout the healthcare continuum. Currently, the NHIN is developing recommendations for standards for a broad audience.

Connecting for Health is a public-private collaborative that includes representatives from more than 100 organizations across the healthcare industry. Its purpose is to provide a catalyst for widespread industry changes needed to implement health IT while protecting a patient's privacy and security.

Connecting for Health's Common Framework approach was selected by the US Department of Health and Human Services as the initial prototype for the nationwide health information network. The Common Framework is composed of a set of technical and policy specifications designed to assist organizations and providers in creating data exchange and expected to require technical standards to support interoperability. One such infrastructure component is a record locator service (RLS). The RLS provides authorized participants of an HIE with the location of patient health information across the multiple participants (e.g., patient John Doe has health records at hospitals A and B and with physician A).

All of these current industry activities and initiatives will require accurate patient identification across multiple databases. The key to accurate and timely information exchange will be an accurate MPI.

MPI Deployment

MPIs are commonly deployed in either an active or passive mode by using existing Health Level Seven International messages, with additional data requirements being defined during the vendor selection process and implementation. An active deployment method implies that the MPI application is at the front end of the registration or scheduling process. Thus, patient identification is undertaken by using the MPI software, which requires integrating the MPI with legacy systems.

The user will identify the patient from a data repository, and at a select point in the identification pathway, the user drops to the facility-level registration or scheduling system. This process is generally transparent to the user.

A passive deployment method does not directly affect the registration or scheduling pathway. Rather, identification is undertaken behind the scenes or at the back end of the registration function. Generally, thresholds are established whereby a person is automatically linked or merged with existing data. If the threshold is not met, the registration data are held in a work queue for later resolution.

Many organizations and enterprises choose to launch MPI software applications in a passive mode initially and then migrate to active mode. Initial business goals, timelines, and budget will determine the deployment method for any given organization.

Both active and passive MPI methods should have the ability to identify persons at an enterprise and organizational level because initial deployment involves loading all databases to facilitate initial duplicate identification. New patient identification policies and procedures must be formulated before launching an MPI, with careful consideration given to how the registrars will search for a patient if the MPI is deployed in an active mode, how to interpret scores and weights, and how to select the correct patient.

Data Elements

Because the MPI is essentially a database that maintains a unique identifier for each patient seen at the organizational or enterprise level, correctly identifying the data elements of the MPI is very important. Linking the correct clinical information from visit to visit and between enterprise activities requires that the core data elements be standardized and clearly defined. Once defined, these core data elements become the basis for matching algorithms, error reports, quality measurements, and staff training initiatives.

With no current healthcare industry standard for required data elements, organizations and HIEs often struggle in determining how much information to include in the MPI. At a minimum, MPI data elements should allow for the accurate matching of patients with a single identifier, facilitate a longitudinal health record, facilitate clinical system linkage, and improve access to patient health information. See **APPENDIX 4A.1** for AHIMA-recommended data elements.

A review of the data elements associated with errors may reveal the need to collect new data elements or enforce the importance of accurately collecting existing data elements. For example, missing data from legacy system conversions or incomplete data collection during registration compromises the registrar's ability to select the correct patient. An important aspect of achieving and maintaining MPI data integrity is evaluating these procedural causes of duplicates and other issues affecting the MPI.

An organization should develop standard definitions of MPI data elements (data dictionary), standards for capturing and recording patient demographic data (naming conventions), and performance standards that hold staff accountable for accuracy. In addition, adherence to formal business processes and work flows will ensure data accuracy.

Algorithms for Identifying Duplicates

Algorithms are mathematical formulas used by an organization or enterprise that combine weighted data elements to determine the probability of a duplicate in order to identify potential duplicate MPI entries (see **APPENDIX 4A.2** for a full list of terms and definitions). The matching algorithm is a critical component of any successful MPI solution.

The algorithm must be sophisticated, powerful, flexible, and accurate. Without a powerful algorithm to support accurate patient identification, the healthcare organization or enterprise will continue to create errors and will be forced to expend considerable time and money on maintenance efforts.

There are three types of matching algorithms available in the industry today: deterministic, rules based (sometimes known as ad hoc weighting), and probabilistic. Most organizations use deterministic, or exact match, algorithms, meaning they require exact matches on a combination of data elements such as name, birth date, sex, and Social Security number (SSN).

Deterministic algorithms are considered only 20 percent to 40 percent accurate in patient identification and often result in a high volume of false matches. Therefore, one could expect less than half of the duplicates to be identified through the deterministic method. Deterministic algorithms are particularly weak in identifying individuals when there is transposition of numbers or letters, name changes, limited data, or large databases.

A more sophisticated technique for record matching uses rules-based algorithms. Rules-based algorithms are sometimes referred to as "fuzzy logic," or even mistakenly called "probabilistic." A rules-based algorithm allows an organization to assign weights, or significance values, to particular data elements and use these weights to compare one record with another. This type of algorithm requires the facility to estimate weights in advance and then apply those weights to the data analysis process.

Because the organization determines the weights for data elements, the accuracy of rules-based algorithms varies widely. Using this method, only 50 percent and 80 percent of the potential duplicate record population may be identified. Usually, several repetitions of trial-and-error analysis on rules-based algorithms are required before an organization achieves acceptable results.

Probabilistic matching is considered to be the most sophisticated technique available, with an accuracy rate of 90 percent or higher. These algorithms are considered more advanced and more complex and able to support large data sets. Probabilistic algorithms are based on complex mathematical formulas that actually analyze the facility-specific MPI data to determine precisely matched weight probabilities for attribute values of various data elements.

For example, consider an MPI file where the name "Jones" appears more frequently than the name "Wheatley." A match on the name "Jones" has lower significance (less likely to be the same person) than a match on the name "Wheatley" (higher probability that a match represents the same person). Supporting digit transpositions and rotations, alternate name cross-referencing, distance editing, and enhanced phonetic searching can further enhance probabilistic algorithms. Therefore, many integrated healthcare delivery systems and HIEs choose probabilistic matching algorithms for enterprise-wide MPI activities.

Once determined, the algorithm is applied to a software application report that identifies potential duplicates. A threshold measure is used to interpret comparison scores based on the number of matches within required data element fields as defined in the algorithm.

For example, an organization has defined five data elements (patient name, date of birth, sex, SSN, and telephone number) as required matches for duplicate identification. The threshold for identification is defined as matching between three and five of the required elements. When scores are below the threshold (e.g., one data element matches), the records are assumed to represent different individuals, and the associated medical record numbers or enterprise identifiers are assumed to be accurate.

If the score is above the threshold (e.g., four of the five elements match), the record is assumed to be duplicative, and further research is required. If the score is between the two thresholds, the record is flagged and the information is placed in a work queue for review, resolution, and potential manual record review by the appropriate staff.

The table below shows an example of a deterministic algorithm. It shows how the exact matches regarding data elements date of birth, sex, SSN, and telephone number are matched by the algorithm to produce a possible duplicate for John A. Smith.

PATIENT NAME	DATE OF BIRTH	SEX	SSN	TELEPHONE NUMBER
John A. Smith	01-01-90	M	444-44-4444	555-555-5555
Johnnie A. Smith	01-01-90	M	444-44-4444	555-555-5555

Data Integrity

Data have integrity if they are complete, accurate, and consistent. A clean MPI contains only one record for each person and begins at registration. The diagram below illustrates how inaccurate information in the MPI has the potential to cascade to the various systems in an organization and can culminate in exporting erroneous information to an HIE:

⇒ MPI

  ⇒ scheduling system

    ⇒ operating room system

      ⇒ computerized physician order entry

        ⇒ clinical documentation system

        ⇒ transcription

        ⇒ radiology

        ⇒ pharmacy

        ⇒ laboratory

        ⇒ pathology

          ⇒ HIM system

            ⇒ encoder

              ⇒ document management

                ⇒ release of information

                  ⇒ HIE

A review of the identified duplicates and overlays often reveals procedural problems that contribute to the creation of errors. Although HIM departments may be the hub of identifying, mitigating, and correcting MPI errors, that information may never be shared with the registration department. If the registration staff is not aware of the errors, how can they begin to proactively prevent the errors from occurring in the first place?

Registration process improvement activities can eventually reduce work for HIM departments. In addition, monitoring new duplicates is a critical process, and tracking reports should be created and implemented. Identifying and reporting MPI errors is important; however, tracking who made the error and why will decrease the number of duplicates.

The HIM, registration, and ancillary departments should establish communications to identify, report, and correct new duplicates, as well as methods for tracking, trending, and retraining individuals who created duplicate medical record numbers. Routine corrections of all identified duplicates must be a core organizational MPI maintenance function.

Calculating MPI Error Rate

Whether the MPI is at a local, enterprise, or HIE level, its primary purpose is to facilitate the link between clinical and administrative information between disparate systems. With so many patient care and industry initiatives at stake, the quality of MPI data can no longer be considered a back-end function.

Errors in MPI databases can lead to billing problems, unnecessary duplicate tests, and potential legal exposure. In addition, duplicates contribute to HIM operational workload and create inefficiencies as each new patient receives a new medical record number, file folder (in the paper world), and staff time in MPI maintenance activities.

Traditionally, MPI maintenance activities may not have received prioritization within the functional assignments of the HIM department for reasons such as chart assembly, analysis, coding, and abstracting. These other functions contributed to the revenue cycle of the organization and were given priority.

As EHRs were adopted and integrated, it became evident that the integrity of the MPI was in jeopardy because of the lack of merging and maintenance priorities. As disparate systems were implemented, an additional burden of correcting duplicates within multiple systems added increased administrative time in clinical departments such as the laboratory.

As the HIM department merges two duplicates together, the source system (laboratory) also must be corrected. This creates new challenges for organizations because merge functionality could be different in each system or module, which in turn creates data redundancy. Addressing ongoing errors within the MPI means an established quality measurement and maintenance program is crucial to the future of healthcare.

Organizations struggle to identify industry benchmarks and standards regarding MPI error percentages. Although no organization expects to have duplicated patient information in the MPI, it is unrealistic to assume that duplicates will never occur. Even though errors may occur at the point of registration, the actual cause of error varies.

Duplicate information can occur as the result of insufficient patient information, clerical typos or transpositions, inability to capture important information (e.g., the patient is unconscious), and EHR system limitations in naming conventions. In addition, several processes also may contribute to duplicate creations.

The following processes can affect the quality of MPI data:

- Decentralized registration

- Converted data

- Lack of standards

- Lack of staff training

- Difficulties associated with registering laboratory specimens

- Acceptance of data from physician offices without verification procedures

- Lack of formal business processes and work flows

The duplicate error rate describes the quality of the MPI data. The error rate is calculated by dividing the total number of duplicate records with the total number of records multiplied by 100. An error rate is assigned to the MPI based on the file size and the number of duplicate records identified.

Industry experts estimate current organizational MPI error rates are between 7 percent and 10 percent and cost between $10 and $20 per duplicate to correct.[1] To put the duplicate MPI problem in proper perspective, if the organization has 300,000 patients in the MPI, there could be 30,000 duplicates, which, in turn, cost the organization $60,000.

Organizations can mitigate increased costs in MPI maintenance by developing MPI policies and procedures that clearly define review and maintenance activities.

Data Ownership

The issue of data ownership is a potentially difficult one that organizations must address early in their planning process, particularly if the corporation that is purchasing the MPI software license does not own all the participating facilities or sites. This challenge is further complicated by HIPAA because organizations must consider the relationship between covered entities, organized healthcare arrangements, business associates, and the obligations for disclosure of information to patients.

Participating for-profit entities of an integrated healthcare delivery system must consider the Gramm-Leach-Bliley Act limitations for sharing data.[2] Furthermore, as different facilities contribute data to the MPI, organizations should develop a comprehensive strategy to address demographic changes and duplicate resolution.

Participation in HIEs also will present challenges when patient-specific information changes. Specifically, organizations, integrated healthcare delivery systems, and HIEs should determine who will have the authority to change what level of data and how data changes will be communicated.

Enterprise and Corporate Identifiers

Inherent in the deployment of an EMPI is the assignment of the enterprise identifier. Although enterprise identifiers can be used for patient care, they are not commonly used by any downstream systems. Instead, they serve as a behind-the-scenes identifier to link and identify persons at a corporate level, with the existing identifiers such as medical record number or account number still providing identification at the local or facility level. However, with the push for more linking of clinical data to facilitate care across an integrated healthcare delivery system, organizations and technology may embrace the propagation of the corporate identifier.

Maintaining the MPI

The management of a high-quality, error-free MPI requires constant maintenance, which includes oversight, evaluation, and correction of errors. The responsibility for MPI maintenance should be centralized under the direction of a qualified professional. Employees responsible for MPI maintenance must be carefully trained, have adequate tools and procedures, and be supervised to ensure their consistent compliance with established guidelines.

A comprehensive maintenance program should include:

- Ongoing processes to identify and address existing errors

- Advanced person search capabilities for minimizing the creation of new errors

- Mechanisms for efficiently detecting, reviewing, and resolving potential errors

- Ability to reliably link different medical record numbers and other identifiers for the same person to create an enterprise view of the person

- Consideration of the types of physical merges (files, film, etc.) and the interfaces and correction routines to other electronic systems that are populated or updated by the EMPI

The personnel performing duplication resolution activities require a foundation in the registration process to facilitate process improvement and ongoing communication between departments. This process includes an overview of the registration work flow, frequent obstacles encountered, and departmental expectations. In addition, training should include knowledge of downstream systems that are affected by duplicate identifiers and resolution activities in source systems.

Staff also should receive in-depth training, be supported by detailed policies and procedures, and be able to demonstrate competency in the areas of duplicate identification and resolution. Ongoing education should include feedback from a well-defined quality program. Updates to the training program should be performed periodically and should be based on a review of the initial training to incorporate system modifications, upgrades, and internal process improvements.

All training should be performed before beginning any duplicate resolution or maintenance activity.

Adequate staffing is needed to maintain and ensure the quality of the MPI. Staff members should have the authority to resolve duplicates, investigate demographic overlays, and link persons across the enterprise. See **APPENDIX 4A.3** for a sample job description.

MPI maintenance policies and procedures also should outline:

- Whether to use the most recent information for each data element or criteria for determining which data elements will be stored as the patient's information

- Identification of duplicate data elements (e.g., prior name or alias)

- Communication of merges to ancillary staff for source system revision

- Regular review of error reports and trending of duplicate percentages

MPI management should be a key strategic activity for any healthcare organization, integrated healthcare delivery system, or HIE as the backbone of the EHR and the support for a longitudinal patient record. The integrity of the MPI is more important now than ever before. MPI maintenance and management requires a leader who possesses a variety of skills and experiences. There are vast opportunities in the healthcare industry today for professionals who can demonstrate knowledge of both information management and technology that supports MPI database integrity.

Notes

1. Hess, Robbi. "Masters of Their Domain." *For the Record* 17, no. 17 (Aug. 15, 2005). Available online at www.fortherecordmag.com/archives/ftr_081505p30.shtml.

2. The Financial Services Modernization Act of 1999, also known as the Gramm-Leach-Bliley Act, requires financial institutions to provide customers with a notice of privacy policies and procedures and to satisfy various disclosure and consumer opt-out requirements.

References

AHIMA. "Reconciling and Managing EMPIs." *Journal of AHIMA* 81, no. 4 (Apr. 2010): 52–57.

AHIMA MPI Task Force. 2004. "Practice brief: Building an Enterprise Master Person Index." *Journal of AHIMA* 75(1):56A–D.

Altendorf, Robin L. "Establishment of a Quality Program for the Master Patient Index." AHIMA's 79th National Convention and Exhibit Proceedings, October 2007. Available online in the AHIMA Body of Knowledge at www.ahima.org.

Brown, Eric, Jim Burke, Erica Foster, and Thea Campbell. "Accurate Patient Identification: The Foundation for EHRs." AHIMA's 78th National Convention and Exhibit Proceedings, October 2006. Available online in the AHIMA Body of Knowledge at www.ahima.org.

Connecting for Health Common Framework. "Correctly Matching Patients with Their Records." April 2006. Available online at www.connectingforhealth.org/commonframework/docs/P4_Correctly_Matching.pdf.

Connecting for Health Common Framework. "Record Locator Service: Technical Background from the Massachusetts Prototype Community." Available online at www.connectingforhealth.org/commonframework/docs/T6_RecordLocator.pdf.

Department of Health and Human Services. "Nationwide Health Information Network: Public Forums and Other Products." Available online at www.hhs.gov/healthit/healthnetwork/forums/.

Dimick, Chris. "Exposing Double Identity at Patient Registration." *Journal of AHIMA* 80, no. 11 (Nov-Dec 2009): Web extra. Available online in the AHIMA Body of Knowledge at www.ahima.org.

Greenwald, Constance Z., and Jason Broad. "Master Patient Index Overlaps (2 Patients, 1 Record): We Don't Know What We Don't Know." 2009 AHIMA Convention Proceedings, October 2009. Available online in the AHIMA Body of Knowledge at www.ahima.org.

Health Level Seven International. "V3 Messaging Standard." Available online at www.hl7.org/implement/standards/v3messages.cfm.

Hewitt, Joseph B., and Michele O'Connor. "Connecting Care through EMPIs." *Journal of AHIMA* 73, no. 10 (Oct. 2002): 32–38.

Hieb, Barry R. "The EMPI Magic Quadrant for 2001: A Maturing Market." Market Analysis, Nunn, Sandra. "Risk-Based MPI Management." *Journal of AHIMA* 79, no. 6 (June 2008): 48–49, 56.

Wheatley, Vicki. "Quality Impact of the Master Patient Index" *Journal of AHIMA* 79, no. 10 (Oct. 2008): 78–79.

Wheatley, Victoria. "Unique Identifiers: Preparing for HIPAA." 2002 AHIMA Convention Proceedings, September 2002. Available online in the AHIMA Body of Knowledge at www.ahima.org.

Appendix 4A.1

Recommended Core Data Elements for EMPIs

DATA ELEMENT	DEFINITION	DATA TYPE*
Internal patient identification	Primary identifier used by the facility to identify the patient at admission (e.g., the medical record number)	Extended composite ID with check digit
Person name	Legal name of patient or person, including surname, given name, middle name or initial, suffixes (e.g., junior, IV), and prefixes (e.g., Father, doctor)	Extended person name
Date of birth	Year, month, and day of birth (e.g., YYYY/MM/DD)	Time stamp
Gender	For example, male, female, unknown, or undetermined	Coded value
Race	Race is a concept used to differentiate population groups largely on the basis of physical characteristics transmitted by descent. Races currently used by the federal government for statistical purposes are American Indian or Alaskan Native, Asian or Pacific Islander, Black, White, Unknown, Other, and Missing.	Coded value
Ethnicity	Ethnicity is a concept used to differentiate population groups on the basis of shared cultural characteristics or geographic origins. Ethnic designations currently used by the federal government for statistical purposes are Hispanic origin, not of Hispanic origin, and Unknown, Other, and Missing.	Coded value
Address	Address or location of patient's residence. Components include the street address, other designation (e.g., apartment number), city, state/province, zip or postal code, country, and type of address (e.g., permanent, mailing).	Extended address
Telephone number	Telephone number at which that patient can be contacted. This may be a home or business telephone number or the telephone number of a friend, neighbor, or relative.	String data
Alias/previous/ maiden names	Any names by which the patient has been known other than the current legal name, including nicknames, maiden name, previous name that was legally changed, etc. All previous names available should be converted and retained.	Extended person name
Social Security number	Personal identification number assigned by the US Social Security Administration	String data
Facility identification	The unique identification number of a facility where patients seek care. (The Centers for Medicare and Medicaid Services has developed a provider ID system for healthcare facilities.)	Person location
Universal patient identifier	Not yet established	N/A
Account/visit number	Number assigned by the facility billing or accounting office for all charges and payments for this encounter or visit	Extended composite ID with check digit
Admission/ encounter/visit date	Date the patient actually arrived for care (e.g., YYYY/MM/DD/HH/SS)	Time stamp
Discharge or departure date	Date the patient actually left the facility or died (e.g., YYYY/MM/DD/HH/SS)	Time stamp

(continued)

Encounter/service type	Categorization of the encounter, such as emergency, inpatient, outpatient, home care, or electronic (e.g., e-mail, Internet, telemedicine)	Coded value
Encounter/service location	Location in which the encounter, visit, or treatment occurred	Coded value
Encounter primary physician	Attending physician for the associated encounter, visit, or treatment, identified with the primary physician's National Provider Identifier	Coded value
Patient disposition	Patient's intended care setting after discharge. Examples include discharge home (not to home health service), acute care hospital, nursing facility, home to be under the care of a home health service provider, or other healthcare facility; left against medical advice; alive, other, or not stated; died; admitted to hospital; admitted for observation; transferred to skilled nursing facility, intermediate care facility, or other facility; or other disposition as dictated by type of MPI	Coded value

*Data types correspond to those described in Health Level Seven International's Application Protocol for Electronic Data Exchange in Healthcare Environments. Version 2.6. Version 2 Messaging Standard.

The table "Additional Recommended EMPI Data Elements" lists additional data elements that can be stored in EMPIs.

Additional Recommended EMPI Data Elements

DATA ELEMENT	DEFINITION	DATA TYPE*
Mother's maiden name	The given, family, or last name of the patient's mother	String data
Marital status	Marriage status of the patient (e.g., never married, married, separated, widowed, divorced, or unknown). Organizations must determine whether marital status will be tied to a visit or just reflect current status and whether historical information for specific visits will be available.	Coded value
Place of birth	City, state, and country of the patient's birth	String data
County	County in which the patient lives	Coded value
Blood type/Rh	Patient's blood type or Rh factor	Coded value
Employer	Name of patient's employer	String value
Work telephone number	Patient's work telephone number	String value
Advance directive and surrogate decision making	An indication that the patient has an advance directive on file. It describes an individual's current preferences about treatment should the person become incompetent or unable to communicate these preferences to medical personnel. Surrogate decision making is an alternative method for medical decision making on the individual's behalf. It is invoked in the absence of an advance directive when the individual is not competent to make an informed decision.	Boolean
Organ donor status	Whether the patient has consented to donate his or her organ(s) in the event of death	Boolean
Emergency contact name	Name of the person whom the patient wishes to be the primary contact if notification is necessary	String data
Emergency contact relationship	Relationship to the patient of the person whom the patient wishes to be the primary contact if notification is necessary	String data

(continued)

DATA ELEMENT	DEFINITION	DATA TYPE*
Emergency contact address	Address of the person whom the patient wishes to be the primary contact if notification is necessary	String data
Emergency contact telephone number	Telephone number of the person whom the patient wishes to be the primary contact if notification is necessary	String data
Guarantor name	Name of the person responsible for the payment of the patient's bill	String data
Guarantor relationship	Relationship of the person responsible for the payment of the patient's bill	String data
Guarantor address	Address of the person responsible for the payment of the patient's bill	String data
Guarantor telephone number	Telephone number of the person responsible for the payment of the patient's bill	String data
Payer information	Type of payer (commercial insurance, Medicare, self, etc), including policy information such as payer name, policy number, etc.	String data, separate fields for each data element
Problem list	Master list of all of a patient's health problems or diagnoses	String data
Encounter primary physician contact address	Encounter primary physician business address	String data
Referring physician	Referring physician for the associated encounter, visit, or treatment, identified with the physician's National Provider Identifier	Coded value
Referring physician contact address	Referring physician's business address	String data
Receipt of notice of privacy practices	Whether the notice of privacy practices been given to the patient	Coded value

*Data types correspond to those described in Health Level Seven International's Application Protocol for Electronic Data Exchange in Healthcare Environments. Version 2.6. Version 2 Messaging Standard.[1]

Note

1. AHIMA. "Reconciling and Managing EMPIs." *Journal of AHIMA* 81, no. 4 (Apr. 2010): 52–57.

Appendix 4A.2

Glossary

Active Deployment: MPI software application deployment that uses a method for identifying patients at the front end of the registration or scheduling process.

Algorithms: MPI algorithms are mathematical formulas that combine weighted data elements to determine the probability of a duplicate. Used to identify potential duplicate MPI entries.

Corporate Identifier: Unique link that identifies and links persons at a corporate or enterprise level.

Data Ownership: Process of defining, within EMPIs, the owner of the individual data contained within the database.

Deterministic Algorithm: MPI algorithm that requires an exact match of combined data elements such as name, birth date, sex, and Social Security number.

Duplicate: More than one unique identifier (e.g., medical record number or person identifier) for the same person in the MPI. This causes one patient to have two or more different medical records within the same facility.

Enterprise Master Patient Index (EMPI): Index referencing of all known patients in two or more facilities (e.g., integrated healthcare delivery system or HIE).

Error Rate: Total number of duplicate patient identifiers within a database. Calculated by dividing the total number of duplicates by the total number of records multiplied by 100.

Integrated Healthcare Delivery System: Coordinated healthcare delivery system that includes physicians and hospitals. Integrated healthcare delivery systems provide a broad range of health services, such as clinic visits, ambulatory surgery, urgent care clinics, inpatient hospitalization, rehabilitative services, and behavioral health services.

Maintenance: Routine actions an organization undertakes to review and correct MPI data errors.

Master Patient Index (MPI): Index referencing of all known patients to a single organization linked together by a common identifier, usually the medical record number (used interchangeably with EMPI).

MPI Data Elements: Key data points within patient demographic information that will be included in the MPI (e.g., patient name, sex, race, date of birth, medical record number, Social Security number).

MPI Error Rate: Percentage assigned to the number of potential duplicates within a given MPI. Calculated by dividing the total number of duplicate records by the total number of records multiplied by 100.

Overlap: More than one unique identifier for the same person across two or more facilities in the enterprise (e.g., patient John Smith has medical record number 12345 at facility A and medical record number 447788 at facility B).

Overlay: One EMPI record for more than one person (e.g., two people sharing the same identifier).

Passive Deployment: MPI software application deployment method—this is behind the scenes or at the back end of the registration function.

Probabilistic Algorithm: MPI algorithm based on complex mathematical formulas that analyzes facility-specific MPI data to determine precisely matched weight probabilities for attribute values of various data elements. Used most often in large databases such as HIEs.

Record Locator Service (RLS): Information service that locates patient health records across the multiple systems that subscribe or participate in HIE. A key piece of infrastructure within the health information environment in which authorized care providers submit a request for information to an HIE. The RLS responds to the request by providing information to the requester regarding pertinent records (e.g., health records for John Doe can be found at hospitals A and B and with physician A).

Resolution: Act of identifying, assigning, correcting, and merging duplicates within the MPI (also called "merging").

Rules-Based Algorithm: MPI algorithm that assigns weights, or significant values, to particular data elements and later uses these weights to compare one record to another.

Appendix 4A.3

Sample Job Description

Department Name:	Cost Center:
Status/Pay Grade:	Effective Date:
Job Title: MPI Coordinator	Reports to:
Hire Date:	Annual Review Date:

Position Summary/General Purpose: The master patient index (MPI) is a critical business function and resource because it links a patient to demographic, clinical, and financial information. For those purposes, the MPI must contain accurate, timely, and complete data that include a single identifier for each patient registered. The MPI coordinator will be responsible for reviewing, analyzing, and maintaining data integrity within the MPI. In addition, this position is responsible for ensuring that the information exchanged between (insert organization name) and health information exchange (HIE) databases is accurate and that corrections are communicated in a timely manner.

Position Requirements/Qualifications:

Licensure/Certification/Registration: RHIA, RHIT, CHDA certification preferred.

Education: Associate or bachelor's degree in health information management preferred.

Experience: Prior healthcare experience preferred. Previous health data analyst experience preferred.

Degree of Supervision: Employee must be able to work independently, effectively, and efficiently on his or her own. This position has no direct reports.

Physical Requirements: Employee must be able to perform the essential functions of this job. This position includes a requirement to walk, climb stairs, balance, and sit. Lifting is limited to health information charts and is not expected to exceed 25 pounds. Vision requirements include the ability to read paper and electronic health records.

Responsibilities:

- Monitor duplicate analysis reports daily to identify potential overlaps and overlays
- Review, prioritize, and facilitate merging of facility and HIE duplicates
- Report monthly MPI data integrity efforts to the appropriate committee
- Provide ongoing training to registration staff on MPI data entry and the importance of MPI data integrity
- Provide training to HIM personnel assigned to resolution and merging activities

- Provide facility-wide training on data-integrity efforts

- Review organizational policies and procedures regarding merging and provide input on key indicators such as which information to retain when merging duplicates

- Coordinate and communicate MPI activities and merges with other departments (e.g., laboratory) for source system resolution

- Retrieve, analyze, and make appropriate MPI changes in both electronic and paper records within the appropriate system

Knowledge/Skills

- Proficient in Microsoft Word, Excel, Access, and PowerPoint

- Ability to present complex information in an understandable and compelling manner

- Knowledge of coding classification systems

- Ability to analyze information to determine appropriate resolutions and merges

- Excellent written and verbal communication skills

- Strong customer service skills

Chapter 5

Clinical Information and Nonclinical Data

Ruthann Russo, PhD, MPH, RHIT

Learning Objectives

- List the types of demographic data collected in health records and explain the purpose of each element

- List the types of administrative information collected in health records and explain the purpose of each element

- Explain the functions of general and special (or informed) consents

- Identify the types of clinical information collected in health records and explain the purpose of each element

- List the data elements collected in the report of history and physical examination and explain their relevance to patient treatment

- Describe the types of services covered in physicians' orders

- List the various types of documentation written by physicians and explain their content and functions

- Explain the conditions under which medical consultations should be ordered

- List the various types of documentation written by nurses and explain their content and functions

- List the data elements that must be included in laboratory reports

- List the data elements that must be included in imaging reports

- Explain the purpose and content of anesthesia assessments and reports

- List the data elements that must be included in operative reports

- List the data elements that must be included in pathology reports

- List the data elements that should be collected in implant and transplantation records

- Explain the function and content of discharge summaries

- Explain the function and content of patient instructions

- List the various types of specialty documentation maintained in acutecare records

- List the data elements that must be collected in emergency and trauma records

- List the uniform data sets that are collected for hospital patients and describe their content

Key Terms

Administrative information

Advance directive

American Recovery and Reinvestment Act (ARRA)

Ancillary services

Attending physician

Autopsy report

Bar Code Medication Administration (BCMA)

Cardiology report

Care plan

Case management

Clinical information

Clinical pathway

Clinical practice guideline

Clinical protocol

Commission on Accreditation of Rehabilitation Facilities (CARF)

Computerized physician order entry (CPOE)

Consent to treatment

Consultation report

Data

Demographic data

Discharge summary

Do-not-resuscitate (DNR) order

Dumping

Emergency Medical Treatment and Active Labor Act (EMTALA)

Encounter note

Expressed consent

Financial data

Flowchart

History

Hospitalist

Imaging report

Implied consent

Information

Informed consent

Interval note

Intraoperative anesthesia record

Labor and delivery record

Laboratory report

Living will

Master patient index (MPI)

Medical staff bylaws

Medication administration record (MAR)

Neurology report

Notice of privacy practices

Nursing assessment

Nutritional assessment

Operative report

Pathology report

Patient assessment instrument (PAI)

Patient's rights

Physician's order

Postoperative anesthesia record

Preoperative anesthesia evaluation

Principal diagnosis

Principal procedure

Progress note

Recovery room record

Standing order

Transfer record

Transfusion record

Uniform Ambulatory Care Data Set (UACDS)

Uniform Hospital Discharge Data Set (UHDDS)

Unique identifier

Visit note

Introduction

A health record is maintained for every patient who receives services in a healthcare facility. The content of the record consists of identifying data about the patient, the patient's reason for seeking services, diagnoses, and the types of services provided to the patient during his stay in the healthcare facility.

This chapter explores the types of data and information in a patient's hospital health record. A patient's health record contains all of the clinical and nonclinical information that pertains to the care the patient received while in the hospital. Each type of information can be further subdivided. For example, clinical information includes the services provided, medications or tests ordered, type of report, and location of care. Nonclinical data can be divided into administrative, demographic, and financial information. This chapter looks at each type or category of information that may be included in a patient's hospital-based health record. For each category, the following questions will be answered:

- When is the information collected?

- Who collects (or records) the information?

- Why is the information collected?

- What data elements are collected?

In addition, samples of each type of information are provided in the chapter. As healthcare systems continue to work toward the electronic health record (EHR), hospitals' health records will include varying degrees of electronic, or digital, information. Most hospitals still use paper-based forms to some extent. In addition, paper-based forms provide a basis for the minimum information that needs to be collected electronically. EHRs are addressed in detail in chapter 6. This chapter focuses on the content of paper-based forms, and chapter 6 focuses on electronic screen design and data capture.

Nonclinical data is the first type explored. First, administrative data, such as that collected during admissions and registration, are described. Second, demographic data, or basic factual information about the patient, are reviewed. The third and last type of nonclinical data discussed is financial data. Financial data that is part of the patient's hospital-based record are primarily health insurance or other information that addresses who is responsible for paying the bill for healthcare services. Each of these types of nonclinical data will be explained in detail in the first part of this chapter.

Consents for treatment and authorizations are another type of information maintained in the patient's health record. Different types of consents for treatment and authorizations are described. The advance directive, also referred to as a **living will**, is described in this section.

Clinical information makes up the greatest portion of the patient's health record. First, the content of the patient history and physical exam, which is one of the first documents recorded in the patient's record, is described. Second, orders for medication, tests, or treatment are explained. Third, documents that describe clinical observations, including observations by physicians, nursing staff, ancillary clinicians, and surgical staff, are explored. Fourth, documentation for outpatient services provided in acute care facilities is reviewed. This includes documentation in emergency department records and for ambulatory surgery and diagnostic or therapeutic services. Specialty care documentation is discussed, and an entire section is dedicated to the discharge summary and the autopsy report.

Every patient record contains a significant amount of information, much of it unstructured. Although the **American Recovery and Reinvestment Act (ARRA)** of 2009 requires that the EHR be implemented in hospitals by 2015, a completely electronic and structured patient health record may not be in place until after that deadline. In the meantime, it is essential to ensure that the massive amount of information included in a patient record can be accurately and reliably represented using some type of shorthand methodology. This is known as data abstracting. In the hospital setting, data should conform to one of two uniform healthcare data sets: the **uniform hospital discharge data set (UHDDS)** for inpatient services and the **uniform ambulatory care data set (UACDS)** for outpatient services. These systems are described at the end of the chapter.

Data Versus Information

Because data and information are at the core of all health records, it is important to define these terms.

Data are the dates, numbers, images, symbols, letters, and words that represent basic facts and observations about people, processes, measurements, and conditions (Johns 2011).

Information is factual data that have been collected, combined, analyzed, interpreted, and/or converted into a form that can be used for a specific purpose (Johns 2011).

While the terms are sometimes used interchangeably, here is a difference. Applying the definitions provided above, data are really very basic facts or elements. And information combines data elements so they can be used for a specific purpose. An example of data in a patient record would be a culture and sensitivity for a urine sample showing greater than 100,000 colonies of *Escherichia coli* bacteria. The finding of greater than 100,000 colonies of *E. coli* bacteria in the patient's urine is the data in this example. That data, when combined with the additional data that that patient has a fever of 102 degrees Fahrenheit, chills, and flank pain, can be used to generate a diagnosis of urinary tract infection.

Administrative Information

Administrative information includes personal data about the patient, such as name, address, birth date, and age. It includes consents for treatment and the use of healthcare information. Administrative information also describes the nature of the patient's admission, or the chief complaint, and the patient's health insurance coverage. Administrative nonclinical data that are included in a patient's health record are generally collected at the time of, or just prior to, the patient's admission to the hospital, during the registration process. The registration staff collects personal information about the patient and information about the patient's health insurance coverage at the time of admission. This is the beginning of the patient health record. Healthcare organizations use a computer-based registration system tied to a database called the **master patient index (MPI)**. The MPI identifies all patients who have been treated in a facility or enterprise and lists the health record numbers associated with the names. If a patient has been treated in the facility in the past, the registration personnel access her personal and health insurance data and check it against her current information to ensure that it is current and correct. The patient's administrative information is recorded on an identification sheet (often called a face sheet). In paper-based record systems, a printout of the identification sheet is used as the front page in the patient's record.

Nonclinical data are collected to ensure that the patient's record can be accurately and easily identified. More importantly, nonclinical data are used to ensure that only data and information relating to that patient are included in that patient's record. Once a record has been created for a patient in a healthcare provider setting, all information relating to that patient should be housed in that record, whether it is an electronic, paper-based, or hybrid record.

Demographic Data

The term *demographics* refers to the study of statistical information about human populations. In the context of healthcare, **demographic data**, collected during the registration process, incorporates basic factual details about the individual patient, including the patient's

- Full name
- Address
- Telephone number
- Gender
- Date and place of birth
- Race or ethnic origin
- Marital status
- Next of kin's name and address
- Social Security number
- Account number (generally a patient is assigned a new account number for each visit)
- Health record number (the patient retains the same health record number for every visit)
- Admission date
- Primary care physician
- Admitting physician

FIGURE 5.1. Health record file illustrating that only one medical record number is assigned to each patient

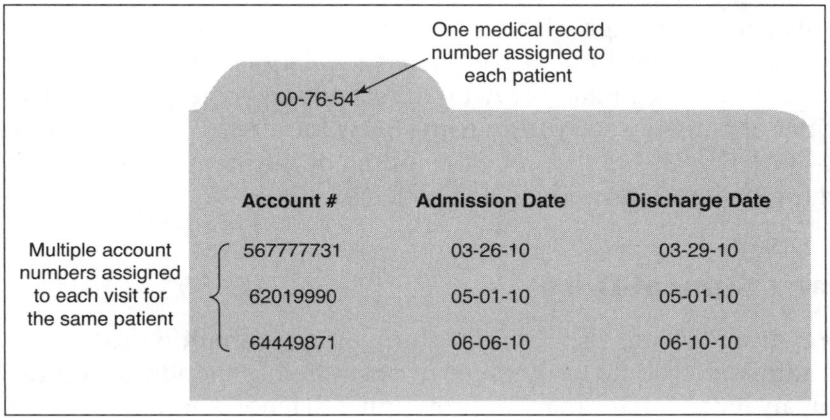

The main purpose of collecting demographic data is to confirm the unique identity of the patient. Hospitals and other healthcare-related organizations also use the demographic data collected from patients as the basis of statistical records, research, and resource planning.

Healthcare facilities assign **unique identifiers** to individual health records to ensure that the information in the records is not misplaced, lost, or confused with the information for another person. For most facilities, the health record number (often called a medical record number) remains constant for each patient. Each time the patient visits the facility, the same medical record number is used; this allows communication between past and present healthcare providers and consistent sharing of information regarding the course of treatment. A unique account number is assigned to each admission. This ensures that treatment specific to each visit can be accessed. **FIGURE 5.1** illustrates the concept of a single medical record number but multiple account numbers for each patient.

Financial Data

The registration and admission staff also collect details about the patient's occupation, employer, and insurance coverage during the patient registration process. These data are used to complete the claims forms that the healthcare provider will submit to third-party payers, who may be either health insurance companies or, in the case of patients who are Medicare or Medicaid recipients, the government.

To ensure that the information is accurate, a copy of the insurance card may be made and kept in the patient's record. Each time a patient has a new admission, the staff must verify financial data to identify any change in health insurance coverage. **Financial data** include the following:

- Patient's name

- Name of the insured party and his or her relationship to the patient if the patient is a dependent of the insured party

- Insured party's member identification number

- Name of the insurance company and the group policy number

- Employer's name and address
- Social Security number (SSN). (Note that although SSNs may be used to help identify patients, using the patient's SSN as a health record number is not recommended. This could be considered a violation of Health Information Portability and Accountability Act [HIPAA] privacy protections Because of this, facilities are moving away from using SSNs for identification purposes. Many now block the SSN so that only the billing department can see it. It is mainly used for insurance processing and collections.)

Preliminary Clinical Data

Preliminary clinical data are also recorded during the registration process. The reason for the patient's admission should be provided or confirmed by the admitting physician. These data generally include a preliminary or provisional diagnosis and the ICD-9-CM code for the diagnosis. In the event that a diagnosis has not been established, the symptom causing the patient's admission to the hospital is recorded, along with the ICD-9-CM code for that symptom. This code ensures that the patient is assigned to the correct nursing unit, supports the medical necessity of the admission, and may be used for future research.

Consents and Acknowledgments

Healthcare providers ask patients or their legal representatives to sign consents. These include a general consent for treatment and specific consents for any treatment that involves significant risk. Patients are also asked to sign a consent form for the use of their health information pursuant to HIPAA. Different types of consents are addressed in the following sections. Acknowledgments usually apply to the patient's confirmation that he has received specific information. All consents, authorizations, and acknowledgments that have been signed by patients or their legal representatives in connection with services to be provided in a hospital should be stored in the patients' health records.

Consents Related to Clinical Care

The need to obtain the patient's consent before performing medical and surgical procedures is based on the legal concept of battery. Battery is the unlawful touching of a person without his or her implied or expressed consent.

Implied consent is assumed when a patient voluntarily submits to medical treatment. The rationale behind this conclusion is that it is reasonable to assume that patients must understand the nature of the medical care or they would not submit to it. **Expressed consent** is permission that is either spoken or written. In the healthcare setting, most expressed consent is given in the form of informed consent to treatment, which is addressed in the next section.

Most healthcare providers ask patients or their legal representatives to sign a general **consent to treatment**. By doing so, the patient agrees to submit to routine clinical procedures and medical and nursing care while she is a patient. Except in emergency situations, patients are usually asked to sign a general consent form during the registration and admissions process. More specific consents, also known as **informed consent** to treatment, are required for procedures that involve significant risk. These specific consents require the physician providing the service to explain the procedure to the patient. (See **Figure 5.2**.)

FIGURE 5.2. Example of a combined consent to treatment and consent to the use and disclosure of protected health information

University of Anystate Hospitals

**CONSENT FOR TREATMENT AND DISCLOSURE
OF PROTECTED HEALTH INFORMATION**
PAGE 1 OF 2

PATIENT LABEL

To the Patient (or his/her parent, guardian, or legal representative):

Before University of Anystate Hospitals and Clinics or any of its departments can provide inpatient or outpatient services to you, you will need to understand the services you are to receive, give the hospital your consent to perform those services, and agree to pay for them. You will also need to understand the ways the hospital uses the information in your health record and agree to allow the hospital to use that information.

Part I of this form covers your consent to treatment and explains other important matters related to your healthcare. Part II explains the use of your personal health information. You may ask a member of the admissions staff to read this form to you, and we encourage you to ask any questions you may have about it. When you fully understand the form's content, please sign it in the place indicated on the back of the form. Thank you very much for helping us to fulfill the hospital's responsibility to you and the rest of the community we serve.

Part I: Treatment-Related Information

Consent to the Treatment

You authorize your physician and/or other qualified medical providers to perform medical treatments and services on your behalf. You also consent to all of the hospital medical and/or diagnostic services ordered for you during your outpatient visit or inpatient stay in the hospital. This consent includes testing for infections such as hepatitis B and HIV and providing blood or body fluids for such tests in order to protect you and/or those who care for you.

Payment for Services and Insurance

You are directly responsible for paying for the services provided during your hospital visit or stay. The hospital will work directly with the third parties who provide coverage of your medical expenses, including health insurance companies, Medicare, Medicaid, Workers' Compensation, and various types of liability, accident, and disability insurance providers. By signing this form, you attest that your insurance coverage is current, valid, and effective and that you will promptly pay any required copayment amounts and unpaid deductibles. If your stay qualifies for Medicare coverage, the benefits you will receive include coverage for the physician services that were performed as part of your hospital care.

You guarantee payment to the hospital for all noncovered services and any unpaid, billed amounts not covered by insurance benefits when your insurance plan allows the hospital to bill you for any unpaid balances. You understand and accept that your physician's orders may include services not paid by insurance plans but will be provided to you by the hospital. Also, you accept that insurance plans may deny payment for what you believed were covered services, resulting in your responsibility for paying for these services. You may be billed for the professional component of any hospital services, such as the professional component for clinical laboratory tests.

Valuables

You accept full responsibility for your valuables, especially money or jewelry. The hospital does not accept any liability for your valuables. The hospital expects you will entrust any valuables to family or friends for safekeeping. Alternatively, you may deposit them in the safe that the hospital provides for that purpose. This is especially important when you are an inpatient, but this responsibility also extends to when you are an outpatient and must change into a hospital gown, remove jewelry, or undergo sedation during a medical procedure.

Special Note for Medicare or CHAMPUS Beneficiaries

You acknowledge and certify by your signature that all of the information you have provided to the hospital for Medicare or CHAMPUS benefits is correct. You also agree to allow the hospital or others who have information on your Medicare or CHAMPUS benefits claim to provide this information to Medicare or CHAMPUS or their agents in order for them to determine your eligibility for benefits. To carry out this activity, the hospital may use a copy rather than the original of this consent form. You also acknowledge that you have received a copy of the *Important Message from Medicare* or the *Important Message from CHAMPUS* form. This acknowledgement does not waive your rights for a review or make you liable for payment.

FIGURE 5.2. (continued)

University of Anystate Hospitals

**CONSENT FOR TREATMENT AND DISCLOSURE
OF PROTECTED HEALTH INFORMATION**
PAGE 2 OF 2

PATIENT LABEL

Part II: Health Record-Related Information

Consent to the Use and Disclosure of Protected Health Information

You agree to honestly, completely, and correctly provide all requested information. You also agree to permit the hospital to share your health record as applicable under the law with your physician, your insurers, Medicare, Medicaid, or their designated agents. They may review your record and copy it in full or in part in order to obtain billing and payment information. Insurers (private or government) may also use your health record to determine whether they cover your services. You agree to allow the hospital to use the record created during this visit to meet any reporting requirements related to your care and to collect payment for the services you received. You agree to allow your physicians to send copies of your health records to other physicians, hospitals, and healthcare facilities as they deem necessary for continuity of care. You also agree to have your name posted on scheduling boards and outside your hospital room.

Specific Uses of Your Protected Information

The hospital originates and maintains health records describing your health history, symptoms, examination and test results, diagnoses, treatment, and any plans for future care or treatment. This information serves as:

- The basis of care planning and treatment

- A means of communication among the many healthcare professionals who contribute to your care

- A source of information for applying diagnosis and surgical information to your bill

- A means by which a third-party payer (usually your insurance company or a government healthcare program) can verify that the services billed were actually provided

- A tool for routine healthcare operations, such as assessing quality and reviewing the competence of healthcare professionals

Your signature acknowledges that you received the *Notice of Information Practices,* which provides a description of information uses and disclosure practices. You accept and understand that:

- You have the right to review the notice prior to signing this consent.

- The hospital reserves the right to change the notice and its information practices, for past, current, or future information. The new notice will contain the effective date on its first page and be made available on our Web site.

- You have the right to object to the use of your health information for the hospital's patient directory.

- You have the right to request restrictions on the use or disclosure of your health information to carry out treatment, payment, or healthcare operations and to correct error(s) in your record. The hospital, however, is not required to agree to the restrictions requested.

- You may revoke in writing the consent that you provide to the hospital. The revocation does not apply to any uses of your information made by the hospital in reliance upon this consent form and on the belief that your consent was still effective.

I certify that I have read (or had read to me) both parts of this form and fully understand and agree to the content.

Patient/Agent: _____ Date: _____

If you are signing as the patient's agent, please state your relationship to the patient (parent, guardian, or legal representative): _____

Witness (when form is accepted verbally,
by telephone, or by electronic means): _____ Date: _____

CONSENT FOR TREATMENT AND DISCLOSURE
000002 (11/2002)

Informed Consent

Special consents, known as informed consent, are required for procedures that involve a significant risk for the patient, such as invasive diagnostic tests, transfusions, and surgical procedures. Medical staff rules and/or hospital policies usually list which types of services always require written documentation of the patient's informed consent. In general, the following types of procedures usually require informed consent:

- Procedures that involve the use of anesthetics

- Treatments that involve the use of experimental drugs

- Surgical procedures that involve the manipulation of organs and tissues

- Procedures that involve a significant risk for complications

- Procedures that involve the use of blood and blood products

In addition, some states require documentation of the patient's written consent for specific types of diagnostic procedures; for example, HIV testing.

It is primarily the responsibility of the patient's physician or surgeon to explain the nature of the specific procedure to be performed. The physician should make sure that the patient or the patient's legal representative understands the procedure's potential risks, complications, and benefits. Patients or their representatives should also be made aware of the comparative risks and benefits of any alternative treatments that are available. Only then should the patient or the patient's representative be asked to sign and date the consent form.

All informed consents become a permanent part of the patient's health record. The content of the consent form varies according to the type of procedure to be performed, but most include at least the following information:

- Patient identification, including name and record number

- Name of the individual providing informed consent to the patient

- Name of the procedure to be performed

- Name of the person who is to perform the procedure, if applicable

- Description of the procedure to be performed in language that the patient can understand

- Benefits and risks associated with the procedure

- Alternatives to the procedure

- Date the procedure is to be performed

- Patient's or representative's signature (with a note on the representative's relationship to the patient)

- Date the consent was signed

Consent in Specific Psychiatric Cases

Generally, the patient decides whether to consent to or forgo treatment. Two assumptions apply, however:

1. The patient is competent under the law.

2. An emergency situation is not present.

In the case of a patient declared incompetent by a court of law, state law provides the order of individuals who may serve to authorize treatment and disclosure.

Consents Related to Confidential Health Information

Since the implementation of the HIPAA (1996), hospitals and other healthcare organizations have been required to provide information to patients about the facility's use of the patient's confidential health information, known as protected health information (PHI). The explanation must be provided in the form of a **notice of privacy practices**. The notice must describe how the patient's health information will be used, and it must provide examples of those uses in hospital treatment, operations, and reimbursement. (See **Figure 5.3**.) HIPAA mandates a minimum set of privacy protections for all patients, including the right to

- Obtain and inspect a copy of the patient's own health record

- Request a correction of inaccurate health information

- Find out where the patient's health information has been shared for purposes other than care, payment, or healthcare administrative uses.

- Request special restrictions on the use or disclosure of the patient's health information

- Receive a notice that tells the patient how health information may be used and shared

The patient keeps the notice of privacy practices for his own reference. However, the patient signs the signature page from the notice, which is then kept on file in his health record as evidence that he received and read the notice of privacy practices.

Advance Directives

The admissions staff is required to ask patients whether they have established advance directives and to inform patients that they have the right to accept or refuse medical treatment. An **advance directive** is a written document that describes the patient's healthcare preferences in the event that she becomes unable to communicate. Advance directives include such items as living wills and statements of the patient's wishes in case of a critical illness (for example, whether the patient would want measures such as life support, ventilator support, and food and hydration administered via feeding tubes).

Hospitals are also required to provide written information to patients explaining hospital policies regarding advance directives. The information must describe the treatment decisions that patients may make and any related hospital policies.

FIGURE 5.3. Example of acknowledgement of notice of privacy practices

Anytown Community Hospital

**ACKNOWLEDGMENT OF NOTICE
OF PRIVACY PRACTICES**

PATIENT LABEL

I understand that as part of my healthcare, this organization originates and maintains health records describing my health history, symptoms, examination and test results, diagnoses, treatment, and any plans for future care or treatment. I understand that this information serves as:

- A basis for planning my care and treatment
- A means of communication among the many health professionals who contribute to my care
- A source of information for applying my diagnosis and surgical information to my bill
- A means by which a third-party payer can verify that services billed were actually provided
- And a tool for routine healthcare operations such as assessing quality and reviewing the competence of healthcare professionals

I understand and have been provided with a *Notice of Information Practices* that provides a more complete description of information uses and disclosures. I understand that I have the right to review the notice prior to signing this consent. I understand that the organization reserves the right to change their notice and practices and prior to implementation will mail a copy of any revised notice to the address I've provided. I understand that I have the right to object to the use of my health information for directory purposes. I understand that I have the right to request restrictions as to how my health information may be used or disclosed to carry out treatment, payment, or healthcare operations and that the organization is not required to agree to the restrictions requested. I understand that I may revoke this consent in writing, except to the extent that the organization has already take action in reliance thereon.

☐ I request the following restrictions to the use or disclosure of my health information:

_____

_____

_____
Signature of Patient or Legal Representative   Date

_____
Witness   Date

_____
Notice Effective Date or Version

☐ Accepted   ☐ Denied

_____ _____ _____
Signature   Title   Date

ACKNOWLEDGMENT OF PRIVACY NOTICE
100093 (1/2002)

When a patient has executed an advance directive or living will, federal law also requires that that fact be noted in the patient's health record. A copy of the document may be included in the record, but this is not required. Documentation by the physician that the patient's physician has discussed the patient's wishes with the patient or the patient's next of kin constitutes sufficient health record documentation.

Patient's Rights Information

The Medicare Conditions of Participation (CMS 2010) require hospitals to provide patients with a **patient's rights** statement at the time of admission. According to the Medicare Patient Bill of Rights, patients have the following rights (Medicare 2010):

- **The Right to Information.** Patients have the right to receive accurate, easily understood information to assist them in making informed decisions about their health plans, facilities, and professionals.

- **The Right to Choose.** Patients have the right to a choice of healthcare providers. This choice must be sufficient to ensure access to appropriate high-quality healthcare, including access for women to qualified specialists such as obstetricians/gynecologists and access to specialists for patients with serious medical conditions and chronic illnesses.

- **The Right to Access Emergency Services.** Patients have the right to access emergency health services when and where the need arises. Health plans should provide payment when a patient presents himself to any emergency department with acute symptoms or pain—symptoms a "prudent layperson" ascertains may seriously impair a person's health if untreated.

- **The Right to Be a Full Partner in Healthcare Decisions.** Patients have the right to fully participate in all decisions related to their healthcare. Consumers who are unable to fully participate in treatment decisions have the right to have parents, guardians, family members, or other conservators represent them. Additionally, provider contracts should not contain any gag clauses that restrict health professionals' ability to discuss and advise patients on medically necessary treatment options.

- **The Right to Care Without Discrimination.** Patients have the right to considerate, respectful care from all members of the healthcare industry under all circumstances. Consistent with policy benefits and legal mandates, healthcare providers may not discriminate against patients in marketing, enrolling, or providing healthcare services based on race, ethnicity, national origin, religion, sex, age, current or anticipated mental or physical disability, sexual orientation, genetic information, or payment source.

- **The Right to Privacy.** Patients have the right to communicate with healthcare providers in confidence and to have the confidentiality of their individually identifiable healthcare information protected. Patients also have the right to review and copy their own health records and request amendments to their records.

- **The Right to Speedy Complaint Resolution.** Patients have the right to a fair and efficient process for resolving differences with their health plans, healthcare providers, and the institutions that serve them, including a rigorous system of internal review and an independent external review

All Medicare beneficiaries receive a copy of the Medicare Patient Bill of Rights. Many states have enacted a Patient Bill of Rights for all patients treated in the state. These states require hospitals to provide all patients with a copy of the state- or hospital-specific Patient Bill of Rights. In some cases, patients may be asked to sign an acknowledgment that they received a copy.

Other Administrative Information

Some hospitals ask patients to sign a release that absolves the facility of any responsibility for the loss or damage of personal property. This form is signed during the admissions process and then becomes part of the patient's health record.

Birth and death certificates are not considered part of the legal health record, although copies may be stored in patients' records. Hospital personnel often prepare this administrative documentation and submit it to state and local departments of health, where the records are stored.

Clinical Information

This section provides an overview of who, in the hospital setting, is responsible for documenting in a patient's health record. The regulations and policies that determine the content are also addressed briefly. Chapter 8 provides a more detailed description of regulatory and accreditation requirements. This introductory information is followed by a detailed description and examples of clinical reports in the patient health record.

Who Documents in the Health Record?

The most important function of the health record is the collection of information on the patient's medical condition and progress throughout her treatment. Every clinician who provides care to the patient must document that care in the patient's health record. The record serves as the primary means of communication among all physicians, clinicians, and other individuals who provide services to the patient during her hospital stay.

The clinicians who most commonly document in a patient's health record include the emergency department physician, if the patient is admitted through the emergency department; the admitting physician (who may also be the patient's primary care physician); specialists such as neurologists and cardiothoracic surgeons; nurses; nurse practitioners; and physician assistants. A detailed list follows of healthcare practitioners likely to document in a patient's health record in the hospital setting.

- **Attending physicians.** The attending physician is responsible for coordinating the patient's overall healthcare during the hospital stay. He orders any necessary consultations with specialists and coordinates care among them. The attending physician is also responsible for documenting orders for the patient's discharge from the hospital. An attending physician in the hospital may be a patient's personal or primary care physician. However, some hospitals employ physicians known as **hospitalists** who are responsible for coordinating the care of patients in the hospital.

- **Surgeons.** If a patient has a surgical procedure, the surgeon is responsible for documenting the reason for surgery, explaining risks of the procedure, and obtaining informed consent from the patient. The surgeon also documents the details of the procedure performed on the patient.

- **Specialists.** Specialist physicians are also called *consulting physicians*. The consultant is an expert in the area in which the patient is suspected to have a problem. Examples of specialists include cardiologists, neurologists, endocrinologists, and gastroenterologists. Generally, a specialist physician will evaluate the patient in response to a request by the patient's attending physician.

- **Mid-Level Practitioners: Nurse Practitioners and Physician Assistants.** The mid-level practitioner is a licensed healthcare provider who provides care that is often at a higher level than what a registered nurse (RN) can provide, but less than what a physician provides. Physician assistants and nurse practitioners are mid-level practitioners. Mid-level practitioners may obtain and document a patient's history and physical. In some states, they may be licensed to order tests and/or medications.

- **Unit nurses.** In the inpatient hospital setting, nurses provide continuity of the patient's care. Present on all hospital units 24 hours a day, they regularly monitor vital signs and implement physician orders, such as administering medication. Nurses provide significant documentation in the patient's record, including times and dosages of medication and observations of the patient's condition.

- **Radiologists.** The radiologist is the physician who reads and interprets X-rays, magnetic resonance imaging (MRI) scans, computed tomography (CT) scans, and other images. He generally does not provide direct treatment to the patient. Rather, he is in direct contact with the X-ray film, MRI reading, or CT scan output. The radiologist reads and interprets each test and then documents his impression or diagnosis in a formal report.

- **Pathologists.** The pathologist is another physician who provides indirect treatment. She works in the laboratory, analyzing tissue or body fluid removed during surgery. If the pathologist does not find any abnormalities, she documents a negative report. If she does find abnormalities, she documents her impression and a suspected or confirmed diagnosis.

- **Therapists.** Like other clinical specialists, therapists evaluate and treat a patient based on the patient's needs and the physician's orders. Examples of therapists include physical therapists, respiratory therapists, speech therapists, and occupational therapists. Each of these clinicians documents his evaluation of the patient's condition in a formal report called a *consultation*. In addition, whenever a therapist provides treatment, he documents the details of the treatment in the patient's record.

Everyone on the patient's healthcare team needs to know about *all* of the diagnoses, treatments, and reports completed by the other members of the team and filed in the patient's record. The health record is the vital instrument containing all healthcare data about the patient.

Who Regulates Health Record Content?

The content of the patient record is regulated by governmental agencies and accrediting bodies. Specifically, the entities that regulate clinical content of the patient health record for acute care hospitals are the federal government, state departments of health, and The Joint Commission. Of these, governmental requirements are mandatory and Joint Commission requirements are mandatory for those hospitals seeking to be accredited by the organization. General information about each entity appears in the following list, and more detail can be found in chapter 8.

- **The federal government:** Centers for Medicare and Medicaid Services via the Medicare Conditions of Participation. The Conditions of Participation are published in the *Federal Register* (CFR), Title 42, and, among other things, identify the minimum clinical content requirements for patient health records. Section 482.24 of the Conditions of Participation address health record services and content. Specifically, the section identifies the minimum content for the patient health record. (See **Figure 5.4**.)

- **The Joint Commission:** The Joint Commission is a not-for-profit, standards-setting organization. It provides accreditation and evaluation services for most types of healthcare provider sites. Joint Commission standards for health record content are found in the "Record of Care, Treatment and Services" section of the accreditation manual. Accreditation by The Joint Commission is voluntary. But because accreditation provides evidence to patients and the community that the hospital meets certain standards of care and patient safety, over 80 percent of hospitals in the United States are currently accredited. Accreditation by The Joint Commission allows for continued participation in the Medicare reimbursement plan without an annual Medicare review.

- **Medical staff bylaws:** These are a collection of guidelines adopted by a hospital's medical staff to govern its business conduct and the rights and responsibilities of its members (LaTour and Eichenwald Maki 2010). The bylaws are approved by the board of trustees or governing body in every type of healthcare facility. In addition to describing the organization's manner of operation, the bylaws outline the content of patient health records, identify the exact personnel who can enter information into the records, and restate applicable Joint Commission and Centers for Medicare and Medicaid Services requirements. In addition, bylaws describe the time limits for completing patient health records. All medical staff personnel are required to abide by the approved bylaws. Bylaws must, at the least, reflect the minimum requirements of federal, state, and local laws, along with Joint Commission standards, if the facility is accredited by the Joint Commission.

FIGURE 5.4. Medicare Conditions of Participation: Medical record content

---

Title 42: Public Health

PART 482—CONDITIONS OF PARTICIPATION FOR HOSPITALS

Subpart C—Basic Hospital Functions

§ 482.24 Condition of Participation: Medical Record Services

The hospital must have a medical record service that has administrative responsibility for medical records. A medical record must be maintained for every individual evaluated or treated in the hospital.

a. *Standard: Organization and staffing.* The organization of the medical record service must be appropriate to the scope and complexity of the services performed. The hospital must employ adequate personnel to ensure prompt completion, filing, and retrieval of records.

b. *Standard: Form and retention of record.* The hospital must maintain a medical record for each inpatient and outpatient. Medical records must be accurately written, promptly completed, properly filed and retained, and accessible. The hospital must use a system of author identification and record maintenance that ensures the integrity of the authentication and protects the security of all record entries.

   1. Medical records must be retained in their original or legally reproduced form for a period of at least 5 years.

   2. The hospital must have a system of coding and indexing medical records. The system must allow for timely retrieval by diagnosis and procedure, in order to support medical care evaluation studies.

   3. The hospital must have a procedure for ensuring the confidentiality of patient records. Information from or copies of records may be released only to authorized individuals, and the hospital must ensure that unauthorized individuals cannot gain access to or alter patient records. Original medical records must be released by the hospital only in accordance with Federal or State laws, court orders, or subpoenas.

c. *Standard: Content of record.* The medical record must contain information to justify admission and continued hospitalization, support the diagnosis, and describe the patient's progress and response to medications and services.

   1. All patient medical record entries must be legible, complete, dated, timed, and authenticated in written or electronic form by the person responsible for providing or evaluating the service provided, consistent with hospital policies and procedures.

      i. All orders, including verbal orders, must be dated, timed, and authenticated promptly by the ordering practitioner, except as noted in paragraph (c)(1)(ii) of this section.

      ii. For the 5 year period following January 26, 2007, all orders, including verbal orders, must be dated, timed, and authenticated by the ordering practitioner or another practitioner who is responsible for the care of the patient as specified under §482.12(c) and authorized to write orders by hospital policy in accordance with State law.

      iii. All verbal orders must be authenticated based upon Federal and State law. If there is no State law that designates a specific timeframe for the authentication of verbal orders, verbal orders must be authenticated within 48 hours.

   2. All records must document the following, as appropriate:

      i. Evidence of—

         A. A medical history and physical examination completed and documented no more than 30 days before or 24 hours after admission or registration, but prior to surgery or a procedure requiring anesthesia services. The medical history and physical examination must be placed in the patient's medical record within 24 hours after admission or registration, but prior to surgery or a procedure requiring anesthesia services.

         B. An updated examination of the patient, including any changes in the patient's condition, when the medical history and physical examination are completed within 30 days before admission or registration. Documentation of the updated examination must be placed in the patient's medical record within 24 hours after admission or registration, but prior to surgery or a procedure requiring anesthesia services.

FIGURE 5.4. (continued)

> ii. Admitting diagnosis.
>
> iii. Results of all consultative evaluations of the patient and appropriate findings by clinical and other staff involved in the care of the patient.
>
> iv. Documentation of complications, hospital-acquired infections, and unfavorable reactions to drugs and anesthesia.
>
> v. Properly executed informed consent forms for procedures and treatments specified by the medical staff, or by Federal or State law if applicable, to require written patient consent.
>
> vi. All practitioners' orders, nursing notes, reports of treatment, medication records, radiology, and laboratory reports, and vital signs and other information necessary to monitor the patient's condition.
>
> vii. Discharge summary with outcome of hospitalization, disposition of case, and provisions for follow-up care.
>
> viii. Final diagnosis with completion of medical records within 30 days following discharge.
>
> 51 FR 22042, June 17, 1986, as amended at 71 FR 68694, Nov. 27, 2006; 72 FR 66933, Nov. 27, 2007.

Source: CMS 2010.

Clinical Reports in Health Records

Many different clinical reports are included in a patient health record. The reports described in the sections that follow are ordered first by the clinician responsible for the documentation of the report. For example, the first reports described are the patient history and physical, which the attending physician is responsible for documenting. Other reports documented by physicians come next, followed by reports documented by nursing staff and ancillary clinicians. The last part of this section contains descriptions of reports based on the location of service in the hospital. Included in this section are emergency department reports, radiology reports, and specialty department reports such as tests performed in the neurology and cardiology departments.

Medical History

The **history** is the first part of the history and physical, which is generally the first clinical document created for the patient's record. The history is a summary of the patient's illness provided by the patient and documented by the attending physician. The admitting physician is usually also the patient's attending physician. However, in teaching hospitals that employ resident physicians, the resident may take the patient's initial history. In some cases, the physical may be obtained by a representative of the admitting physician—either a physician assistant or a nurse practitioner. In every case, however, the attending physician is ultimately responsible for the content of the history and physical.

When a patient is unable to communicate and the history is provided by a second party, that fact should be recorded in the health record. Similarly, documentation should note that no history could be taken in cases where the patient is alone and unable to communicate. However, a history can be obtained in these cases from exam records from physicians who previously treated the patient.

The purpose of documenting the patient's medical history is to gather background information about the patient's condition. (See **FIGURE 5.5**.)

The physician uses the history and the physical exam to determine her approach to assessing and treating the patient. Generally, all clinicians treating the patient reference the history and the physical exam.

FIGURE 5.5. Example of a history report

University of Anystate Hospitals and Clinics

PATIENT LABEL

HISTORY

Order of Recording:

1. Chief complaint
2. History of present illness
3. History of past illness
4. Family history
5. General history
6. System review:
   Skin
   HEENT
   Neck and thyroid
   Lymphatics
   Respiratory
   Cardiovascular
   Gastrointestinal
   Genitourinary
   Neuropsychological
   Musculoskeletal
   Endocrine
7. Allergies (medications and drugs)

For Children and Adolescents:

8. Evaluation of developmental age
9. Immunization status

Physician Signature: _____ Date:_____

HISTORY
000005 (11/2002)

The physician gathers information for the patient's history by asking a series of questions about the patient's current and past health-related problems and circumstances, such as the following:

- What brought you to the hospital/office today?

- How long have you had these symptoms?

- What were you doing when you first experienced the problem?

- Have you ever had this problem before?

- What medications are you taking?

- Are you experiencing any other symptoms?

The physician attempts to record the patient's responses in the patient's own words to create a subjective account of the illness. Health record documentation of the patient's medical history usually includes the following elements:

- **Chief complaint:** a subjective description of the reason the patient is seeking medical treatment

- **Present illness:** a subjective description of the development of the patient's illness

- **Past medical history:** a subjective account of current and past illnesses, injuries, surgeries, and hospitalizations, including information on current medications and allergies

- **Social and personal history:** a subjective description of the patient's occupation, marital status, personal habits, and living conditions

- **Family medical history:** a subjective description of illnesses that occurred among close family members

- **Review of systems:** a subjective description of other symptoms or illnesses organized by body system

TABLE 5.1 provides examples of the information collected in a complete medical history.

Report of Physical Examination

Generally, the physician or clinician who obtains the patient's history also conducts the physical exam. As with the history, this may be the attending physician or his or her designee (who may be a resident, physician assistant, or nurse practitioner). Regardless of who conducts the initial physical exam, however, the attending physician is ultimately responsible for the content and quality of the exam and its documentation.

The physical exam provides objective information on the patient's condition. The initial physical exam includes an assessment of the main body systems. The physician gathers this information by observing the patient's physical condition and behavior, palpating (touching) the patient's body, tapping the patient's chest and abdomen, listening to the patient's breath and heart sounds, and taking the patient's vital signs. **TABLE 5.2** shows the types of information usually documented for a physical examination. (See also **FIGURE 5.6**.)

TABLE 5.1. Information typically included in a complete medical history

Components of the History	Complaints and Symptoms
Chief complaint	Nature and duration of the symptoms that caused the patient to seek medical attention as stated in his or her own words
Present illness	Detailed chronological description of the development of the patient's illness, from the appearance of the first symptom to the present situation
Past medical history	Summary of childhood and adult illnesses and conditions, such as infectious diseases, pregnancies, allergies and drug sensitivities, accidents, operations, hospitalizations, and current medications
Social and personal history	Marital status; dietary, sleep, and exercise patterns; use of coffee, tobacco, alcohol, and other drugs; occupation; home environment; daily routine; and so on
Family medical history	Diseases among relatives in which heredity or contact might play a role, such as allergies, cancer, and infectious, psychiatric, metabolic, endocrine, cardiovascular, and renal diseases; health status or cause and age at death for immediate relatives
Review of systems	Systemic inventory designed to uncover current or past subjective symptoms that includes the following types of data: • *General*: Usual weight, recent weight changes, fever, weakness, fatigue • *Skin*: Rashes, eruptions, dryness, cyanosis, jaundice; changes in skin, hair, or nails • *Head*: Headache (duration, severity, character, location) • *Eyes*: Glasses or contact lenses, last eye examination, glaucoma, cataracts, eyestrain, pain, diplopia, redness, lacrimation, inflammation, blurring • *Ears*: Hearing, discharge, tinnitus, dizziness, pain • *Nose*: Head colds, epistaxis, discharges, obstruction, postnasal drip, sinus pain • *Mouth and throat*: Condition of teeth and gums, last dental examination, soreness, redness, hoarseness, difficulty in swallowing • *Respiratory system*: Chest pain, wheezing, cough, dyspnea, sputum (color and quantity), hemoptysis, asthma, bronchitis, emphysema, pneumonia, tuberculosis, pleurisy, last chest X-ray • *Neurological system*: Fainting, blackouts, seizures, paralysis, tingling, tremors, memory loss • *Musculoskeletal system*: Joint pain or stiffness, arthritis, gout, backache, muscle pain, cramps, swelling, redness, limitation in motor activity • *Cardiovascular system*: Chest pain, rheumatic fever, tachycardia, palpitation, high blood pressure, edema, vertigo, faintness, varicose veins, thrombophlebitis • *Gastrointestinal system*: Appetite, thirst, nausea, vomiting, hematemesis, rectal bleeding, change in bowel habits, diarrhea, constipation, indigestion, food intolerance, flatus, hemorrhoids, jaundice • *Urinary system*: Frequent or painful urination, nocturia, pyuria, hematuria, incontinence, urinary infections • *Genitoreproductive system*: Male—venereal disease, sores, discharge from penis, hernias, testicular pain, or masses; female—age at menarche, frequency and duration of menstruation, dysmenorrhea, menorrhagia, symptoms of menopause, contraception, pregnancies, deliveries, abortions, last Pap smear • *Endocrine system*: Thyroid disease; heat or cold intolerance; excessive sweating, thirst, hunger, or urination • *Hematologic system*: Anemia, easy bruising or bleeding, past transfusions • *Psychiatric disorders*: Insomnia, headache, nightmares, personality disorders, anxiety disorders, mood disorders

TABLE 5.2. Information typically documented in the report of a physical examination

Report Components	Content
General condition	Apparent state of health, signs of distress, posture, weight, height, skin color, dress and personal hygiene, facial expression, manner, mood, state of awareness, speech
Vital signs	Pulse, respiration, blood pressure, temperature
Skin	Color, vascularity, lesions, edema, moisture, temperature, texture, thickness, mobility and turgor, nails
Head	Hair, scalp, skull, face
Eyes	Visual acuity and fields; position and alignment of the eyes, eyebrows, eyelids; lacrimal apparatus; conjunctivae; sclerae; corneas; irises; size, shape, equality, reaction to light, and accommodation of pupils; extraocular movements; ophthalmoscopic exam
Ears	Auricles, canals, tympanic membranes, hearing, discharge
Nose and sinuses	Airways, mucosa, septum, sinus tenderness, discharge, bleeding, smell
Mouth	Breath, lips, teeth, gums, tongue, salivary ducts
Throat	Tonsils, pharynx, palate, uvula, postnasal drip
Neck	Stiffness, thyroid, trachea, vessels, lymph nodes, salivary glands
Thorax, anterior and posterior	Shape, symmetry, respiration
Breasts	Masses, tenderness, discharge from nipples
Lungs	Fremitus, breath sounds, adventitious sounds, friction, spoken voice, whispered voice
Heart	Location and quality of apical impulse, trill, pulsation, rhythm, sounds, murmurs, friction rub, jugular venous pressure and pulse, carotid artery pulse
Abdomen	Contour, peristalsis, scars, rigidity, tenderness, spasm, masses, fluid, hernia, bowel sounds and bruits, palpable organs
Male genitourinary organs	Scars, lesions, discharge, penis, scrotum, epididymis, varicocele, hydrocele
Female reproductive organs	External genitalia, Skene's glands and Bartholin's glands, vagina, cervix, uterus, adnexa
Rectum	Fissure, fistula, hemorrhoids, sphincter tone, masses, prostate, seminal vesicles, feces
Musculoskeletal system	Spine and extremities, deformities, swelling, redness, tenderness, range of motion
Lymphatics	Palpable cervical, axillary, inguinal nodes; location; size; consistency; mobility and tenderness
Blood vessels	Pulses, color, temperature, vessel walls, veins
Neurological system	Cranial nerves, coordination, reflexes, biceps, triceps, patellar, Achilles, abdominal, cremasteric, Babinski, Romberg, gait, sensory, vibratory
Diagnosis(es)	

FIGURE 5.6. Example of a physical examination report

University of Anystate Hospitals and Clinics

PHYSICAL EXAMINATION

PATIENT LABEL

Date: _____ Age: _____ Sex: _____ Height: _____ Weight: _____

T: _____ P: _____ R: _____ BP: _____

Order of Recording:
1. General appearance
2. Skin
3. HEENT
4. Lymph glands
5. Neck
6. Breasts
7. Chest
8. Heart
9. Abdomen
10. Genitalia
11. Musculoskeletal
12. Neurological
13. Rectal
14. Vaginal

Impression: _____

_____

_____

_____

Course of Action Planned: _____

_____

Physician Signature: _____ Date: _____

PHYSICAL EXAMINATION
000006 (11/2002)

Medicare Conditions of Participation (CMS 2010) require that admitting physicians perform an initial physical examination within 24 hours of admission. Documentation of medical history, consents, and the physical examination must be available in the patient's record before any surgical procedures may be performed (Reynolds and Bowman 2010). To ensure that a facility is meeting all of the time requirements of a history and physical examination, the health information professional should check the state regulations, federal regulations, and medical staff bylaws. Reviewing agencies will hold a facility to the strictest time frame.

The physical examination may also be performed before a planned admission, usually in the physician's office. However, the Medicare Conditions of Participation for Hospitals require that the examination be performed no more than seven days before admission. In addition, a legible copy of the results of the preadmission physical examination must be included in the patient's health record.

Patients are sometimes readmitted to the same hospital for treatment of the same condition. When the readmission occurs within 30 days of the previous discharge, the admitting physician may add an interval note to the patient's record in place of a complete history and physical. An **interval note** includes information about the patient's current complaint, any relevant changes in his or her condition, and the physical findings since the last admission. However, when the patient is admitted for treatment of a different condition, a complete history and physical must be performed and documented. If a patient is admitted more than 30 days after the previous discharge for the same condition, a complete history and physical must be obtained.

Physician's Orders

Physician's orders are the instructions the physician gives to the other healthcare professionals who perform diagnostic and therapeutic procedures, provide nursing care, formulate and administer medications, and provide nutritional services to the patient. (See **FIGURES 5.7** and **5.8**.) These orders may be for medications, diagnostic tests, therapeutic services, ancillary medical services, or medical devices. They may also be for the use of seclusion or restraints. Health record documentation must support the medical necessity of the services and materials ordered. The Joint Commission record of care, treatment, and services guidelines require that orders contain the reason for the order. Orders are changed and updated as the patient's condition progresses.

Hospital-based diagnostic and therapeutic services are provided under the direction of the patient's physician or physicians. In most states, only licensed physicians are allowed to issue orders. In some states, however, physician's assistants, certified nurse practitioners, and psychologists are also allowed to write orders under limited conditions.

State regulations and hospital medical staff policies also stipulate which healthcare professionals may receive and execute physicians' orders. For example, only licensed nurses and pharmacists are allowed to receive and fulfill medication orders in most states. However, most allied health professionals are allowed to accept physicians' orders for services within their area of practice. Examples include nurse anesthetists, physical therapists, and respiratory therapists. Many hospitals permit physicians to communicate verbal orders via telephone. In such cases, state regulations and the hospital's medical staff bylaws stipulate which healthcare practitioners are allowed to accept and carry out verbal orders and how such orders are to be authenticated.

Many hospitals use electronic order-entry systems. The systems include safeguards that ensure the authenticity, accuracy, and completeness of physicians' orders. Such

FIGURE 5.7. Example of a physician's order sheet

University of Anystate Hospital

PHYSICIAN ORDERS

PATIENT LABEL

Drug Allergies

Date and Time	RN Signature	

PHYSICIAN ORDERS
000122 (02/2003)

FIGURE 5.8. Example of a physician's order in electronic format

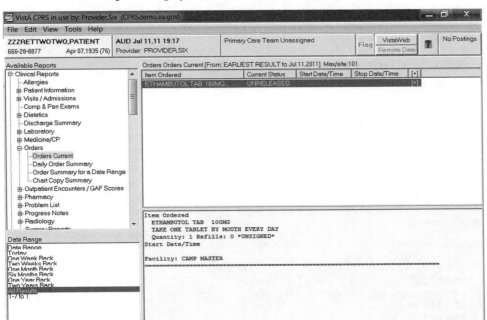

Source: VistA.

computer-based order-entry systems, known as **computerized physician order entry (CPOE)**, are an integral part of EHR systems. CPOE is addressed in detail in chapter 6.

Standing orders are routine physicians' orders that have been established by individual physicians or by the hospital's medical staff. (See **FIGURE 5.9**.) Each standing order applies to a specific diagnosis or procedure. For example, a standing order might be established for the postoperative care to be provided to all patients who have undergone an appendectomy. Some facilities allow nurses to implement standing orders that have been previously approved by the medical staff. Others require physicians to specifically order the implementation of standing orders for their patients, and others may allow an RN to initiate standing orders preapproved by medical staff (Reynolds and Bowman 2010).

At a minimum, physicians' orders must contain

- Date and time of order

- Reason for the order (such as diagnosis, symptom, abnormal test result)

- Instructions/details of the order (for example, medication and dose; X-ray and site)

- Ordering physician's (or clinician's) signature (manual or electronic if CPOE)

- If the order is given verbally or via telephone to an RN, the nurse must sign and the ordering physician must cosign the order, generally within 24 to 48 hours

Physicians' orders, including the physician's signature, must be legible. In addition, an abbreviation may only be used in the order if the abbreviation is included in the list of approved abbreviations for the facility.

FIGURE 5.9. Example of a physician's standing order

Midwest Medical Center

HEPARIN ORDER: REGULAR UNFRACTIONATED HEPARIN FOR ADULTS

PATIENT LABEL

Diagnosis: _____

Allergies: _____

Total Body Weight: _____lb = _____kg

Warning: Due to an increased risk of serious bleeding, patients should not receive both regular heparin and low-molecular-weight heparin.

Patients should also be evaluated for continuance of other medications such as aspirin, clopidogrel, and NSAID therapy.

---

1. Check baseline PTT, PT/INR, heme panel

---

2. Check the appropriate bolus regimen according to diagnosis/disease
   a. ☐ No initial bolus
   b. ☐ Acute coronary syndrome—heparin bolus 75 units/kg = _____ units IV
      (round to the nearest 1000 units—maximum bolus = 10,000 units)
   c. ☐ In combination with thrombolytic therapy for acute MI (TNKase, Retavase, TPA)
      ☐ 5000 units bolus if 65 kg or greater
      ☐ 4000 units bolus if less than 65 kg
   d. ☐ Treatment of DVT/PE—heparin bolus 80 units/kg = _____ units IV
      (round to the nearest 1000 units—maximum bolus = 10,000 units)

---

3. Following bolus, begin IV heparin infusion (check the appropriate regimen):
   • Premixed IV bag contains heparin 25,000 units in 250 ml of D5W (100 units/ml)
   • Maximum initial infusion rate not to exceed 2000 units/h
   ☐ All cardiology regimens: 16 units/kg/h = _____ ml/h
   ☐ Treatment of DVT or PE: 18 units/kg/h = _____ ml/h

---

4. Check PTT 6 hours after initiation of heparin infusion

---

5. Adjust heparin based on guidelines below
   (document all changes on MAR and physician's orders sheet):

PTT (seconds)	Bolus Dose	Rate Changes	Repeat PTT after Each Dosage Change
PTT <35	Bolus 4000 units	Increase rate 200 units/h	6 h
PTT 35–45	Bolus 3000 units	Increase rate 200 units/h	6 h
PTT 46–70	No bolus	No rate change	Next a.m.
PTT 71–90	No bolus	Decrease rate 100 units/h	6 h
PTT 91–100	No bolus	Hold infusion 1 h, then decrease rate by 200 units/h	6 h
PTT >100	No bolus	Hold infusion 1 h, then decrease rate by 300 units/h	6 h

---

6. Check PTT and heme panel every morning (while patient is on heparin protocol).

---

7. Check stools daily for occult blood and notify physician if positive.

---

8. Notify physician for bleeding, hematoma, or heart rate above 120 bpm.

Physician Signature: _____ Date/Time:_____

RN Signature: _____ Date/Time:_____

HEPARIN ORDER
000013 (11/2002)

Special Orders

Two types of special orders are relatively common in healthcare facilities: do-not-resuscitate orders and orders for restraint and seclusion. **Do-not-resuscitate (DNR) orders** are issued when the patient or the patient's legal representative decides that if the patient is near death, no resuscitation attempts should be made when the patient stops breathing. In addition to the order, health record documentation must indicate that the decision to withhold resuscitation efforts was discussed with the patient or the patient's legal representative, when the decision was made, and who took part in making the decision. The patient can make this decision at any time prior to the critical time. When the patient has made the decision and has documented it formally, that document is the patient's living will, as discussed earlier in this chapter.

See chapter 13 for information about restraints and seclusion.

Discharge Orders

Only the patient's attending physician can decide when the patient is ready to be discharged from the hospital. Discharge orders must be documented. When a patient leaves the hospital against medical advice, a note describing the situation should be included in the patient's health record. Similarly, when a patient dies, a note should be added to the health record in lieu of a discharge order. (See **Figure 5.10.**)

Progress Notes

Progress notes are the records of clinical observations of the patient in the hospital. In the ambulatory setting, the terms *encounter* or *visit note* are used. They are recorded in chronological order by every physician and clinician who sees or treats the patient. Generally, notes from all physicians and clinicians treating a patient are recorded in the same section of the record. When notes of different types of clinicians are recorded in the same section, these are known as interdisciplinary progress notes. The purpose of this documentation is to create a chronological record of the patient's condition and response to treatment during his entire hospital stay or episode of care. The progress notes also allow clinicians to efficiently communicate their observations to other members of the healthcare team.

The collection of information on the patient's progress is also required for reimbursement purposes. This information justifies the patient's continued stay and treatment, and it supports the medical necessity of the services provided. The progress notes should indicate why medical intervention was required and why that intervention needed to be performed in a specific type of setting. They should support the logic behind the patient's care and demonstrate how the services were planned and coordinated.

The rules of the hospital's medical staff specify which healthcare professionals are allowed to enter clinical documentation into the health record. Typically, the patient's principal physician, consulting physicians, house medical staff, nurses, dietitians, social workers, and clinical therapists are authorized to create and access health record documentation. Like physicians, nurses and allied health professionals sign and date all of their record entries and include their credentials after their names. (See **Table 5.3**.)

Progress notes include the following types of information:

- Patient's health status on admission and discharge

- Findings of physical examinations

FIGURE 5.10. Example of a discharge order

University of Anystate Hospitals

PHYSICIAN ORDERS

PATIENT, PETUNIA P.
000000001
DOB: 08/14/1949

Drug Allergies: *Codeine*

Date/Time	RN Signature	Physician Order/Physician Signature

10/11/200X
 	
6:00 a.m.
	Claire Barton, RN	(1) Admit via surgery (2) NPO
		(3) CBC, urinalysis (4) BCP 8
		(5) Prothrombin time, PTT (6) Type and screen
		(7) PA chest X-ray
		(8) EKG
		  (9) Prep abdomen
		(10) Start IV fluids: 1000 cc D5LR at 125 cc/h via 18g Jelco
		(11) Mefoxin 2 g IV at 7:45 a.m.
		        Myron P Gynsurg MD 10/11/200x

10/11/200X 10:00 a.m.	Claire Barton, RN	(12) Morphine sulfate 2 mg PCA IV RR q.1.0-1.5.h. (13) Mefoxin 2 g IV in 8 h then discontinue (14) D5LR 1000 cc at 125 cc/h (15) Liquid diet (16) Bed rest (17) Vital signs every 4 h Myron P Gynsurg MD 10/11/200x
10/11/200x 2:00 p.m.	Nancy Nurse, RN	Telephone order from Dr. Gynesurg: (18) Morphine sulfate 2 mg IV push Myron P Gynsurg MD 10/12/200x
10/11/200x 3:00 p.m.	Nancy Nurse, RN	Telephone order from Dr. Gynesurg: (19) Temporarily discontinue PCA pump until vital signs return to normal (20) Vital signs every hour Myron P Gynsurg MD 10/12/200x
10/12/200x 12:05 p.m.	Nancy Nurse, RN	(21) Remove Foley (22) Begin to ambulate (23) Soft diet (24) Vital signs every 4 h Myron P Gynsurg MD 10/12/200x
10/13/200x 12:15 p.m.	Nancy Nurse, RN	(25) Discontinue morphine (26) Darvacet-N 100 mg, one or two tablets q.4h. as needed for pain (27) Solid diet Myron P Gynsurg MD 10/13/200x
10/14/200x 8:00 a.m.	Nancy Nurse, RN	(28) Discontinue IVs (29) Discharge to home—see discharge instruction sheet Myron P Gynsurg MD 10/12/200x

PHYSICIAN ORDERS
000010 (11/2002)

TABLE 5.3. Clinical credentials of healthcare professionals who write health record documentation

Credential	Abbreviation	Health Record Documentation
Registered nurse	RN	Nursing assessments, progress notes, medication records, vital signs, care plans, transfer records, flowcharts
Licensed practical nurse or licensed vocational nurse	LPN or LVN	Nursing assessments, progress notes, medication records, vital signs, transfer records, flowcharts
Nurse-anesthetist	CRNA	Anesthesia records
Nurse-midwife	CRNM	Obstetrical records
Nurse-practitioner	NP	Records associated with specialized nursing practice (pediatric, geriatric, obstetric, and others)
Clinical social worker	LSW	Psychosocial assessments, progress notes
Respiratory therapist	CRT	Records of respiratory therapy, progress notes
Occupational therapist	OT	Records of occupational therapy, progress notes
Speech therapist or speech–language pathologist	SLP	Records of speech therapy, progress notes
Physical therapist	PT	Records of physical therapy, progress notes
Dietitian	RD	Nutritional assessments and plans
Physician assistant	PA	Records of assessments and patient education
Surgeon assistant	SA	Records of assessments and patient education
Pharmacist	RPh	Records of pharmaceuticals and intravenous solutions formulated and dispensed
Clinical psychologist	PhD	Reports of psychological assessments, progress notes
Medical physician	MD	Records of history and physical, orders, progress notes, discharge summaries
Surgeon	MD	Reports of history and physical; orders; progress notes; discharge summaries; and preoperative, intraoperative, and postoperative reports
Radiologist	MD	Records of radiotherapy (nuclear medicine) and imaging results
Pathologist	MD	Records of pathology results and laboratory results and blood bank records
Osteopathic physician	DO	Reports of history and physical, orders, progress notes, and discharge summaries
Oral surgeon	MD/DDS	Records of oral surgery (preoperative, intraoperative, and postoperative reports), orders, progress notes, and discharge summaries

- Observations of vital signs, including pain assessments

- Chronological record of the patient's course, including his or her response to treatment

- Results of laboratory and imaging procedures, along with interpretations and plans for follow-up

- Requests for consultations and reasons for the requests

- Records of patient and family education

- Reports of procedures or operations after the procedure is complete

Documentation of Physicians' Services

In addition to the history and physical exam, physician services are primarily documented in the form of progress notes and consultation reports. Other physician documentation, such as operative reports, reports of diagnostic testing, and the patient discharge summary, are described later in this chapter. This section focuses on progress notes and consultation reports.

Physicians' Progress Notes

All physicians who treat or visit with a patient must record a progress note in the patient's health record as evidence of that encounter. There is no specific requirement for how a progress note is formatted. However, many physicians learn the SOAP (subjective, objective, assessment, plan) format in medical school and residency and may use it when documenting their progress notes. Using the SOAP acronym, the physician may document subjective aspects of the patient's current status (such as the patient's statement of current pain), objective aspects of the patient's current status (such as diagnostic test results), the physician's current assessment of the patient, and the plan for the patient.

The admitting physician assesses the patient's condition early in the hospitalization or episode of treatment .The initial progress note is often referred to as the initial assessment and can be treated as the history and physical until the formal history and physical are transcribed and filed in the patient's record. After the initial assessment note, the physician's clinical decision making is documented in additional progress notes.

Physicians must document a progress note every time they visit with or provide treatment to the patient, and progress notes should be documented at least daily. Progress notes may include any or all of the following, depending upon the patient's current clinical status:

- Current status or daily progress

- Reactions to treatment

- Results of diagnostic tests

- Revisions in treatment plans

- Conversations with the patient or the patient's family

The final progress note provided by the physician is the discharge note, and it describes the patient's status at discharge along with any special instructions for post-discharge care.

Consultation Reports

Physicians often seek the advice of physician specialists before making final diagnostic and therapeutic decisions. For example, a family practice physician may request a consultation from a cardiologist for a patient with acute chest pain. The patient's attending physician documents the consultation request in the patient's record in the form of an order. The consulting physician then documents his or her examination of the patient in a consultation report, which becomes part of the patient's record. The consulting physician may discuss the case with the requesting physician to arrive at a mutual diagnostic decision or treatment plan. The consultant's follow-up findings and recommendations may also be documented in progress notes in the patient's record.

Consultation reports usually contain the following types of information (see **Figure 5.11** for an example):

- Name of the physician who requested the consultation and the reason for the consultation

- Date and time the consultant examined the patient

- Pertinent findings of the examination

- Consultant's opinion, diagnosis, or impression

- Recommendations for diagnostic tests and/or treatment

- Signature, credentials, and specialty of the consultant

The Medicare Conditions of Participation (CMS 2010) require the hospital's medical staff to create internal rules regarding consultations. Although, in general, the attending physician decides when or if a patient needs a consultation, some hospitals have very specific requirements that define additional circumstances under which a consultation may be required. For example, consultations may be required on every patient who is critically ill. Physicians responsible for the following types of cases usually choose to request consultations:

- Patients who are not good risks for surgery

- Patients whose diagnoses are unclear

- Patients whose physicians are not sure which treatment regimen would have the most favorable results

- Patients whose illnesses or injuries may be the result of criminal activities

Medical staff rules may also categorize the types of consultations. For example, consultations that allow the consultant to write orders may be considered materially different from consultations that do not allow the consultant to write orders. Medical staff rules also determine whether partners in multispecialty group practices may provide care to another's patients without going through a formal consultation process (Glondys 1999, 59–61).

Documentation of Nursing Services

RNs and licensed practical or vocational nurses maintain chronological records of the patient's vital signs (blood pressure, heart rate, respiration rate, and temperature) and level of discomfort throughout the patient's hospital stay. They also maintain medication records, write progress

FIGURE 5.11. Example of a consultation report

Anytown Community Hospital

CONSULTATION REPORT
PAGE 1 OF 2

PATIENT, BLUTO P.
070095111
DOB: 04/01/1930

I was asked by Dr. Doctor to evaluate Mr. Patient for consideration of left VATS talc pleurodesis.

CHIEF COMPLAINT: Shortness of breath

HISTORY OF PRESENT ILLNESS: Mr. Patient is a 73-year-old male who has a history of metastatic pancreatic cancer. He was found to have left pleural effusion and underwent thoracentesis. He returned with a recurrent effusion. He was admitted on 05/12/200x and underwent left chest tube thoracostomy and an attempt at talc pleurodesis through the chest tube. He has had residual pneumothorax and continues to drain from the left chest tube. He was referred for the purpose of left VATS talc pleurodesis.

PAST SURGICAL HISTORY: His past surgical history is remarkable for Whipple procedure.

PAST MEDICAL HISTORY: His past medical history is remarkable for prostate cancer and pancreatic cancer.

MEDICATIONS: Avalide and pancrease

ALLERGIES: He has no known drug allergies.

FAMILY/SOCIAL HISTORY: Remarkable for being married. He drinks socially.

REVIEW OF SYSTEMS: Remarkable for no history of seizure or stroke, no history of previous pneumonia, no history of previous myocardial infarction, no history of previous liver failure, renal failure. He has had no swelling in his legs.

PHYSICAL EXAMINATION: He is 5 feet 6 inches tall. He weighs 158 pounds. His blood pressure is 126/70. His pulse is 62. His respiratory rate is 20. His temperature is 97.1. His neurological exam is remarkable for a normal affect. He is oriented × 3. His gross motor examination is 5/5 in all four extremities. His head and neck exam is remarkable for no icteric sclerae. He has no oral lesions. His neck demonstrates no cervical or supraclavicular adenopathy. He has no carotid bruits. His chest exam is remarkable for no use of accessory muscles, no dullness to percussion. He has a left chest tube in place with no air leak. He has serous-appearing drainage from his left chest tube. His breath sounds are remarkable for a slight decrease in breath sounds in the left lateral lung. His cardiovascular exam is remarkable for no lift, heave, or thrill. He has a normal S1, S2 without murmurs. Abdomen is remarkable for well-healed Whipple incision. His abdomen is nontender, nondistended without evidence of masses or organomegaly. His extremities are without clubbing, cyanosis, or edema.

His chest CT shows a loculated left pneumothorax with small residual effusion. He has chest tube in place. This is a small caliber tube. His chest X-ray shows loculated left pneumothorax.

FIGURE 5.11. (continued)

Anytown Community Hospital

CONSULTATION REPORT
PAGE 2 OF 2

PATIENT, BLUTO P.
070095111
DOB: 04/01/1930

His laboratory studies are further remarkable for urinalysis that is normal, an EKG that is normal sinus rhythm, sodium of 133, potassium 3.8, chloride 95, BUN 19, creatinine 1.1, PPTT of 11.8, INR of 0.9, PTT of 29.

My impression is that Mr. Patient is a 73-year-old male with metastatic pancreatic cancer status post Whipple. He has a recurrent left pleural effusion. He has undergone previous tube thoracostomy and pleurodesis and now has a residual left pneumothorax and residual chest tube drainage from his malignant effusion.

I have recommended to Mr. Patient that we proceed with left VATS talc pleurodesis today. He understands that his risks include, but are not limited to, death (1–2%), bleeding requiring blood transfusion, infection, prolonged air leak from the cut surface of his lung, and a 30% chance of recurrent effusion. Understanding these risks as well as the alternative of continued drainage, he wishes to proceed today with left VATS talc pleurodesis.

Thank you very much for allowing me to participate in his care.

Signature:

James W. Medman, MD   5/17/200x
                                        Date

d: 05/17/200x
t: 05/20/200x
JWM, MD/mc

notes, and document patient assessments. In hospitals that employ patient-care technicians and nursing assistants, RNs verify any information provided by unlicensed patient-care staff before it becomes part of the permanent health record.

Nursing Assessments

An initial **nursing assessment** is always performed to obtain clinical and personal information about the patient shortly after she has been admitted to the nursing unit. State, Joint Commission, and federal guidelines require nursing assessments within 24 hours. At a minimum, the initial nursing assessment summarizes the date, time, and method of admission and the patient's current condition, symptoms (including level of pain), and vital signs. Most hospitals develop and use a nursing assessment instrument to collect additional information about the patient's physical condition and psychosocial status at admission. The instruments are designed to solicit the following types of information from the patient (see **FIGURE 5.12**):

- Reason for being in the hospital

- Current and past illnesses

- Current medical condition, including the condition of the skin and the level of pain

- Current cognitive status, including ability to communicate and to understand and follow instructions

- Current functional status, including level of physical activity and ability to walk, move, and perform personal care

- Current psychosocial status, including marital status, living arrangements, personal habits (such as smoking, alcohol consumption, and use of illegal drugs), and occupation

- Family history, including information about parents, children, and siblings and their current health status or cause of death

- Current nutritional status, including ability to feed herself and any special dietary requirements or food allergies

- Known drug allergies, including any sensitivity to latex products

- Current medications

- Need for special discharge planning

Care Plans

Current accreditation standards and the Medicare Conditions of Participation (CMS 2010) require hospitals to develop patient-specific care plans. A **care plan** is a multidisciplinary tool for organizing the diagnostic and therapeutic services to be provided to a patient. Care plans are also required in the long-term care setting and other inpatient environments. The purpose of the care plan is to ensure the efficacy and efficiency of patient services and the quality of patient outcomes. Care plans usually include the following elements:

- Initial assessment (medical and nursing) of the patient's immediate and long-term needs

- Statement of treatment goals based on the patient's needs and diagnosis

FIGURE 5.12. Example of an initial nursing assessment

Midwest Medical Center

INITIAL NURSING ASSESSMENT

PATIENT LABEL

Baseline Information

Date:	Time:	Age:	Arrived: AMB WC Stretcher EMS Carried Other:	Primary MD:

Initial/Chief Complaint/History of Present Illness:

T: PO R TM	P:	R:	BP: R L	⊕ O₂ Sats %	Sex: M F	Height:	Weight: Actual: Stated:

⊕ Tetanus/Immunizations:	Pneumococcal Vaccine ☐ No ☐ Yes Most Recent Date:
⊕ Pregnant ☐ No ☐ Yes LNMP:	Influenza Vaccine ☐ No ☐ Yes Most Recent Date:

Allergies: ☐ None ☐ Medications ☐ Latex ☐ Food ☐ Anesthesia ☐ Other

List Names and Reactions:

TB Assessment (Initiate airborne isolation if 4 or more criteria are checked yes)

Persistent Cough > 2 weeks ☐ No ☐ Yes	Abnormal Chest X-Ray ☐ No ☐ Yes	Respiratory Isolation
Fever > 100.4 (night sweats) ☐ No ☐ Yes	Physician Order for AFB (smear/culture) ☐ No ☐ Yes	Ordered ☐ No ☐ Yes
Unexplained Weight Loss ☐ No ☐ Yes	Recent Exposure to Person with Suspected TB or +PPD ☐ No ☐ Yes	

RN/LPN Signature: _____

☐ See Home Medication Orders   Medication/Over the Counter/Herbal History   ☐ Investigation Drugs/Devices

Medication	Dose	Freq	Last Dose	Medication	Dose	Freq	Last Dose

Hospitalizations/Surgeries:

Medical History

Neurological	☐ No	☐ Yes		Sensory Impairment	☐ No	☐ Yes
Cardiovascular	☐ No	☐ Yes		Endocrine	☐ No	☐ Yes
Hypertension	☐ No	☐ Yes		Blood Disorder	☐ No	☐ Yes
Respiratory	☐ No	☐ Yes		Cancer	☐ No	☐ Yes
Gastrointestinal	☐ No	☐ Yes		Psychological	☐ No	☐ Yes
Renal/Urological	☐ No	☐ Yes		Tobacco Use	☐ No	☐ Yes
Gynecological	☐ No	☐ Yes		Alcohol/Drug Use	☐ No	☐ Yes
Musculoskeletal	☐ No	☐ Yes		Infectious Disease	☐ No	☐ Yes
Integumentary	☐ No	☐ Yes		Cough/Cold Past 2 Weeks	☐ No	☐ Yes
EENT	☐ No	☐ Yes		Anesthesia	☐ No	☐ Yes

Source of Information ☐ Patient ☐ Family ☐ Unable to Obtain ☐ Other ☐ Medications Sent Home with Patient: _____

Arrival Date:	Arrival Time:	T: PO R TM	P:	R:	BP: R L	O₂ Sats %: (If applicable)

RN Initial: _____ RN Signature: _____ Date: _____ Time: _____ Unit: _____

RN Initial: _____ RN Signature: _____ Date: _____ Time: _____ Unit: _____

INITIAL NURSING ASSESSMENT
000039 (10/2002)

- Description of the activities planned to meet the treatment goals

- Patient education goals

- Discharge planning goals

- Timing of periodic assessments to determine progress toward meeting the treatment goals

- Indicators of the need to reassess the plan to address the patient's response to treatment and/or the development of complications

Clinical Practice Guidelines and Protocols

Several types of clinical tools are available to support clinical decision making, ensure clinical quality, and facilitate interdisciplinary-care planning. EHRs use computerized clinical decision support tools, which are addressed in chapter 6. Clinical tools include the following:

- **Clinical practice guidelines:** Detailed step-by-step guides used by healthcare practitioners to make knowledge-based clinical decisions directly related to patient care. Clinical practice guidelines are developed with the goal of standardizing clinical decision making. Practice guidelines are based on scientific evidence and research and are issued by authoritative organizations such as medical societies, professional associations, and government agencies (HHS 1996).

- **Clinical protocols:** Treatment recommendations that are often based on clinical practice guidelines.

- **Clinical pathways:** Structured plans of care that help organizations implement clinical guidelines and protocols. Sometimes known as critical paths, care paths, or care maps, they are widely used by institutions hoping to reduce costs and improve quality through decreased variation in practices.

Case Management Reports

In many hospitals, RNs called case managers prepare patient assessments and care plans. Most clinical case managers are highly experienced nurses, many of whom hold advanced degrees. In some hospitals, clinical social workers are responsible for case management functions. **Case management** involves a process of ongoing and concurrent review performed to ensure the medical necessity and effectiveness of the clinical services being provided to the patient. Case managers are involved in care planning prior to and at the time of admission, review the progress of care while the patient is hospitalized, and conduct discharge planning to facilitate appropriate placement of the patient upon discharge.

Nurses' Progress Notes

The nursing staff begins writing progress notes in the patient's health record soon after the patient is admitted to the nursing unit. Because nurses have frequent contact with patients, the progress notes written by nurses provide a complete record of the patient's care and response to treatment. Nurses also ensure the continuity of patient care by confirming that all physicians' orders have been carried out and appropriately documented.

Nurses usually record the patient's vital signs at least every shift, or three times in a 24-hour period. (See **FIGURE 5.13**.) Intensive-care nurses provide continuous patient

FIGURE 5.13. Example of vital signs documentation in graphic format

University of Anystate Hospitals

GRAPHIC VITAL SIGNS

PATIENT LABEL

Date																										
Hospital Day/Postop																										
Hour			a.m.			p.m.			a.m.			p.m.			a.m.			p.m.			a.m.			p.m.		
	°C	°F	12 (2400)	4 (0400)	8 (0800)	12 (1200)	4 (1600)	8 (2000)	12 (2400)	4 (0400)	8 (0800)	12 (1200)	4 (1600)	8 (2000)	12 (2400)	4 (0400)	8 (0800)	12 (1200)	4 (1600)	8 (2000)	12 (2400)	4 (0400)	8 (0800)	12 (1200)	4 (1600)	8 (2000)
Temperature	40.0	104																								
	39.5	103																								
	38.9	102																								
	38.4	101																								
	37.8	100																								
	37.2	99																								
	36.7	98																								
	36.1	97																								
	35.6	96																								

P	
R	
BP	

S&As	a.m.
(time/results)	p.m.

Height: _____ Weight: _____

_____ Bed/Chair/Stand   _____ Bed/Chair/Stand   _____ Bed/Chair/Stand   _____ Bed/Chair/Stand   _____ Bed/Chair/Stand

Stool

		Shift	7-3	3-11	11-7	24-H Total	7-3	3-11	11-7	24-H Total	7-3	3-11	11-7	24-H Total	7-3	3-11	11-7	24-H Total	7-3	3-11	11-7	24-H Total
Intake	Tube Feedings																					
	Oral																					
	Intravenous																					
	Piggyback																					
	Blood																					
	Shift Total																					
Output	Voided																					
	Catheter																					
	Gastric																					
	Emesis																					
	Shift Total																					

GRAPHIC VITAL SIGNS
000029 (11/2002)

FIGURE 5.14. Example of nursing progress notes

University of Anystate Hospitals

PROGRESS NOTES
PAGE 1 OF 2

PATIENT LABEL

Barriers to Patient Education

☐ No Barriers   ☐ Language
☐ Physical   ☐ Reading Difficulties
☐ Cognitive   ☐ Lacks Readiness
☐ Emotional   ☐ Lacks Motivation
☐ Other _____

Patient/Family Instructions		Outcome	Initials	Discipline
☐ Nutrition	P/F			
☐ Medications	P/F			
☐ Activity/Rehabilitation	P/F			
☐ Safety	P/F			
☐ Signs/Symptoms	P/F			
☐ Wound/Skin Care	P/F			
☐ Pre/Postop Care	P/F			
☐ Equipment	P/F			
☐ Procedures	P/F			
☐ Treatments	P/F			
☐ Pain Management	P/F			
☐ PEARLS	P/F			
☐ Other	P/F			

Outcome Key:
1. Able to state understanding and/or return demonstration.
2. Unable to state understanding and/or return demonstration. Continue to reinforce. (See progress notes.)

Date	Time	Discipline	PROGRESS NOTES

Key
CM = Case Manager
CR = Cardiac Rehabilitation
DTC = Diabetes Treatment Center
ETN = Enterostomal Nurse
FSR = Financial Services Representative
HCC = Home Care Coordinator

NSG = Nursing
NSPY = Neuropsychology
OT = Occupational Therapy
PC = Pastoral Care
PHM = Pharmacy
PT = Physical Therapy

RD = Registered Dietitian
RT = Respiratory Therapy
SLP = Speech/Language Pathologist
SW = Social Worker
TR = Therapeutic Recreation

FIGURE 5.15. Example of progress notes in electronic format

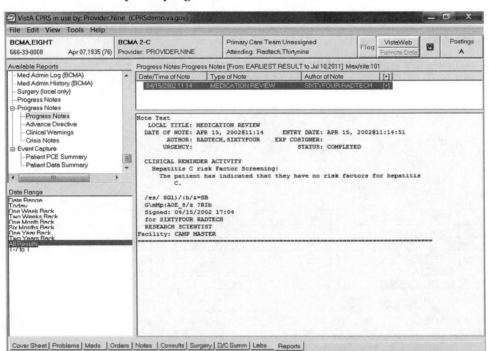

Source: VistA.

monitoring. A complete assessment of the patient's condition is performed every time the nursing shifts change (Reynolds and Bowman 2010). When problems are noted, a member of the nursing staff contacts the patient's physician to determine the appropriate action.

Nursing progress notes are written in a narrative style (**FIGURE 5.14**). They are handwritten in paper-based health records. Many hospitals that have implemented EHRs provide bedside computer terminals to make documentation more efficient and timely (**FIGURE 5.15**).

Medication Administration Records

Nurses keep a separate log for each patient's medications. The **medication administration record (MAR)** includes all of the medications administered to the patient while the patient is in the nursing unit.

The medication record indicates the date and time each drug was administered, the name of the medication, the form of administration, and the medication's dosage and strength. The entry for each medication is signed or initialed and dated by the person who administered the drug.

Surgical patients and others who experience severe levels of pain are sometimes treated with patient-controlled analgesics such as morphine. The medications are administered through a pump that delivers continuous doses controlled manually by the patient. Monitoring equipment automatically records the patient's respiration rate, level of sedation, pain level, pump volume, dose received, and cumulative dosage since the beginning of the monitoring period. (See **FIGURE 5.16**.)

FIGURE 5.16. Example of a patient-controlled analgesia record

Midwest Medical Center

PATIENT-CONTROLLED ANALGESIA FLOWCHART

PATIENT LABEL

Physician Order:

_____	Morphine	1 mg/ml = 50 mg/50 ml
_____	Mependine	10 mg/ml = 500 mg/50 ml
_____	Hydromorphone	1 mg/ml = 50 mg/50 ml

Customized

_____ _____ mg/ml = ___ /50 ml

List Medication   List Concentration

Order Date	Dose	Delay	Basal	1-H Limit	Load	Bolus		Physician
	mg	mg	mg	mg	mg	mg	q. _____ h.	
	mg	mg	mg	mg	mg	mg	q. _____ h.	
	mg	mg	mg	mg	mg	mg	q. _____ h.	
	mg	mg	mg	mg	mg	mg	q. _____ h.	
	mg	mg	mg	mg	mg	mg	q. _____ h.	

Start Date:_____ Signature (MD/RN): _____
Time:_____a.m./p.m. Cosignature: (RN): _____

☐ Check if syringe change only. **Initial Baseline Vital Signs:** BP: _____ P: _____ R: _____ 15 min. after administration: BP: _____ P: _____ R: _____

Date	Time	· R	Sedation Level	Pain Level (greater than or equal to 5 × 2 requires documented intervention)	O₂ Sat. (peds required; adults only if ordered)	Total Given	Syringe Volume Infused	Syringe Infused (syringe volume Infused × concentration)	Loading or Bolus Dose	Initials
	a.m. p.m.						mg	cc	mg	mg	
	a.m. p.m.						mg	cc	mg	mg	
	a.m. p.m.						mg	cc	mg	mg	
	a.m. p.m.						mg	cc	mg	mg	
	a.m. p.m.						mg	cc	mg	mg	

Vital Signs: Date: _____ Time: _____ BP: _____ P: _____ R: _____ *Document additional boluses on BP graphic sheet.*
15 Min. after Rebolus: Date: _____ Time: _____ BP: _____ P: _____ R: _____

Initials	Signature	Initials	Signature	Initials	Signature	Initials	Signature	Initials	Signature

Pain Scale: For the Conscious Patient

0	5	10
no pain	bad pain	worse pain

For Adult Patients: Stop infusion and call physician for respiratory rate of 10/minute or less.
For Pediatric Patients: Stop infusion and call physician for oxygen saturation less than 94% and/or respiratory rate of 14/minute or less.

Pain Scale: For the Pediatric Patient
Wong-Baker FACES Pain Rating Scale

0 NO HURT	2 HURTS LITTLE BIT	4 HURTS LITTLE MORE	6 HURTS EVEN MORE	8 HURTS WHOLE LOT	10 HURTS WORST

Pain Scale: For the Cognitively Limited

Observe	Criteria	Points	Observe	Criteria	Points
Emotion	Smiling	0	Facial Cues	Relaxed, calm expression	0
	Anxious/irritable	1		Drawn around mouth and eyes	1
	Almost in tears	2		Facial frowning, wincing	2
Movement	None	0	Positioning/Guarding	Relaxed body	0
	Restless/slow or decreased movement	1		Guarding/tense	1
	Immobile, afraid to move	2		Fetal position/jumps if touched	2
Verbal Cues	States no pain	0			
	Whining/whimpering/moaning	1			
	Screaming, crying out	2			

Sedation Level: Modified Ramsay Scale
1. Patient anxious, agitated, or restless
2. Patient cooperative, oriented, and tranquil
3. Patient responds to commands only
4. Patient responds to gentle shaking
5. Patient responds to noxious stimulus
6. Patient has no response to firm nail bed pressure or other noxious stimuli

PATIENT-CONTROLLED ANALGESIA FLOW CHART
000031 (10/2002)

Medication errors are not uncommon in healthcare facilities, and such mistakes can have serious consequences. Every medication error must be described fully in the patient's health record. The time the incorrect medication was administered and the names of the correct and incorrect medications involved must be included in the documentation. The patient's response to the incorrect medication must also be documented, along with any treatment interventions performed to address the effects of the medication and the patient's response to the interventions.

Adverse reactions to drugs administered correctly or incorrectly must be documented in a progress note and reported to the patient's principal physician. Most hospitals have policies that dictate reporting of adverse reactions and medication errors to the risk management and performance improvement departments.

New requirements from The Joint Commission (2006) focus on medication reconciliation within the health record. Medications must be reconciled on admission to include name of medication, route, and dosage. Medication reconciliation must include any over-the-counter medications the patient may be taking in addition to medications prescribed by a physician. In addition, medications must be reconciled on moving from one level of care to another, such as from the intensive care unit (ICU) to a step-down unit and at discharge.

Many hospitals have begun to use electronic medication administration record technology (EMAR) to decrease medication errors. **Bar code medication administration (BCMA)** is one such technology. BCMA makes use of a centralized computer system and specific bar code identifiers for each medication. The nursing staff use a scanning device when administering medications to patients to ensure that the right patient receives the right medication. Chapter 6 provides more detail on BCMA and EMAR.

Flowcharts

Flowcharts are graphic illustrations of data and observations. They make it easy to visualize patterns and identify abnormal results and are often used in addition to narrative progress notes for recording the patient's fluid consumption (input) and elimination (output) patterns. Input and output records are especially important in pediatric patients because medications are often based on the patient's weight and may affect input and output. Blood glucose records for patients with diabetes are also maintained as flowcharts. Pain assessments can be charted as well. (See **FIGURE 5.17** for an example of a flowchart.)

Transfer Records

Patients can be transferred from one hospital department to another, for example, from their rooms to the surgery department, and from one facility to another. Nurses maintain records of these patient transfers. (See **FIGURE 5.18**.) **Transfer records** are created whenever a patient is transferred from one facility to another. The records contain a summary of the care provided in the facility from which the patient is being transferred as well as the reason for transfer. A copy of the transfer record is kept in the record of each facility. Transfer records are important to the continuum of care because they document communication between caregivers in multiple settings. It is important that a patient's treatment plan contain accurate and consistent information as the patient moves through the healthcare delivery system.

Diagnostic and Therapeutic Reports

Patients may undergo a variety of diagnostic and therapeutic procedures, depending on the nature of their illnesses. Some procedures are performed as a part of general patient

FIGURE 5.17. Example of a flowchart form

Midwest Medical Center

VASCULAR FLOWCHART

PATIENT LABEL

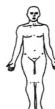 Use diagram to identify graft site

		Date												
Key	RL/LL = Right Leg/Left Leg													
	RA/LA = Right Arm/Left Arm **Time**													
	Graft Site = A, B, C **Extremities**													
Pain	Pain Level (0–10)													
	Homan's Sign (+ or −)													
Sensation	N = Normal NB = Numbness T = Tingling A = Absent													
P	0 = No Pulse 1+ = Diminished 2+ = Normal 3+ = Bounding DM = Doppler Monophasic DB = Doppler Biphasic													
Color	R = Red PK = Pink PL = Pallor MOT = Mottled CY = Cyanotic													
T	H = Hot W = Warm C = Cool CD = Cold													
Capillary Refill	N = Normal (1–3 sec) S = Sluggish (>3 sec) B = Brisk (<1 sec)													
Edema	A = Absent 1+, 2+, 3+, 4+													
Two-Pt. Discrim.	1–10 mm (normal = 3–5 mm)													
Vital Signs	T													
	P													
	R													
	BP													
	Initials													

Initial	Signature	Comments

Signature: _____ Date/Time: _____

VASCULAR FLOWCHART
000032 (10/2002)

FIGURE 5.18. Example of an interdepartmental transfer record

Anycity General Hospital

INTERDEPARTMENTAL TRANSFER RECORD

PATIENT LABEL

Admit/Transfer to Room #: _____ From: _____ Via ☐ Stretcher ☐ Wheelchair

Time Report Given: _____

Date: _____ Diagnosis: _____

☐ Falls prevention protocol must be initiated on unit.

Vital Signs (within 30 min): T: _____ P: _____ R: _____ BP: _____   Pain Scale: _____

Valuables: ☐ N/A ☐ Given to Patient ☐ Given to Family ☐ Other: _____

Assessment

Cardiovascular

Rhythm: _____

Edema: ☐ Yes ☐ No

Where: _____

Amt.: _____

Pulses × 4 3 2 1

☐ Other: _____

_____

Respiratory

☐ Lungs Clear

☐ Lung Sounds Abnormal

Explain: _____

_____

Oxygen Sat. _____ % on room air

Oxygen at _____ liters/min via:

☐ N/C ☐ Mask ☐ Other: _____

☐ Other: _____

Neurological

Responds: ☐ Alert/Oriented × 3 2 1
☐ Verbal
☐ Pain
☐ Unresponsive

Pupils: ☐ ERLA ☐ Other: _____

Weakness: ☐ Yes ☐ No

Where: Right: _____
Left: _____

☐ Other: _____

Gastrointestinal

Abd: ☐ Soft, nontender
☐ Distended
☐ Tender

Bowel Sounds:
☐ All quadrants
☐ Absent
☐ Other: _____

☐ Other: _____

Renal

☐ Incontinent

☐ Foley Size: _____

☐ Dialysis

Type: _____

Intake: _____

Output: _____

☐ Other: _____

Musculoskeletal

☐ Fracture: _____

☐ Dislocation: _____

Immobilization:
☐ Cast ☐ Splint
☐ Traction

Neurovascular Status:
☐ Intact
☐ _____

☐ Other: _____

Integumentary

☐ Intact ☐ Ecchymosis/Redness: _____ ☐ Decubitus/Breakdown: _____ ☐ Wounds: _____

Interventions

IV Access ☐ N/A

☐ INT ☐ IV ☐ Implanted Port

Size: _____ Site: _____

Fluid: _____ Amount: _____ Rate: ____

Other: _____

Drip Infusions ☐ N/A

_____ Rate: _____

_____ Rate: _____

_____ Rate: _____

_____ Rate: _____

Medications ☐ N/A

_____ @ _____

_____ @ _____

_____ @ _____

_____ @ _____

Labs ☐ N/A

☐ CBC ☐ Heme Panel
☐ B/CMP ☐ Fingerstick Glucose
☐ CIP ☐ PT/PTT
☐ UA ☐ Urine Dip ☐ HCG
☐ Hemoccult ☐ Amylase ☐ Lipase

Other: _____

Abnormals: _____

_____

Procedures ☐ N/A

☐ EKG

☐ X-rays ☐ CXR ☐ KUB

☐ Other: _____

☐ Tube Insertion

Type: _____ Size: ____ Location: ____

Type: _____ Size: ____ Location: ____

Other: _____

Miscellaneous ☐ N/A

_____

_____

Infection Control ☐ N/A

☐ Contact ☐ Droplet ☐ Airborne

Equipment Needed in Room ☐ N/A

☐ Oxygen ☐ IV Pump ☐ Suction

☐ Monitor ☐ Other: _____

Nurse Preparing Report

Unit Phone #: _____

Nurse Receiving Patient

☐ Agree with Above Assessment
☐ See Nurses' Notes

INTERDEPARTMENTAL TRANSFER RECORD
000102 (10/2002)

management; for example, basic blood and urine analyses. Other procedures, such as brain scans, are performed to determine the extent and nature of a patient's illness. Surgical interventions are performed to determine the extent and nature of the patient's disease as well as to provide definitive treatment; breast cancer surgery would be one example.

The most common diagnostic and management procedures performed by hospitals include routine laboratory analyses of blood and other bodily fluids, X-ray examinations, and other imaging procedures. Surgical procedures such as biopsies, endoscopic examinations, surgical explorations, excisions, and resections are performed for both inpatients and outpatients. Every diagnostic and therapeutic test or procedure must be ordered by a physician. A report of the test or procedure must be included in the patient's health record.

Ancillary Services

Ancillary services are diagnostic or therapeutic services provided to hospital patients *other than* those provided by physicians or nurses. Diagnostic ancillary services include laboratory, nuclear, radiology, and some cardiology and neurologic testing. Examples include routine blood tests, MRI, electrocardiograms (EKGs), and electroencephalograms (EEGs). Therapeutic ancillary services include services provided by physical, occupational, and speech therapists as well as pharmacy and dietary services. Documentation addressed in this section focuses on diagnostic ancillary services. Therapeutic ancillary services documentation is addressed later in the chapter.

Laboratory Reports: Clinical laboratories routinely examine samples of blood, urine, spinal fluid, and other fluids and substances collected from patients. Laboratory tests require a physician's order. The samples for testing are usually collected from patients by nurses or phlebotomists (technicians specially trained to draw blood samples) and then delivered to the laboratory.

When the samples are received in the laboratory, a medical technologist or another laboratory specialist performs the standardized testing procedures ordered. Medical technologists receive training in four-year college programs, where they learn a combination of manual and automated biochemical analysis techniques. Large clinical laboratories may also employ bacteriologists, biologists, and other scientists to conduct more complex analyses, such as genetic testing.

In hospitals, the results of most routine laboratory procedures are generated automatically by electronic testing equipment. Laboratory computer systems generate reports on the test results, which are returned to the physician who ordered the tests. Paper or electronic copies of the results are also placed in the patient's health record. (See **Figure 5.19.**) Reports of laboratory results include the following information:

- Patient identification, including name and record number

- Name of the test performed

- Date the test was performed and time in and out of the laboratory

- Manual or electronic signature of the laboratory technologist or scientist who performed the test

- Name of the laboratory where the test was performed

- Results of the test

FIGURE 5.19. Example of a laboratory report

Midwest Medical Center

**LABORATORY SERVICES REPORT:
COAGULATION**

PATIENT, WYLIE C.
090241237
DOB: 10/10/1928

ADMISSION DATE:	05/14/20XX
ADMITTING PHYSICIAN:	M. D. Doctor
SPECIMEN DATE:	05/20/XX
COLLECTED TIME:	4:55 p.m.
WEEKDAY:	Tuesday

——ROUTINE COAGULATION——		UNITS	REFERENCE	
PT	**17.6 H**	SEC	11.2–13.8	
INR	1.9			(1)
PTT	32.0	SEC	22.1–32.5	(2)

H = High

Footnotes

(1) The INR therapeutic range (1.5–4.0) for patients on warfarin therapy will depend on the clinical disorder being treated.

(2) Effective August 19, 20XX, the suggested therapeutic range may vary from 40.9–68.3 sec for inpatients on heparin therapy.

In hospitals with clinical computer systems, laboratory test results are available to physicians and nurses as soon as they are generated by the laboratory reporting system. A laboratory summary is available electronically throughout the patient's hospital stay, and a final summary is available soon after the patient's discharge. When health records are paper based, copies of summaries are filed in the paper record.

Imaging Reports: Most hospital imaging departments are equipped to perform X-ray examinations, CT scans, MRI, and positron-emission tomography. Some imaging procedures require radiopharmaceuticals, or radioactive contrast media, to be administered to the patient before or during the procedure to make it possible to visualize physiological processes and tissues more clearly.

Imaging procedures require a physician's order. Most imaging procedures are performed by specially trained radiology technicians. However, the interpretation of scans and images must be performed by a radiologist. The radiologist's written report, signed and dated, becomes part of the patient's permanent record. (See **FIGURE 5.20**.) The original scans and images are generally stored in the radiology department rather than in patient records. However, most EHR systems are capable of storing copies of diagnostic scans and images for easy reference.

Imaging reports generally include the following information:

- Patient identification, including name and record number

- Image identification data, including image number and hospital number

- Physician's order for the test, signed and dated

- Name of the test performed

- Date the test was performed

- Type and amount of radiopharmaceutical administered, if applicable

- Radiologist's interpretation of the images, authenticated by date and signature

Specialty Diagnostic Services

Several diagnostic tests are performed by clinical specialists rather than as ancillary services. The most common are tests related to cardiac and neurological functioning. In every case, the patient's attending physician must order the specialty diagnostic procedure, and the physician interpreting the test results must document the findings in a report that is included in the patient's health record. Specialty diagnostic reports generally include the following information:

- Patient identification, including name and record number

- Physician's order for the examination, signed and dated

- Name of the test performed

- Date the test was performed

- Specialist's interpretation of the test results, dated and signed

Invasive diagnostic examinations, such as angiocardiography and image-guided surgical procedures, require recordkeeping and informed consents similar to those required

FIGURE 5.20. Example of an imaging services report

Midwest Medical Center

IMAGING SERVICES REPORT

OUTPATIENT, OLIVE O.
121212000
DOB: 02/27/1942

EXAM DATE: 5/12/20XX

REFERRING PHYSICIAN: B. Interary

Check-in #: 62

Order #: 1201

Exam #: 36080

FXR: Chest Single View

DIAGNOSIS: V72.84

PA AND LATERAL CHEST: 5/12/20XX

COMPARISON: 6/8/98

FINDINGS: The lungs are clear. The heart and mediastinum are normal in size and configuration. There are minor degenerative changes of the lower thoracic spine.

CONCLUSION: Minor degenerative change of the lower thoracic spine; otherwise negative chest.

Signature: _N~DR~/_   _5/12/20xx_

Norman D. Radiol, MD   Date

d: 05/12/200x
t: 05/14/200x
NDR, MD/na

for regular surgical procedures. Procedures that involve conscious sedation require documentation of the sedatives administered and the patient's period of recovery. The physicians who perform these procedures must write short discharge progress notes in addition to full reports of the procedures and any findings. For procedures performed under general anesthesia, documentation is required for the entire perioperative period. The facility should establish a list of the imaging procedures that require special consents and documentation.

Cardiology Reports: Cardiologists perform and report on a number of different cardiac diagnostic tests performed in the hospital on both inpatients and outpatients. Many patients being treated primarily for noncardiac diagnoses may also have preexisting cardiac conditions that need monitoring through routine electrocardiography. (See **FIGURES 5.21** through **5.23**.) Specialized tests that must be performed and interpreted by cardiologists include the following:

- Exercise and pharmacological stress tests

- Tilt-table tests

- Holter monitoring

- Pacemaker checks

- Echocardiography

- Cardiac radionuclide imaging

- Myocardial imaging

- Cardiac catheterization

Cardiac catheterizations may also include treatment interventions such as the insertion of stents and balloons.

Neurology Reports: Neurologists are often called upon to evaluate the neurological status of patients. Sometimes these patients are being treated for other types of illnesses. For example, neurological dysfunction is common among patients suffering from systemic disorders such as alcoholism, cancer, cerebrovascular and cardiovascular disease, and autoimmune disease. It can be difficult to distinguish neurological impairment from psychiatric illness, so psychiatrists sometimes ask for neurological evaluations of patients with ambiguous symptoms. In addition, because critically ill patients can be maintained indefinitely on cardiopulmonary support after their other systems have shut down, neurologists may be called upon to perform an examination to confirm brain death. (See **FIGURE 5.24**.)

Common diagnostic tests that must be performed or interpreted by neurologists include the following:

- Mental status examinations

- Echoencephalography

- Cerebral angiography

- Myelography

- Lumbar puncture

FIGURE 5.21. **Example of a cardiac catheterization report**

Midwest Medical Center

PATIENT, SYLVESTER Q.
00999067
DOB: 01/03/1960

CARDIAC CATHETERIZATION REPORT
PAGE 1 OF 2

DATE: 05/17/20XX

REFERRING PHYSICIAN(S): M. D. Doctor

PROCEDURES PERFORMED:

1. Left heart catheterization
2. Selective coronary artery study
3. Left ventriculography
4. Insertion of an intra-aortic balloon pump

DESCRIPTION OF PROCEDURE: The patient was brought over from Anyplace General Hospital, where he had been admitted last week with acute respiratory failure. It was felt that it was on the basis of an acute myocardial event. The above procedures were performed. He was taken to the cardiac diagnostic unit at Midwest Medical Center, where the right groin was prepped and draped in the usual sterile manner. One percent Xylocaine was instilled in the region surrounding the right femoral artery. An 18-gauge needle was advanced into the right femoral artery area. Using exchange guide wire technique, a #5 French sheath was placed. This was later exchanged for a #8 French sheath when the intra-aortic balloon pump was placed.

Hemodynamic Data: (1) ascending aortic pressure was 188/62; (2) left ventricle was 188/23-35.

With the patient in the right anterior oblique position, 12 cc of Isovue was injected into the left ventricular chamber. The ejection fraction is approximately 50–55%.

Selective coronary arteriography was performed of both the right and left coronary arteries in multiple oblique projections.

Left Main Coronary Artery: The left main coronary artery was markedly narrowed. The ostium was very significantly obstructed. As the catheter tip barely entered the main coronary artery, the pressure dipped to near 0%. This was confirmed on two further very careful positionings of the catheter. Direct injection into the left main coronary artery was not possible.

Left Anterior Descending Artery: The very proximal portion of the left anterior descending artery shows very high-grade near-total occlusion. The distal vessel is irregular, however, free of high-grade occlusions. There is a large intermediate branch.

Left Posterior Circumflex Coronary Artery: The left posterior circumflex coronary artery was nearly totally occluded at its origin. Minor disease is noted throughout the system.

Right Coronary Artery: The right coronary artery was irregular; however, there was no evidence of significant obstructive disease.

FIGURE 5.21. (continued)

Midwest Medical Center

CARDIAC CATHETERIZATION REPORT
PAGE 2 OF 2

PATIENT, SYLVESTER Q.
00999067
DOB: 01/03/1960

At the conclusion of the procedure, Dr. Surgeon was contacted regarding the possibility of urgent surgery. With Dr. Doctor and Dr. Surgeon consulting by phone, it was elected to place an intra-aortic balloon pump.

The intra-aortic balloon pump was placed without difficulty. Its position was confirmed by fluoroscopy. It appeared to be functioning normally.

During the procedure when the intra-aortic balloon pump was put in, the patient was given 5000 units intravenous heparin and will be on an intravenous heparin drip.

IMPRESSIONS:

1. Relative preservation of left ventricular systolic function at rest with ejection fraction of approximately 50%.
2. Coronary artery disease—three vessels involved
   a. Near-total occlusion of left main coronary artery
   b. High-grade near-total occlusion of the left anterior descending artery proximally
   c. High-grade near-total occlusion of the left posterior circumflex coronary artery proximally
   d. Mild diffuse disease, right coronary artery, as described above
3. Placement of intra-aortic balloon pump in patient with left main coronary artery disease and history of flash pulmonary edema.

Signature:

M. Dennis Heartmann

M. Dennis Heartmann, MD

5/17/20xx

Date

d: 05/17/200x
t: 05/18/200x
MDH, MD/dq

FIGURE 5.22. Example of an echocardiography report

Anytown Community Hospital

ECHOCARDIOGRAPHIC REPORT

TEST, PATIENT
009999999
DOB: 04/01/1930

DATE: 06/02/20XX

REFERRING PHYSICIAN: Dr. Doctor

INDICATION FOR STUDY: Murmur

TAPE: House 528

Outpatient Study

Two-dimensional and M-mode echocardiograms were performed

The left atrium is at the upper limits of normal size at 3.7 cm compared to an aortic root diameter of 2.9 cm. The left ventricle is at the upper limits of normal size with a normal internal dimension of 5.6 cm in diastole and 3.3 cm in systole. There is normal wall thickness. There is hyperdynamic left ventricular systolic performance. The ejection fraction is estimated at greater than 70%. No specific regional wall motion abnormalities were identified. The cardiac valves appear structurally normal. No intracardiac masses were identified and a pericardial effusion was not visualized.

Conventional as well as color-flow Doppler imaging was performed. There are findings of mitral regurgitation which is estimated to be at least moderate to severe, if not severe. There is tricuspid regurgitation with peak right ventricular systolic pressure of 31 mmHg. No other significant valvular stenoses or regurgitation were identified.

IMPRESSION:

1. The left atrium and left ventricle at the upper limits of normal size with a hyperdynamic left ventricular systolic performance.

2. There is evidence of mitral regurgitation which is at least moderate to severe. Would consider transesophageal echocardiography to further assess the severity of the mitral regurgitation as well as potentially its etiology.

Signature:

_____
Philip Default, MD

6/2/20XX
_____
Date

d: 06/02/20XX
t: 06/02/20XX

FIGURE 5.23. Example of an electrocardiography report

University of Anystate Hospitals

GRAPHIC EKG REPORT

PATIENT, PETUNIA P.
000000001
DOB: 08/14/1949

NAME: Patient, Petunia

TECHNICIAN: SKH

PROCEDURE DATE/TIME: 10/06/20XX 9:59:02

CARDIOLOGIST: Julius W. Cardiolini, MD

SEX/RACE: Female, White

REPORT DATE: 10/08/20XX

REQUESTED BY: M. Gynesurg, MD

RESULTS: Normal EKG

PR	200	Normal sinus rhythm rate: 59
QRST	73	
QT	407	
QTc	403	
Axes		
P	28	
QRS	36	
T	35	

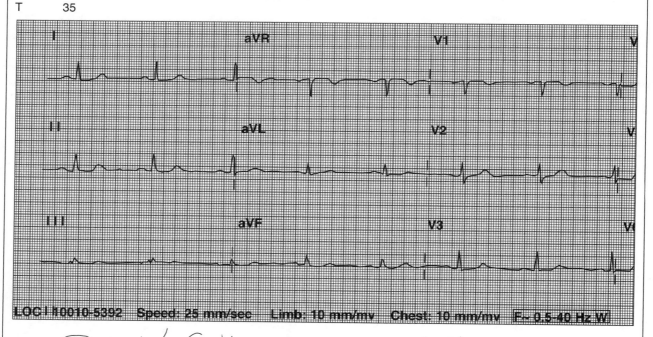

LOC I 0010-5392   Speed: 25 mm/sec   Limb: 10 mm/mv   Chest: 10 mm/mv   F~ 0.5-40 Hz W

Julius W Cardiolini
_____
Julius W. Cardiolini, MD
Cardiologist

_10/8/200x_
_____
Date

FIGURE 5.24. Example of a neurological assessment form

University of Anystate Hospitals

**NEUROLOGICAL ASSESSMENT
AND REASSESSMENT**

PATIENT LABEL

			Date and Time																		

Glasgow Coma Scale

Eye Opening	Spontaneous	=	4														**C** = Eyes Closed by Swelling
	To Voice	=	3														
	To Pain	=	2														
	None	=	1														
Verbal Response	Oriented	=	5														**T** = Endotracheal Tube or Tracheostomy
	Confused	=	4														
	Inappropriate Words	=	3														
	Incomprehensible Words	=	2														**A** = Aphasia
	None	=	1														
Motor Response	Obeys Command	=	6														
	Localizes Pain	=	5														
	Withdraws	=	4														Record Best Arm Response
	Flexion	=	3														
	Extension	=	2														
	None	=	1														
Total Score		3–7 = Severe 8–13 = Moderate 13+ = Mild																

Limb Movement

Grade limb movement either spontaneous or to command. Do not rate reflex movement. Use scale below.

RA															
RL															
LA															
LL															

Limb Movement Scale: 0 = No Response 1 = Flicker or Trace of Movement 2 = Active Movement without Gravity
3 = Active Movement against Gravity 4 = Active Movement against Gravity with Limited Resistance 5 = Normal Power

Pupils	**Reaction**															
Size	C = Closed by swelling	Size	R													
1 mm 2 mm 3 mm 4 mm 5 mm 6 mm 7 mm 8 mm	B = Brisk S = Sluggish F = Fixed		L													
	Shape	Reaction	R													
			L													
	R = Round O = Oval K = Keyhole I = Irregular	Shape	R													
			L													

Ventriculostomy Data	ICP															
	CSF Output															
Key: CL = Clear R = Red	Color															
Y = Yellow PK = Pink CLO = Cloudy	Character															
Vital Signs	Temperature															
	Pulse															
	Respirations															
	Blood Pressure															

Other: _____

Other: _____

Comments: _____

Signature: _____ Date/Time: _____

NEUROLOGICAL ASSESSMENT
000080 (10/2002)

Surgical Services

Hospital-based surgery departments provide services to inpatients and outpatients, although many hospitals maintain separate preoperative and recovery areas for outpatients. The documentation requirements for outpatient surgery (also called ambulatory surgery and same-day surgery) are the same as for inpatient surgical procedures.

Preoperative History and Physical Reports

Except in emergency situations, every surgical patient's chart must include a report of a complete history and physical (discussed earlier in the chapter) conducted no more than seven days before the surgery is to be performed. This requirement is the same for inpatient and outpatient procedures. The report must be present in the patient's chart before surgery can begin. Ideally, advance directives and organ donation forms should also be placed in the chart before surgery.

Anesthesia Evaluations and Records

The anesthesia and/or sedation administered to patients during surgical procedures represent a significant risk independent of the risks involved in the surgery itself. Regulations and accreditation standards require anesthesiologists (who are physicians) and certified nurse anesthetists (advanced practice nurses who work under the direction of anesthesiologists) to perform and document a **preoperative anesthesia evaluation** (preprocedure record and preoperative checklist) for every patient to whom anesthesia is administered. The evaluation, which includes information on the patient's medical history and current physical and emotional condition, becomes the basis for an anesthesia plan that stipulates the type of anesthesia to be used; addresses the patient's risk factors, allergies, and drug usage; and considers the patient's general medical condition. (See **FIGURES 5.25** and **5.26**.)

The professional who is to administer anesthesia to the patient must also perform a reevaluation of the patient's condition immediately before the procedure to confirm that it is safe to begin the operation. The timing and dosage of any preanesthesia medications should also be documented at this point. This reevaluation is part of the preoperative anesthesia record.

The professional administering anesthesia must also maintain an **intraoperative anesthesia record** and vital signs report. The intraoperative record is created while the procedure is being performed. (See **FIGURES 5.27** and **5.28**.) The record describes the entire surgical process and includes the following information:

- Patient identification, including name and record number
- Name of the anesthesiologist or nurse anesthetist
- Type and amount of anesthesia administered
- Induction mechanisms
- Medication log, including medical gases and fluid administration
- Usage of blood products
- Placement of lines and monitoring devices
- Patient's reaction to anesthesia
- Results of continuous patient monitoring, including vital signs and oxygen saturation levels

FIGURE 5.25. Example of a preprocedure record

University of Anystate Hospitals

PREPROCEDURE RECORD
PAGE 1 OF 2

PATIENT LABEL

Preprocedure Care (Day of Procedure)

Date: _____ Time: _____

☐ NPO Since: _____ Voided? ☐ Yes ☐ No

Valuables (check if present, put O if removed)?
☐ Clothing ☐ Dentures ☐ Glasses ☐ Contact
☐ Hearing aid ☐ Hair piece/wig ☐ Jewelry Lenses
☐ Other: _____
☐ Patient was informed hospital is not responsible for lost valuables
Signature of Person Responsible for Valuables
_____

Disposition if no one is present: _____
☐ Responsible adult available to accompany patient at discharge
☐ TED Hose ☐ SCDs/plexi pulse
☐ Skin prep: _____ By: _____

Medication Given Prior to Procedure:

_____ Time: _____ Initials: ____
_____ Time: _____ Initials: ____
_____ Time: _____ Initials: ____
_____ Time: _____ Initials: ____
_____ Time: _____ Initials: ____
_____ Time: _____ Initials: ____
_____ Time: _____ Initials: ____

Douche/Enema: _____ Time: _____ Initials: ____
☐ IV gauge #: _____ Site: _____ Fluid: _____ Rate: _____ Initials: _____
☐ IV gauge #: _____ Site: _____ Fluid: _____ Rate: _____ Initials: _____

Completed by _____

Operating Room Checklist (initial when completed)

_____ ID Bracelet Correct
_____ Informed Consent
_____ H&P
_____ Operative Plan
_____ Site/Procedure Verified with Schedule/MD Order, Consent, and Patient/Representative
_____ Procedure Site Marked
_____ Procedure and Site Verified with Available Imaging Studies by MD, if Applicable (procedure staff)
_____ Patient, Procedure, and Site Verified Verbally Immediately prior to Start by Procedural Team (final "time out") (procedure staff)

For Moderate Sedation and Anesthesia Patients:
_____ Preanesthesia Assessment
_____ Anesthesia Plan of Care

Completed by: _____

Diagnostic Studies
(O if ordered, checkmark if on chart)
☐ CBC ☐ Sed. Rate ☐ Heme
☐ Chemistry ☐ Urine C&S ☐ Potassium
☐ PT, PTT ☐ U/A ☐ Creatinine
☐ EKG ☐ X-rays ☐ T+S
☐ T&C _____ Units Available

☐ Pregnancy ☐ _____
Bedside Glucose: _____
☐ Abnormal Results Called to MD

Completed by: _____

Assessment

Alert and Oriented: ☐ Yes ☐ No (see supplemental nurses' notes)
Suspected Abuse: ☐ No ☐ Yes (see supplemental nurses' notes)
Learning Barriers: ☐ No Barriers ☐ Physical ☐ Religious ☐ Cultural ☐ Cognitive ☐ Emotional ☐ Language (see supplemental nurses' notes)
Pain: ☐ No Pain ☐ Yes, Location: _____ ☐ Onset: _____ ☐ Duration: _____ ☐ Intensity: ____ (1–10) Qual/Characteristics/Pattern: _____
Alleviating Factors: _____ Aggravating Factors: _____ Effects on ADL: _____ Relieved by: _____
Diabetic/Special Diet? ☐ No ☐ Yes (see supplemental nurses' notes)
Recent Mobility Limitation? ☐ No ☐ Yes (see supplemental nurses' notes)

Nursing Assessment (Inpatient) Initiated

Completed by: _____ **RN**

Plan of Care

Potential for Fear and/or Anxiety Goal: Reduction of Fear and Anxiety	☐ Goal Met

☐ Procedures Explained to Patient and Family
☐ Patient and Family Encouraged to Verbalize Concerns and Questions
☐ Patient and Family's Questions Answered
☐ Age-Appropriate Emotional Support Provided

Knowledge Deficit Relating to Procedure Goal: Demonstrates and/or Verbalizes Knowledge	☐ Goal Met

☐ Patient's Level of Learning Assessed and Instructions Modified to Meet Needs
☐ Reviewed Printed Discharge Instructions with Patient and Family
☐ Cough, Turn, Deep-Breathe
☐ PRN Pain Medications/Pain Scale
☐ Patient/Family Verbalize Understanding of Instructions
☐ Age-Appropriate Approach Used in Education

Initials/Signature:
_____
_____

Clinical Pathway Initiated

Potential for Injury Goal: Patient Is Free from Injury	☐ Goal Met

Side Rails Up: ☐ × 2 ☐ × 4 Bed Position: ☐ Low ☐ High
☐ Instructed Patient to Call for Assistance

Potential for Alteration in Fluid Volume Goal: Fluid Volume Is within Normal Limits	☐ Goal Met

☐ IV Access Present, No Infiltration Noted

Privacy/Confidentiality Goal: Privacy/Confidentiality Maintained	☐ Goal Met

☐ Confidentiality of Patient Records, Diagnosis, Procedure Maintained
☐ Patient Minimally Exposed during Preparation

Potential Alteration in Cardiovascular Function Goal: Hemodynamically Stable	☐ Goal Met

☐ Continuous Cardiac Monitoring ☐ Continuous Heart Rate Monitoring

Potential Alteration in Gas Exchange Goal: Adequate Air Exchange	☐ Goal Met

☐ Continuous Pulse Oximetry in Use ☐ Oxygen Therapy Initiated as Ordered

Initials/Signature:
_____
_____

PREPROCEDURE RECORD
000019 (11/2002)

FIGURE 5.25. (continued)

University of Anystate Hospitals

PREPROCEDURE RECORD
PAGE 2 OF 2

PATIENT LABEL

Pediatrics (Neonate through 17 Years of Age)

☐ Grade in School _____

☐ Developmental Milestones Appropriate for Age
   ☐ Yes ☐ No

☐ Security Object/Toys _____

☐ Immunizations Current ☐ Yes ☐ No

Signature: _____

Feeding ☐ Breast ☐ Bottle/Formula ☐ Solids

Type of Formula _____

Primary Caregiver _____

Interaction between Caregiver and Child _____
☐ Calming ☐ Agitative

Signature: _____

Head Circumference _____
        (infants under 1 year of age only)

Further Assessment

Cardiac Rhythm: _____

Preprocedure Peripheral Pulses (Absent, 1+, 2+, 3+, 4+, Doppler)
R DP: _____ L DP: _____ R PT: _____ L PT: _____ R Rad.: _____ L Rad.: _____ Other: _____

Other: _____

Signature: _____

Supplemental Nurses' Notes: _____
_____
_____
_____

Preprocedure Preparation

Type of Procedure: _____ Date Called: _____ Time Called: _____

Date of Procedure: _____ Time of Procedure: _____ Arrival Time: _____

Instructions Given To: _____

Via: ☐ Phone ☐ Appointment ☐ Left Phone Message ☐ Unable to Reach

☐ No Makeup, Jewelry, Perfume, Nail Polish, or Valuables ☐ Medications A.M. of Procedure with a Sip of Water

☐ NPO Status/Time _____

☐ Instructions for: _____
_____
_____
_____
_____

☐ Bring Medications/Inhalers/List to Hospital

☐ Preadmission Diagnostic Tests Done:
   Date: _____ Location: _____

☐ Date/Location Previous CXR: _____

☐ Date/Location Previous EKG: _____

☐ Informed that responsible adult must accompany patient to hospital, transport home, and remain with patient after the procedure

Name of Responsible Person after Procedure: _____

Signature: _____ RN/LPN

PREPROCEDURE RECORD
000019 (11/2002)

FIGURE 5.26. Example of a preoperative checklist

University of Anystate Hospitals

PREOPERATIVE CHECKLIST

PATIENT LABEL

(It is the responsibility of the unit nurse to see that this is completed before the patient goes to the operating room.)

Vital Signs Taken prior to Transfer

Date: Time: BP: T: P: R: O$_2$Sat: Weight: Height:

	Yes	No	Initials		Yes	No	Initials		Yes	No	Initials
Side Rails Raised?	☐	☐	____	Instructed Not to Smoke?	☐	☐	____	Instructed to Stay in Bed?	☐	☐	____

	Yes	No	N/A	Initials
Dentures Removed?	☐	☐	☐	____
Contact Lens Removed?	☐	☐	☐	____
Jewelry Removed?	☐	☐	☐	____
Jewelry Disposition _____	☐	☐	☐	____
Hair Piece, Pins, Clamps Removed?	☐	☐	☐	____
Hearing Aid(s) Removed?	☐	☐	☐	____
Hospital Gown?	☐	☐		____
ID Name Band on Patient?	☐	☐		____
Fenwal ID Band on Patient?	☐	☐	☐	____

Prep Site: _____
By Whom: _____ Checked By: _____
NPO Since: _____ a.m./p.m.
Voided: _____ cc Catheter: _____ cc
Bedside Glucose: _____ Time: _____

If Ordered to Operating Room with Patient

	Yes	No	N/A	Initials		Yes	No	N/A	Initials
X-rays?	☐	☐	☐	____	Meds?	☐	☐	☐	____
Old Charts?	☐	☐	☐	____					
SCDs/TEDs	☐	☐	☐	____					

On Chart

		Initials
Site/procedure verified with schedule/MD order, consent, and patient/representative		____
Procedure site marked		____

	Yes	No	Initials
Informed Consent?	☐	☐	____
History and Physical?	☐	☐	____
Operative Plan?	☐	☐	____
Patient Labels?	☐	☐	____
MARS?	☐	☐	____
Clinical Pathway, if applicable?	☐	☐	____

OR/Procedure Staff Use Only   Initials

	Initials
Procedure and site verified with available imaging studies by MD, if applicable	____
Patient, procedure, and site verified verbally immediately prior to start by procedural team (final "time out")	____
Preanesthesia/moderate sedation assessment completed	____
Anesthesia/moderate sedation plan completed	____

Results on Chart: Preop Diagnostics

	Yes	No	N/A	Initials		Yes	No	N/A	Initials
T&C/T+S ____ Units available	☐	☐	☐	____	EKG	☐	☐	☐	____
CBC	☐	☐	☐	____	X-ray reports	☐	☐	☐	____
Chemistry	☐	☐	☐	____	PT/PTT	☐	☐	☐	____
Urinalysis	☐	☐	☐	____	Physician notified of abnormal results?	☐	☐	☐	____

Preop Medications/IV Therapy

☐ IV gauge # ____ Site ____ Fluid ____ Rate ____ Initials ____

☐ IV gauge # ____ Site ____ Fluid ____ Rate ____ Initials ____

Preop Meds   **Time Given/Initials**

_____   _____

_____   _____

Plan of Care	Clinical Pathway Initiated

Privacy/Confidentiality Goal: Privacy/Confidentiality Maintained ☐ Goal Met

☐ Patient Minimally Exposed during Preparation

Potential for Alteration in Fluid Volume Goal: Fluid Volume Is within Normal Limits ☐ Goal Met

☐ IV Access Present, No Infiltration Noted

Potential for Fear and/or Anxiety Goal: Reduction of Fear and Anxiety ☐ Goal Met

☐ Procedures Explained to Patient and Family
☐ Patient and Family Encouraged to Verbalize Concerns and Questions
☐ Patient and Family's Questions Answered
☐ Age-Appropriate Emotional Support Provided

Potential for Injury Goal: Patient Is Free From Injury ☐ Goal Met

Bed Position: ☐ Low ☐ High
Side Rails Up ☐ × 2 ☐ × 4
☐ Instructed to Call for Assistance

Knowledge Deficit Relating to Procedure Goal: Demonstrates and/or Verbalizes Knowledge ☐ Goal Met

☐ PEARLS for Progress Reviewed with Patient
☐ Cough, Turn, Deep Breath
☐ PRN Pain Medications/Pain Scale
☐ Patient/Family Verbalize Understanding of Instructions
☐ Age-Appropriate Approach Used in Education

Location of Family during Surgery _____

Report Called: Yes ☐ No ☐ N/A ☐ Called to: _____
Miscellaneous Information: _____

Signature of Nurse Transferring Patient to Operating Room

____ Initials _____
____ Initials _____

____ Initials _____
____ Initials _____

PREOPERATIVE CHECKLIST
000018 (11/2002)

FIGURE 5.27. Example of an intraoperative anesthesia record

University of Anystate Hospitals

INTRAOPERATIVE RECORD

PATIENT LABEL

OR #: _____ ☐ SDA ☐ Outpatient
Date: _____ ☐ Inpatient ☐ Add-On (day of surgery)

Preoperative Assessment Reviewed
☐ Agree with Assessment
☐ See Additional Notes

☐ **Patient Confirms Surgical Site**
☐ Yes
☐ See Additional Notes

Allergies: _____

Preprocedure Diagnosis: _____
Postprocedure Diagnosis: _____
Procedure Performed: _____

Times: Room In/Room Out_____ / _____
Anesthesia Start _____ / _____
Procedure Start/Stop _____ / _____

Transferred to/Discharge: ☐ PACU ☐ ICU ☐ Room # _____ ☐ Home
Method of Transfer: ☐ Stretcher ☐ Bed ☐ Other: _____ ☐ Report Called: _____
Condition on Discharge: ☐ Satisfactory ☐ Other_____

Anesthesia:
☐ General
☐ MAC
☐ Regional
  ☐ Epidural
  ☐ Spinal
  ☐ Axillary Block
  ☐ Bier Block
☐ IV Sedation
☐ Local
☐ Other: _____

Personnel Role:
MD: _____
Circ.: _____
Scrub: _____
Anes.: _____
Other: _____
Role: _____

Relief: _____ Time: _____
Relief: _____ _____
Rad. Tech.: _____
Perfusionist: _____

☐ **Potential for Fear and Anxiety**	**Goal: Reduction of Fear and Anxiety**

☐ Perioperative Events Explained
☐ Intraop Family Communication   Time: _____   ☐ Goal Met

☐ **Potential for Injury**	**Goal: Patient Free From Injury**

Intraop Position: ☐ Goal Met
☐ Supine
☐ Prone
☐ Lithotomy
☐ Lateral R
☐ Lateral L
☐ Jackknife
☐ Beach Chair
☐ Other: _____

Safety Strap =
Arm Position →
ESU Pad ∅
Padding #
Pulse Oximeter ☐
EKG ●
BP Cuff X

Positional Aids: ☐ None
☐ Donut
☐ Pillow
☐ Eggcrate Pad
☐ Bean Bag
☐ Lami Rolls
☐ Chest Roll
☐ Axilla Roll
☐ Shoulder Roll
☐ Sand Bag
☐ Stirrups
  ☐ Candy Cane
  ☐ Bierhoff
  ☐ Allen
☐ Knee Holder
☐ Mayfield Headrest
☐ Lami-Frame
☐ Shoulder Holder
☐ Beach Chair Attachment
☐ Fracture Table
☐ Surgita Headrest
☐ Other: _____

Equipment: ☐ None
☐ ESU #: _____ PAD #: _____
  Coagulation: _____ Cut: _____
  Post Op Site: _____
☐ Bipolar #: _____
  Setting: _____
☐ C-Arm/OEC
☐ Phaco #: _____
☐ Cryo #: _____
☐ Laser #: _____
☐ Ultrasound #: _____
☐ CUSA #: _____
☐ Bair Hugger #: _____
☐ Seq. Comp. Mach. #: _____
  Settings _____
☐ Tourniquet #: _____
  ☐ Arm ☐ Leg ☐ R ☐ L
  Applied by: _____
  Pressure: _____ mm Hg
  Time Up: _____
  Time Down: _____

Final Counts:
☐ Correct ☐ Incorrect

Circ. Signature: _____

☐ **Patient Privacy**	**Goal: Privacy Maintained**

☐ Patient Minimally Exposed during Positioning, Prepping, and Draping

☐ **Potential for Infection**	**Goal: Sterile Technique Maintained**

Skin Preparation: ☐ None
☐ Shave _____
☐ Clip _____

Prep: ☐ Goal Met
☐ Iodophor Prep
☐ Iodophor Scrub
☐ Iodophor Gel
☐ Dura-Prep
☐ Other: _____

Skin Condition:
Before Surgery: ☐ Normal ☐ Other: _____
After Surgery: ☐ Normal ☐ Other: _____

Cultures: ☐ None
☐ Aerobic—Site:
☐ Anaerobic—Site:
☐ AFB—Site:
☐ Fungus—Site:

Wound Class:
☐ I
☐ II
☐ III
☐ IV

Lines/Drains: ☐ None
☐ JP/Hemovac/Blake
☐ Chest Tube
☐ Foley
☐ Arterial
☐ CVP/Swanz
☐ NG Tube
☐ Other: _____

Dressings: ☐ Yes ☐ No
_____
_____
☐ Splint _____
☐ Cast _____
☐ Other: _____
☐ **Packing:** ☐ Yes ☐ No

☐	**Miscellaneous**

Meds: _____
_____
_____

Blood Products: ☐ None
☐ PRC _____ Units
☐ FFP _____ Units
☐ Cryo _____ Units
☐ Cell Saver _____

Specimens: ☐ None
☐ Gross Only—Site: _____
☐ Frozen—Site: _____
☐ Fresh—Site: _____
☐ Routine—Site: _____

Irrigation Type: _____
☐ Heparin Amount: _____
☐ NS Amount: _____
☐ LR Amount: _____
☐ Triple Amount: _____
☐ H_2O Amount: _____
☐ Glycerin Amount: _____
☐ Other: _____
CCs Infused: _____

INTRAOPERATIVE RECORD
000020 (11/2002)

FIGURE 5.28. Example of an intraoperative vital signs report in graphic format

University of Anystate Hospitals

ANESTHESIA RECORD
PAGE 1 OF 2

PATIENT LABEL

Date: _____   Time: _____
Age: _____ Sex: _____ Height: _____ Weight: _____ BP: _____ P: _____ R: _____ T: _____
Lab: _____   Status: _____
Allergies: _____   Last Intake: _____
Premedication: _____

☐ **Patient reassessed immediately prior to induction. Condition satisfactory for planned anesthesia.**

Vital Signs

Time		Machine Check
		Initials
		Patient Position

Systolic ∨ — 240
Diastolic ∧ — 220
— 200
Pulse ∧∧ — 180
Respiration ○ — 160
Spon ● — 140
Assist ⊙ — 120
Controlled — 100
Surgery Start/End ⊗ — 80
— 60
Anesthesia Start/End X — 40
Anesthesia Start — 20
— 15
— 10
Anesthesia End — 5

☐ General
☐ Regional
☐ Local
☐ Monitored
☐ IVs (spinal/EPI needle)

Position
Prep
Site
Agent
Paresthesia
Catheter
Sensory Block TO

☐ Heat/Moisture Exchanger
☐ Warming Blanket
☐ Fluid Warmer
☐ Bair Hugger

Endotracheal Tube
Cuff Inflated
Laryngoscope Blade
Stylet
Direct Vision
Blind

FIGURE 5.28. (continued)

University of Anystate Hospitals

ANESTHESIA RECORD
PAGE 2 OF 2

PATIENT LABEL

Monitors
☐ NIBP ☐ R ☐ L
☐ APB   ☐ R ☐ L
☐ T (site): _____
☐ Pulse oximeter (site): _____
☐ ECG (lead): _____
☐ Airway gas monitor
☐ FiO$_2$ analyzer
☐ Pulmonary artery
☐ CVP
☐ EEG
☐ Stethoscope (site): _____
☐ SSEP
☐ Peripheral nerve stimulator
☐ Capnography

Remarks

Fluid		Fluid		Fluid		Fluid		Fluid		Fluid	
Start	Finish	Start	Finish	Start	Finish	Start	Finish	Start	Finish	Start	Finish

Operation

Surgeon   Anesthesiologist   Date

Recovery Room   Time: _____
BP
P   T   °F   Endotracheal
                                   In ☐ Out ☐
Condition   SpO$_2$ %

Preanesthesia Evaluation

Review of Clinical Data

☐ Yes ☐ No   Patient Medical History Reviewed
☐ Yes ☐ No   Current Medications Reviewed
☐ Yes ☐ No   Allergies Reviewed
☐ Yes ☐ No ☐ N/A Lab Results Reviewed
☐ Yes ☐ No ☐ N/A CXR Results Reviewed
☐ Yes ☐ No ☐ N/A EKG Results Reviewed

Pertinent Physical Exam

	Normal	Abnormal	Comments
EENT			
Respiratory			
Cardiac			
Mental Status			

Anesthesia History

☐ Yes ☐ No Past Hx of Anesthesia Complications
☐ Yes ☐ No Family Hx of Anesthesia Complications
☐ Yes ☐ No History of Malignant Hyperthermia

ASA Classification

1   2   3   4   5   E

Airway Evaluation

Dentures: ☐ None ☐ Upper ☐ Lower
Capped Teeth: ☐ None ☐ Yes
Condition of Teeth: ☐ Good ☐ Fair ☐ Poor
Estimated Intubation Difficulty:
☐ Normal ☐ Moderately Difficult ☐ Difficult

Anesthesia Plan

☐ General   ☐ Rapid Sequence Intubation
☐ Spinal   ☐ MAC
☐ Epidural   ☐ Epidural for POPM
☐ Regional Block

☐ Alternatives, risks of anesthesia, and potential complications were discussed. Patient and/or guardian state understanding and acceptance of anesthesia plan.

Comments:

_____   _____
Anesthesiologist   Date

ANESTHESIA RECORD
000017 (11/2002)

The **postoperative anesthesia records** contain information on any unusual events or complications that occurred during surgery. It also documents the patient's condition at the conclusion of surgery and after recovery from anesthesia. (See **Figures 5.29** and **5.30**.)

Transfusion Records

Surgical and emergency patients sometimes require transfusions of whole blood or blood products. Blood transfusions carry an inherent risk of complications. Except in emergency situations, the patient's physician should discuss the relative risks and benefits with the patient and/or the patient's family before the procedure is performed. This discussion and patient consent must be documented in the patient's health record.

A **transfusion record** includes information on the type and amount of blood products the patient received, the source of the blood products, and the patient's reaction to the transfusion. It also documents the blood group and Rh status of the patient and the donor, the results of cross-matching tests, and a description of the transfusion process. Every adverse reaction to a transfusion must be fully documented in the patient's health record.

Postoperative Progress Notes

The surgeon primarily responsible for the case must write a brief postoperative progress note in the patient's record immediately after surgery and before the patient leaves the operative suite. The purpose of the note is to communicate postoperative-care instructions to recovery room nurses. The note should also indicate the presence or absence of anesthesia-related complications or other postoperative abnormalities in addition to the patient's vital signs and general condition at the conclusion of the operation. Surgeons may also document progress notes and postoperative orders. (See **Figures 5.31** and **5.32**.) In the absence of or in a delay in obtaining a dictated operative report, the postoperative progress note should serve as the communication between the surgeon and other care providers.

Recovery Room Records

Postsurgery patients are monitored in a dedicated recovery room until the effects of the anesthesia are completely reversed. Recovery room nurses monitor postsurgery patients very carefully until the patients are well enough to be moved to surgical intensive care or their regular rooms. (See **Figure 5.33**.) Same-day surgery patients receive the same level of care and observation as inpatients do until they are ready to leave the hospital.

Most hospitals have developed a **recovery room record** form that is used by nursing staff to document the patient's reaction to anesthesia and condition after surgery. Nurses document information on the patient's level of consciousness, overall medical condition, vital signs, and medications and intravenous fluids when the patient enters the recovery room. The same information is documented when the patient is ready to be transferred or discharged. The status of any surgical dressings, catheters, tubes, and drains is also recorded.

The patient's surgical record should also include documentation that demonstrates that the patient met the facility's discharge criteria before being discharged or transferred. The name of the physician or surgeon who was responsible for the discharge must be included on the discharge order.

Operative Reports

Surgical procedures involve substantial medical, legal, and financial risks for patients, surgeons, and hospitals. For this reason, it is especially important that surgical documentation be complete, accurate, and timely. In addition to anesthesia and recovery room records,

FIGURE 5.29. Example of a postoperative anesthesia record

Midwest Medical Center

POSTANESTHESIA RECORD
PAGE 1 OF 2

PATIENT LABEL

Date: _____
PACU Admission Time: _____ a.m./p.m.   Anesthesia End Time: _____ a.m./p.m.
Procedure: _____
Surgeon: _____ Anesthetist: _____
Anesthesia: ☐ General   ☐ Regional   ☐ Local Only   ☐ Spinal   ☐ Epidural   ☐ Local w/Sedation
☐ Chart Orders Checked   Allergies: _____
Admitting Nurse(s): _____

Assessment

LOC: ☐ Drowsy ☐ Alert   ☐ Oriented ☐ Sleeping while
                                                                                    undisturbed
Respiratory Quality: ☐ Deep   ☐ Shallow ☐ Labored
Circulatory: ☐ Pink   ☐ Warm   ☐ Cool   ☐ Mottled
Circulation Check: ☐ N/A   ☐ Pink   ☐ Warm   ☐ Cool   ☐ Mottled
Operative: ☐ Pulse Palpable ☐ Unable to Palpate Due to Dressing
Extremity: ☐ Capillary Refill Adequate ☐ Other (see notes)
Dressing/Operative Site: _____ ☐ Dry and Intact ☐ Other (see notes)
IV Therapy: Fluid: _____ Site: _____ Amt.: _____ cc
☐ Patent, No Redness or Edema Noted   ☐ Other (see notes)
Level of Pain: _____ Init. _____

Vital Signs									
Time	BP	Pulse	Resp.	Pain Level	Time	BP	Pulse	Resp.	Pain Level

Dressing Check: ☐ Time: ☐ Dry and Intact ☐ Other (see supplemental notes)
                         ☐ Time: ☐ Dry and Intact ☐ Other (see supplemental notes)

Medications				
Medicine	Dosage	Route	Time Given	Initials

PACU Scoring						
Time						
Activity						
R						
Circulation						
LOC						
Skin T						
Total						

Discharge Evaluation

☐ Vital Signs at Preoperative Level
☐ Meets PACU Score of 10 OR   ☐ Return of Preoperative Level
☐ Minimal or No Pain
☐ Minimal or No Nausea
☐ Dressing Dry and Intact
☐ Ambulates with Minimal Assistance
☐ Responsible Adult Present to Accompany Patient Home
Initials: _____ Signature: _____
Initials: _____ Signature: _____
Initials: _____ Signature: _____

Plan of Care/Interventions

Potential Alteration in Mental Status	**Goal: Return to Pre-Op Status**

☐ Reoriented to time and place   ☐ Goal Met
☐ Other: _____

Potential for Fear and/or Anxiety	**Goal: Reduction of Fear and Anxiety**

☐ Oriented to Environment   ☐ Goal Met
☐ Encouraged to Verbalize Concerns
☐ Age-Appropriate Emotional Support Provided
☐ Family at Bedside
☐ Patients and/or Family's Questions Answered
☐ Other: _____

Potential Alteration in Comfort	**Goal: Decrease Level of Pain**

☐ Patient Repositioned for Comfort   ☐ Goal Met
☐ Pain Scale Used According to Verbal Communication Level
☐ Medication Given as Ordered
☐ Other: _____

Potential for Injury	**Goal: Create a Safe Environment**

☐ Siderails Elevated   ☐ Goal Met
☐ Ambulated with Assistance
☐ Family at Bedside
☐ Other: _____

Potential Alteration in Fluid Volume	**Goal: Adequate I/O**

☐ PO Fluids Given   ☐ IV Discontinued   ☐ Voided   ☐ Goal Met
☐ Antiemetic Medication Administered
☐ Other: _____

Knowledge Deficit/Potential for Postop Complications at Home	**Goal: Exhibits Knowledge of Postop Care**

☐ Need for Home Care Assistance Assessed   ☐ Goal Met
Assistance Needed:
☐ No   ☐ Yes If Yes: ☐ Physician   ☐ Case Management Notified
☐ Written Discharge Instructions Given
☐ Prescriptions Given to Patient/Family
☐ Other: _____

Other Problems/Needs

_____
_____
_____

Discharge to		**Phase II Recovery**

Discharge _____ MD
Discharge to ☐ Home ☐ Room #: _____ Postop Contact #: _____
Discharged @: _____ Via ☐ Wheelchair ☐ Ambulance ☐ Stretcher
                                    ☐ Other _____
RN Signature: _____

FIGURE 5.29. (continued)

Midwest Medical Center

POSTANESTHESIA RECORD
PAGE 2 OF 2

PATIENT LABEL

PACU Scoring Guide

Activity

2 = Able to move 4 extremities
1 = Able to move 2 extremities
0 = Able to move 0 extremities

Respirations

2 = Clear, unsupported (strong cry, if pediatric)
1 = Obstructed, supported (spontaneous respiration may be shallow or slow)
0 = Apneic/mechanical ventilation/ Ambu

Circulation
(adults and children)

2 = BP ± 20 of preanesthesia level
1 = BP ± 20-50 of preanesthesia level
0 = BP ± 50 or more of preanesthesia level

Infants

2 = Radial pulse easy to palpate
1 = Axillary pulse palpable, radial pulse weak
0 = Carotid is only palpable pulse

Consciousness

2 = Awake—Oriented to time and place (preop level)
1 = Drowsy—Able to be aroused on name calling or gentle stimuli
0 = Unresponsive

Skin Temperature

2 = Warm, dry, pink
1 = Warm, dry, pale
0 = Cool, clammy, mottled

Supplemental Nursing Notes

_____
_____
_____
_____
_____
_____
_____
_____
_____
_____
_____
_____
_____
_____

Postprocedure Followup

Date: _____ Time: _____

☐ Patient Contacted ☐ No Answer ☐ Answering Machine

Dressing: ☐ Dry and Intact ☐ Drainage Present (see comments)
☐ Redness Present (see comments)

Comfort: ☐ No Discomfort ☐ Mild Discomfort
☐ Moderate Discomfort ☐ Severe Discomfort (any discomfort, see comments)

N/V: ☐ None ☐ Minimal ☐ Moderate ☐ Severe

Fever: ☐ No ☐ Yes:_____°F

Instructions: ☐ Easily Understood ☐ Further Instructions Needed (see comments)

Comments:
_____
_____
_____
_____
_____
_____
_____
_____

Signature: _____

POSTANESTHESIA RECORD
000024 (11/2002)

FIGURE 5.30. Example of a postoperative record

University of Anystate Hospitals

POSTOPERATIVE RECORD
PAGE 1 OF 2

PATIENT LABEL

Type of Procedure: _____ Date: _____ Time Arrive on Unit: _____
Arrived Via: ☐ Bed   ☐ Stretcher   ☐ Wheelchair

Postprocedure Assessment

Level of Consciousness ☐ Alert ☐ Responds to Painful/Verbal Stimuli ☐ Drowsy ☐ Unresponsive	**IV Therapy**
Oxygen ☐ Room Air ☐ Nasal Cannula ☐ Other @ _____ liter/min	#1 Fluid: _____ Site: _____ Rate: _____ ☐ No Redness or Swelling at Site ☐ Other: _____
Respiratory Quality ☐ Regular ☐ Irregular ☐ Other	#2 Fluid: _____ Site: _____ Rate: _____ ☐ No Redness or Swelling at Site ☐ Other: _____
Breath Sounds ☐ Clear all Fields ☐ Other: _____	#3 Fluid: _____ Site: _____ Rate: _____ ☐ No Redness or Swelling at Site ☐ Other: _____

Cardiac ☐ Regular ☐ Irregular ☐ Dysrhythmia

GI ☐ N/A ☐ Hypo Bowel Sound ☐ Hyper Bowel Sound ☐ Absent Bowel Sound
☐ Firm ☐ Distended ☐ Tender ☐ Protuberant

Drainage Tubes: ☐ N/A
Type: _____ ☐ Patency Checked Drainage: _____
Type: _____ ☐ Patency Checked Drainage: _____
Type: _____ ☐ Patency Checked Drainage: _____

Skin Color ☐ Pink ☐ Pale ☐ Mottled ☐ Cyanotic

Skin Condition ☐ Warm ☐ Dry ☐ Cold ☐ Clammy

Puncture Site: ☐ N/A
Location: _____
Sand Bag Intact: ☐ Yes ☐ No   Bleeding: ☐ Yes ☐ No
Hematoma: ☐ Yes ☐ No   Sheath Sutured: ☐ Yes ☐ No ☐ N/A

Circ. √ Distal to Site ☐ N/A ☐ Warm ☐ Pink
☐ Cyanotic ☐ Mottled ☐ Cool

Sheath Removal Date: _____ Time: _____ Initials: _____
Assessment Unchanged from Postprocedure ☐ Yes ☐ See Notes
Verbalizes Understanding of Sheath Removal ☐ Yes ☐ See Notes

Peripheral Pulses (absent, +1, +2, +3, +4, Doppler) _____ N/A
_____ R Rad _____ R DP _____ R PT _____ Other
_____ L Rad _____ L DP _____ L PT

Site Check Post Sheath Removal

Sandbag Intact	☐ Yes	☐ No
Hematoma	☐ Yes	☐ See Notes
Pain	☐ Yes	☐ See Notes
Loss of Distal Pulse	☐ Yes	☐ See Notes
Compression Device in Use	☐ Yes	☐ See Notes
Uncontrolled Bleeding	☐ Yes	☐ See Notes
Vasovagal Reaction	☐ Yes	☐ See Notes

Dressing/Operative Site: _____ ☐ Dry and Intact
Dressing/Operative Site: _____ ☐ Dry and Intact

RN Signature: _____

Plan of Care   Clinical Pathway Continued

☐ **Potential for Alteration and Ventilation**
Goal: Adequate Air Exchange   ☐ Goal Met
☐ Continuous Pulse Oximetry in Use
☐ Coughing and Deep Breathing Encouraged
☐ O₂ Therapy Initiated as Ordered
☐ Incentive Spirometry Initiated as Ordered
☐ Other: _____

☐ **Potential Alteration Cardiovascular Function**
Goal: Hemodynamically Stable   ☐ Goal Met
☐ Continuous Cardiac Monitoring in Use
☐ Other: _____

☐ **Potential Alteration in Mental Status**
Goal: Return to Preop Status   ☐ Goal Met
☐ Reoriented to Time and Place
☐ Other: _____

☐ **Potential for Fear and/or Anxiety**
Goal: Reduction of Fear and Anxiety   ☐ Goal Met
☐ Oriented to Environment
☐ Encouraged to Verbalize Concerns
☐ Age-Appropriate Emotional Support Provided
☐ Family at Bedside
☐ Patients/Families Questions Answered
☐ Other: _____

☐ **Potential for Injury**
Goal: Create a Safe Environment   ☐ Goal Met
☐ Side Rails Raised
☐ Ambulated with Assistance
☐ Family at Bedside
☐ Call Bell within Reach
☐ Bed in Low Position
☐ Other: _____

☐ **Knowledge Deficit/Potential for Postprocedure Complications at Home**
Goal: Exhibits Knowledge of Postprocedure Care   ☐ Goal Met
☐ Need for Home Care Assistance Assessed
☐ If Assistance Needed, Notify: ☐ Physician ☐ Case Manager
☐ Written Discharge Instructions Reinforced. Copy to Patient.
☐ Prescription Given to Patient/Family with Instructions on Usage
☐ Explained Procedure for Transferring to Inpatient Unit
☐ Other: _____

☐ **Potential Alteration in Fluid Volume**
Goal: Adequate I/O   ☐ Goal Met
☐ IV Hydration Initiated
☐ Antiemetic Medication Administered
☐ PO Fluids Given without Nausea/Vomiting
☐ Other: _____

☐ **Potential Alteration in Comfort**
Goal: Decrease Level of Pain   ☐ Goal Met
☐ Patient Repositioned for Comfort
☐ Pain Level (0–10)
☐ Wong-Baker Face Scale for Pediatrics—Face Score: _____
☐ Reevaluation of Pain after Medication—Level of Pain: _____
☐ Medication Given as Ordered
☐ Other: _____

☐ **Other Problems/Needs**   ☐ Goal Met
_____
_____
_____

RN Signature: _____ Date: _____

FIGURE 5.30. (continued)

University of Anystate Hospitals

POSTOPERATIVE RECORD
PAGE 2 OF 2

PATIENT LABEL

Postprocedure Record (page 2)

IV Site	Date	7–3	3–11	11–7	Date	7–3	3–11	11–7

Date: _____

0 NO HURT	2 HURTS LITTLE BIT	4 HURTS LITTLE MORE	6 HURTS EVEN MORE	8 HURTS WHOLE LOT	10 HURTS WORST

Pain Management (scale 0–10 for adults—Wong/Baker Faces for Pediatrics)

Time	Pain Scale	Medication/Dose	Initials	Response/Pain Scale	Time	Initials

Vital Sign Postprocedure/Sheath Removal

Time	LOC	T	BP	P	RR/O₂ Sat.	Pain Level	Peripheral Pulse	Site Check	Initials

Daily Care Record

Shift: Date	7–3	3–11	11–7	7–3	3–11	11–7
Bedrest						
Ambulating						
R or L Leg Straight						
SCD						
Antiembolism Hose						
PCA Pump						
Traction						
Telemetry						
Type of Diet						
Amount Eaten						
Bath/Shower/Bed						
Complete—Self/Assist.						
Oral Care/P.M. Care						
Other:						

Level of Consciousness (LOC) Scale
2 = Awake—Oriented to Preop Time and Place
1 = Drowsy—Able to Arouse with Name Calling or Gentle Stimuli
0 = Unresponsive—Unable to Arouse Except with Painful Stimuli

Date/Time	Notes:

Initials	Signature	Initials	Signature	Initials	Signature

POSTOPERATIVE RECORD
000022(11/2002)

FIGURE 5.31. Example of a postoperative progress note

Midwest Medical Center

POSTOPERATIVE PROGRESS NOTE

PATIENT LABEL

Procedure(s) Performed:

_____

_____

_____

_____

_____

Name of Primary Surgeon:

_____

Assistant(s):

_____

_____

Findings:

_____

_____

_____

_____

_____

_____

Technical Procedures Used:

_____

_____

_____

_____

_____

Specimens Removed:

_____

_____

_____

Estimated Blood Loss:

_____

Postoperative Diagnosis:

_____

_____

_____

_____

Physician Signature: _____ Date: _____

POSTOPERATIVE PROGRESS NOTE
000025 (11/2002)

FIGURE 5.32. Example of postoperative orders

Midwest Medical Center

POSTOPERATIVE ORDERS

PATIENT LABEL

Date:

Postoperative Diagnosis:

Operation:

Orders: Allergies:

Date/Time	RN Signature	Postop Orders Begin Here
		1. Position of Patient
		2. Ambulate
		3. Leg Exercises
		4. Medication for Pain
		5. Medication for Nausea
		6. Medication for Sleep
		7. Other Medications—Include Previous Orders to Be Continued
		8. Antibiotic
		9. Oral Intake
		10. IV Fluids (include blood)
		11. Tubes to Be Connected
		A. Nasogastric
		B. T Tube
		C. Thoracotomy
		D. Foley
		E. Other
		12. Catheterize
		13. Care of Dressing
		14. Drains
		15. Respiratory Care
		16. IPPB Freq. Duration Pressure Drug
		17. Vital Signs
		18. Intake and Output
		19. Lab Studies
		20. Other:

RN Signature: _____ Date: _____

Physician Signature: _____ Date: _____

POSTOPERATIVE ORDERS
000026 (11/2002)

FIGURE 5.33. Example of a postanesthesia nursing record

University of Anystate Hospitals

POSTANESTHESIA NURSING RECORD
PAGE 1 OF 4

PATIENT LABEL

Procedure: _____ Date: _____

Surgeon: _____ Anesthetist: _____
Anesthesia: ☐ General ☐ Regional ☐ Local Only ☐ Epidural ☐ Local w/Sedation
☐ Chart Orders Checked Allergies: _____

PACU Admission Time: _____ a.m./p.m.
Anesthesia End Time: _____ a.m./p.m.

Phase I Assessment

Arrived Via:	☐ Stretcher	☐ Bed	☐ Infant Carried by Anesthetist	☐ Crib
LOC:	☐ Drowsy	☐ Reacting	☐ Alert ☐ Disoriented	☐ Unresponsive

Circulatory:
Skin:	☐ Pink	☐ Warm	☐ Cool	☐ Mottled	☐ Cyanotic
Extremities:	☐ Pink	☐ Warm	☐ Cool	☐ Mottled	☐ Cyanotic ☐ SCD _____

Airway Support: ☐ None ☐ Oral ☐ Nasal ☐ Chin Lift ☐ Jaw Thrust ☐ ET Tube ☐ Tracheostomy
Oxygen Ventilation: ☐ None ☐ 40% ☐ ____% ☐ Mask ☐ Cannula ☐ T-Bar ☐ LMA
☐ Adequate Exchange ☐ Ambu ☐ Ventilator ☐ Other ☐ Tent
Respiratory Quality: ☐ Deep ☐ Shallow ☐ Snoring ☐ Stridor ☐ Labored ☐ Tachypnea
☐ Regular ☐ Irregular
Breath Sounds: ☐ Clear All Fields ☐ Equal Bilat. ☐ Rates ☐ Rhonchi ☐ Wheezing ☐ Other
Cardiac: ☐ Regular Rhythm: _____ ☐ Irregular Rhythm:_____
Abdomen: ☐ Soft ☐ Firm ☐ Distended

Dressing/Operative Site: _____ ☐ Dry and Intact ☐ Other: _____
☐ Peripad ☐ Dry and Intact ☐ Other: _____
☐ Cast ☐ Dry and Intact ☐ Damp ☐ Other: _____
☐ Epidural ☐ Dry and Intact ☐ Other: _____
☐ Packing Site: _____

Drains: ☐ None ☐ CBI Fluid: _____ Amt. on Admisssion: _____ ☐ Other:
☐ Foley Cath. ☐ Suprapubic ☐ Patent Color of Drainage: _____ ☐ JP Site: _____ ☐ Patent Color of Drainage: _____
☐ Hemovac Site: _____ ☐ Patent Color of Drainage: _____ ☐ NG Site: _____ ☐ Patent Color of Drainage: _____
☐ Chest Tube Site: _____ ☐ Patent Color of Drainage: _____ ☐ Penrose Site: _____ ☐ Patent Color of Drainage: _____

IVs: ☐ None #1 Site: _____ Fluid: _____ Amount: _____ ☐ Patent, Dressing Dry and Intact, No Redness or Edema Noted ☐ Other
#2 Site: _____ Fluid: _____ Amount: _____ ☐ Patent, Dressing Dry and Intact, No Redness or Edema Noted ☐ Other
#3 Site: _____ Fluid: _____ Amount: _____ ☐ Patent, Dressing Dry and Intact, No Redness or Edema Noted ☐ Other
☐ A-Line Site:_____ ☐ Calibrated to Monitor ☐ Heparin Flush ☐ Appropriate Waveform ☐ Other: _____
☐ Swan Site:_____ ☐ Calibrated to Monitor ☐ Heparin Flush ☐ Appropriate Waveform ☐ Other: _____

Physician Orders

PACU Orders

O$_2$ 3 LNC for O$_2$ Sat. < _____ for 24 hours
_____
_____
_____
_____
_____

Diagnostic Studies
_____
_____
_____
_____
_____
_____
_____
_____

Pain Control **As Needed for Pain**

Meperidine IV: Dosage ☐ 6.25 mg ☐ 12.5 mg ☐ 25 mg ☐ Other: _____
Frequency ☐ q.5min. ☐ q.10min. ☐ q.15min. ☐ Other: _____
Maximum Dosage: _____ mg

Morphine IV: Dosage ☐ 1.0 mg ☐ 2.0 mg ☐ 5 mg ☐ Other: _____
Frequency ☐ q.5min. ☐ q.10min. ☐ q.15min. ☐ Other: _____
Maximum Dosage: _____ mg

Antiemetics **As Needed for Nausea, Vomiting**

Phenergan IV: Dosage ☐ 6.25 mg ☐ 12.5 mg ☐ Other: _____
Frequency ☐ q.5min. ☐ q.10min. ☐ Other: _____
Maximum Dosage: _____ mg/h

Inapsine IV: Dosage ☐ 0.25 cc ☐ Other: _____
Frequency: _____ Maximum Dosage: _____

Anzemet: Dosage ☐ 12.5 meq ☐ Other: _____
Frequency: _____

Signature of MD: _____

Discharge after Score (≥) 8

_____MD

Discharge

_____MD

FIGURE 5.33. (continued)

University of Anystate Hospitals

POSTANESTHESIA NURSING RECORD
PAGE 2 OF 4

PATIENT LABEL

Ongoing Assessment/Evaluations/Documentation

Postop V/S: _____

Neurovascular/ Orthopedic Surgery Pulse Checks	R
	L

Palpable=1+, 2+, 3+
√ = Yes X = No
B = Brisk S = Sluggish
W = Warm C = Cool
D = Doppler
U = Unable to palpate due to dressing/cast

Time

Site

Movement

Sensation

T

Cap Refill

P

☐ See vascular flow sheet
☐ See neuro flow sheet

Sensory Chart
T-4 = Nipple line
T-6 = Xiphoid process
T-8 = Costal margin
T-10 = Umbilicus
T-12 = Iliac arrest
L-2, 3 = Thigh
S-2, 5 = Perineum

Site Code
A = L upper arm
B = R upper arm
C = L hip (LUOQ)
D = R hip (RUOQ)
E = L thigh
F = R thigh
G = Abdomen

IV Site Code
1 = R Extremity
2 = L Extremity
3 = Central Line
4 = Other (i.e., scalp)

Time
Activity
Respirations
Circulation
Consciousness
Temperature
Total
Pulse Oximetry
Temperature
CVP
Pap
Spinal Level
Epidural Level

Cuff ▽   250
BP △   240
                 230
                 220
A-Line ▼   210
       ▲   200
                 190
NBP ∨   180
    ∧   170
                 160
Pulse ●   150
                 140
                 130
Warm   120
Blanket B   110
                 100
                 90
Temperatures   80
Tympanic,   70
unless   60
indicated: 50
R = Rectal   40
O = Oral   30
A = Axillary   20
                 10
                 0

Respirations
Dressing _____
Pain Level

Activity
2 = Able to move 4 extremities
1 = Able to move 2 extremities
0 = Able to move 0 extremities

Respirations
2 = Clear, unsupported (strong cry if pediatric)
1 = Obstructed, supported (spontaneous respiration may be shallow or slow)
0 = Apneic/mechanical (ventilation/ambu)
Mandatory Score = 2 in Respiratory

Circulation
Adults and Children
2 = BP plus or minus 20 of preanesthesia level
1 = BP plus or minus 20-50 of preanesthesia level
0 = BP plus or minus 50 or more of preanesthesia level
Infants
2 = Radial pulse easy to palpate
1 = Axillary pulse palpable, radial pulse weak
0 = Carotid is only palpable pulse

Consciousness
2 = Awake—Oriented to time and place (preop level)
1 = Drowsy—Able to be aroused with name calling or gentle stimuli
0 = Unresponsive

Temperature
2 = Tympanic T > 96° F, R= > 97°, 0= > 96°, A= >96°
1 = Tympanic T 95–96° F, R=96-97°, 0=95–96°, A=94–96°
0 = Tympanic T < 95°, R= < 96°, 0= < 95°, A= < 94°

Dressing
0 = Dry
* = See note

Miscellaneous
* = See note

Medication	Amount	Route	Site	Time/Initials					Time Started	Fluid, Amount, Additives	Initials

Ongoing Assessment Nurse: _____ RN _____ RN _____ RN

FIGURE 5.33. (continued)

University of Anystate Hospitals

POSTANESTHESIA NURSING RECORD
PAGE 3 OF 4

PATIENT LABEL

Plan of Care/Interventions

☐ **Potential for Alteration in Ventilation**   **Goal: Adequate Air Exchange**
☐ Continuous pulse oximetry in use   ☐ Goal Met
☐ Coughing and deep breathing encouraged
☐ O₂ therapy initiated as ordered
☐ Airway out @ _____   ☐ Extubated @ _____
☐ O₂ discontinued @: _____
☐ O₂ reapplied @: _____ via mask @ _____ %
☐ O₂ reapplied @ _____ via nasal cannula @ _____ l/m
☐ Other: _____

☐ **Potential Alteration in Cardiovascular Function   Goal: Hemodynamically Stable**
☐ Continuous cardiac monitoring   ☐ Goal Met
☐ Other: _____

☐ **Potential Alteration in Mental Status**   **Goal: Return to Preop Status**
☐ Reoriented to time and place   ☐ Goal Met
☐ Other: _____

☐ **Potential for Fear and/or Anxiety**   **Goal: Reduction of Fear and Anxiety**
☐ Oriented to PACU environment
☐ Encouraged to verbalize concerns
☐ Age-appropriate emotional support provided
☐ Family at bedside
☐ Patient's and/or family's questions answered
☐ Other: _____

☐ **Potential for Injury**   **Goal: Create a Safe Environment**
☐ Side rails elevated   ☐ Goal Met
☐ Family at bedside
☐ Other: _____

☐ **Potential Alteration in Comfort**   **Goal: Decrease Level of Pain**
☐ Patient repositioned for comfort   ☐ Goal Met
☐ Medication given as ordered
☐ Scale used according to verbal communication level
☐ Other: _____

☐ **Potential Alteration in Body Temperature**   **Goal: Return to Preop Status**
☐ Bair hugger applied   ☐ Goal Met
☐ Warm blanket applied
☐ Warmed IV fluids given
☐ Other: _____

☐ **Potential Alteration in Tissue Perfusion   Goal: Adequate Vascular Perfusion**
☐ Capillary refill monitored on operative limb   ☐ Goal Met
☐ Circulation of operative limb monitored
☐ Other: _____

☐ **Potential Alteration in Fluid Volume**   **Goal: Adequate I/O**
☐ IV infusing   Goal Met
☐ Antiemetic medication administered
☐ Other: _____

☐ **Other Problems/Needs**
_____
_____
_____

Phase I Discharge Assessment

	Intake				Output				
Time	IV	Blood	PO	CBI	Urine ☐ Foley ☐ Voided	☐ NG ☐ CT	Emesis	☐ Hemovac ☐ JP	Other
OR I/O									
PACU I/O									
Total I/O									

Discharge IV Fluid

Type: _____   Amount: _____

Type: _____   Amount: _____

Type: _____   Amount: _____

Type: _____   Amount: _____

LOC   ☐ Drowsy ☐ Alert ☐ Oriented ☐ Sleeping While Undisturbed
Circulatory:
  Skin   ☐ Pink   ☐ Warm ☐ Cool   ☐ Mottled
  Extremities ☐ Pink   ☐ Warm ☐ Cool   ☐ Mottled
Oxygen   ☐ Room Air ☐ O₂ @ _____ % _____ ☐ Vent
Respiratory
  Quality   ☐ Deep   ☐ Regular   ☐ Other: _____
Breath
Sounds   ☐ Clear All Fields   ☐ Equal Bilat.   ☐ Rales
        ☐ Rhonchi ☐ Wheezing
Cardiac   ☐ Regular Rhythm ☐ Cardiac Monitoring ☐ Rhythm: _____
Dressing/Operative Site: _____ ☐ Dry and Intact ☐ Other: _____
Drains   ☐ None   ☐ Secure and Patent
IV Sites   ☐ Patent, Dressing Dry and Intact, No Redness or Edema Noted
        ☐ Other (see nurses' notes)
  ☐ A-Line: ☐ To Monitor ☐ Heparin Flush ☐ Appropriate Waveform
  ☐ Swan: ☐ To Monitor ☐ Heparin Flush ☐ Appropriate Waveform
Comfort   ☐ Comfortable ☐ Other
Discharged
To: ☐ Phase II Recovery ☐ Room #: _____ ☐ Side Rails Up

☐ Prescription on Chart _____
_____
_____

Discharge Time: _____ a.m./p.m.
☐ Family Notified ☐ Unable to Reach
Report Called to: _____ Transported by: _____

RN Signature: _____

☐ Patient Reassessed—Agree with PACU Discharge   V/S: _____
_____ a.m./p.m.
RN Receiving Patient   Time

FIGURE 5.33. (continued)

University of Anystate Hospitals

POSTANESTHESIA NURSING RECORD
PAGE 4 OF 4

PATIENT LABEL

Rhythm Strips

Supplemental Nursing Notes

POSTANESTHESIA NURSING RECORD
000023 (11/2002)

an operative report must be prepared for every surgical procedure performed outside the patient's room. Joint Commission regulations require that the operative report be written or dictated before the patient is transferred from the recovery room to the next level of care.

An **operative report** is a formal document prepared by the principal surgeon to describe the surgical procedure(s) performed for the patient. (See **FIGURE 5.34**.) Each report includes the following information:

- Patient identification, including name and record number

- Patient's preoperative and postoperative diagnoses and indications for surgery

- Descriptions of the procedures performed

- Descriptions of all normal and abnormal findings

- Descriptions of any specimens removed

- Descriptions of the patient's medical condition before, during, and after the operation

- Estimated blood loss

- Descriptions of any unique or unusual events that occurred during the course of the surgery

- Names of the surgeons and their assistants

- Date and duration of the surgery

- Signature of principal physician along with credentials, dated

- Date the report was written or dictated

Operating room nurses maintain a record of the number of ligatures, sutures, packs, drains, sponges, instruments, and needles used during a procedure. This information may also be included in the surgeon's operative report.

The operative report should be written or dictated immediately after surgery and filed in the patient's health record as soon as possible. Some hospitals may require surgeons to include brief descriptions of the operations in their postoperative progress notes when delays in dictation or transcription are unavoidable. Other caregivers can then refer to the progress note until the final operative report becomes available.

Pathology Reports

Pathology examinations must be performed on every specimen or foreign object removed or expelled from a patient during a surgical procedure. Each examination includes a microscopic and macroscopic (or gross) evaluation of the specimen, which is fully described in a **pathology report**. Some hospitals have established medical staff rules that exempt some types of specimens from microscopic examination. Examples include normal placentas, tonsils, and foreign bodies such as bullets.

Pathology reports must be prepared by pathologists, specialty physicians who analyze surgical specimens, perform autopsies, and supervise other laboratory services. Pathology reports on surgical specimens must be authenticated by the pathologist who performed the examination and then placed in the surgery section of the patient's health record.

FIGURE 5.34. Example of an operative report

Midwest Medical Center

OPERATIVE REPORT
PAGE 1 OF 2

PATIENT, TWEETY PYE
00555066
DOB: 02/18/1948

DATE: 06/02/20XX

SURGEON: Douglas Default

ASSISTANT: Stanley Cutter

ANESTHETIC: Spinal

PREOPERATIVE DIAGNOSES:

1. Intrauterine pregnancy, term, previous cesarean section, voluntary repeat cesarean section
2. Multiparity, voluntary sterilization

POSTOPERATIVE DIAGNOSES:

1. Intrauterine pregnancy, term, previous cesarean section, voluntary repeat cesarean section
2. Multiparity, voluntary sterilization
3. Delivery of viable unengaged 6 pound 2 ounce female, APGAR 8–9

OPERATION:

1. Low-segment transverse cesarean section
2. Bilateral partial salpingectomy

COMPLICATIONS: None

DRAINS: One Foley catheter in urinary bladder

ESTIMATED BLOOD LOSS: Approximately 500 to 600 cc

PACKS: None

DESCRIPTION OF OPERATION: After satisfactory level of spinal anesthesia was obtained, the patient was placed in the dorsal supine position with mild left lateral uterine displacement. The lower abdominal skin tissues were prepped with a Hibiclens solution. She was then draped with sterile drapes in a sterile manner.

There was a previous transverse skin scar on the lower abdominal skin. A repeat transverse skin incision was made very carefully with sharp dissection. The fascia of the anterior abdominal wall was incised in a lateral crescentic manner exposing the rectus muscles, which were then bluntly divided in the midline exposing the peritoneum, which was then carefully incised in a vertical manner. There was a wetting amount of peritoneal fluid. The peritoneum reflection over the lower anterior uterine segment was then incised in a superficial transverse manner, and the "bladder flap" was gently pushed off the lower segment without difficulty.

FIGURE 5.34. (continued)

Midwest Medical Center

OPERATIVE REPORT
PAGE 2 OF 2

PATIENT, TWEETY PYE
00555066
DOB: 02/18/1948

A transverse uterine incision was made very carefully with both sharp and blunt dissection. The myometrium was noted to be only 2 to 3 mm in thickness. The amniotic fluid was clear. The unengaged vertex was delivered through the uterine and abdominal incision without difficulty. The nasal and oropharynx were suctioned with bulb suction prior to the newborn's initial inspiration. The remainder of the delivery was accomplished without difficulty. The cord was clamped and severed, and the newborn was handed crying and in good condition to the awaiting nursery personnel.

The placenta was then manually removed from a fundal location showing a central insertion of a three-vessel cord. There were no visible extensions of the uterine incision. Both tubes and ovaries appeared normal for pregnant state. The uterine incision was then closed with a running interlocking #1 chromic suture.

With the patient's strong desire for permanent sterilization, approximately 1 to 1.5 cm segment of the isthmic portion of each fallopian tube was isolated with Babcock clamps, doubly ligated and excised, and sent to the laboratory labeled as portion of left and right fallopian tube, respectively. Hemostasis was deemed adequate. Both tubes appeared occluded.

The abdominal cavity was irrigated with copious amounts of warm normal saline. The first sponge, needle, and instrument counts were correct. The parietal peritoneum was then closed with a running 0 chromic suture. Hemostasis was deemed adequate in the subfascial space. The fascia was then approximated with running 0 PDS suture. Hemostasis was deemed adequate in the subcutaneous tissue. The skin was then approximated with running 3-0 Vicryl subcuticular suture. Sterile dressing was placed upon the incision.

The patient tolerated the procedure quite well and was sent to the recovery room in good condition. The newborn was taken to the nursery by the nursery personnel in good condition. The second and third sponge, needle, and instrument counts were corrected.

Signature:

Douglas D Default   6/2/03

Douglas D. Default, MD   Date

d: 06/02/20XX
t: 06/04/20XX
DDD, MD/sf

(See **Figure 5.35** for an example of a pathology report.) The following basic information is usually included in pathology reports:

- Patient identification, including name and record number

- Date of examination

- Description of the tissue examined

- Findings of the microscopic and macroscopic examination of the specimen

- Diagnosis or diagnoses

- Name, credentials, and signature of the pathologist

Preliminary pathology results are sometimes communicated to the surgical team while the procedure is still in progress. The purpose of the preliminary report is to provide information about the characteristics of any neoplasms or other abnormalities that have been removed for examination. The information allows the surgeons to modify their operative scope when the condition is more or less widespread than originally estimated.

Implant Information

Millions of Americans have undergone surgery for the implantation of artificial joints, heart valves, cardiac pacemakers, ocular lenses, and other medical devices in the past few decades. Although most of these devices are safe, there have been periodic product alerts and recalls.

The International Implant Registry, created in 1988, collects information about patients who have received implants worldwide. Since 1991, federal regulations have required manufacturers to number and track many types of implantable devices so that patients and their physicians can be notified of potential safety concerns. In addition, the Food and Drug Administration (FDA 1998) requires hospitals and other healthcare organizations to report deaths and serious illnesses that appear to have been the result of malfunctioning medical devices. Some hospitals maintain their own implant registries in addition to taking part in the International Implant Registry.

Information about the type of medical device, its manufacturer, and any product numbers on the device should be included in the operative report for the implantation procedure. In addition, for medical devices that require batteries, such as pacemakers, the operative report should also indicate how often the device must be replaced to ensure patient safety.

Transplantation and Organ Donation Records

Thousands of patients every year receive kidneys, livers, hearts, and lungs salvaged from healthy patients who died of injuries and other causes. Organ donations from live donors have also become quite common, and it is not unusual for a family member to donate a kidney or part of his or her liver to a child or sibling. Bone marrow transplants from live donors have also saved the lives of thousands of cancer patients when other treatments failed.

Living donors must undergo surgery to remove bone marrow, kidneys, and other organs for transplantation to another patient. The surgical teams for the donor and the recipient must prepare operative reports for both patients, and the reports must follow the same standards as any other operative record.

Because of a shortage of transplantable organs and the difficulty of matching donors to recipients, transplantation entails a number of ethical problems. To ensure that the

FIGURE 5.35. Example of a surgical pathology consultation report

Midwest Medical Center

SURGICAL PATHOLOGY CONSULTATION

PATIENT, SWEETPEA C.
007770021
DOB: 12/18/1931

ADMITTING PHYSICIAN: M. D. Doctor

CONSULT PHYSICIAN 1:

CONSULT PHYSICIAN 2:

ACCESSIONED IN LAB: 05/20/20XX

ACCESSION #: S-03-010101

DATE OF SURGERY: 5/20/20XX

SPECIMEN: A-Vag Mucosa

CLINICAL DATA: Cystocele/rectocele, stress incontinence

GROSS: Received are four wrinkled, variegated, pink/tan portions of vaginal mucosa, which are 7 × 6 × 1 cm in aggregate dimension. Representative portions of each are submitted for microscopic evaluation. M/1/pg.

MICROSCOPIC COMMENT: Sections are of squamous mucosa. There are no atypia.

DIAGNOSIS: Squamous mucosa, multiple portions exhibiting no atypia (vaginal)

Signature:

Watts Q. Pathman   5/20/03
_____   _____
Walter Q. Pathman, MD   Date

d: 05/20/20XX
t: 05/23/20XX
WQP, MD/jt

available organs are going to the most suitable recipients, the national Organ Procurement and Transplantation Network was implemented. Patients who need transplants are placed on a national waiting list. The application for the waiting list reports information about the patient, such as race, ethnicity, and geographic location.

The Medicare Conditions of Participation (CMS 2010) require hospitals to provide organ donation information to the families of potential organ donors. When a patient is near death and the family has decided to donate his organs, documentation that shows that the transplantation network has been notified must be placed in the patient's record. Arrangements should be made to harvest the patient's organs soon after death, and those procedures should also be documented in the patient's health record.

Outpatient Services Provided in Acute Care Facilities

Hospital-based outpatient services, provided in several departments of the hospital, are services that require the patient to be in the hospital for less than 24 hours. A physician's order must accompany the patient to the hospital to provide a diagnosis and confirm medical necessity before the service is rendered. The contents of outpatient records depend on the type of procedures provided. At a minimum, the outpatient record will include the same type of administrative, demographic, and financial information as an inpatient record as well as a complete report of findings from the tests or procedures performed in the outpatient setting. Outpatient services include the following:

- Sleep lab testing
- Outpatient radiology exams
- Pulmonary function testing
- Radiation therapy
- Physical therapy
- Occupational therapy
- Speech therapy

Emergency and Trauma Care

Hospital emergency departments provide emergent diagnostic and therapeutic services to patients who have potentially life-threatening medical conditions or traumatic injuries that need immediate attention. The patients treated in emergency departments are considered outpatients. Some emergency patients require inpatient care after their conditions have been diagnosed and stabilized. At that time, the patient is transferred to the inpatient hospital and the patient's emergency room record becomes part of her inpatient record.

Most states require emergency-care facilities to maintain a chronological record of every patient who was treated at the facility, including those who were dead on arrival or those who left the facility against medical advice. The records in most states must include at least the patient's name, the date and time of arrival, and the patient's health record number.

In accordance with the **Emergency Medical Treatment and Active Labor Act (EMTALA)** (CMS 2006), emergency departments must complete a medical screening examination prior to collecting any information regarding the patient's ability to pay for the services.

Records of Emergency Services

The health records maintained for emergency services contain the same basic information as inpatient records. Emergency physicians take a medical history and perform a physical examination soon after each patient is admitted to the department. Nurses also perform a nursing assessment for each new patient. Physicians' orders, progress notes, and reports from ancillary services are documented throughout the patient's stay in the emergency department.

The emergency health record usually includes the following information:

- Patient identification, including name and record number

- Time of arrival

- Means of arrival (ambulance, private automobile, or police vehicle)

- Name of the person or organization that transported the patient to the emergency department

- Consent to treatment

- Pertinent history, including chief complaint and onset of injury or illness

- Significant physical findings

- Laboratory, X-ray, EEG, and EKG findings

- Treatment rendered and results

- Conclusions at termination of treatment

- Disposition of patient, including transfer, admission, or discharge home

- Condition of patient at discharge or transfer

- Diagnosis upon discharge

- Instructions given to the patient or family regarding care and follow-up

- Signatures and credentials of caregivers

Emergency services records may be filed separately or incorporated into the patient's inpatient record when the patient is admitted to the same facility. When the records are filed separately, the emergency record must be made available when the patient is readmitted or appears for care in the future.

Emergency Department Transfer Records

State regulations specifically require emergency facilities to maintain records of the screening examinations performed on patients who were subsequently transferred to other facilities. Similarly, federal legislation passed in 1986 and implemented in 1990 contains provisions intended to curtail the practice known as patient dumping. As stated in EMTALA, **dumping** refers to the once-common practice among private hospitals of transferring indigent patients to the emergency departments of nearby public hospitals solely to avoid providing emergency treatment to patients who were uninsured or underinsured and could not pay for the services themselves. Basically, state and federal regulations require emergency facilities to thoroughly document the reasons for patient transfers to confirm that they were not related to the patient's ability to pay for treatment or the source of payment.

To avoid the appearance of dumping, it is particularly important that the records of emergency-care patients include enough information to justify each patient's disposition. In addition, when a decision is made to transfer a patient to another facility, the physician primarily responsible for the patient's care must document in detail the reason for the transfer and the results of the patient's screening examination. Specifically, the patient's record for the encounter must contain documentation that confirms that the following actions were taken (Glondys 1999, 215):

- The physician explained to the patient why the transfer was appropriate and what the risks and benefits of the transfer would be.

- Emergency department nursing and medical staff monitored the patient's medical condition from the time the patient came to the department for treatment until the time the patient was transferred.

- Emergency department staff recorded the patient's time of arrival and time of transfer.

- A screening examination was performed and clinical findings were analyzed to support the physician's initial diagnosis.

- Appropriate treatment was provided to stabilize the patient's medical condition before and during the transfer.

- On-call physicians were consulted as appropriate, the timing of the calls and responses was noted, and the on-call physicians' recommendations were documented.

- The hospital documented the patient's informed consent for the transfer if the patient decided to refuse the screening examination or the recommended care and treatment.

- If the patient requested a transfer, the request was documented, and it was specifically noted that the transfer was not requested by a healthcare provider.

- The transferring hospital sent a copy of the patient's emergency record with the patient to the second facility. The record described the reason the patient sought treatment, the results of any diagnostic examinations or tests, and the treatments provided, including any medications that were administered. The record also included a copy of the patient's informed consent for the transfer or the physician's certification that the transfer was appropriate.

- Prior to transfer, the patient was clinically stable and consented to the transfer. In addition, the transferring hospital contacted the receiving hospital and obtained approval to transfer. This conversation was documented on the transfer form.

Ambulatory Surgery

The records of outpatients who receive surgical services in an ambulatory surgery unit of the hospital must meet the same documentation requirements as inpatient surgical cases. (Surgical services were discussed earlier in this chapter.) The outpatient records of patients who require inpatient admission after ambulatory surgery are combined with the patients' inpatient records.

Specialty-Care Documentation

Specialty care in this section refers to care provided by clinicians with training in a unique clinical area. (Note: Services are listed in alphabetical order, not in order of complexity or importance.) In some cases, such as obstetrics or psychiatry, that care may be provided in specialized areas of the hospital. Specialty-care records often include information that is not required in general medical and surgical records. Government regulations, accreditation standards, and professional practice standards dictate unique content requirements for several types of specialty-care records. These requirements are over and above the basic content and documentation required for general health records.

Chemotherapy Services

Chemotherapy involves the administration of oral and intravenous pharmaceuticals for the treatment of many forms of cancer. The type of disease determines the exact type of chemotherapeutic agent administered. Chemotherapy is the primary treatment for diseases that are inoperable or cannot be treated surgically, such as leukemia. Chemotherapy is also performed in combination with surgery, radiotherapy, or both. The treatment goals of chemotherapy, like all treatments for cancer, may be to cure the disease, control it, or relieve its symptoms.

Intravenous forms of chemotherapy are usually performed in hospital oncology departments. Services may be performed on an inpatient or outpatient basis. Most patients, however, receive chemotherapy as outpatients either before or after surgical interventions to remove their tumors.

The health records of chemotherapy patients include the following information:

- Patient identification, including name and record number

- Diagnosis

- Name of the agent and method of administration

- Dates the procedure was performed

- Findings or results of the treatment procedure

- Date of report and signature of the oncologist who oversaw the treatment

Minors Seeking Services

Additional documentation requirements are in place when the patient is a minor. Consent for treatment or release of information is required from the custodial parent or legal guardian. This applies until the minor reaches the age of majority or becomes emancipated in the eyes of the law. Documentation in the record must establish whether the patient is an emancipated minor.

Common conditions of emancipation include evidence that the minor is one of the following:

- Married

- On active duty with the US armed forces

- Self-supporting and living away from home

- Unmarried and pregnant

Neonatal Services

The health records of newborn infants are maintained separately from their mothers' records. For normal deliveries, the neonatal record usually duplicates much of the information documented in the mother's record in addition to a general assessment of the newborn's condition at birth. (See **Figure 5.36**.) In some cases, a discharge progress note is acceptable for a normal newborn's record.

Much more extensive documentation is required for premature infants and other infants who require intensive care after birth. Some infants require months of treatment in the neonatal ICU before they are strong enough to go home with their parents. The records of these babies require full documentation, including admission and discharge assessments, operative reports when applicable, and discharge summaries.

Some hospitals do not offer neonatal intensive care services. Infants born at these hospitals require immediate transfer to another facility equipped to handle their needs. In such cases, the neonatal record maintained by the hospital where the infant was born should include admission and discharge information and documentation of the reason for the child's transfer to the other facility.

For those newborns who are born and die shortly after delivery a unique health record number and account number should be assigned and a separate record generated by the hospital. A common guideline for creating newborn records is to review the Apgar score; if a newborn is born with an Apgar score of one or above, an individual record for the newborn should be generated, regardless of how long the newborn survives.

If a newborn is born with no Apgar score or an Apgar score of zero, the birth is considered a stillbirth. Hospitals may choose in this instance to combine the newborn record with that of the mother and not generate a separate health record number and account number for the newborn.

Nutritional Services

Nutritional services are provided by registered dietitians in response to an order from the patient's attending physician. A nutritional-care plan is based on an initial **nutritional assessment** performed by the registered dietitian. The assessment includes the patient's diet history, weight and height, appetite and food preferences, and information on food sensitivities and allergies. Nutritional care plans usually include the following information:

- Confirmation that a diet order for the patient was issued within 24 hours of admission

- Summary of the patient's diet history and/or the nutritional assessment performed upon admission

- Documentation of nutritional therapy and/or dietetics consultation

- Timely and periodic assessments of the patient's nutrient intake and tolerance of the prescribed diet

FIGURE 5.36. Example of a neonatal assessment record

Anytown Community Hospital

NEONATAL ASSESSMENT RECORD
PAGE 1 OF 2

PATIENT LABEL

	Within Normal Anatomical Limits	
Development		Birth Date _____ Type of Delivery ☐ Vaginal ☐ C-Section Gender _____ Head Circumference _____ Birth Weight _____ Birth Length _____

		Within Normal Anatomical Limits	

Neurological/Musculoskeletal

Pupil Size
R ____ L ____

Yes	No
☐	☐

LOC	Movement	Pupils
☐ Lethargic	☐ ↓ RA	☐ Nonreactive
☐ Unresponsive	☐ ↓ RL	☐ Sluggish
☐ Irritable	☐ ↓ LA	☐ Constricted
☐ Responds Only to Stimuli	☐ ↓ LL	☐ Fixed

Comments:

Heart/Vascular

Yes	No
☐	☐

Heart	Edema	Vascular (0, 1, 3, 4)
☐ Skips	☐ Generalized	R Radial + _____ ☐ Dop ☐ Abs
☐ Palpitations	Location _____	L Radial + _____ ☐ Dop ☐ Abs
☐ Valve Click	Degree (1–4) _____	R Pedal + _____ ☐ Dop ☐ Abs
☐ Murmur		L Pedal + _____ ☐ Dop ☐ Abs
		R Brach + _____ ☐ Dop ☐ Abs
		L Brach + _____ ☐ Dop ☐ Abs

Comments:

Pulmonary/Lungs

Yes	No
☐	☐

Respirations		Breath Sounds	Right	Left
☐ Orthopnea	☐ Retractions	☐ Crackles	☐	☐
☐ Dyspnea	☐ Shallow	☐ Rhonchi	☐	☐
☐ Apnea	☐ Cough	☐ Wheezes	☐	☐
☐ Labored	☐ Nasal Flaring	☐ Diminished	☐	☐
☐ Tachypnea		☐ Absent	☐	☐

Comments:

Gastrointestinal

Last BM _____
Pattern _____

Yes	No
☐	☐

Bowel Sounds	Abdomen	Bowel Habits
☐ Hypo	☐ Firm	☐ Frequency
☐ Hyper	☐ Protuberant	☐ Diarrhea
☐ Absent	☐ Distended	
	☐ Tender	

Comments:

Nutritional

☐ Breast Feeding Frequency _____ Feeding Length _____
☐ Bottle Feeding Frequency _____ Formula _____ Amount _____

Genitourinary/Reproductive

Yes	No
☐	☐

Urinary		Reproductive
☐ Hematuria	☐ Frequency	☐ Undescended testicles
☐ Oliguria	☐ Dysuria	R ☐ L ☐

Comments:

EENT

Yes	No
☐	☐

Problem	Hearing	Sight
☐ Swallowing ☐ Choking	↓☐ R ↓☐ L	↓☐ R ↓☐ L

Comments:

FIGURE 5.36. (continued)

Anytown Community Hospital

NEONATAL ASSESSMENT RECORD
PAGE 2 OF 2

PATIENT LABEL

	Within Normal Anatomical Limits			
	Yes	No		
Skin Integumentary	☐	☐	**Problem** Location ☐ Bruise _____ ☐ Burn _____ ☐ Rash _____ ☐ Oral Mucosa _____ ☐ Dry ☐ Thrush ☐ Lesions Comments:	**Problem** Location ☐ Wound _____ ☐ Ulcer _____ ☐ Bleeding _____ ☐ Other _____ **Problem** ☐ Pale ☐ Jaundice ☐ Mottled ☐ Tugor ☐ Tenting ☐ Dry
Emotional/ Mental	Yes ☐	No ☐	☐ Lethargic ☐ Fussy ☐ Withdrawn ☐ Inconsolable Crying Comments:	
Sleep Pattern			Bedtime _____ Naptime _____	
Family Information			Primary Caretaker _____ Siblings? How many and what are their ages? _____	
Pain	Yes ☐	No ☐		

Neonatal/Infant Pain Scale (NIPS) (A score greater than 3 indicates pain)

Observe	Criteria	Points
	Relaxed Muscles—restful face, neutral expression	0
	Grimace—tight facial muscles, furrowed brow, chin, jaw (negative facial expression nose, mouth, and brow)	1
	No Cry—quiet, not crying	0
	Whimper—intermittent	1
	Vigorous Cry—loud scream, rising, shrill, continuous (note: silent cry may be scored if baby is intubated as evidenced by obvious mouth and facial movement)	2
	Relaxed—usual pattern for this infant	0
	Change in Breathing—indrawing, irregular, faster than usual, gagging, breath holding	1
Arms	Relaxed/Restrained—no muscular rigidity, occasional random movements of arms	0
	Flexed/Extended—tense, straight legs, rigid and/or rapid extension, flexion	1
Legs	Relaxed/Restrained—no muscular rigidity, occasional random leg movement	0
	Flexed/Extended—tense, straight legs, rigid, and/or rapid extension, flexion	1
State of Arousal	Sleeping/Awake—quiet, peaceful sleeping or alert random leg movement	0
	Fussy—alert, restless, and thrashing	1
	Total Score	

Or
Nonverbal Assessment

Observe	Criteria	Points
	Anxious/Irritable	1
	Almost in Tears	2
	None	0
	Restless/Slow or Decreased Movement	1
	Immobile	2
Verbal Cues	Whining/Whimpering/Moaning	1
	Screaming, Crying Out	2
Facial Cues	Relaxed, Calm Expression	0
	Drawn Around Mouth and Eyes	1
	Facial Frowning, Wincing	2
Positioning/ Guarding	Relaxed Body	0
	Guarding/Tense	1
	Fetal Position/Jumps If Touched	2
	Total Points	

Comments:

RN Initials: _____ RN Signature: _____ Date: _____ Time: _____ Unit: _____

RN Initials: _____ RN Signature: _____ Date: _____ Time: _____ Unit: _____

NEONATAL ASSESSMENT RECORD
000060 (10/2002)

- Nutritional discharge plan and patient instructions

- Documentation that a copy of the plan was forwarded to the facility to which the patient was transferred after discharge from the hospital, if applicable

- Dietitian's signature, credentials, and date

Observation Services

Physicians can admit a patient for observation from the emergency department or other outpatient department of the hospital. Patients are admitted to observation to rule out an acute condition when they present with a symptom. Common reasons for admission to observation include chest pain and shortness of breath. Observation patients are considered outpatients, and they generally stay in the hospital for less than 24 hours. The health records for observation patients must include a physician's order for admission to an observation bed or unit and the time and date of the patient's admission and discharge. Other documentation should include vital signs, medication records, and physicians' and nurses' progress notes. A discharge summary or note should describe the patient's condition and disposition at discharge.

Third-party payers have strict rules on reimbursement for observation services. Therefore, complete documentation of the medical necessity and length of observation services is particularly important.

Case managers can be of particular assistance in monitoring observation admissions and ensure that medical necessity is met. The case manager can also avoid potential inappropriate observation admissions by communicating with the physician to ensure that the patient is placed in appropriate status.

Obstetrical Services

The hospital records for pregnant women admitted for labor and delivery contain elements similar to general health records with additional assessments and monitoring of the labor and delivery process. The obstetrician's records of prenatal care constitute documentation of the patient's preadmission history and physical. At admission, the physician also prepares a note describing the patient's progress since he or she last saw her for prenatal care. (See **Figure 5.37**.) For normal deliveries, a **labor and delivery record** takes the place of an operative report. (See **Figure 5.38**.)

Cesarean deliveries are operative procedures, and as such, they require documentation of the patient's informed consent. Obstetricians who perform cesarean deliveries must prepare complete operative reports. Similarly, sterilization procedures performed after a cesarean or normal delivery are considered separate procedures that must be fully documented.

Discharge summaries are not required for normal deliveries. A preprinted discharge form or discharge progress note is considered sufficient discharge reporting for mother and child. Complete discharge summaries, however, are required for surgical and complicated deliveries.

The health records of the mother and her newborn infant or infants must be maintained separately. An exception is made for cases of stillbirth. Information on the stillborn infant can be incorporated into the mother's record.

Every labor and delivery record should contain the following information:

FIGURE 5.37. Example of a maternal/prenatal care summary

Anytown Community Hospital

MATERNAL/PRENATAL CARE SUMMARY

PATIENT LABEL

Mother's Name: _____

Mother's Age: _____ Gravida: _____ Term: _____

Premature: _____ Abnormal: _____ Living: _____

Expected Delivery Date: _____

Prenatal Labs: _____

Maternal/Prenatal/Family History: _____

_____

_____

Social Problems: _____

_____

Type of Delivery: ☐ Vaginal

☐ C-Section

Type of Anesthesia: _____

Tubal Ligation: ☐ Yes ☐ No

Apgars: 1 min __ 5 min __ 10 min __

Complications of Labor and Delivery: _____

_____

_____

Transfer From: _____

Date: _____

Delivery Weight: _____

Last Weight: _____

Service Notified: _____

Date and Time: _____

Person Notified: _____

Examined: _____

Void: ☐

Stool: ☐

Circumcision: ☐ Yes ☐ No

Done: _____

Date: _____

Metabolic Screen: ☐ Yes ☐ No

Done: _____

Date: _____

Hearing Screen: ☐ Yes ☐ No

Done: _____

Date: _____

Pass/Refer:

Follow-up Appointment
Made: _____

Vitals: _____

Glucoses: _____

Breast: _____

Formula: _____

IVF _____ @ _____

UAC _____ @ _____

UVC _____ @ _____

Mother's Blood Type and RH: _____

Cord Blood: _____

COOMBS: _____

Cord Bili: _____

Baby Safe Signed: ☐

Gift Bags Given: ☐

Hepatitis B Vaccine:
☐ Yes   ☐ No

Orders:

_____

_____

_____

_____

_____

_____

_____

_____

_____

_____

Medications: _____

_____

_____

_____

Messages: _____

_____

Obstetrician	Delivery Date	Delivery Time	Baby's Gender
Mother's Room Number		Pediatrician	

FIGURE 5.38. Example of a labor and delivery summary

Anytown Community Hospital

LABOR AND DELIVERY SUMMARY
PAGE 1 OF 5

PATIENT LABEL

LABOR SUMMARY

G	T	Pt	A	L	Blood Type and Rh	EDD
						/ /

Prenatal Events ☐ None

☐ No Prenatal Care

☐ Preterm Labor (≤37 Weeks)

☐ Postterm Labor (≥42 Weeks)

☐ Previous Cesarean

☐ Prenatal Complications

☐ Other_____

Maternal Intrapartal Events

☐ None
☐ Febrile (≥100.4°F/38°C)
☐ Bleeding—Site Undetermined
☐ Preeclampsia: ☐ Mild ☐ Severe
☐ Seizure Activity
☐ Medications: ☐ None

Date	Time	Medication	Dose	Route

☐ Transfusion _____ units
   Blood Component _____
☐ Other _____

Amniotic Fluid

☐ SROM ☐ AROM Date ____ Time ____

☐ Premature ROM ☐ Prolonged ROM

☐ Clear

☐ Meconium-Stained (Describe) _____

☐ Bloody

☐ Foul Odor

  ☐ Cultures Sent _____ Time _____

☐ Polyhydramnios

☐ Oligohydramnios

☐ Other_____

Placenta

☐ Placenta Previa

☐ Abruptio Placenta

☐ Other_____

Labor

☐ Precipitous Labor (<3 h)

☐ Prolonged Labor (≥20 h)

☐ Prolonged Latent Phase

☐ Prolonged Active Phase

☐ Prolonged 2nd Stage (>2.5 h)

☐ Secondary Arrest of Dilatation

☐ Induction:

  ☐ None   ☐ AROM
  ☐ Oxytocin   ☐ Other_____

☐ Augmentation:

  ☐ None   ☐ AROM
  ☐ Oxytocin   ☐ Other_____

FIGURE 5.38. (continued)

Anytown Community Hospital

LABOR AND DELIVERY SUMMARY
PAGE 2 OF 5

PATIENT LABEL

LABOR SUMMARY (Continued)

Fetus

Gestational Age (Weeks): _____ By Dates _____ By Ultrasound

Presentation: **Position:**

☐ Vertex ☐ Face/Brow

☐ Breech: ☐ Frank ☐ Complete ☐ Single Footing ☐ Double Footing

☐ Transverse Lie: ☐ Back Up ☐ Back Down

☐ Compound

☐ Unknown

☐ Cephalopelvic Disproportion (CPD)

☐ Cord Prolapse

Monitor: ☐ None ☐ External FHR ☐ External UC
☐ Internal FHR ☐ Internal UC

STV: ☐ Present ☐ Absent

☐ LTV _____

☐ Fetal Bradycardia

☐ Fetal Tachycardia

☐ Sinusoidal Pattern

☐ Accelerations: ☐ Spontaneous ☐ Uniform

☐ Decelerations: ☐ Early ☐ Late ☐ Variable ☐ Prolonged

☐ Scalp pH ≤ 7.2

☐ _____

FM Discontinued _____ Time _____

FHR Prior to Delivery _____ bpm Time _____

Signature _____ Date _____

DELIVERY SUMMARY

Support Person Present: ☐ Yes ☐ No

Location: ☐ LDR ☐ LDRP ☐ DR ☐ OR ☐ Birthing Room ☐ Other _____

Method of Delivery: Vaginal

☐ VBAC (Number _____)

☐ Vertex

   ☐ Spontaneous

   ☐ Assisted **Position:** ___ to ___ **Position:** ___

   ☐ Manual Rotation

   ☐ Forceps (Type) _____)

      ☐ Outlet ☐ Low ☐ Mid

   ☐ Vacuum Extraction Duration ___ min.
      Degree of Suction _____ kg/cm²

☐ Breech (Type _____)

   ☐ Spontaneous ☐ Partial Extraction (Assisted) ☐ Total Extraction

   ☐ Forceps Assist

      ☐ Piper ☐ Other _____

Episiotomy

☐ None ☐ Midline ☐ Mediolateral L   R

Laceration/Episiotomy Extension:

☐ None ☐ Periurethral ☐ Vaginal ☐ Cervical ☐ Uterine

☐ Perineal ☐ 1" ☐ 2" ☐ 3" ☐ 4"

Repair Agent Used _____

☐ Vagina Free of Sponges

Placenta

☐ Spontaneous ☐ Expressed ☐ Manual Removal

☐ Adherent (Type _____)

☐ Uterine Exploration

☐ Curettage

Configuration

☐ Normal

☐ Abnormal _____

Weight _____ g

Disposition _____

Cord

☐ Nuchal Cord (× _____) ☐ True Knot Length _____ cm

☐ 2 Vessels ☐ 3 Vessels

Cord Blood ☐ To Lab ☐ Refrig ☐ Discard

Lab ☐ Type + Rh ☐ Cultures ☐ COOMBS

☐ pH ☐ _____

Signature _____ Date _____

FIGURE 5.38. (continued)

Anytown Community Hospital

LABOR AND DELIVERY SUMMARY
PAGE 3 OF 5

PATIENT LABEL

DELIVERY SUMMARY (Continued)

Method of Delivery: Cesarean

☐ Scheduled ☐ Emergency ☐ Primary ☐ Repeat (× —————) ☐ Other _____

Operative Indication: ☐ Previous Uterine Surgery ☐ Failure to Progress ☐ Placenta Previa ☐ Abruptio Placenta

☐ Fetal Malpresentation _____ ☐ Nonreassuring FHR Pattern _____

☐ Other_____

Uterine Incision: ☐ Low Cervical, Transverse ☐ Low Cervical, Vertical ☐ Classical

Hysterectomy: ☐ Yes ☐ No **Tubal Ligation:** ☐ Yes ☐ No

Skin Incision: ☐ Vertical ☐ Pfannenstiel

Surgical Data

Sponge Counts Correct: ☐ NA ☐ Yes ☐ No _____

Needle Counts Correct: ☐ NA ☐ Yes ☐ No _____

Vaginal Pack Count Correct: ☐ NA ☐ Yes ☐ No _____

Estimated Blood Loss _____ *cc*

Anesthesia: ☐ None ☐ Local ☐ Pudendal ☐ General ☐ Epidural ☐ Spinal

Date	Time	Medication	Dose	Effect

Complications of Anesthesia: ☐ Yes _____ ☐ None

Medications: ☐ None

Date	Time	Medication	Dose	Route Site	Initials

Chronology

	Date	Time		
EDD				
Admit to Hospital				
Membranes Ruptured				
Onset of Labor			Total Time H/Min	
Complete Cervical Dilation				I
Delivery of Infant				II
Delivery of Placenta				III
				Total Labor

Signature _____ Date _____

FIGURE 5.38. (continued)

Anytown Community Hospital

LABOR AND DELIVERY SUMMARY
PAGE 4 OF 5

PATIENT LABEL

NEONATAL SUMMARY

Birth Data

Time of Birth _____ ☐ Male ☐ Female

ID Band # _____

Condition: ☐ Alive ☐ Antepartum Death ☐ Intrapartum Death ☐ Neonatal Death

Birth Order _____ of _____

Apgar Score	1 min	5 min	10 min
Heart Rate			
Respiratory Effort			
Muscle Tone			
Reflex Irritability			
Color			
Total			

Signature _____

Airway
☐ Bulb Suction
☐ Suction Catheter   Size _____ Fr
   ☐ Mouth   Pressure _____ mm Hg
   ☐ Nose   ☐ At Delivery
   ☐ Pharynx
☐ Endotracheal Tube Size _____ Fr
   ☐ Meconium Below Cords Times _____

Breathing
☐ Spontaneous
☐ O_2 _____ Liters   Time Initiated
   ☐ Free Flow   _____
   ☐ PPV
      ☐ Bag/Mask   _____
      ☐ ET Tube Size _____ Fr   _____
      ☐ CPAP _____ *mm*
_____ Minutes to First Gasp
_____ Minutes to Sustained Respiration

Circulation
☐ Spontaneous
☐ External Cardiac Massage
   Time Initiated _____ Time Completed _____
_____ Minutes for HR >100
   Heart Rate (bpm)
      _____ Time _____
      _____ Time _____
      _____ Time _____

IV Access
☐ Umbilical Catheter
☐ Peripheral Line

Person Managing Reuscitation
_____

Medications: ☐ None

Date	Time	Medication	Dose	Route Site	Initials

Laboratory Data: ☐ None

Blood Gases	Sent	Umb Art	Umb Vein
pH			
pO_2			
pCO_2			
HCO_3			

Test	Result
Dextrostix	_____

FIGURE 5.38. (continued)

Anytown Community Hospital

LABOR AND DELIVERY SUMMARY
PAGE 5 OF 5

PATIENT LABEL

NEONATAL SUMMARY (Continued)

Initial Newborn Exam

Weight _____ g _____ lb _____ oz ☐ Deferred
Length _____ cm _____ in ☐ Deferred
Head _____ cm _____ in ☐ Deferred
Chest _____ cm _____ in ☐ Deferred
Abdomen _____ cm _____ in ☐ Deferred
T _____ ☐ Rectal ☐ Axillary
AP _____ R _____ BP _____
☐ No Observed Abnormalities
☐ Abnormalities Noted
☐ Meconium Staining ☐ Cephalhematoma
☐ Petechiae ☐ Other
Describe _____
_____
_____

Intake ☐ None
  Breast Feed: ☐ Yes ☐ No
Output ☐ None
  ☐ Urine ☐ Stool (Type_____)
  ☐ Gastric Aspirate _____ cc
Examined By _____
Transfer: ☐ With Mother
        ☐ To Newborn Nursery
        ☐ To NICU
        ☐ Other_____
Date ___ / ___ / ___ Time _____
Mode of Transport_____

Delivery Personnel

RN (1)_____
    (2)_____
Anesthesiologist/CRNA _____
CNM _____
Physician—Attending _____
Physician—Assist (1) _____
        (2) _____
Pediatric Provider _____
☐ Notified ☐ Present at Birth

Remarks

_____

_____	_____	
Signature	Date	LABOR AND DELIVERY SUMMARY 200366 (6/2004)

- Patient's married and/or maiden name(s)

- Patient's record number

- Delivery date

- Gender of the infant

- Names and credentials of the physician and any assistants

- Descriptions of any complications that developed

- Type of anesthesia

- Name of the person who administered the anesthesia

- Names of other persons who witnessed the delivery

Psychiatric Services

Psychiatric services are generally provided on distinct units of hospitals that are designated for psychiatric care or in psychiatric hospitals. Inpatient psychiatric hospitals and psychiatric units within acute-care hospitals maintain documentation similar to that of other inpatient units as well as documentation unique to psychiatric care. The following list includes the elements of minimum documentation for psychiatric patient records established by accreditation standards, federal regulations, and Medicare Conditions of Participation (CMS 2010):

- Demographic data

- Source of referral

- Reason for referral

- Patient's legal status

- All appropriate consents for admission, treatment, evaluation, and aftercare

- Admitting psychiatric diagnoses

- Psychiatric history

- Record of the complete patient assessment, including the complaints of others regarding the patient and the patient's comments

- Medical history, report of physical examination, and list of medications

- Provisional diagnoses based on assessment that includes other current diseases and psychiatric diagnoses

- Written, individualized treatment plan

- Documentation of the course of treatment and all evaluations and examinations

- Multidisciplinary progress notes related to the goals and objectives outlined in the treatment plan

- Appropriate documentation related to special treatment procedures, such as the use of physical and chemical restraints and seclusion techniques to control dangerous patient behavior

- Updates to the treatment plan as a result of ongoing assessments detailed in the progress notes

- Records of multidisciplinary case conferences and consultation notes, which include the dates of the conferences or consultations, the recommendations made, and the actions taken

- Information on any unusual occurrences, such as treatment complications, accidents or injuries to the patient, death of the patient, and procedures that placed the patient at risk or caused unusual pain

- Correspondence related to the patient, including all letters and dated notations of telephone conversations relevant to the patient's treatment

- Discharge or termination summary

- Plan for follow-up care and documentation of its implementation

- Individualized aftercare or post treatment plan

See chapter 13 for additional information about behavioral healthcare.

Radiotherapy Services

Like chemotherapy, radiotherapy (also called radiation therapy) is performed as a primary or adjuvant (supporting) treatment for neoplastic disease and many forms of cancer. Physicians specializing in nuclear medicine work with oncologists and other specialty physicians to develop treatment plans targeted to reach specific types of lesions. Radiation therapy equipment is precisely calibrated to deliver radiation to the abnormal tissue while sparing the patient's normal tissue as much as possible. Individual patients may undergo weeks of daily radiation therapy to achieve partial or complete relief of their symptoms. Radiation therapy also prevents the recurrence of the disease in many cases.

Radiotherapy is usually performed in hospital nuclear medicine or radiology departments. Services may be performed on an inpatient or outpatient basis. Most patients, however, receive radiotherapy as outpatients either before or after surgical interventions to remove their tumors.

The health records of radiotherapy patients include the following information:

- Patient identification, including name and record number

- Diagnosis

- Name and site of the procedure

- Dates the procedure was performed

- Findings or results of treatment procedure

- Date of report and signature of the radiologist who oversaw the treatment

Rehabilitation Services

Rehabilitation services may be provided in certain units of a hospital or in a rehabilitation hospital. In addition, rehabilitation services can be provided in an inpatient or outpatient setting. Patients are admitted to rehabilitation care after being treated in an acute hospital following trauma or an acute condition that resulted in impaired functioning. For example, a patient with a cerebrovascular accident with residual hemiparesis might be admitted to rehabilitation to improve speech or manual dexterity.

Rehabilitation services include a number of different therapies designed to build or rebuild the patient's ability to perform the **activities of daily living (ADLs)**. ADLs include the basic activities of self-care, including the ability to communicate with others, feed oneself, bath and dress oneself, use the toilet, and move within one's environment. Rehabilitation services include physical therapy, occupational therapy, speech therapy, and treatment by physicians who specialize in rehabilitation and the use of orthotics, known as physiatrists.

Physical therapists help patients build or rebuild their muscle strength and respiratory and circulatory capacities. Physical therapists work with patients who have been disabled by illnesses (stroke and heart disease are the most common), injuries, and birth defects.

Occupational therapists help patients restore their ability to read and write and to perform self-care activities after they have been disabled by illness or injury. Similarly, speech therapists conduct dysphasia evaluations and help disabled patients regain their ability to communicate.

Inpatient rehabilitation hospitals and rehabilitation units within acute care hospitals are subject to a Medicare prospective payment system that is based on documentation. A standardized assessment tool called the **patient assessment instrument (PAI)** must be completed shortly after the patient's admission and on discharge. Payment level is based on the patient's medical condition and diagnostic profile as well as the services provided.

The Joint Commission's *Comprehensive Accreditation Manual for Hospitals* (2006) and the Medicare *Conditions of Participation for Hospitals* (CMS 2010) both require that the records of rehabilitation services include documentation of a preliminary patient assessment and a written rehabilitation plan. The plan must be developed by qualified professionals on the basis of the patient's needs. (See **Figure 5.39**.)

Many rehabilitation facilities are accredited through the **Commission on Accreditation of Rehabilitation Facilities (CARF)**. CARF requires rehabilitation facilities to maintain a single case record for every patient they admit. The documentation standard for health records includes the following requirements:

- Patient identification data
- Pertinent history
- Diagnosis of disability
- Rehabilitation problems, goals, and prognosis
- Reports of assessments and individual program planning
- Reports from referring sources and service referrals
- Reports from outside consultations and laboratory, radiology, orthotic, and prosthetic services
- Designation of a manager for the patient's program

FIGURE 5.39. Example of a rehabilitation care plan

University of Anystate Hospital

REHABILITATION PLAN OF CARE
PAGE 1 OF 4

PATIENT LABEL

Date Developed/Updated: _____ Anticipated Discharge: _____

Rehab Diagnosis: _____ Prognosis: _____

Anticipated Discharge Disposition: _____

Patient/Caregiver Goals: _____

Medical Status: _____

Self-Care/Events	TD	RD	Interventions	Person(s) Responsible
1. Upper extremity dressing with: _____			1. ADL program	OT, Nursing
2. Lower extremity dressing with: _____			2. ADL program	OT, Nursing
3. Bathing with: _____			3. ADL program	OT, Nursing
4. Toileting with: _____			4. ADL program	OT, Nursing
5. Grooming with: _____			5. ADL program	OT, Nursing
6. Eating with: _____			6. ADL program	OT, Nursing, SLP

Discharge Outcome(s): ADLs with: _____

Mobility/Events	TD	RD	Interventions	Person(s) Responsible
1. Transfers with: _____			1. Transfer training	PT, Team
2. Tub/shower transfers with: _____			2. Transfer training	OT, Team
3. Toilet transfers with: _____			3. Transfer training	OT, Team
4. Bed mobility with: _____			4. Rolling, bridging, supine-sit	PT, Team
5. Wheelchair propulsion: _____ ft with: _____			5. Wheelchair skills training	PT, Team
6. Ambulation: _____ ft using: _____ with: _____			6. Gait training	PT, Team
7. Up and down: _____ stairs with: _____			7. Real-life room, flight of stairs	PT, TR
8. Community surfaces/barriers: _____			8. RLR, outing	TR, Team

Discharge Outcome(s): Transfer with: _____ Ambulation with: _____

Wheelchair propulsion with: _____ Up/down stairs with: _____

FIGURE 5.39. (continued)

University of Anystate Hospital

REHABILITATION PLAN OF CARE
PAGE 2 OF 4

PATIENT LABEL

Communication/Events	TD	RD	Interventions	Person(s) Responsible

Discharge Outcome(s): Effective communication skills with: _____

Bio-Psycho-Social Functioning/Events	TD	RD	Interventions	Person(s) Responsible
Redirect pain complaints with: _____			Peer interaction, relaxation techniques	TR
Interact with peers/staff with: _____			Group and individual socialization	TR

Discharge Outcome(s): Adjust to lifestyle changes and to disability; to participate in community activities at level of functioning

Cognitive/Events	TD	RD	Interventions	Person(s) Responsible
Alert and oriented X: _____			Reorientation	SLP, Team
Adaptive leisure skills with: _____			Assistive devices, resources, body awareness	TR
				SLP, Team

Discharge Outcome(s): Increase cognition to within functional limits for basic self-care with good safety awareness and judgment

Patient/Caregiver Education/Events	TD	RD	Interventions	Person(s) Responsible
1. Patient/caregiver able to relate use and frequency of medications			1. Medication teaching	Nursing
2. Patient/caregiver able to assist patient with activities of daily living and transfers			2. ADL program, transfer training	Team
3. Patient/caregiver able to relate bowel and bladder programs			3. Bowel and bladder programs	Nursing
4. Patient/caregiver able to demonstrate skin care			4. Turning, pressure relief, skin assessment, skin care, signs of infection	Team
5. Patient/caregiver able to relate nutrition and hydration requirements			5. Dietary teaching	Nursing
6. Patient/caregiver able to relate safety issues/ management precautions			6. Demonstration, discussion, activities of daily living, mobility	Team

Discharge Outcome(s): Caregiver able to safely and appropriately assist patient; patient able to manage own care

FIGURE 5.39. (continued)

University of Anystate Hospital

REHABILITATION PLAN OF CARE
PAGE 3 OF 4

PATIENT LABEL

Environmental/Discharge Planning/Events	TD	RD	Interventions	Person(s) Responsible
Discharge planning			Patient/caregiver teaching, DME assessed and ordered, patient–caregiver conference, home healthcare	Team
Identify resources and complete appropriate applications			Leisure education, transportation resources	TR

Discharge Outcome(s): Safe discharge home with caregiver and support from community resource

Other Areas of Concern/Events	TD	RD	Interventions	Person(s) Responsible
1. Preadmission bowel status			1. Bowel program	Nursing
2. Preadmission bladder status			2. Bladder program	Team
3. Skin free of breakdown			3. Pressure relief measures	Nursing
4. Wound free of infection; facilitate healing			4. Wound care: per MD; D/C staple: per MD; ET consult PRN	Physician, Nursing, ET
5. Pain less than or equal to level 3			5. Medicate prior to therapy and PRN; cold pack PRN; relaxation techniques; position Δ	Team
6. Preadmission nutritional status			6. I&O, dietary consult, monitor caloric intake	Team
7. UE strength:			7. UE exercise program	OT
8. LE strength:			8. LE exercise program	PT
9. Endurance:			9. Endurance activities	Team

Discharge Outcome(s): No fall or injury during rehabilitation stay; reestablish appropriate bowel elimination; reestablish appropriate urinary elimination; skin intact; no signs of infection; patient/caregiver able to manage wound/skin care; adequate management of pain; adequate nutritional status; maximize UE/LE strength to perform ADLs

FIGURE 5.39. (continued)

University of Anystate Hospital

REHABILITATION PLAN OF CARE
PAGE 4 OF 4

Functional Independence Measure

	ADM	CURR		ADM	CURR			
Eating			Transfer: Tub/Shower					
Grooming			Locomotion: Walk		FT	SLS	US	FIM
Bathing			Locomotion: Wheelchair		FT	SLS	US	FIM
Dressing—Upper			Stairs					
Dressing—Lower			Comprehension					
Toileting			Expression					
Bladder Management			Social Interaction					
Bowel Management			Problem Solving					
Transfer: Bed, Chair, Wheelchair			Memory					
Transfer: Toilet								

Communication with patient/caregiver prior to team conference	NSG	OT	PT	PSY	SLP	TR	SW
Progress discussed with patient/caregiver							
Patient/caregiver input for treatment goals given and discussed							
Patient/caregiver input for treatment goals given/discussed; progress related							

N/A = Patient unable to provide input toward goals due to deficit

_____   _____

Physician Signature   Date

_____   _____

Patient/Caregiver Signature   Date

_____ Initials of person reviewing team conference with patient/caregiver

Signature	Date/Time	Signature	Date/Time

REHABILITATION PLAN OF CARE
0000205 (10/2002)

- Evidence of the patient's or family's participation in decision making

- Evaluation reports from every service

- Reports of staff conferences

- Patient's total program plan

- Plans from each service

- Signed and dated service and progress reports

- Correspondence pertinent to the patient

- Release forms

- Discharge report

- Follow-up reports

Renal Dialysis Services

Renal dialysis services are provided to patients who are diagnosed with renal failure. The only cure for renal failure is a kidney transplant, but dialysis performed on a regular basis (for example, three times per week) can treat the illness's symptoms. Dialysis is the process of removing toxins from the blood directly or indirectly. Hemodialysis works by gradually removing the patient's blood and pumping it through an external filtering system before the blood is returned to the body via a vascular port. Peritoneal dialysis works by instilling an electrolyte solution into the patient's peritoneum. Periodically, the fluid is drained to remove the fluid and accumulated toxins.

Hemodialysis is performed in hospital-based units and dedicated ambulatory care centers. Although it is less effective than hemodialysis, peritoneal dialysis is a simpler procedure and may even be performed in the patient's home.

The health records of dialysis patients include the following information (**Figure 5.40**):

- Patient identification, including name and record number

- Diagnosis

- Name of the procedure

- Duration of the procedure

- Dates the procedure was performed

- Findings or results of the procedure

- Names, credentials, and signatures of the nurses or physicians who oversaw the procedure

Respiratory Services

Respiratory therapy is administered by respiratory therapists, nurses, and pulmonologists (physicians who specialize in the diagnosis and treatment of respiratory illness). Patients with acute or chronic respiratory conditions, such as pneumonia and asthma, often

FIGURE 5.40. Example of a hemodialysis record

Anycity General Hospital

HEMODIALYSIS RECORD

PATIENT LABEL

Machine Serial #: _____

| Orders | Duration | Concentrate
K+ | Cell Type | Heparinization
Systemic: _____
ACT Range: _____ |

Blood Flow	Desired Weight Loss	BP Support		Blood TXM: _____ Transfuse: _____
		Saline	Albumin	

Predialysis Labs: _____   Postdialysis Labs: _____

_____
_____
_____

Assessment: _____ kg, Weight: _____ Time: _____

_____
_____
_____
_____
_____
_____

Plan:

_____

Abbreviations

ACT	= Activated clotting time	Pres = Pressure
		Seq = Sequential
Art	= Arterial	TMP = Transmembrane pressure
BF	= Blood flow	
DLSC	= Dual Lumen subclavian catheter	UF = Ultrafiltration

Vital Signs	Post: ____	Pre: ____	Post: ____
Weight			
BP Supine			
BP Standing			
P			
T			
Edema			
Lungs/R			

Time	BP	Blood Flow	Dialysate Flow	Arterial Pressure	Venous Pressure	Dialysate Pressure	UF / TMP	ACT / Heparin	NS / Albumin	Weight	Interventions/Comments:
											_____
											_____
											_____
											_____
											_____
											_____
											_____
											_____
											_____
											_____

Evaluation/Goal Achievement: _____ kg   Weight: _____   Cell: _____   Total Heparin Dose: _____ units   Total Saline: _____ cc   Total Albumin: _____ g

☐ Goals and/or plan of care revised/reviewed with patient/family

Physician Signature: _____ Date: _____ RN Signature: _____ Date: _____

HEMODIALYSIS RECORD
000140 (10/2002)

require respiratory therapy. Emergency respiratory therapy is often provided in hospital emergency departments when patient-administered treatments are not effective.

Basic treatments include the administration of aerosol medications and humidified oxygen. When breathing problems become life threatening, physicians administer cardiopulmonary resuscitation and/or place the patient on mechanical ventilation.

Hospitals also provide a number of diagnostic services related to respiratory conditions. Common services include pulmonary function testing and blood gas analysis. Respiratory therapists and nurses work directly with patients to provide coughing and breathing exercises and therapeutic percussion and vibration to clear the lungs of fluid and mucus.

Respiratory therapy services must be ordered by the patient's physician. Respiratory assessments and treatment plans contain information about the patient's diagnosis, the services to be provided, and the goals of treatment. (An example of a respiratory therapy report is provided in **Figure 5.41**.)

Discharge Summaries

The **discharge summary** is a concise account of the patient's illness, course of treatment, response to treatment, and condition at discharge. (Other terms for this type of documentation include *discharge abstract* and *clinical resume*.) The summary states the patient's reason for admission and gives a brief history explaining why he or she needed to be hospitalized. Pertinent laboratory, X-ray, consultation, and other significant findings, as well as the patient's response to treatment or procedures, are included. In addition to a description of the patient's condition at discharge, the discharge summary delineates specific instructions given to the family for future care, including information on medications, referrals to other providers, diet, activities, follow-up visits to the physician, and the patient's final diagnoses. The discharge summary must be authenticated and dated by the physician (LaTour and Eichenwald Maki 2010).

The physician principally responsible for the patient's hospital care generally dictates the discharge summary. However, a resident, physician assistant, or nurse practitioner who is being supervised by the attending physician may complete this task. Regardless of who documents it, the attending is responsible for the content and quality of the summary and must sign and date it. The summary must be completed within 30 days of discharge for most patients but within 24 hours for patients transferred to other facilities. Discharge summaries are not always required for patients who were hospitalized for less than 48 hours. (See **Figures 5.42** and **5.43**.)

The functions of the discharge summary include the following:

- Ensuring the continuity of future care by providing information to the patient's primary care physician and any consulting physicians

- Providing information to support the activities of the medical staff review committee

- Providing concise information that can be used to answer information requests from authorized individuals or entities

Each facility adopts different formats for the discharge summary. However, at a minimum, the patient's discharge summary should include:

- Name of the attending physician

- Date and time of discharge

FIGURE 5.41. Example of a respiratory therapy record

Midwest Medical Center

VENTILATOR FLOW SHEET

PATIENT LABEL

Diagnoses: _____

Physician: _____

Current Settings: _____

DATE				
TIME				
INITIALS				
MODE				
SET VT				
ACTUAL VT				
PS/SPONT VT				
MINUTE VOLUME				
SET RATE/TOTAL RATE				
WAVE FORM/PF				
FIO_2/FIO_2 ACTUAL				
PRESSURE SUPPORT				
PEEP/CPAP				
PEAK PRESSURE				
SENSITIVITY				
PIP ALARM				
LIP ALARM				
LOW-PEEP ALARM				
LOW-VT ALARM				
LOW/SET VE ALARM				
HIGH-RR ALARM				
HME				
AMBU BAG/MASK				
HHN/MDI MED				
RESTRAINTS				
HR/PULSE O_2				
CUFF PRESSURE				
ET SIZE/PLACE CM				
BREATH SOUNDS R LUNG				
L LUNG				
SUCTION SITE				
SPUTUM AMOUNT				
COLOR				
APNEA ALARMS	Sec/VT	RR/PF/FIO_2	PIP/Itime	I:E/H PR

Breath Sounds:	1. Rhonchi	2. Rales	3. Wheezing	4. Diminished	5. Clear	6. Other _____
Sputum Amount:	1. Scant	2. Small	3. Moderate	4. Large	5. Copious	
Sputum Color:	1. Beige	2. Yellow	3. Blood-tinged	4. White	5. Clear	6. Other _____

Therapist Signature: _____   Date: _____

VENTILATOR FLOW SHEET
000035 (10/2002)

FIGURE 5.42. Example of a discharge summary

Midwest Medical Center

DISCHARGE SUMMARY

SAYLORMEN, POPEYE T.
333333333
DOB: 02/09/1961

PHYSICIAN/SURGEON: Philip P. Heartstopper, MD

DATE OF DISCHARGE: 05/18/20XX

PRINCIPAL OPERATION AND PROCEDURE: OPCAB × 3, left internal mammary artery of the LAD, saphenous vein graft to D-1, and saphenous vein graft to OM-1

HISTORY OF PRESENT ILLNESS: Mr. Saylormen was seen at the request of Dr. Doctor regarding surgical treatment of ischemic heart disease. He is a 42-year-old male with a family history of coronary artery disease. He smokes a pipe and had a previous myocardial infarction approximately three years ago. His current status is postangioplasty. While working on a construction project, he developed anginal-type symptoms and was seen in the emergency room and then admitted to the hospital for further evaluation.

ADMITTING DIAGNOSIS: Coronary artery disease

HOSPITAL COURSE: The patient underwent cardiac catheterization and was found to have significant three-vessel coronary artery disease. It was felt that he would benefit from undergoing an OPCAB procedure. On 05/14/200x, the patient underwent OPCAB × 3 as described above. The patient tolerated the procedure well and returned to the Cardiothoracic Intensive Care Unit hemodynamically stable. On postoperative day one, he was weaned from mechanical ventilation, extubated, and transferred to the Cardiothoracic Step-Down Unit, where he continued on a progressive course of recovery. On postoperative day four, he was up and about in his room and the halls without difficulty. Upon discharge, he was tolerating his diet well. His lungs were clear. His abdomen was soft, and his incisions were unremarkable. His vital signs were stable. He was in normal sinus rhythm. His heart rate was in the 70s and 80s. Blood pressure had been running consistently in the low 110s/60s. He was afebrile. Oxygen saturations on room air were reported at 97%.

LABORATORY DATA AT DISCHARGE: BUN 14, Creatinine 0.9, H&H 8.8 and 25.4

MEDICATIONS AT DISCHARGE: Lisinopril 5 mg q.d.; Lipitor 80 mg q.d.; metoprolol 50 mg q.d.; aspirin 81 mg q.d.; Darvocet-N 100—one to two tablets every 4–6 hours as needed for pain; iron sulfate 325 mg q.d. × 30 days; and Colace 100 mg b.i.d. × 30 days

DIET: He may follow a regular diet.

FINAL DIAGNOSIS: Coronary artery disease

DISPOSITION: No lifting greater than 10 pounds. No driving for 4–6 weeks. He may shower but he should not take a tub bath. Follow up with Dr. Doctor in 1–2 weeks.

_____
Philip P. Heartstopper, MD

5/18/200x
_____
Date

d: 05/18/20XX
t: 05/19/20XX
PPH, MD/mb

FIGURE 5.43. Example of a short-form discharge summary

Anytown Community Hospital

SHORT-FORM DISCHARGE SUMMARY

PATIENT LABEL

DATE OF DISCHARGE: _____

REASON FOR HOSPITALIZATION: _____

_____

_____

SIGNIFICANT FINDINGS: _____

_____

_____

CONDITION/CONCLUSIONS AT DISCHARGE: _____

_____

_____

PROCEDURES AND TREATMENT: _____

_____

_____

INSTRUCTIONS TO PATIENT/FAMILY: _____

_____

_____

DISCHARGE DIAGNOSIS(ES): _____

_____

_____

Physician Signature: _____ Date: _____

SHORT-FORM DISCHARGE SUMMARY
0034632 (02/2002)

- Principal and secondary diagnoses

- Diagnostic and therapeutic procedures and the dates on which the procedures were performed

- Name of the surgeon or surgeons who performed the surgical procedures, if applicable

- Disposition of the patient (for example, was the patient transferred to a subacute facility, a rehabilitation facility, or discharged to home?)

- Medications and instructions upon discharge.

Discharge Instructions

The discharge summary usually includes specific instructions for patient care after discharge. The instructions for aftercare may be given directly to the patient or to her caregiver at the time of discharge. Discharge instructions usually include the primary physician's recommendations for diet and activity levels, prescriptions for any needed medications, and referrals for follow-up care. Many hospitals also provide standardized aftercare instructions to patients who underwent inpatient or outpatient surgical procedures or received other relatively common therapeutic services (for example, chemotherapy).

To ensure patient safety after hospital treatment, it is vital that the patient receive clear, concise discharge instructions. Ideally, patient instructions should be communicated both verbally and in writing. The healthcare professional (usually the patient's primary nurse) who delivers the instructions to the patient or the caregiver should also complete health record documentation that indicates that he explained the instructions before the patient left the facility. In addition, the person receiving the instructions should be asked to sign a form verifying that she understands the instructions. A copy of the written instructions should then be filed in the patient's health record. (See **Figure 5.44** for an example of patient instructions.)

When someone other than the patient assumes responsibility for the patient's aftercare, the record should indicate that the instructions were given to the party responsible for the patient. Documentation of patient education may be accomplished by using forms that prompt the person providing instruction to cover specific information.

Autopsy Reports

A hospital **autopsy report** is a description of the examination of a patient's body after he has died. Autopsies are usually conducted when there is some question about the cause of death or when information is needed for educational or legal purposes. The purpose of the autopsy is to determine or confirm the cause of death or to provide more information about the course of the patient's illness. (See **Figure 5.45** for an example of an autopsy report.)

When local authorities suspect that a patient's death may have been the result of a crime, a local medical examiner may conduct the autopsy rather than a hospital pathologist.

FIGURE 5.44. Example of patient discharge instructions

University of Anystate Hospitals

PATIENT/FAMILY INSTRUCTIONS
PAGE 1 OF 2

PATIENT LABEL

This is a guide for your care. Call your doctor for any problems or changes that concern you.

Diet

Diet: _____ If on special diet and have questions, call dietitian.

Managing Your Meds Discussed
(Place a checkmark if medication handouts given) ↓

Medications (list all medications)

Name/Dose	How to Take	

Activities/Special Care

Activities (Check as indicated)
- ☐ Crutches/walker
- ☐ Walk with assistance
- ☐ Gradually resume normal activity
- ☐ Bedrest
- ☐ Other _____

Dressing and Wound Care
(Report increased pain, redness, swelling, drainage, or fever)
- ☐ Doctor to change dressing
- ☐ Keep dressing dry
- ☐ If no dressing, keep incision clean and dry
- ☐ Clean wound and change dressing

Additional Instructions (PEARLS)

Follow Up (appointments/equipment/referrals)

Agency	Phone	Arrangements (instructions provided by agency)

Dr. _____   Date/Time _____ ☐ Call for an appointment
Dr. _____   Date/Time _____ ☐ Call for an appointment
Dr. _____   Date/Time _____ ☐ Call for an appointment

I understand the above instructions and have the ability to carry these out after discharge. I am aware of the importance of medical follow-up with my doctor.

Patient/Patient Rep. Signature: _____   Date: _____

RN Signature: _____   Date: _____

FIGURE 5.44. (continued)

University of Anystate Hospitals

PATIENT/FAMILY INSTRUCTIONS
PAGE 2 OF 2

PATIENT LABEL

Discharge Date: _____ Time: _____ Mode: _____

Discharged With:

☐ Family member ☐ Friend ☐ By self ☐ Other: _____

Escorted by: ☐ Hospital Attendant ☐ Ambulance Attendant

RN Discharge Assessment

_____

_____

_____

_____

_____

_____

Continuing Care Assessment		
Care Plan	☐ All goals resolved on IPOC/clinical path/plan of care. Exceptions documented.	
Discharge with:	☐ Self/family care	• Patient and/or family verbalized an understanding of instructions. Person (s) to assist if needed: _____
Discharge with:	☐ Support services	• Patient will receive follow-up with a referral agency or extended care facility. See front of form.
Discharge to:	☐ Home ☐ Home with home health ☐ Extended care facility ☐ Other: _____	

☐ Patient Expired   Date: Time: Valuables Given to: ☐ Family ☐ Funeral Home ☐ Security
☐ Patient Left without Permission   Date: Time:

RN Signature: _____ Date: _____

PATIENT INSTRUCTIONS
5435680 (03/2002)

FIGURE 5.45. Example of an autopsy report

Lincoln County Hospital

O'PATIENT, RENATA H.
4378802133524
DOB: 02/18/1958

AUTOPSY REPORT
PAGE 1 OF 4

ACCESSION NUMBER:	1-121320XX		
DATE OF DEATH:	12/13/20XX	**DATE OF AUTOPSY:**	12/15/20XX
ADMITTING PHYSICIAN:	Nelda Oncodoct, DO	**PATHOLOGIST:**	Frank Reeper, MD
CONSULTING PHYSICIAN #1:	Leo Kardiovsky, MD	**PROSECTOR:**	Nelda Oncodoct, DO
CONSULTING PHYSICIAN #2:	NA	**ATTENDANT:**	Georges Helper

FINAL ANATOMICAL DIAGNOSES

CLINICAL DIAGNOSES:

1. Metastatic sarcoma

2. Possible sepsis

3. History of thyroid carcinoma

4. Hypocalcemia

5. Hypokalemia

6. Cortical nodules, right adrenal gland

7. Angiolipoma, left kidney

8. Myocardial hypertrophy, left ventricle

9. Diverticulosis, colon

PATHOLOGICAL DIAGNOSES:

1a. Possible primary osteosarcoma of superior sternum/anterior rib cage with superior mediastinal extension

1b. Metastatic osteosarcoma involving lungs extensively and T5 vertebral body with pathologic fracture

2a. Hemorrhagic bronchopneumonia

2b. Premortem sputum culture positive for Staphylococcus aureus (cocci identified in inflamed areas of lung at autopsy)

2c. Diffuse alveolar damage syndrome, lungs (shock lung)

3. No evidence of recurrent thyroid carcinoma, examination of neck not included

4. No anatomic correlate

5. No anatomic correlate

INCIDENTAL FINDINGS:

Signature: _Frank G Reeper, MD_   _12/15/200x_
PATHOLOGIST   DATE

FIGURE 5.45. (continued)

Lincoln County Hospital

AUTOPSY REPORT
PAGE 2 OF 4

O'PATIENT, RENATA H.
4378802133524
DOB: 02/18/1958

CASE HISTORY: This 45-year-old, white female was admitted to the Medical ICU at County Hospital on 12/12/2003 after presenting earlier that day at Dr. Oncodoct's office with profound general weakness and difficulty breathing. The patient's past medical history indicated a history of thyroidectomy for tall-cell variant papillary carcinoma. She was treated postthyroidectomy with I-131 and external beam radiation because of multiple lymph node metastases. She had been diagnosed last month with metastatic sarcoma, which presented as a symptomatic T5 vertebral compression fracture. She had also developed progressive swelling of the legs, but a CT scan of the abdomen and pelvis performed several days before admission showed no evidence of venous thrombosis.

On admission, she had a potassium level of 2.5, calcium of 4.8, and phosphorus of 7.3. She was initially treated with two amps of calcium gluconate and potassium chloride administered intravenously. A chest X ray performed upon admission showed extensive masses within the lung fields, consistent with metastatic disease. Other studies performed after admission showed a free T-4 of 4.04 ng per deciliter (0.71 to 1.85). Shortly after admission, the patient was intubated and placed on a ventilator. A cardiology consultant noted pump failure secondary to tumor burden. The patient was febrile at admission, and her hypotension was thought to be secondary to sepsis. She was treated with antibiotics, but despite supportive measures, she died on the second hospital day (12/13) at 3:55 p.m. An autopsy limited to the chest and abdomen was performed on 12/15.

GROSS EXAMINATION

GENERAL INSPECTION: The body was that of a slightly malnourished female who looks like her stated age of 45 years. The body was identified as that of Renata H. O'Patient according to the ID band on her left wrist and the ID tag on her right big toe. The irises were hazel and the hair was brown, with normal female distribution. Oral and nasal tubes were present and in place. There was a single-lumen catheter in the right neck. A 9-cm, well-healed, longitudinal scar was also present on the anterior neck. There was also a full-lumen catheter in the right antecubital fossa. A Foley catheter was present. Postmortem lividity was present posteriorly, and marked edema was noted.

BODY CAVITIES: The organs of the thorax and abdomen were in their normal anatomic relationships. There was 10 ml of straw-colored serous fluid in the right and 15 ml of straw-colored serous fluid in the left pleural cavities. The pericardial sac contained 10 ml of serous fluid. The great vessels and chambers of the heart were in a normal anatomic relationship. Firm areas of gray and tan tumor involved the mediastinum. Tumor was identified and involved the upper sternum, skeletal muscle, anterior rib cage, and mediastinum. There was no fluid within the peritoneal cavity. The cranial cavity and neck organs were not examined due to permit restrictions.

CARDIOVASCULAR SYSTEM: The heart weighed 510 g and was of a normal configuration. The epicardium was normal. The heart was opened in the plane of the atrioventricular groove. Neither ventricle appeared dilated. The myocardium was reddish brown and firm. The right ventricular wall was 0.6 cm in thickness, and the left ventricular wall was 2.1 cm in thickness. The left ventricle appeared hypertrophic. No significant abnormalities were found in the valves, and the endocardium was normal. The coronary arteries had a normal anatomic distribution, with the right coronary artery being predominant. The arteries were sectioned in 0.2- to 0.3-cm intervals. The proximal right coronary artery, the main left coronary artery, the left anterior descending coronary artery, and the left circumflex coronary artery showed no calcific atherosclerosis. The aorta also showed no calcific atherosclerosis, ulceration, or mural thrombi.

RESPIRATORY SYSTEM: The mucosa of the trachea was unremarkable. The right lung weighed 1100 g and the left lung 1050 g. The pleura was glistening and nodular with multifocal gray and tan, firm lesions. The lung was fresh cut. The cut surfaces showed greater than twenty nodules within the parenchyma. The largest nodule was 8 by 6 by 3 cm, and it was located within the base of the left lower lobe. In addition, the parenchyma was congested and hemorrhagic. The bronchial walls were thickened and the mucosa reddened. The pulmonary arteries showed no atherosclerosis or thromboemboli. The hilar and bronchial lymph nodes had tumor and were enlarged.

FIGURE 5.45. (continued)

Lincoln County Hospital

AUTOPSY REPORT
PAGE 3 OF 4

O'PATIENT, RENATA H.
4378802133524
DOB: 02/18/1958

DIGESTIVE SYSTEM: The esophagus was unremarkable. The stomach contained approximately 10 ml of semi-liquid, tan material. The mucosa was markedly reddened. The small intestine was unremarkable. The large intestine contained brown fecal material, and scant colonic diverticula were noted. The appendix was present and unremarkable. The liver weighed 2300 g, and the capsular surface was smooth and glistening. On section, the parenchyma was reddish brown with central lobular congestion. The gallbladder contained approximately 35 ml of brown-green bile. The mucosa showed prominent yellow streaks. No stones were identified. The common bile duct was unremarkable. The pancreas appeared normal and was normal in consistency.

GENITOURINARY SYSTEM: The right kidney weighed 210 g, and the left kidney weighed 220 g. The capsule was stripped with difficulty, and the underlying cortical surfaces were coarsely granular and pitted. A 0.3-cm, firm, tan-colored nodule was noted on the left kidney. On section, the cortex measured 0.8 cm in thickness. The cortex was markedly hyperemic. The renal arteries showed no atherosclerosis. The urinary bladder showed no mass lesions. Mucosal hemorrhages were absent. The endocervical canal and os appeared unremarkable. The endometrium was pale yellow. No leiomyomas were present. The myometrium was unremarkable. The ovaries were pale yellow and without cysts.

HEMATOPOIETIC SYSTEM: The thymus was not identified. The spleen weighed 250 g and had a dull-gray capsule. On section, the spleen was dark red and firm. Systemic lymph nodes were grayish tan and enlarged. The bone marrow was reddish brown.

ENDOCRINE SYSTEM: The adrenal glands were slightly enlarged. Two separate nodules were present within the right adrenal gland. Each nodule was about 1 cm in diameter.

MUSCULOSKELETAL SYSTEM: The vertebral column showed no osteopenia. A fracture was identified along the vertebral column at T5. The fracture site was surrounded by firm areas of tan to gray tumor.

CASSETTE SUMMARY: (1) Left lung, lower lobe and tumor; (2) left lung, upper and middle lobes and tumor; (3) right lung, upper lobe and tumor; (4) right lung, middle and lower lobes; (5) T5 soft-tissue mass; (6) upper sternum and mediastinal mass; (7) T5 vertebra; (8) liver and gallbladder; (9) spleen; (10) right kidney and adrenal gland with mass; (11) left kidney and adrenal gland with cortical nodule; (12) uterus, cervix, right tube and ovary; (13) pancreas and bladder; (14) stomach, small and large intestines; (15) right and left ventricles of heart.

MICROSCOPIC EXAMINATION

GENERAL TUMOR DESCRIPTION: Sections of the tumor masses show a neoplasm characterized by highly cellular proliferations of spindle cells with generally indistinct cytoplasm and marked nuclear pleomorphism. Best demonstrated in slide A1 from a metastatic site and A6, a possible primary site, there is prominent, irregular osteoid formation characteristic of osteosarcoma. Infiltration of subchondral bone is present in the latter area. Sections of the T5 vertebra show extensive necrosis of the neoplasm within the bone with no morphologically intact residual tumor seen. The adjacent soft-tissue mass, however, shows large zones of intact neoplasm associated with areas of necrosis.

RESPIRATORY SYSTEM: In addition to the metastatic osteosarcoma, the uninvolved lung tissue shows numerous areas of an exudate of neutrophils within the alveolar spaces associated with focal areas of hemorrhage. Numerous colonies of coccoid bacteria are present within these zones of inflammation. In addition to the extensive broncho-pneumonia, other areas show vascular congestion, prominent alveolar lining cells, and focal hyaline membrane formation consistent with shock lung (diffuse alveolar damage syndrome).

FIGURE 5.45. (continued)

Lincoln County Hospital

AUTOPSY REPORT
PAGE 4 OF 4

O'PATIENT, RENATA H.
4378802133524
DOB: 02/18/1958

GENITOURINARY SYSTEM: Sections of the nodule in the left kidney show a lesion composed of spindle cells with a prominent vascular network mixed with fat cells. Spindle cells show fibrillar eosinophilic cytoplasm characteristic of smooth-muscle differentiation. This lesion represents an angiomyolipoma. There is no evidence of metastatic sarcoma. Elsewhere, the kidney shows pigment casts within tubules but no other significant findings.

ENDOCRINE SYSTEM: Sections confirm the presence of adrenal cortical nodules.

GENERAL: Sections of the other organs sampled show no additional significant findings or confirmed the gross impressions.

CASE SUMMARY: This 45-year-old white woman with a history of tall-cell variant of papillary carcinoma had been treated with I-131 and external beam radiation therapy because of multiple lymph node metastases and an aggressive primary tumor. Her course had been complicated by hypoparathyroidism. Recently, she had developed a compression fracture of the T5 vertebral body and on further evaluation was found to have a widely metastatic sarcoma involving the lungs and bones of the chest. Mediastinal tumor was noted on imaging studies. On the day before her death, the patient presented with a febrile illness and hypotension secondary to sepsis. Despite treatment, she died on the second hospital day.

Autopsy documented extensive metastatic sarcoma involving the lungs, and the large samples available at autopsy showed osteoid formation within several areas characteristic of osteosarcoma. A relatively large mass involving the superior sternum, anterior rib cage, and superior mediastinum suggested a possible primary tumor in this site. This finding raised the possibility of a postradiation sarcoma. Autopsy documented extensive pulmonary metastases involving nearly half of the lung parenchyma bilaterally. There was a large soft-tissue extension surrounding the vertebral body metastasis, and there was extensive necrosis of the bone tumor in this site consistent with recent radiation therapy.

The immediate case of death was hemorrhagic bronchopneumonia secondary to *Staphylococcus aureus*, which was cultured postmortem from the sputum. Other findings in the lungs were consistent with diffuse alveolar damage syndrome secondary to shock and sepsis (shock lung).

Other findings of an incidental nature are documented in the final diagnoses.

In such cases, the patient's body is generally moved to a county facility for autopsy. In most states, medical examiners are required to issue provisional autopsy reports within three days of the autopsy and final reports within 60 days.

Authorizations for autopsy, signed by the patients' next of kin or by law enforcement officials, should also be filed in the patients' permanent health records. Copies of hospital autopsy reports should also be stored in the patients' records.

Clinical Information as the Basis for Uniform Data Sets

The clinical information in the patient's record is primarily used to treat the patient. However, when clinical information from many patient records is combined, it can be used to help the larger groups of patients through research and public health data analysis. Clinical information in the patient record can be standardized through the use of uniform data sets.

Uniform data sets are groups of data elements that are the minimum accepted level of information to be collected for a specific purpose, along with uniform definitions (LaTour and Eichenwald Maki 2010) These data result from the manual abstracting of information in the patient health record. One example of a data element in a uniform data set is the ICD-9-CM code assigned to a patient's **principal diagnosis**.

Two data sets developed by the National Committee on Vital Health Statistics (NCVHS) for hospital use are the UHDDS and the UACDS, which were created in 1985 and 1989, respectively. The UHDDS contains 20 data elements, and the UACDS contains eight. The NCHVS recommends that every hospital use the uniform data sets to voluntarily submit data to the federal government for large-scale analyses for public health and research purposes. To date, 40 states submit at least some of the data elements from their hospital and ambulatory stays for analysis. Each state determines whether hospital data will be abstracted and submitted to the state department of health. The HIM professional should be aware of the specific requirements for submitting discharge data using the uniform data set in the state where he or she practices. For those states that require mandatory reporting, the data sets collected by different hospitals can be compared, and the data can be combined for national analysis and healthcare delivery planning.(See **Figures 5.46** and **5.47**)

An example of a data element from the UHDDS is data element No.13, "other diagnoses." To ensure uniformity when abstracting data from the patient record for reporting purposes, the UHDDS defines other diagnoses as "all conditions that coexist at the time of admission or that develop subsequently or that affect the treatment received and/or the length of stay. Diagnoses that relate to an earlier episode and have no bearing on the current hospital stay are to be excluded." Further clarification is found in data element No.14, "qualifier for other diagnoses," which UHDDS explains as follows: "a qualifier is given for each diagnosis coded under 'other diagnoses' to indicate whether the onset of the diagnosis preceded or followed admission to the hospital. The option 'uncertain' is permitted."

In 1996, ten years after the creation of the UHDDS guidelines, NCVHS issued a report on core uniform health data elements (NCHVS 1996). The report said,

FIGURE 5.46. UHDDS data elements

Data Element	Definition/Descriptor
01. Personal identifier	The unique number assigned to each patient within a hospital that distinguishes the patient and his or her hospital record from all others in that institution.
02. Date of birth	Month, day, and year of birth. Capture of the full four-digit year of birth is recommended.
03. Sex	Male or female
04. Race and ethnicity	04a. Race American Indian/Eskimo/Aleut Asian or Pacific Islander Black White Other race Unknown 04b. Ethnicity Spanish origin/Hispanic Non-Spanish origin/Non-Hispanic Unknown
05. Residence	Full address of usual residence Zip code (nine digits, if available) Code for foreign residence
06. Hospital identification	A unique institutional number used across data collection systems. The Medicare provider number is the preferred hospital identifier.
07. Admission date	Month, day, and year of admission.
08. Type of admission	Scheduled: Arranged with admissions office at least 24 hours prior to admission Unscheduled: All other admissions
09. Discharge date	Month, day, and year of discharge
10. & 11. Physician identification • Attending physician • Operating physician	The Medicare unique physician identification number (UPIN) is the preferred method of identifying the attending physician and operating physician(s) because it is uniform across all data systems.
12. Principal diagnosis	The condition established, after study, to be chiefly responsible for occasioning the admission of the patient to the hospital for care.
13. Other diagnoses	All conditions that coexist at the time of admission or that develop subsequently or that affect the treatment received and/or the length of stay. Diagnoses that relate to an earlier episode and have no bearing on the current hospital stay are to be excluded.
14. Qualifier for other diagnoses	A qualifier is given for each diagnosis coded under "other diagnoses" to indicate whether the onset of the diagnosis preceded or followed admission to the hospital. The option "uncertain" is permitted.
15. External cause-of-injury code	The ICD-9-CM code for the external cause of an injury, poisoning, or adverse effect (commonly referred to as an E code). Hospitals should complete this item whenever there is a diagnosis of an injury, poisoning, or adverse effect.
16. Birth weight of neonate	The specific birth weight of a newborn, preferably recorded in grams.
17. Procedures and dates	All significant procedures are to be reported. A significant procedure is one that is: • Surgical in nature, or • Carries an anesthetic risk, or • Carries a procedural risk, or • Requires specialized training. The date of each significant procedure must be reported. When more than one procedure is reported, the principal procedure must be designated. The principal procedure is one that is performed for definitive treatment rather than one performed for diagnostic or exploratory purposes or was necessary to take care of a complication. If two procedures appear to be principal, the one most closely related to the principal diagnosis should be selected as the principal procedure. The UPIN must be reported for the person performing the principal procedure.
18. Disposition of the patient	• Discharged to home (excludes those patients referred to home health service) • Discharged to other healthcare facility • Discharged to acute-care hospital • Left against medical advice • Discharged to nursing facility • Alive, other; or alive, not stated • Discharged home to be under the care of a home health service (including a hospice) • Died All categories for primary and other sources are: • Blue Cross/Blue Shield • Health maintenance organization (HMO) • Other health insurance companies • CHAMPUS • Other liability insurance • CHAMPVA • Medicare • Other government payers • Medicaid • Self-pay • Worker's Compensation • No charge (free, charity, special research, teaching) • Self-insured employer plan • Other
19. Patient's expected source of payment	Primary source Other sources
20. Total charges	All charges billed by the hospital for this hospitalization. Professional charges for individual patient care by physicians are excluded.

FIGURE 5.47. UACDS data elements

Data Element	Definition/Descriptor
Provider identification, address, type of practice	Provider identification: Include the full name of the provider as well as the unique physician identification number (UPIN).
	Address: The complete address of the provider's office. In cases where the provider has multiple offices, the location of the usual or principal place of practice should be given.
	Profession: • Physician, including specialty or field of practice • Other (specify)
Place of encounter	Specify the location of the encounter: • Private office • Clinic or health center • Hospital outpatient department • Hospital emergency department • Other (specify)
Reason for encounter	Includes, but is not limited to, the patient's complaints and symptoms reflecting his or her own perception of needs, provided verbally or in writing by the patient at the point of entry into the healthcare system or in the patient's own words recorded by an intermediary or provider at that time.
Diagnostic services	All diagnostic services of any type.
Problem, diagnosis, or assessment	Describes the provider's level of understanding and the interpretation of the patient's reasons for the encounter and all conditions requiring treatment or management at the time of the encounter.
Therapeutic services	List, by name, all services done or ordered: • Medical (including drug therapy) • Surgical • Patient education
Preventive services	List, by name, all preventive services and procedures performed at the time of encounter.

Disposition	The provider's statement of the next step(s) in the care of the patient. At a minimum, the following classification is suggested:
	
	 1. No follow up planned
	 2. Follow up planned
	    • Return when necessary
	    • Return to the current provider at a specified time
	    • Telephone follow up
	    • Return to referring provider
	    • Refer to other provider
	    • Admit to hospital
	    • Other

The identification, definition, and implementation of standardized data in the health care and health care information fields are long overdue. Information is collected by a wide range of users and in a myriad of different formats. Work has been undertaken in the past to try to bring some semblance of order to selected areas of health data collection, especially in the areas of hospital inpatients and physician office visits. The ever-expanding sites of care, combined with the increasing use of electronic data, make it imperative that all health data collection activities, where possible, utilize standardized data elements and definitions. Standardized data elements will be vitally important in the evolving managed care field, where there is a need to follow individuals through a continuum of care and at multiple sites. Performance monitoring and outcomes research are two additional areas that are currently hampered by the inability to link data sets from various sources due to varying data elements and definitions.

In many ways, the NCVHS's realization almost 30 years ago that there was a need to pull standardized information from patient records and classify the elements into national, uniform data sets to benefit patients, the healthcare industry, and society in general was quite visionary. Uniform data sets are, in many ways, the early precursors of EHR standards, which see a future far beyond the current limitations of the 20 UHDDS and eight UACDS data elements obtained through manual review and abstraction of a patient's record.

Summary

The primary purpose of a health record is to facilitate medical care provided to the patient. To fulfill this purpose, health records must contain complete and accurate documentation of the care provided to the patient, the rationale for that care, patient reactions to treatment, and patient diagnoses. This chapter explores widely accepted standards for documentation for each report type found in health records. The content for the most commonly used forms is included, along with some specialty requirements.

Documentation is compiled throughout a patient's treatment. It begins with admission to a service and concludes with discharge from care. The four categories of information are administrative, demographic, financial, and clinical. The required elements can be collected in a paper-based or electronic system. In both cases, it is imperative that complete information be documented to facilitate quality and continuity of care for a patient and to serve the legal, statistical, and reimbursement needs of the facility and healthcare provider. The health information professional must be familiar with requirements for each type of clinical report in a patient's record. This includes federal government requirements, state departments of health requirements, The Joint Commission's requirements (if the hospital is accredited), and the hospital's own medical staff bylaws requirements for health record content.

Once a patient is discharged and his health record is complete, information in the record is abstracted, or pulled out of the record by manual reviewers or health record coders. This abstracting process should follow the structure recommended by the NCHVS in the UHDDS for inpatient discharges and the UACDS for ambulatory care discharges.

References

AHIMA. 2005. *Documentation and Reimbursement for Behavioral Healthcare Services.* Chicago: AHIMA.

AHIMA Association Ambulatory Care Section. 2001. *Documentation and Reimbursement for Ambulatory Care,* rev. ed. Chicago: AHIMA.

Centers for Medicare and Medicaid Services (CMS). 2010. Conditions of Participation for Hospitals; Final rule. 42 CFR Part 482. *Federal Register* 71(227):68672–68695. http://ecfr.gpoaccess.gov/cgi/t/text/text-idx?c=ecfr&sid=dee029e8667b45b65efaf4c6b967bb9c&rgn=div8&view=text&node=42:5.0.1.1.1.3.4.4&idno=42.

Centers for Medicare and Medicaid Services (CMS). 2006. Provider Agreements and Supplier Approval; Special Responsibilities of Medicare Hospitals in Emergency Cases; Final Rule. 42 CFR Part 489.24. *Federal Register* 71(160):48143. http://www.access.gpo.gov/nara/cfr/waisidx_06/42cfr489_06.html.

Food and Drug Administration (FDA). 1998. Medical Device Reporting; Final Rule. 21 CFR 803. *Federal Register* 63(91):26069. http://www.access.gpo.gov/nara/cfr/waisidx_06/21cfr803_06.html.

Glondys, B. 1999. *Documentation Requirements for the Acute Care Patient Record.* Chicago: AHIMA.

Johns, M., ed. 2011. *Health Information Management Technology: An Applied Approach.* Chicago: AHIMA.

Health Insurance Portability and Accountability Act (HIPAA) of 1996. Public Law 104-191. http://www.gpoaccess.gov/cfr/index.html.

The Joint Commission. 2006. *2006 Comprehensive Accreditation Manual for Hospitals: The Official Handbook (CAMH).* Oakbrook Terrace, IL: The Joint Commission.

LaTour, K., and S. Eichenwald Maki. 2010. *Health Information Management: Concepts, Principles, and Practice,* 3rd ed. Chicago: AHIMA.

Reynolds, R., and E. Bowman. 2010. Paper-Based and Hybrid Health Records. In *Health Information Management: Concepts, Principles, and Practice,* 3rd ed., edited by K. LaTour and S. Eichenwald Maki. Chicago: AHIMA.

Medicare. 2010. *Medicare and You.* http://www.medicare.gov/Publications/Pubs/pdf/10050.pdf.

National Center for Injury Prevention and Control. 1997. Data Elements for Emergency Department Systems, release 1.0. Atlanta, GA: Centers for Disease Control and Prevention. http://www.cdc.gov/ncipc/pub-res/pdf/deeds.pdf.

National Committee on Vital and Health Statistics (NCVHS). 1996. Core Health Data Elements. http://www.ncvhs.hhs.gov/ncvhsr1.htm.

National Guideline Clearinghouse. 2007. *About NGC.* http://www.guideline.gov/about/index.aspx.

Shaw, P., C. Elliot, P. Isaacson, and E. Murphy. 2010. *Quality and Performance Improvement in Healthcare: A Tool for Programmed Learning,* 4th ed. Chicago: AHIMA.

US Department of Health and Human Services (HHS). 1996. Public Health Service, AHCPR. Clinical practice guidelines number 19. Rockville, MD: US Department of Health and Human Services.

Chapter 6

Health Record Design

Ruthann Russo, PhD, MPH, RHIT

Learning Objectives

- Compare the format, functionality, and features of three different paper-based health record formats

- List the limitations of paper-based health records

- Explain the different definitions for the electronic health record (EHR) and list the elements that are common to all definitions

- Define data, information, and knowledge and give examples of each

- Describe the federal policies and legislation driving national EHR implementation

- Describe the benefits and barriers to EHR implementation

- List the ten components of the EHR

- Describe HITECH Act criteria for meaningful use of the EHR and list criteria for stages 1, 2, and 3

- List the organizations that provide guidance toward a standardized National Health Information Network (NHIN) and EHRs

- Describe the different technical standards used to ensure consistency in EHRs

- List and define the different standard clinical terminologies and identify which one will likely be used for EHRs and the NHIN

- Define the term *data dictionary*, explain its purpose, and describe the basic steps involved in developing one

- Define the term *database* and explain the concept of database integration in EHR development

- Explain electronic form design concepts and their impact on the functionality of EHRs

- Explain the functions of clinical decision support systems included in EHRs

- Define the hybrid health record and the challenges it presents

- Describe the different types of electronic document management systems (EDMSs)

- Explain the Veterans Administration EHR system, VistA, and how it facilitates both patient care and healthcare research

- Define the term *authentication* within the context of health records and discuss some of the tools used to achieve it

- Explain the process for correcting errors in paper-based records and EHRs

- Identify four areas of concern when working to prevent fraud in the EHR environment

- Identify and explain three concepts important to developing a litigation response plan for e-discovery

- Define the term *disaster recovery planning* and outline the points an EHR disaster-recovery plan should address

Key Terms

Agency for Healthcare Research and Quality (AHRQ)

American Recovery and Reinvestment Act (ARRA)

American Society for Testing and Materials (ASTM)

Authentication

Clinical data repository

Clinical decision support (CDS) systems

Computer output laser disk/enterprise report management (COLD/ERM) technology

Data exchange standards

Database

Database management system

Digital information

EHR Collaborative

Electronic document management system (EDMS)

Electronic health record (EHR)

Functionality standards

Health information exchange (HIE)

Health Level Seven (HL7)

Institute of Medicine (IOM)

Integrated health record

Meaningful use criteria

Messaging standard

National Committee on Vital and Health Statistics (NCVHS)

National health information infrastructure (NHII)

National Health Information Network (NHIN)

National network for health data exchange

National Resource Center for Health Information Technology

Office of the National Coordinator for Health Information Technology (ONC)

Problem list

Problem-oriented health record

Prohibited abbreviations

Source-oriented health record

Structure and content standards

Technical standards

Veterans Health Information Systems and Technology Architecture (VistA)

Vocabulary standards

Introduction

The design of health records is at a crossroads. The passage of the **American Recovery and Reinvestment Act of 2009 (ARRA)** amended the Health Information Privacy and Accountability Act of 1996 (HIPAA) privacy and security rules. The goal of having a complete electronic health record (EHR) by 2015 for all Americans ensures a National Health Information Network (NHIN). Prior to ARRA, healthcare organizations that solely used paper-based records could choose from among a few standard formats. Once the organization chose a format, it could create and use organization-specific forms. As a result, the format varied from one organization to the next, and standardization was impossible.

A key goal of ARRA is to create a national standard for the configuration and content of health records so that health information can be easily shared among providers in different organizations to ensure the best possible care for all patients. Today, most healthcare organizations use a hybrid record, which includes both paper and electronic elements. Although the goal of a nationwide health information network is still many years away, the ARRA incentives to health care providers beginning in 2011 and ending in 2015 bring us one step closer.

This chapter starts by exploring paper-based health records as the precursors to the EHR. Paper formats include the source-oriented, the problem-oriented, and the integrated health record. Until ARRA, no single rule existed for arranging the content of a health record. Healthcare organizations were free to select the arrangement that best suited their needs as long as their systems fulfilled the requirements of state laws, federal regulations, and accreditation standards. With the transition to the EHR, the paradigm shifts from format and filing to standardization and the ability to access meaningful, digital health information.

The federal government has regulated healthcare since the passage of Medicare legislation in 1964. However, the regulations generally focused on outcomes—for example, the federal government limited how much it would reimburse an organization for healthcare. Under ARRA, the government regulates the day-to-day operations of healthcare providers through incentive payments. These policies, the legislation driving national EHR legislation, reimbursement incentives for providers and organizations that demonstrate meaningful use of EHRs, the benefits of and barriers to EHR implementation, and the ten components of an EHR are all discussed in the chapter.

The role of national standardization activities is also described. First, organizations such as the Certification Committee on Health Information Technology (CCHIT) and others whose primary aim is to guide the transition to a standard EHR to facilitate information exchange are discussed. Second, standards used to ensure technical consistency for EHRs, such as Health Level 7 (HL7) and ANSII, are described. Finally, systems used to ensure consistent use of clinical terminology, such as MUMPS and SNOMED, are discussed.

The chapter goes on to discuss the role of the hospital or healthcare system in ensuring a high-quality EHR. In addition to meeting meaningful use criteria, every healthcare provider must ensure that the EHR is effective. This involves creating a data dictionary, integrating all databases within the organization, incorporating clinical decision support systems, designing electronic forms, and educating providers, especially physicians, to use the EHR properly.

The next section addresses guidelines for preventing fraud in the EHR. A national, standardized EHR presents many opportunities for privacy violations that must be prevented. Authentication (authorship integrity) of health record entries is discussed, and documentation integrity and specific issues in protecting patient identification and demographic data are explored. Because it is important to preserve health record documentation in certain formats for legal purposes, e-discovery and the development of a litigation response plan are also addressed in this section.

The final section is a look at Veterans Health Information Systems and Technology Architecture (VistA). The first national EHR system, VistA has been in place since the mid-1990s. VistA is the EHR for the Veterans Administration (VA) Healthcare System. It has been used to increase quality, decrease costs, and promote health for patients of the VA health system over the past 15 years.

Last the hybrid record, which uses both paper-based and electronic formats, is described. Common formats and challenges of the hybrid record are illustrated. Finally, the storage of all three types of health records (paper based, electronic, and hybrid) is addressed.

Paper-Based Health Records

Most healthcare facilities currently follow one of three formats for paper-based health records: the source-oriented health record, the problem-oriented health record, or the integrated health record. However, no hard-and-fast rules exist for arranging the elements of a health record. Facilities are free to select the arrangement that best suits their needs, as long as their systems fulfill the requirements of state laws, federal regulations, and accreditation standards described in chapters 5 and 8.

Source-Oriented Health Records

In the **source-oriented health record**, documents are grouped according to their point of origin. That is, laboratory records are grouped together, radiology records are grouped together, clinical notes are grouped together, and so on. Thus, physicians' progress notes for a single episode of patient care are arranged, usually in reverse chronological order, and filed together in the patient's health record. Similarly, notes prepared by nursing services, social services, and other clinical services are grouped according to service and arranged sequentially.

Under this format, the individuals charged with filing reports in paper-based records can do so simply by looking at the source and date of the report. However, the users of information filed in this type of record have more trouble. To follow or document information on the patient's course of treatment, they must search by date of occurrence in each of the sections (that is, laboratory, radiology, and every group of clinical notes). The more departments a hospital has, the more sections the source-oriented health record can have. The end user must tie together information from the various sections of the record to get a full picture of the patient's course of treatment.

Problem-Oriented Health Records

The **problem-oriented health record** is easier to use. This format is arranged according to a **problem list**. A problem list is an itemized description of the patient's past and present social, psychological, and medical problems. Each problem is indexed with a unique number, and reports and clinical documentation are keyed to the numbers representing the problems they address. The documentation is arranged in chronological or reverse chronological order. (See **FIGURE 6.1**.)

FIGURE 6.1. Example of a problem list

Anytown Community Hospital

**INTERDISCIPLINARY PROBLEM LIST
AND PLAN OF CARE**

PATIENT LABEL

Category:

Subcategory:

Problem List:

☐

☐

Discharge Outcomes

Target Date/ Initials	Key Interventions	Discipline	Start Date/ Initials	Stop Date/ Initials

Initials	Signature	Discipline	Initials	Signature	Discipline

Key

CM = Case Manager	NSG = Nursing	RD = Registered Dietitian
DTC = Diabetes Treatment Center	OT = Occupational Therapist	RT = Respiratory Therapist
ETN = Enterostomal Nurse	PC = Pastoral Care	SLP = Speech/Language Pathologist
FSR = Financial Services Representative	PHM = Pharmacy	SW = Social Worker
HCC = Home Care Coordinator	PT = Physical Therapist	

Origin:

INTERDISCIPLINARY PROBLEM LIST
000100 (10/2002)

In addition to the problem list, the problem-oriented health record contains the prescribed set of patient data, an initial care plan, and progress notes. Content of the problem-oriented health record includes the following:

- Chief complaint
- Present illness(es)
- Social history
- Medical history
- Physical examination
- Diagnostic test results

The initial care plan serves as an overall guide for addressing each of the patient's problems. The services described in the plan are numbered to correspond to the problems they address.

The patient's caregivers use progress notes to document how the patient's problems are being treated and how the patient is responding to treatment. Each progress note is labeled with the number of the problem it is intended to address. This problem-indexing system allows the clinician to easily follow the patient's course of treatment. Ideally, other elements of the health record (such as physicians' orders) are also numbered according to the problems they address. Information in the progress notes is organized using a sequence referred to as SOAP—an acronym that reminds the provider to address all four areas of patient care:

1. **S**ubjective information (such as patient complaint)
2. **O**bjective data (such as diagnostic test results)
3. **A**ssessment (diagnosis)
4. **P**lan (treatment)

Many physicians are trained in the use of SOAP notes during medical school and may use the SOAP format regardless of the health record format employed by the hospital. The biggest shortcoming of problem-oriented records is the inconsistent application of problem numbers to every piece of documentation.

Integrated Health Records

The third format used for paper-based acute-care records is the **integrated health record**. The integrated health record is arranged so that the documentation from various sources is intermingled and follows a strict chronological or reverse chronological order. The advantage of the integrated format is that it is easy for caregivers to follow the course of the patient's diagnosis and treatment. The disadvantage is that it is difficult to compare related information or even to locate specific information

Limitations of Paper-Based Health Records

The format, data structure, and organization are important factors in meeting the required function of health records. The traditional paper-based health record has many limitations:

- **Chart order**: Paper-based health records need to adhere to a strict record format, sometimes referred to as "chart order." Because paper-based records are lengthy, it is often challenging to retrieve information when it is needed. Healthcare facilities organize records according to a specific format that must be followed by every user. The greater the number of users, the more important it is that the records follow strict format guidelines.

- **Viewing capability**: Paper-based health records can be viewed by only one user and in only one place at a time. Therefore, the valuable information documented in health records is often unavailable.

- **Updating**: Paper-based health records are difficult to update. An active record of a patient receiving care moves from provider to provider within the healthcare facility. Individuals responsible for updating record content must hand-deliver paper documents to the record's location or wait until the record is returned to them to file the information. Updates and reports may be delayed or misplaced as a result.

- **Impermanence**: Paper-based health records are fragile. They are susceptible to damage from water, fire, and the effects of daily use. For most hospitals, maintaining duplicate copies as backups for paper records is prohibitively expensive. Consequently, paper-based health records are always at risk for being misplaced, misfiled, or damaged.

Electronic Health Records

All healthcare providers in the United States are currently involved in a transition from paper based to EHRs. The primary reason for the transition is to improve the quality of patient care. The primary expected benefit is significant cost savings.

It is and will continue to be essential to use systems that ensure structure, consistency, and efficiency in the EHR. Part of the discussion in this section addresses the historical basis for EHR processes and policies. While some initial policies may not have focused on structure, consistency, and efficiency, these characteristics are paramount under the ARRA and Health Information Technology for Economic and Clinical Health Act (HITECH) Act requirements. If healthcare providers expect to receive incentive payments for their EHR efforts, they will need to meet these criteria.

Definition of the Electronic Health Record

A number of different terms have been used to refer to health records created and maintained in a digital environment. Computer-based patient record (CPR), electronic medical record (EMR), and electronic patient record (EPR) are some of the most common. The preferred term is **electronic health record** or **EHR**. The American Health Information Management Association (AHIMA) reserves the term *EHR* for record systems that fulfill the Institute of Medicine's (IOM) vision for computer-based records (Dick, Steen, and Detmer 1997). The IOM provides health and science policy guidance to all sectors of society.

In its landmark report *The Computer-Based Patient Record: An Essential Technology for Health Care*, the IOM defined the EHR as "an electronic patient record that resides in a system specifically designed to support users by providing accessibility to complete and accurate data, alerts, reminders, clinical decision support systems, links to medical knowledge, and other aids" (Dick, Steen, and Detmer 1997, 55)

The IOM has identified eight key capabilities of an EHR system. The 10 components of an EHR, discussed later in the chapter, incorporate many of the IOM's eight key capabilities. The eight key capabilities are

1. Health information and data

2. Results management

3. Order entry/management

4. Decision support

5. Electronic communication and connectivity

6. Patient support

7. Administrative processes

8. Reporting and population health management

It is widely accepted that EHRs integrate data from multiple sources, capture data at the point of care, and assist the provider in the decision-making process.

The Agency for Healthcare Research and Quality (AHRQ) defines the EMR as a set of databases that contains the health information for patients, including laboratory data, pharmacy data, patient registration data, radiology data, surgical procedures, clinic and inpatient notes, preventive care delivery, emergency department visits, and billing information. An EHR extends the concept of an EMR to include cross-institutional data sharing. The EHR is patient focused, spanning episodes of care rather than just one encounter.

The National Alliance for Health Information Technology (NAHIT) defines the EMR as "an electronic record of health-related information on an individual that can be created, gathered, managed, and consulted by authorized clinicians and staff *within* one health care organization," and the EHR as "an electronic record of health-related information on an individual that conforms to nationally recognized interoperability standards and that can be created, managed, and consulted by authorized clinicians and staff *across* more than one health care organization" (*Healthcare Informatics* 2008) [emphasis added].

The Healthcare Information and Management Systems Society (HIMSS) defines EHR as

A longitudinal electronic record of patient health information produced by encounters in one or more care settings. Included in this information are patient demographics, progress notes, problems, medications, vital signs, past medical history, immunizations, laboratory data, and radiology reports. The EHR automates and streamlines the clinician's workflow. The EHR has the ability to independently generate a complete record of a clinical patient encounter, as well as supporting other care-related activities such as decision support, quality management, and clinical reporting

(HIMSS EHR Association Membership Committee 2006).

While the IOM's definition for the EHR prevails, all definitions have the following common elements:

1. Access to clinical decision support

2. Data collection at the point of care

3. Electronic order entry

4. Accessibility to information across organizations (also known as longitudinal data)

These definitions embrace the ideal EHR. However, few organizations have implemented the ideal EHR; most are still hard at work on achieving this goal. The majority of US hospitals are in the early stages. HIMSS divides EHR transformation into eight stages, from zero to seven. These stages correspond to the activities that healthcare organizations are most likely to undertake in logical sequence when implementing an EHR. HIMSS estimated that as of the second quarter of 2010, about 11 percent of US hospitals were at stage 0 (HIMSS 2010b). Stage 0 means that some clinical automation may be present, but none of the three major ancillary department systems for laboratory, pharmacy, and radiology have been implemented. Roughly 7 percent of hospitals are still in stage 1, 16 percent are in stage 2, 50 percent are in stage 3, 10 percent are in stage 4, and 3 percent each are in stages 5 and 6. Less than 1 percent of hospitals in the HIMSS analytics database were at stage 7 at the time the study was conducted. Stage 7 means the hospital has a paperless shared electronic health record (SEHR) environment with a mixture of discrete data, document images, and medical images. (HIMSS 2010b). The HIMSS Eight Stages of EHR adoption are provided in **TABLE 6.1**.

Many hospitals and other healthcare organizations currently use computerized health record systems that store information as images rather than as individual data elements. In other words, many existing computer-based records are scanned images of paper documentation. Because scanned images cannot be accessed digitally, these health records still have many of the same limitations as paper-based records.

The goal for all EHRs is to ensure that all data and information in the record is in a computer-readable format. Analog data or information is not represented in an encoded, computer-readable format. An example of analog data would be handwritten progress notes in their original or scanned form. Digital refers to the data or information represented in an encoded, computer-readable format.

TABLE 6.1. HIMSS eight stages of EMR adoption

STAGE	CAPABILITIES (CUMULATIVE)	2010 Q2
7	Complete EMR; CCD transactions to share data; data warehousing; data continuity with ED, ambulatory, OP	0.8%
6	Physician documentation (structured templates), full CDSS (variance and compliance), full R-PACS	2.6%
5	Closed-loop medication administration	3.2%
4	CPOE, clinical decision support (clinical protocols)	9.7%
3	Nursing/clinical documentation (flow sheets), CDSS (error checking) PACS available outside radiology	50.2%
2	CDR, controlled medical vocabulary, CDS, may have document imaging, HIE capable	15.5%
1	All ancillaries—lab, radiology, pharmacy— have been installed	6.8%
0	None of the three ancillaries have been installed	11.2%

Source: HIMSS 2010b.

Health record systems that contain all scanned images make patient information more widely accessible, but most lack the decision support capabilities and links to expert medical resources that are characteristic of fully functional EHRs. In addition, documents are often scanned after discharge so that records are not available in electronic form at the point of care, which would have the greatest impact on the quality of patient care. Scanning technology is addressed later in the chapter, in the section on hybrid health records.

Data, Information, and Knowledge

Because data, information, and knowledge are at the core of all health records, definitions of these terms precede the substantive discussion of the EHR.

Data are the dates, numbers, images, symbols, letters, and words that represent basic facts and observations about people, processes, measurements, and conditions (Johns 2011).

Information is factual data that have been collected, combined, analyzed, interpreted, and/or converted into a form that can be used for a specific purpose (Johns 2011).

An EHR is composed of data and information. It uses knowledge to capture or refine data and information. Users can generate knowledge from the data and information in an EHR. An example of data in an EHR would be the lab values for a patient's hemoglobin and hematocrit. An example of information in an EHR would be a physician's statement in the progress notes that, based on lab values, blood in the stools over a two-week time frame, and results of a colonoscopy, the patient has anemia due to a bleeding ulcer. The physician reflects on his clinical education and his experience with other, similar patients and determines that the best way to treat this patient is with a surgical repair of the ulcer, blood transfusion, and dietary modifications. This treatment plan is knowledge about this patient's condition. **FIGURE 6.2** illustrates this movement from data to information to knowledge. One of the benefits of the EHR is the ability to capture expert knowledge and use it in clinical decision support systems.

Benefits of and Barriers to the EHR

The benefits of the EHR can be generally divided into clinical benefits and economic benefits. The clinical benefits can be further divided into benefits to the individual patient

FIGURE 6.2. From data to knowledge

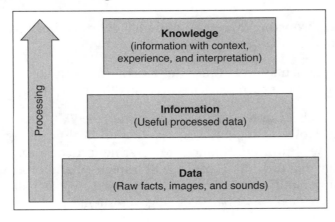

and benefits to all patients. EHR implementation will benefit individual patients because of the following types of changes to the patient health record:

1. Accessibility and availability. The record is available, when it is needed, to any clinician treating the patient. In addition, multiple clinicians can access a patient's record simultaneously.

2. Evidence-based medicine guidelines available at the point of care. Eventually, all EHR systems will have embedded clinical decision support systems that will make clinical alerts and evidence-based medicine guidelines—essentially expert knowledge—available to the clinicians treating the patient.

3. Patient education. The EHR supports patient education by providing electronic discharge instructions and medication information.

4. More clinician–patient face time. The EHR allows healthcare providers to spend more time with patients since most documentation occurs at the bedside (Amatayakul 2007).

Healthcare quality benefits to all of society as a result of a fully implemented NHIN include:

1. Accessibility of data for clinical trials research. The quality and quantity of data available for clinical trials and other research will significantly improve. In addition, manual data abstracting by research staff will be eliminated, increasing the quality of the data.

2. Accessibility of data for public health reporting. The quality and quantity of data available for public health reporting will significantly improve. This includes public reporting for cancer registries and reportable diseases, as well as (nonidentifiable) patient health information that can be used to improve the current and future health of the population.

Economic benefits can be found in elimination of

1. The need to re-run tests because results cannot be accessed

2. Manual patient record retrieval costs

3. Record retention costs (such as scanning, converting to microfilm, or storing records)

4. Manual data abstracting for research, public reporting, healthcare planning, and other administrative purposes

Barriers to EHR implementation fall into the general categories of cost, technology, and fear. Additional detail about each barrier is described in the list that follows.

1. Cost of initial EHR implementation. Over time, the EHR will bring significant costs savings. However, the initial investment for healthcare organizations is quite high. The Healthcare Financial Management Association (HFMA) estimates conservatively that the initial cost of EHR implementation to a hospital is likely to range from $1 million to $10 million (HFMA 2010). Details of these estimates are provided in **TABLE 6.2**. The federal government's payments to healthcare

TABLE 6.2. HFMA estimates for initial hospital implementation of an EHR

BED SIZE	INITIAL INVESTMENT	ANNUAL MAINTENANCE FEES
Less than 100	$1 million to $2 million	$100,000
100 to 200	$3 million to $10 million	$200,000 to $300,000
300 or more	$10 million to $1 billion	more than $1 million

Source: HFMA 2010.

providers to implement EHRs will offset some of these costs, but not all of them. For example, in 2005, AHRQ found that the average EHR implementation cost per physician was $32,606, with costs as high as $37,204 per physician for smaller practices. On top of those costs, AHRQ estimates a monthly upkeep and training cost of $1,500.

2. Availability of appropriate technology. The federal government's payments to healthcare providers to implement the EHR require that only certified EHR companies (addressed later in the chapter) be used. While this requirement ensures some degree of consistency, it is still unclear whether the technology needed to get providers through the entire transition is available. And even if it is, there may not be enough vendors to provide the initial implementation and ongoing technical support.

3. Availability of adequate standardization policies. For EHRs of all healthcare providers to "talk" to each other as the NHIN envisions, the technology and clinical terminology used in EHRs will need to be standardized. Several standards are currently available; a single standard for technology and one standard for terminology have not yet been mandated. Without this standard, many of the benefits of the EHR will be either unavailable or much less effective.

4. Cost of training clinicians to use the EHR. Clinicians must be trained to use the EHR while providing the same quality of care as they did prior to the change.

5. Fear of change and change management. It is natural for human beings to resist change. The fear of change and the resistance that occurs as a result is a barrier that needs to be recognized and managed by the healthcare provider.

Components of the EHR

There are 10 components to the EHR, driven primarily by the IOM's report on the EHR. Consolidating these functions into one system allows health information in the EHR to be used in ways that are impossible in a paper-based health record. The first three components are related to orders and/or medication administration.

1. *Computerized physician/provider order entry system (CPOE).* The CPOE is an electronic methodology for entering a physician order. The term "physician/ provider" is used in the CPOE to differentiate physician documentation from documentation provided by other healthcare professionals caring for the patient and documenting in the patient record. As noted in chapter 5, healthcare providers other than physicians, such as nursing staff, can enter physician orders

so long as the physician validates them within a specified time frame. In the optimal EHR environment, the CPOE is used for all orders. The CPOE requires standardization in the order process that is not required in a paper record. For example, the CPOE will not allow an order to be placed without all of the required data elements being entered into the system. In the paper record, if the physician forgot to document the reason for the order, for example, the order could still be placed. The CPOE also contains alerts specific to the patient. For example, the patient's allergy list and other medications are linked up with the CPOE logic. If a physician attempts to order a medication to which the patient is allergic or a medication that would have an unfavorable interaction with another medication that the patient is taking, the system will not allow the order to be placed and will alert the physician as to the reasons. Finally, the CPOE allows treating clinicians to easily view data about any patient's order history.

2. *Order communication/results retrieval.* Once the physician has used the CPOE to place an order, the order communication system notifies clinical departments, such as the laboratory, radiology, the pharmacy, and the dietary department. The fact that the process is computerized ensures greater effectiveness and efficiency than a paper-based process that relies on the unit nurse to place a call to the correct department for the order. In the same vein, the results of the test or service are automatically sent to the patient's record as part of a complete EHR system. The paper-based record requires the individual providing the service to physically find the record and manually enter the information.

3. *Electronic medication administration record (EMAR).* The EMAR automates the processes involved in administering medications to a patient. Typically, medication administration systems have different levels of automation. Ideally, once the medication arrives at the nursing station, bar codes are used to identify the patient and the medication. The EMAR can also provide alerts for the timing of the medication and reference material about the drugs being administered.

4. *Electronic document/content management (ED/CM).* An ED/CM system is any electronic system that manages both analog and digital documents and content to improve work processes (LaTour and Eichenwald Maki 2010). These technologies include document-imaging technology, document management technology, electronic records management technology, **computer output laser disk/enterprise report management** (COLD/ERM) technology, automated forms processing (e-forms) technology, and digital signature management technology. Many of these systems are discussed in the section of this chapter that describes the hybrid record.

5. *Patient care charting.* Patient care charting in the EHR may use bedside terminals, personal digital assistants, and other wireless devices to allow the clinician to enter data into the patient record while they are she is obtaining information from or treating the patient (LaTour and Eichenwald Maki 2010). Patient care charting systems generally allow the entry of both structured and unstructured data. **Structured data** are generally found in checkboxes, drop-down boxes, and other data entry means whereby the user chooses from options already built into the system. **Unstructured data**, also called narrative data, can be entered in a free text format by the user, usually by typing (Amatayakul 2007). Structured

FIGURE 6.3. Example of structured data in a drop-down menu

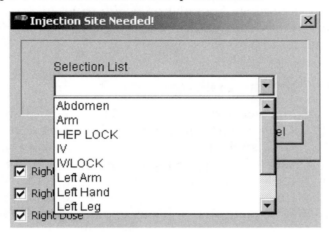

data are usually more easily searched than unstructured data and can be utilized for applications such as computer-assisted coding. Unstructured data can be searched, but only when all users document in the same manner. For example, "CHF," "Congestive Heart Failure," and "Congestive HF" would not be viewed as the same diagnosis in an unstructured data environment. **FIGURE 6.3** is an example of structured data needing to be selected from a drop-down menu.

6. *Clinical messaging.* Clinical messaging is the secure transmission of clinical information from one entity to another, including providers to providers, patients to providers, payers to providers, and among members of a healthcare community, such as within a regional health information organization (Amatayakul 2007).

7. *Clinical decision support (CDS) system.* Computer-based CDS systems can be defined as the use of computers to bring relevant knowledge to bear on the healthcare and well-being of a patient. The result of CDS is to perform some action, usually to make a recommendation. CDS systems are described later in the chapter.

8. *Patient provider portal.* A patient provider portal is a secure method of communication between the healthcare provider and the patient, just the providers, or the provider and the payer. The patient provider portal may include secure e-mail or remote access to test results and may provide patient monitoring.

9. *Personal health record (PHR).* The PHR is an application designed for the patient to manage her own health information for personal maintenance purposes and to provide it to healthcare providers for complete and accurate history information. The PHR may be linked to the EHR through a patient provider portal. PHRs are discussed in chapter 1.

10. *Population health.* Population health is the capture and reporting of healthcare data that are used for public health purposes. This component allows the healthcare provider to report infectious diseases, immunizations, cancer, and

other reportable conditions to public health officials. The use of technology to facilitate the reporting of population health issues increases the efficiency and reliability of the data and the process and can result in improved quality of care.

Federal Policies Driving EHR Implementation

The vision for a **national network for health data exchange** began more than a decade ago with the IOM's report *The Computer-Based Patient Record* (Dick, Steen, and Detmer 1997). In that study, the institute recommended a major, coordinated national effort, with federal funding and strong private-sector advisory support, to accelerate the adoption of computerized health records. In the years that have followed, consensus has emerged that the nation's medical information system must replace its outdated and frequently error-plagued, paper-based approach to information management.

Another early champion of EHRs was the **National Committee on Vital and Health Statistics (NCVHS).** In 1997, NCVHS began to explore the concept of a **national health information infrastructure (NHII)**, a framework that would support the appropriate and secure exchange of health information among organizations throughout the nation.

The current surge in activity began with President Bush's January 2004 state of the union address, which mentioned the benefits of computerized health records. This was followed in spring 2004 by an executive order creating the **Office of the National Coordinator for Health Information Technology (ONC)** within the Department of Health and Human Services (HHS). One of the coordinator's duties was to oversee development of an NHII. Within 90 days of its creation, ONC released *The Decade of Health Information Technology*, which became better known as the "Strategic Framework" (Thompson and Brailer 2006). Soon after, NHII disappeared as ONC referenced the national health information network (NHIN). The following year, the title was revised and *national* switched to *national*, reflecting an integration of locally managed networks rather than a single, national database.

Much of the activity in health information technology concerning the private sector is managed by HHS. The **Agency for Healthcare Research and Quality (AHRQ)**, one of the HHS agencies, provides funding and information for health information technology projects, including grants to state and regional **health information exchange (HIE)** initiatives. The **National Resource Center for Health Information Technology** provides technical assistance. The Centers for Medicare and Medicaid Services (CMS), also housed within HHS, began to manage the demonstration projects for implementation of EHRs in physician offices in 2007. The HHS plays an active role promoting industry discussion, research, and demonstrations.

President Obama signed ARRA into law in February 2009. The HITECH provisions of ARRA detail economic incentives for healthcare providers who implement EHRs according to meaningful use criteria. HITECH has five goals for meaningful use of the EHR by healthcare providers. The five broad goals of ARRA and HITECH are that all EHR activity must:

1. Improve patient care quality, safety, and efficiency

2. Engage patients in their care

3. Increase coordination of care

4. Improve the health status of the population

5. Ensure privacy and security

All criteria that HITECH requires providers to implement to receive incentive payments must be tied back to one of these goals. For example, providers must implement clinical decision support rules, which are tied back to the goal of improving quality, safety, and/or efficiency of care. **TABLE 6.3** provide a summary of federal policies and legislation affecting EHR implementation.

EHR Meaningful Use Criteria

Meaningful use criteria is the term used by the federal government to describe the requirements healthcare providers must meet to receive incentive payments for implementing different phases of an EHR between 2011 and 2015. For an EHR technology to be eligible for certification, it must first meet the ONC's definition of a qualified EHR, as follows (HHS 2010):

TABLE 6.3. Federal policies affecting EHR implementation

YEAR	EHR POLICY ACTIVITY
1997	The IOM's report on the computer-based patient record states the EHR must provide "alerts, reminders, clinical decision support systems, links to medical knowledge and other aids."
1997	The National Committee on Vital and Health Statistics begins to explore the concept of a national health information infrastructure.
1999	The American Society for Testing and Materials (ASTM) develops a standard for EHRs titled "Standard Practice for Content and Structure of the Electronic Health Record."
2003	HL7, a healthcare standards development organization, completes the initial work on a functional model for EHRs.
2004	The ONC is created and charged with overseeing the development of an NHII.
2004	The EHR Collaborative, composed of allied health and trade associations, votes to adopt the proposed HL7 model.
2006	The AHRQ begins funding several health information technology projects.
2008	The CMS Demonstration Project for the implementation of EHRs in physician practices is created.
2009	ARRA, signed by President Obama, includes HITECH to provide incentive payments for healthcare providers to implement certified EHR technology.
2010	CMS proposes a definition for "meaningful use criteria" for providers to quality for incentive payments. Final proposed rule published in the March 15, 2010, *Federal Register*.
2011–2014	Beginning and ending time frame for incentive payments to healthcare providers to adopt EHRs according to meaningful use criteria.

Qualified EHR means an electronic record of health-related information on an individual that

1. Includes patient demographic and clinical health information, such as medical history and problem lists; and

2. Has the capacity (a) to provide clinical decision support; (b) to support physician order entry; (c) to capture and query information relevant to health care quality; and (d) to exchange electronic health information with, and integrate such information from, other sources.

This definition is somewhat less comprehensive than the definitions provided by organizations like the IOM, CCHIT, and HIMSS, discussed at the beginning of the chapter. ONC anticipates that definitions and meaningful use will evolve over time. Currently, meaningful use is a three-stage process over a five-year period. This is the preliminary definition that will be in place for at least Stage 1 criteria. The following is a summary of the EHR activities by stage that providers must have in place to receive incentive payments from CMS.

- **Stage 1**—The stage 1 meaningful use criteria focuses on electronically capturing health information in an encoded format; using that information to track key clinical conditions and communicate that information for care coordination purposes (whether the information is structured or unstructured—but in structured format whenever feasible); implementing clinical decision support tools, in a manner consistent with other provisions of Medicare and Medicaid law, to facilitate disease and medication management; and reporting clinical quality measures and public health information

- **Stage 2**—Stage 2 meaningful use criteria encourage the use of health information technology (IT) for continuous quality improvement at the point of care and the exchange of information in the most structured format possible, such as the electronic transmission of orders entered using CPOE and the electronic transmission of diagnostic test results (such as blood tests, microbiology, urinalysis, pathology tests, radiology, cardiac imaging, nuclear medicine tests, pulmonary function tests, and other such data needed to diagnose and treat disease).

- **Stage 3**—Expands on stage 2. Stage 3 meaningful use criteria focus on promoting improvements in quality, safety, and efficiency; using decision support for national high-priority conditions; ensuring patient access to self-management tools; providing access to comprehensive patient data; and improving population health.

Stage 1 of the meaningful use criteria focuses on ensuring that all data and information in the patient's record is encoded or in a computer-readable format. Encoding the data will ensure that EHR information can be used without the need for human intervention to interpret its meaning. Stage 1 also requires providers to implement clinical decision support tools (at least five measures are required in stage 1). Stage 2 focuses on implementation and use of CPOE systems. And stage 3 focuses on implementing clinical decision support tools in a more comprehensive manner. Stage 3 also requires that patients be given access to self-management tools to increase the patient's control over his or her own health issues.

FIGURE 6.4. Entities exchanging data as part of the National Health Information Network exchange

Exchange of summary patient records for The Social Security Administration disability determination purposes:

- Social Security Administration
- MedVirginia

Exchange of summary patient records for the Virtual Lifetime Electronic Record (VLER):

- Veterans Administration
- Department of Defense
- Kaiser Permanente

Biosurveillance and case reporting:

- Centers for Disease Control and Prevention
- Regenstrief Institute

Source: ONC 2010.

National Infrastructure for the EHR

To achieve the ultimate vision of the NHIN, EHRs must be guided by standards that ensure consistency among all health records. Currently, a national infrastructure is not in place. The organizations exchanging data under the NHIN are listed in **Figure 6.4**. Some estimate that the long-term cost savings produced by a NHIN could reach $77.8 billion each year from reductions in medical errors, diagnostic test duplication, and administrative expenses (Walker 2005).

However, the structure has been refined over the past few years, and we are likely to see resolution by the time healthcare providers implement stage 3. In the meantime, it is important to be familiar with the organizations that provide guidance for making decisions about standardization, the current technology standards available, and the current clinical terminology standards available. The following terms are basic concepts that are helpful in understanding standardization of the EHR and the NHIN:

- **Structure and content standards** establish and provide clear and uniform definitions of the data elements to be included in EHR systems. They specify the type of data to be collected in each data field, the length of each data field, and the attributes of each data field, all of which are captured in data dictionaries.

- **Functionality standards** define the components an EHR needs to support the functions for which it is designed. HL7 draft standards for an EHR were developed in 2004 and, at the time of publication, were being tested in the healthcare industry.

- **Technical standards** complement content and structure, and **vocabulary standards** are also required to make interoperability possible. Technical standards provide the rules, often called protocols, for how these data are transmitted from one computer system to another.

Standards Development Organizations

Certification Commission for Health Information Technology (CCHIT) is a non-profit organization with the public mission of accelerating the adoption of health IT. Founded in 2004, and certifying EHRs since 2006, the commission established the first comprehensive, practical definition of what capabilities were needed in these systems. The certification criteria were developed through a voluntary, consensus-based process engaging diverse stakeholders, and the commission was officially recognized by the federal government as a certifying body.

American National Standards Institute (ANSI). ANSI is a private, nonprofit organization originally founded in 1918 to coordinate the US census systems. Today, ANSI approves official American national standards and includes membership from all sectors, not just healthcare. ANSI helps standards developers and users from the private sector to reach consensus on the need for standards. ANSI is responsible for accrediting healthcare standards development organizations (SDOs) in the United States. Health Level 7, discussed below, is an example of an SDO accredited by ANSI. To be approved, a standard must be open, be voluntary, and have input from stakeholders.

Health Care Informatics Standards Board (HISB). HISB was formed by ANSI in 1995 to oversee healthcare standards work in the United States The scope of HISB includes standards for

1. EHRs

2. Interchange of healthcare data, images, sounds, and signals within and between organizations and practices

3. Healthcare codes and terminology

4. Communication with diagnostic instructions and healthcare devices

5. Representation and communication of healthcare protocols, knowledge, and statistical databases

6. Privacy, confidentiality, and security of medical information

American Society for Testing and Materials (ASTM). ASTM was founded in 1898 as a scientific and technical organization for the development of standards. ASTM is the largest nongovernment source of standards in the United States. ASTM is also a charter member of ANSI. ASTM Committee E31 on Computerized Systems is responsible for developing health information standards and is addressed later, in the section on functionality.

Workgroup for Electronic Data Interchange (WEDI). WEDI was formed in 1991 to promote greater healthcare electronic commerce and connectivity. The organization brings together industry leaders to identify ways to reduce administrative costs in healthcare through electronic data interchange. WEDI is one of four organizations named in HIPAA to be consulted in the development of healthcare standards that would meet HIPAA requirements.

International Standards Organization (ISO) Technical Committee 215—Health Informatics. This ISO committee, with both US and European representation, was formed in 1989. The committee is made up of six working groups addressing health records, messaging and communications, health concept representation, security, smart cards, and ePharmacy. In 2000, ISO and the Institute of Electrical and Electronics Engineers (IEEE) formed ISO/IEEE, in which IEEE standards (addressed later in the chapter) would be moved directly to ISO for approval as ISO standards.

Specific Data Interchange Standards

As healthcare increasingly depends on the connectivity within an organization, a system, or a geographic area, the ability to interchange data in a seamless manner becomes critical (Shortliffe and Cimino 2006). Data interchange standards address both technical and functional components of the EHR and are addressed by the following standards that have been created or refined in the past decade.

Health Level Seven. HL7, the most widely implemented healthcare data-messaging standard, is in use at over 1,500 healthcare facilities in the United States. HL7 was built on ASTM protocols and is an ANSI-accredited SDO. It completed the initial work on a functional model for EHRs in late 2003. In early 2004, industry stakeholders, led by the EHR Collaborative, voted to adopt a proposed model.

American Society for Testing and Materials. ASTM has also developed a standard for EHRs. Currently titled Standard Practice for Content and Structure of the Electronic Health Record, this standard has been revised several times since its initial release in 1999. The current standard, E1384-07, was revised in October 2007. The standard covers the content and structure of EHRs and provides guidelines for healthcare organizations planning and implementing new systems.

Digital Imaging and Communications in Medicine (DICOM). DICOM has developed a standard method for transferring images and associated information between devices manufactured by different vendors that display a variety of digital image formats. The use of DICOM standards allows images to be transferred between systems from different vendors, ultimately allowing imaging in the picture archival and communication systems to share information with clinical information systems and the EHR (Giannangelo 2011).

Institute of Electrical and Electronics Engineers. IEEE is an international organization that is a member of both ANSI and ISO. IEEE 107 is a standard for medical device communications. It is designed for bedside devices in the intensive care unit, operating room, and emergency department.

ANSI X12. ANSI X12 is an independent organization accredited by ANSI. It has developed a group of standards related to providing advice on claims, benefits, and claim payment. The standards support exchange of eligibility and other related information between providers and payers.

National Council for Prescription Drug Programs (NCPDP). NCPDP is an ANSI-accredited SDO. NCPDP creates data-interchange standards for pharmacy services. These standards control data to be shared for new prescriptions, refills, and other communications between physicians and pharmacies. NCPDP is mandated by HIPAA for pharmacy reimbursement and insurance transactions (Giannangelo 2011).

Clinical Terminology Standards

Currently, several different medical terms can be used to describe the same condition. For example, angiohemophilia may also be called von Willebrand's disease, von Willebrand's syndrome, constitutional thrombopathy, or vascular hemophilia. As a result, text searches using one of the synonyms for this condition would likely yield only a small portion of the information that is actually available. To address this problem, healthcare industry groups are working together to develop standardized, controlled medical vocabularies. Of these, the Systematized Nomenclature of Medicine–Clinical Terms (SNOMED-CT) is most likely to be adopted universally. Listed below are the current clinical terminologies in use, including SNOMED.

Systematized Nomenclature of Medicine. SNOMED is intended to be a general-purpose, comprehensive, computer-processable terminology that represents virtually all of the events found in the medical record (Cote et al. 1993). SNOMED was developed and maintained by the College of American Pathologists until recently, when the responsibility was transitioned to the International Health Terminology Standards Development Organization. The current version, SNOMED-CT, is designed to capture detailed clinical information, which then makes it possible to share and aggregate data. SNOMED is used for the EHR and for research and clinical decisions. SNOMED captures information such as diagnoses, procedures, signs, symptoms, and cause of injury in over 350,000 different concepts in description tables with more than 900,000 language description or synonyms (LaTour and Eichenwald Maki 2010). These relationships are important to data retrieval. **TABLE 6.4** provides a short example of how clinical information is coded in SNOMED-CT.

Unified Medical Language System (UMLS). UMLS links the major international terminologies into a common structure, providing a translation mechanism between them. It permits the linkage of different information systems, such as EHRs, bibliographic databases, and CDS systems.

Logical Observations, Identifiers, Names, and Codes (LOINC). LOINC is a laboratory vocabulary that is used to order and report laboratory tests and record clinical observations for use in patient care, outcomes management, and research. Laboratory terms in LOINC include blood chemistry, hematology, and serology. LOINC assists in the electronic transmission of laboratory data between laboratories, providers, and payers.

National Drug Codes (NDCs). NDCs were developed by the Food and Drug Administration (FDA) as a universal unique identifier for human drugs. An NDC identifies the vendor, product, and trade package size and is one of the codes mandated for use by HIPAA.

TABLE 6.4. SNOMED Classification example

NOMENCLATURE	CLASSIFICATION				
Axis	T	+M	+L	+F	+D
Term	Lung	Granuloma	+*Mycobacterium tuberculosis*	+Fever	=Tuberculosis
Code	T-2800	+M-44000	+L-21801	+F-03003	+DE-14800

Massachusetts General Utility Multi-Programming System (MUMPS). MUMPS is a specialized programming language that was specially developed for use in medical applications in the 1970s at Massachusetts General Hospital. For many years, MUMPS was the most widely used language for medical record processing. Under its new name, **MUMPS**, it is still in widespread use (Shortliffe and Cimino 2006).

Healthcare Providers and the Infrastructure for EHRs

In the preceding sections, we discussed national standards that are in the process of being finalized. In the meantime, healthcare providers must use certain internal standards when implementing an EHR. Using these standards will ensure that, at least within their system, all clinicians will have a consistent understanding of the terminology used, and data and information will be used efficiently and effectively. The internal standardized processes that are addressed in this section include the development of a data dictionary, database development and use, implementation of clinical decision support systems, and training physicians to use the EHR.

Data Dictionaries

A data dictionary is a centralized repository of information about data that includes such as elements as meaning, relationships to other data, origin, usage, and format (IBM 1993). The purpose of the data dictionary is to standardize definitions and ensure consistency of use. Standardizing data enhances use across systems. Communication is improved in clinical treatment, research, and business processes through a common understanding of terms.

Standardization provides developers with a common road map to promote consistency across applications. All of the national standards described in the preceding section contain data dictionaries. However, until the decision is made regarding the national standard, healthcare systems will need to either choose one of the data dictionaries in available or customize one (usually with the help of an IT vendor) for their organization. The data dictionary an organization chooses must be designed to accept modifications in anticipation of the national standard.

Lack of a sound data dictionary can cause problems within and across organizations. Organizations may call the same data element by different names, or they may call different data elements by the same name across an enterprise. As a result, an organization may not collect all of the information it needs, or it may be unable to combine or map data across systems. A worse possibility is that an organization may combine data elements it believes to be equivalent and draw incorrect inferences from the invalid data. Multiple users entering data may have different definitions or perceptions of what goes into a data field, thereby confounding the data. For example, are "reason for visit" and "chief complaint" the same or different?

Large, complex systems with multiple stakeholders (internal and external) often need to use multiple, differing data sets. Variances among these data sets that are not recognized across the system can affect the information flow and the workflow. Maintaining expansive, overlapping data sets costs time and money and affects the organization's ability to provide quality care. The organization will not be positioned to harmonize information at the regional or national level.

One purpose of the data dictionary is to provide consistency and understanding of common data across applications. The process requires collecting data or metadata (data about the data) on each data element found to be common across domains. Examples of metadata include name of element, definition, application in which the data element is found, locator key, ownership, entity relationships, date first entered system, date terminated from system, and system of origin. A metadata registry is an authoritative source of reference information about the representation, meaning, and format of data collected and managed by an enterprise. It does not contain the data itself but the information that is necessary to clearly describe, inventory, analyze, and classify the data.

The data dictionary should be designed to accommodate changes resulting from clinical or technical advances and regulatory changes. There should be a plan for future expansion, such as expanding a data field from one element to multiple elements. This becomes problematic when comparing data across time if the meaning of a particular element has changed while its name or representation has not. If a data element is completely revamped, document when that specific data element went into effect and when it was deactivated. If the data element expands into something new, do not migrate the old concept; create a new element to move forward.

Consider future needs to collapse and expand values to accommodate mapping from a larger to a smaller or a smaller to a larger number of values within a field definition. When setting up the information system, consider how to accommodate multiple systems and how to go from one code system to another. For example, race or ethnicity is frequently defined with different values. One data set has four items; another has six. The mainframe or core system needs the maximum amount of values. The mapper needs to know the rules to use when collapsing six values into four. Migrating four to six is usually impossible, which creates other issues.

Examine the nationally recognized standards, and normalize field definitions across data sets to accommodate multiple end-user needs. Define all data characteristics to be included for each data element, for all domains. This includes specifying domain boundaries and identifying links across domains and will require extensive discussion and agreement among all stakeholders. The ideal is a common integrated data and terminology model. Terminologies should be coordinated to eliminate overlaps, redundancies, and inconsistencies. This will eliminate the need for mapping among terminologies. **FIGURE 6.5** illustrates EHR data types and their sources as the very first step in creating a data dictionary.

Databases and Database Management Systems

A **database** is an organized collection of data that have been stored electronically for easy access. **Database management systems (DBMSs)** are an integrated set of programs that helps users store and manipulate data easily and efficiently (Shortliffe and Cimino 2006). DBMSs make it possible to create, modify, delete, and view the data in a database.

Most health record systems are organized according to one of two database models—the centralized or the distributed—or a hybrid of the two models. In the centralized system, all of the organization's patient health information and data are stored in a single system. In the distributed model, patient health information and data are distributed in department-based systems or subsystems that are able to exchange information with one another.

The centralized system, using an electronic format, is frequently built around a clinical data repository. A **clinical data repository** is a centralized database that captures, sorts, and processes patient data and then returns them to the user. These functions demand specialized database management capabilities. The most common type of DBMS in use today is the relational database, which uses data tables to organize information. New types of DBMSs are in development and will probably speed up processing time in the future.

FIGURE 6.5. EHR data types and their sources as the first step in developing a data dictionary

<u>Structured</u>

Document image data

    Handwritten notes

    Drawings

    Signed patient consent forms

Discrete, structured ASCII data

    Laboratory orders/results

    Medication orders/MARs

    Online charting and documentation

    Detailed charges

<u>Unstructured</u>

Text data

    Radiology reports

    Transcribed reports

    UBs and itemized bills

Video data

    Ultrasound and cardiac catheterization examinations

Audio data

    Heart sounds

    Voice dictations and annotations

Signal tracing data

    EKG/EEG/fetal monitoring

Diagnostic image data

    Pathology images

    Nuclear medicine

In decentralized systems, health record information is retained in separate departmental computer systems or databases. Data are then exchanged among departmental systems as needed (for example, between the clinical laboratory's system and the obstetrics unit's system).

The decentralized system can work relatively well when all or most of the facility's computers use the same proprietary operating system. However, all of the organization's departments must follow established **messaging standards**, also called interoperability standards or **data exchange standards**, which ensure that all of the organization's data are structured and formatted in the same way (Amatayakul 2007, 242). However, decentralized systems are often not integrated. Or, if they are integrated, managing multiple interfaces is a labor-intensive activity that requires careful review of source information when corrections are made to information.

FIGURE 6.6 is an example of a distributed DBMS.

Electronic Forms Design

Forms management is critical in both electronic data-management systems and traditional paper-based record systems. The standardization of data-capture tools ensures the

FIGURE 6.6. Physical and logical data repositories for EHR systems

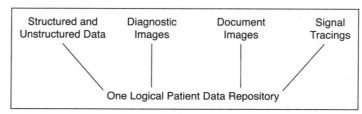

quality and completeness of health record content in paper-based and computer-based environments Most acute care organizations have established forms committees to oversee the development, review, and control of the facilities' data-capturing tools, including all paper forms and on-screen views and interface. The committee should include information users from the following departments (Cerrato and Roberts 2011, 416):

- Health information management (HIM)
- Medical staff
- Nursing staff
- Purchasing
- Information services
- Performance improvement
- Support and ancillary departments

The forms committee or a representative of the committee usually works directly with commercial vendors to develop health record forms or electronic data-capture systems that fulfill the information needs of the organization. The design of on-screen views and the data entry interface are two of the most important considerations in developing EHR systems. Electronic systems allow individual users to choose the way data are presented, so designers should understand how clinicians and other users prefer to receive information. For example, physicians generally prefer to find all of the information they need in one place. Therefore, putting as much information as possible on each view meets their needs better than creating less crowded views that require users to scroll down to see the information or to proceed through multiple views.

In both electronic and paper-based health record systems, the most important step in the standardization of forms and views is to establish the information needs of health information users. Every form or view must fulfill its intended purpose by including all of the data required in an appropriate and easy-to-use format.

For example, when the purpose of a form is to provide patient instructions for aftercare, the data elements on the form must provide all of the information the patient will need in language that the patient can understand. Similarly, when the form is meant to be completed by hand, the response areas on the form must allow enough space for handwritten information. When the purpose of a view is to provide clinicians with an update on the patient's condition, the view should contain all of the pertinent information in a format that can be reviewed at a glance.

Following thoughtful design practices may not always ensure the overall effectiveness of the organization's documentation and data entry tools. Duplication and redundancy can also frustrate users and yield conflicting information. Forms design and management processes should ensure that only one version of each form is available for use at any one time. Processes should also look at the number of different forms in use to determine whether the same information is being collected on multiple forms or views in more than one way.

Standardization of Acronyms, Abbreviations, and Symbols

To avoid ambiguity, facilities should standardize the abbreviations, acronyms, and symbols that are used in health record documentation. Hospital health record policies and medical staff rules should determine which symbols, acronyms, and abbreviations the clinicians who author health record entries may use, and the rules should be enforced. As an alternative method, some hospitals develop lists of prohibited acronyms, symbols, and abbreviations rather than approved lists.

In 2003, The Joint Commission published six patient safety goals, one of which requires healthcare organizations to designate the abbreviations that should never be used in health records (The Joint Commission 2003). In general, **prohibited abbreviations** are those that have more than one meaning or can easily be misinterpreted in handwritten form, with potentially dangerous results for patients. The Joint Commission now requires hospitals to prohibit the use of the following abbreviations in all handwritten, patient-specific documentation:

- **U** (for unit)
- **IU** or **iu**
- **QD** or **qd**
- **QOD** or **qod**
- **.0** (zero after a decimal point)
- **0.** (zero before a decimal point)
- **MS, MSO4, MgSO4**

The Institute for Safe Medication Practices (ISMP) has created a List of Error-Prone Abbreviations, Symbols, and Dose Designations. The list is quite extensive and includes abbreviations that have been identified by the ISMP's program as frequently misinterpreted and involved in harmful medication errors. The list can be found on ISMP's website. Although not required by The Joint Commission, organizations contemplating an EHR or CPOE introduction or upgrade should strive to eliminate the use of dangerous abbreviations, acronyms, symbols, and dose designations from the software.

Symbols, acronyms, and abbreviations should be limited to those that are the most widely applicable and unambiguous. The list should include the accepted definition of each entry, and ideally, each abbreviation, acronym, or symbol should have only one meaning. When illustrations, forms, or other complex materials use numerous or unusual abbreviations, the author should provide a legend to explain what the abbreviations mean.

Because of space limitations, symbols, acronyms, and abbreviations are more likely to be used in on-screen, EHR data entry. This can lead to interpretation problems. To solve this problem, developers should consider creating a feature that makes definitions available when users click an abbreviation, symbol, or acronym.

Clinical Decision Support Systems

Clinical decision support (CDS) is defined broadly as a clinical system, application, or process that helps health professionals make clinical decisions to enhance patient care. Clinical knowledge of interest could range from simple facts and relationships to best practices for managing patients with specific disease states, new medical knowledge from clinical research, and other types of information (HIMSS 2010a). CDS systems help physicians and other clinicians make diagnostic and treatment decisions. A CDS system automatically analyzes health record data and searches for unusual patterns. When it identifies a potential problem (for example, a drug interaction), the system issues an alert or a reminder that includes a recommendation for specific corrective action. Decision support is most effective when provided at the point of care, while the physician is formulating his assessment of the patient's condition and making ordering decisions (Shortliffe and Cimino 2006). Research results can take years to be disseminated throughout the medical community. The use of CDS systems ensures timely receipt of the newest information by all clinicians using such systems.

FIGURE 6.7. Example of a patient-specific clinical suggestion generated from a CDS system

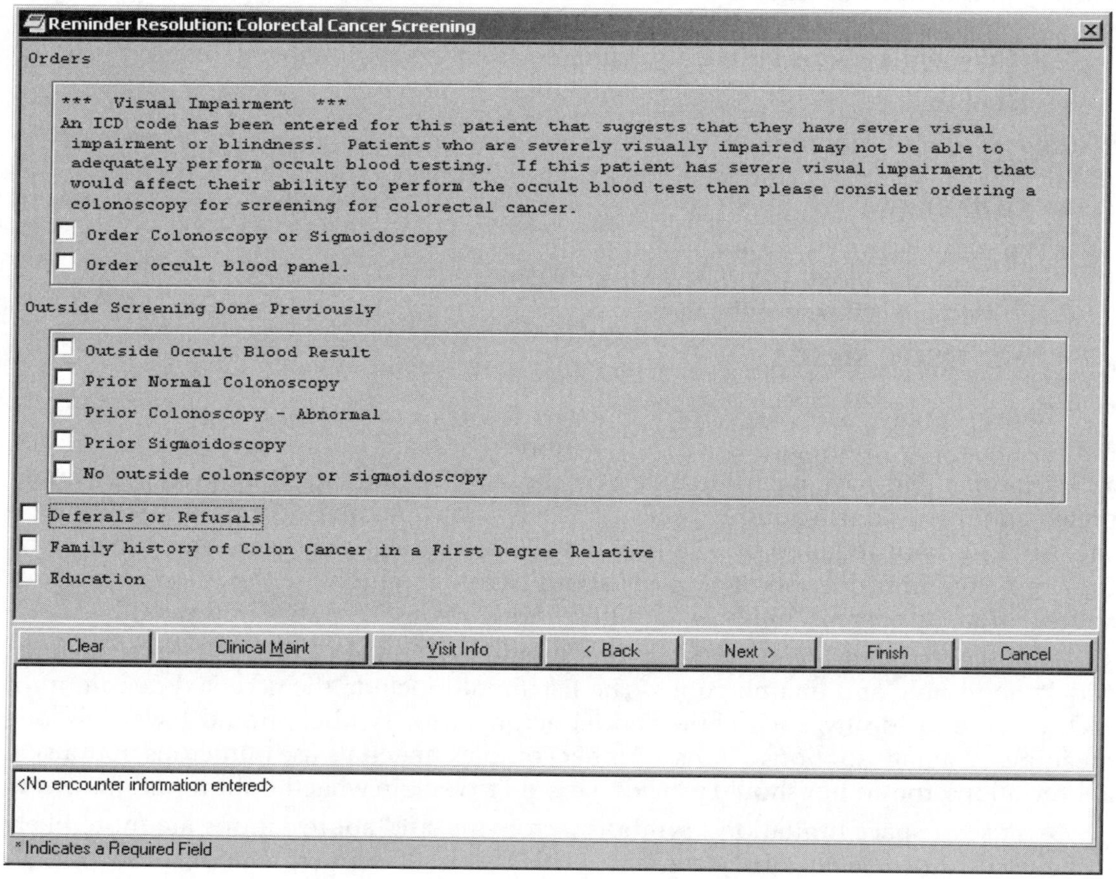

Source: VistA.

Under stage 1 meaningful use criteria, hospitals are required to implement at least five computerized CDS alerts. And under stage 3 requirements, hospitals must implement a comprehensive CDS system. Because CDS systems improve care and reduce errors, they appear to be a good investment for every healthcare provider.

The technology that supports the functions of CDS systems may be categorized as rules engines, statistical analyses, search engines, and expert systems that incorporate a variety of analytical tools (Amatayakul 2007, 396). A CDS system may include alerts and reminders, clinical guidelines, order sets, patient data reports and dashboards, documentation templates, diagnostic support, reference information delivered, and other tools to support decisions within clinical workflow. A CDS system can prevent errors or adverse events. CDS interventions can

- Detect and help prevent potential safety and quality problems

- Foster the greater use of evidence-based medicine principles and guidelines

- Ensure that clinicians and patients use the best clinical knowledge and recommendations

The concept of alert fatigue should be considered when using CDS tools to avoid physicians becoming immune to alerts. One of the ways healthcare systems can ensure appropriate use of the alerts is to monitor the numbers and types of alerts as well as whether the alert has modified the physician behavior. HIM or clinical professionals can provide this monitoring.

FIGURES 6.7 and **6.8** are examples of clinical suggestions and reminders generated for a specific patient based on diagnoses or test findings. These are among the many types of decision support concepts embedded in a CDS system.

FIGURE 6.8. **Example of patient-specific clinical reminders generated from the CDS system**

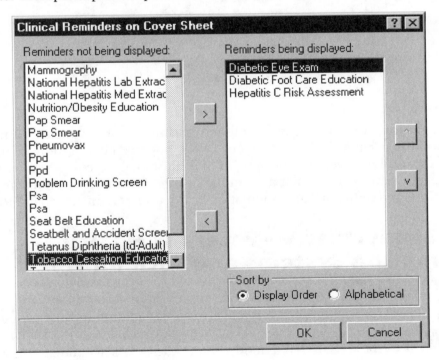

Source: VistA.

327

FIGURE 6.9. Three areas of EHR data standardization and integration

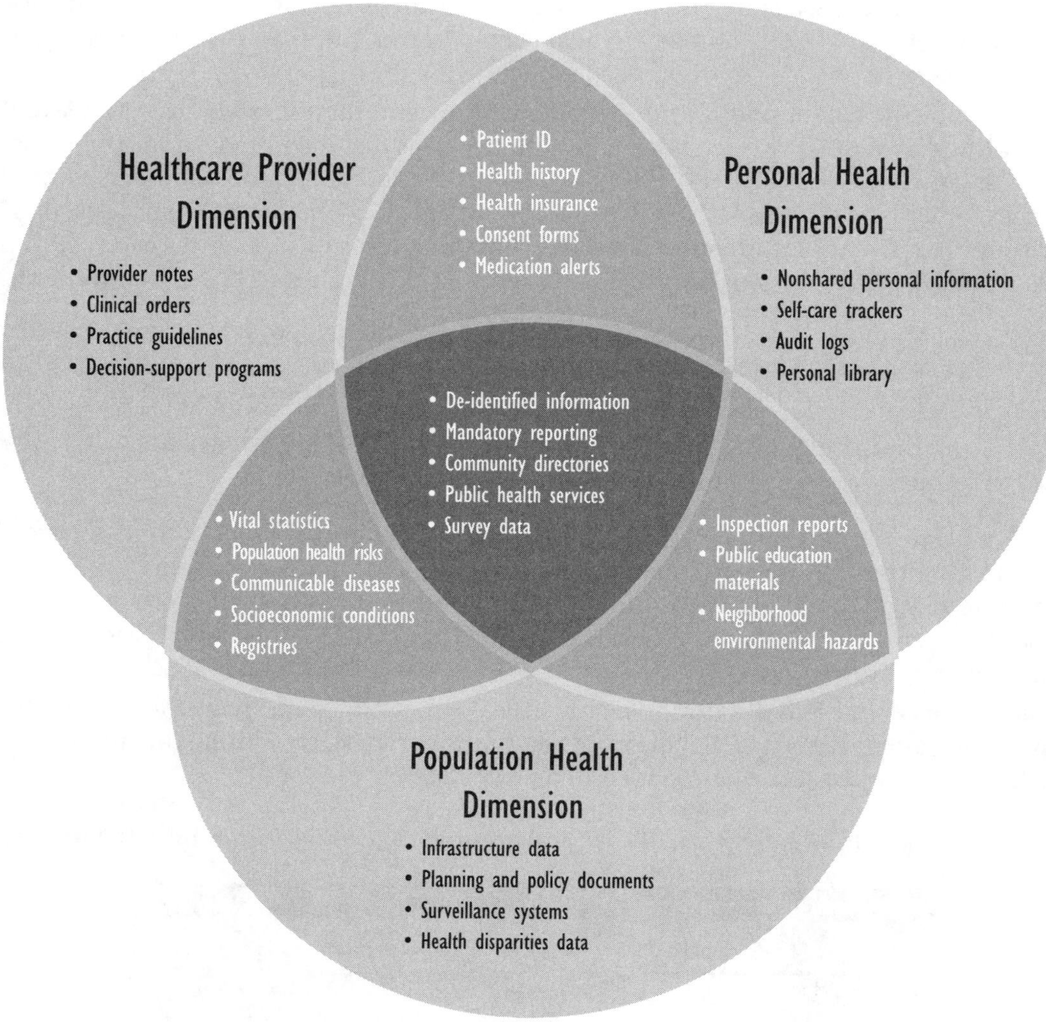

Source: NCVHS 2011.

In this section, we have looked at the responsibilities of hospitals and healthcare systems working together with SDOs to ensure the improvement of individual patients' quality of care and the overall improvement of healthcare for the population. The latter will be achieved through research and public health efforts. The relationship between hospital efforts and individual and population health impact is illustrated in **FIGURE 6.9**.

Case Study: VistA—Veterans Health Information Systems and Technology Architecture

VistA is a microcosm of the NHIN. The Veterans Health Administration (VHA) has achieved on a smaller scale what the nation is working toward with the NHIN and EHR. The following excerpt appeared in a 2006 *Time Magazine* article entitled "How Veterans Hospitals Became the Best in Healthcare" (Waller):

Outside an elderly patient's room, the attending physician gathers her residents around a wireless laptop propped on a mobile cart. [The physician] accesses the patient's entire medical history—a stack of paper in most private hospitals. And instead of trekking to the radiology lab to view the latest X-ray, she brings it up on her computer screen. While [the physician] is visiting the patient, a resident types in a request for pain medication, then punches the SEND button. Seconds later, the printer in the hospital pharmacy spits out the order. The druggist stuffs a plastic bag of pills into what looks like a tiny space capsule, then shoots it up to the ward in a vacuum tube. By the time [the physician] wheels away her computer, a nurse walks up with the drugs.

The VHA runs the largest integrated healthcare system in the country, with 153 hospitals and more than 1,000 clinics and nursing homes employing 14,800 doctors and 61,000 nurses serving 5.3 million veterans. The roots of the VHA's health record transformation began in 1994, when President Clinton appointed a new VHA under secretary. Patient records were transferred to a system-wide computer network. When a veteran is treated, the physician has the patient's complete medical history on a laptop, eliminating the problem of needing to repeat tests because the results of earlier tests are inaccessible. In addition, the VHA was one of the first organizations to implement a bar-code system for medication administration.

VistA Overview

VistA is an integrated system of software applications that directly supports patient care at VHA healthcare facilities. VistA connects VHA facilities' workstations and PCs with nationally mandated and locally adapted software applications that are accessed by end users through a graphical user interface known as the computerized patient record system (CPRS). Each VistA application generates at least one data file. These files contain the clinical, administrative, and computer infrastructure–related data that support day-to-day operations and contain patients' medical and healthcare utilization histories.

Within the VistA system, each active patient is assigned an integration control number (ICN) as a unique identifier. Patient files include data on demographics, episodes of care, medicines, practitioner information, diagnoses, procedures, and other clinical information. All patients treated at VHA medical centers are included in the files, which are updated continuously at the point of care or as part of administrative processes. Data are entered into VistA by way of manual entry, bar codes, and automated instrumentation. Some data are derived from central financial, personnel, and operational systems and distributed to local facilities' VistA files. (US DVA 2010)

VistA for Patient Care

The VA website contains detailed documentation about and for the VistA EHR (US DVA 2010). The content of the VistA files is expansive. This analysis focuses on the three EHR topics of the problem list, vital signs, and medication administration. Together, these topics encompass seven of the ten components of the EHR: order communications/results retrieval, electronic document/content management, clinical messaging, patient care charting, computerized physician/provider order entry system, electronic medication administration reporting, and CDS system.

One of the key elements of the EHR's patient charting component is the problem list. The VistA problem list contains the following features:

- Allows one problem list for a given patient

- Is tied to a coding system

- Requires minimal data entry

- Is linked to other sections of the health record, such as CPRS and Health Summary

- Supports import of problem information from other clinical settings outside the immediate VAMC

- Uses a common language of terminology, the Lexicon Utility, in which each term is well-defined and understandable (a user, site, or application may substitute a preferred synonym)

- Allows reformulation of a problem

- Can be interfaced with a customized encounter form

The problem list is a content management tool because it tracks and updates current problems. It involves clinical messaging and patient care charting because it identifies current problems as well as allergies and reactions. This information creates alerts to providers that act as a basic CDS tool.

A sample screenshot of a problem list from the VistA EHR system can be found in **FIGURE 6.10**, CPRS problem list. From the screenshot, you can also see that the user has access to tabs for meds, orders, notes, consults, D/C sum, labs, and reports for each visit.

Vital signs recorded by the nursing staff are displayed in the VistA system in both summary and graphic format. **FIGURE 6.11** shows a patient Vital Signs screenshot with the data for temperature, pulse, and respiration in both tabular and graphic format. The graphic view allows a healthcare provider to determine quickly if there has been any deviation from the patient's normal values. Vital sign screens contain results retrieval, content management, clinical messaging, and CDS system components.

The VHA pioneered bar code medication administration (BCMA) in the late 1990s. Since then, this system has significantly reduced medication errors. **FIGURE 6.12** contains a screenshot of a patient medication record. The screenshot shows that the medication tab is subdivided into three different areas, Unit Dose, IVP/IVPB, and IV, for the route of administration of the medication. The bottom left-hand corner of the screenshot contains the Scanner Status with the word "Ready" above a green bar. Before the nurse can administer the medication to the patient, she must scan the bar code of the medication, and the scanner status must show green. If the medication should not be administered, the scanner status will show red and an error message like the one in **FIGURE 6.13** will appear. The error message may contain more details, such as the patient's allergy status, incorrect dose, or other errors, depending on the circumstances. The Bar Code Medication Administration section of the VistA EHR represents order communication, content management, clinical messaging, patient care charting, order entry systems, electronic medication administration reporting, and CDS components of the EHR.

FIGURE 6.10. Example of a VistA CPRS problem list

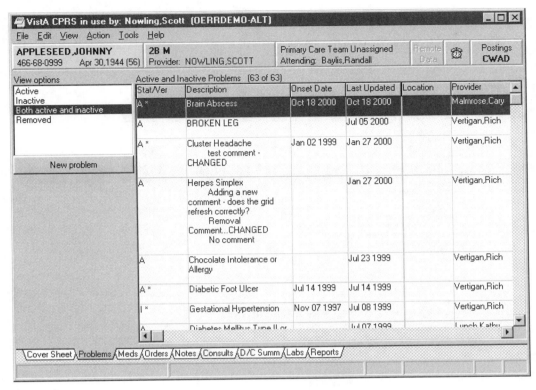

Source: VistA.

FIGURE 6.11. Example of VistA CPRS vital signs

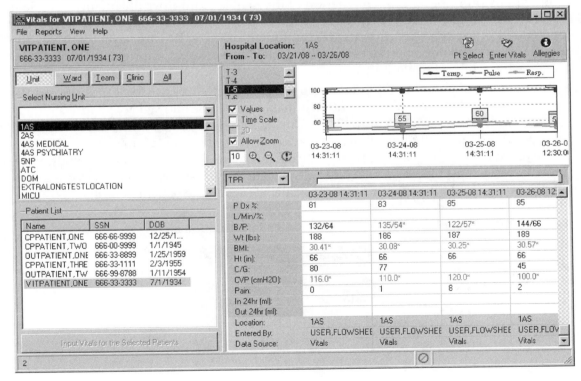

Source: VistA.

FIGURE 6.12. Example of a VistA medication administration record

Stat.	Ver	Hsm	Ty.	Active Medication	Dosage	Route	Admin Time	Last Action
G	xxx		C	ASCORBIC ACID TAB ASCORBIC ACID 100MG TAB take as needed on daily basis	100MG, Q2H	ORAL	11/14@1000	GIVEN: 11/14/2008@16...
	xxx		C	BETHANECHOL TAB BETHANECHOL 25MG TAB	50mg, Q6H	ORAL	11/14@0900	GIVEN: 10/9/2008@1903
	xxx		P	CORTISONE CREAM,TOP HYDROCORTISONE CREAM 1% (BULK/OZ)	.20oz, Q2H	TOPICAL		
	xxx		P	DACARBAZINE INJ DACARBAZINE 100MG INJ take sparingly	100MG/1VIAL, Q6H PRN	INTRAVENOUS INTRAMUSCULAR		GIVEN: 10/13/2008@18...
	xxx		C	FUROSEMIDE TAB FUROSEMIDE 40MG TAB	40MG, Q2H	ORAL	11/14@1000	GIVEN: 10/9/2008@1504
	xxx		C	NITROGLYCERIN OINT,TOP NITROGLYCERIN 2% OINT 20GM TUBE	.2mg, Q2H	TOPICAL	11/14@1000	GIVEN: 10/9/2008@1509
	xxx		C	VITAMIN E CAP,ORAL VITAMIN E 200 IU CAP take with care	200 IU, Q2H	ORAL	11/14@1000	

Source: VistA.

VistA for Research

The primary purpose for implementation of the EHR is to improve the quality of patient care. However, a secondary purpose is to facilitate healthcare research. This purpose is embedded in the population research component of the EHR (Amatayakul 2007). The VistA EHR, as explained on the VHA website, facilitates research through comprehensive database searches (US DVA 2010).

First, researchers must be working on a project approved by the local Institutional Review Board (IRB) for access to patient-identifiable data to be allowed access to VistA data. VistA includes no analytic software. Therefore, data to be analyzed must first be extracted from VistA and transferred to a different platform. Researchers must know the specific data elements that will enable them to access the most accurate population for their study. VistA provides several avenues to access and extract data. New Care Management software includes a query tool for sorting and exporting data for multiple patients simultaneously.

FIGURE 6.13. Example of a bar code medication administration alert

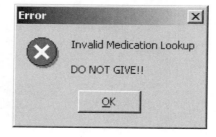

The database management program used to access and manage VistA data contains a data dictionary. Complex data requests can be accomplished more efficiently using **MUMPS**, the primary programming language of the VistA environment.

Care Management software provides a query tool that makes it possible to export data for multiple patients directly from VistA. The query tool can identify a cohort of patients, based on filters such as a membership in a local disease registry, primary care provider, abnormal test results, or a date range. These fields can be exported to a tab-delimited text file for analysis on another platform.

Care Management searches in the Orders file, the Visit/Appointment file, and the Text Integration Utilities document file (for example, progress notes, consults, or procedures) and displays critical elements such as consult status, test results, significant findings, and events admissions, transfers, discharges, and outpatient visits. Data elements that may be displayed in a query report appear in **TABLE 6.5**.

A health summary is a report that presents information gleaned from various VistA applications for an individual patient or group of patients. Some nationally available, standard health summaries focus on topics such as allergies, clinical procedures, active medical problems, current orders, demographics, discharge summaries, future appointments, initial assessments, perioperative assessments, reminders due, surgery reports, selected laboratory results, and detailed vitals. New health summaries can be

TABLE 6.5. VistA data elements displayable in query reports

PATIENT INFORMATION	DOCUMENTS
Name	Reference Date/Time
	Title
SSN (last four digits only)	Author
Age	Status
Ward Location	Expected Cosigner
ORDERS AND CONSULTS	**VISITS/APPOINTMENTS**
Order Date/Time	
Ordering Provider	
Order Text	
	Date/Time
Order Status	
	Location
Signature Status	
	Visit Status
Result Flag (abnormal, critical, significant)	
Significant Finding	

TABLE 6.6. VistA data elements for researchers

Outpatient Pharmacy	Order Entry/Results Reporting
Allergy Tracking System	Patient Care Encounter
Clinical Reminders	Problem List
Consults	Progress Notes
Dietetics	Radiology
Discharge Summary	Registration
Inpatient Medications	Scheduling
Lab	Social Work
Medicine	Surgery
Mental Health	VistA Imaging
Nursing (Vital Signs)	Automated Medical Information Exchange

custom designed by users, either by amending an available health summary or building it entirely from scratch. The VistA applications that can provide data elements for a health summary that will allow researchers to identify certain types of patient records are included in **TABLE 6.6**.

The Hybrid Health Record

Most healthcare entities are in transition from paper-based health records to EHRs. The speed of this transformation varies from entity to entity based on a variety of internal and external factors. The often-lengthy transition forces healthcare facilities to manage and maintain a hybrid health record.

Definition of the Hybrid Health Record

A hybrid health record is a system with functional components that includes both paper and electronic documents and uses both manual and electronic processes. Managing health information in this hybrid environment is challenging, particularly given the transition management requirements. Nevertheless, customer quality of care may be adversely affected for any organization if the transition from a paper-based environment to an electronic environment is not effectively managed. See **APPENDIX 6A** for the AHIMA practice brief "Managing the Transition from Paper to EHRs."

Format of the Hybrid Health Record

In essence, the hybrid health record is a transitional health record. It is dynamic in nature, and the format and content continuously change as healthcare facilities work toward a fully electronic health record.

Hybrid records are positive steps toward the EHR, but they create special challenges. Both manual and computer processes must be supported, policies and procedure are needed for both types of systems, and appropriate safeguards must be in place to ensure the privacy and security of both systems. A definition of what constitutes a record in each system must be developed. As the transition occurs, it is also important to regularly update system descriptions, including the location of all care documents, so that patient health information remains readily available to users. The AHIMA practice brief (**Appendix 6A**) suggested a matrix for this step. See **Appendix 6A**, **Table 6A.2**, for an example.

Image Processing and Storage Technology

Many hospitals incorporate documents into their EHR systems using image-processing technology. Digital scanners create images of handwritten and printed documents that are then stored in health record databases as electronic files. Using scanned images solves many of the problems associated with traditional paper-based health records. Digital files can be backed up frequently, which helps solve the problem of lost paper and microfilm records. In addition, because digital files are always under the control of a system administrator, access and confidentiality can be protected simultaneously. Digital imaging also makes it possible for more than one clinician to view the same document at the same time from distant locations. However, as noted previously, clinical documentation stored as digital images can only be accessed visually; that is, it cannot be searched electronically.

Traditional paper-based health records include few photographs and diagnostic images. With the introduction of clinical imaging devices, it is now possible to combine health record text files with digital diagnostic images (X-rays, CT scans, and so on) and digital photographs. With this technology, clinicians at different locations can view the same images at the same time and then compare their diagnostic interpretations.

Data Retrieval Technology

Retrieving specific data elements from a paper record can require a lot of time and effort. Many organizations have attempted to improve retrieval processes by using color-coded file folders, flags, tabs, and automated record-tracking systems. Data content required for reporting is often abstracted from the paper chart and entered into a computer system for processing. Although such methods are helpful, they have not completely resolved the problem of inefficient information retrieval. Abstracting data is expensive.

The ultimate goal of every health record-keeping system is the fast and secure delivery of accurate and complete health information to authorized recipients when and where they need it. To be effective, data retrieval systems must be based on the needs of the users.

Database systems that use query language applications allow users to perform text searches of EHR data. The ability to identify key words and phrases in textual data makes it easier to find and retrieve key pieces of patient information from health records.

Health Record Storage Systems

Paper-based records and EHRs have different storage requirements. As discussed earlier in the chapter, EHRs are stored digitally in centralized or departmental clinical data repositories. The storage options for paper and mixed-media records include paper-based storage systems, microfilm-based storage systems, and digital image–based storage systems.

Paper-Based Storage Systems

No matter what type of identification system a facility uses, most use color coding on health record folders to make storage and retrieval more efficient. Color-coded file folders are available from suppliers, and color-coded labels can also be used.

Paper-based health record files can be stored in vertical or lateral filing cabinets, open-shelf files, or compressible file systems. Vertical file cabinets are difficult to access and are rarely used to store health records. Lateral file cabinets are easier to access but are used only in low-volume areas of the hospital.

Hospitals usually use open-shelf or compressible files for housing paper-based health records. Open-shelf filing units resemble open bookshelves. Some are always open, and others have recessed doors that can be closed and locked.

Compressible file systems take up less space than fixed storage units. Compressible file systems are similar to open-shelf systems. The difference is that the shelving units are not fixed. In one type of compressible system, the units are mounted on permanent tracks in the floor so that they can be moved. Another type of compressible system is made up of horizontal or vertical carousels. The horizontal, open-shelf carousel contains files that revolve around a central spine or track. The vertical carousel brings all files or records directly to a workstation. Vertical carousel systems are often used to store master patient indexes.

Microfilm-Based Storage Systems

Paper-based health records require a huge amount of storage space, but alternative storage options can significantly reduce space needs. Storing images of paper reports and documentation on microfilm is an effective option for inactive or infrequently used health records. Microfilm records are also acceptable as courtroom evidence, because they are difficult to alter (Johns 2011).

The process of microfilming involves making special photomicrographs of the original paper documents. These tiny negative film images are then archived for long-term storage. Anyone who is interested in accessing the stored records must use a special microfilm reader, which magnifies the images.

Image-Based Storage Systems

Another solution for health records storage is an **electronic document management system (EDMS)**. Source documents are scanned to create digital images. The digital documents can then be stored electronically on optical disks. Some digital scanners can process hundreds or even thousands of documents per day. Access to images stored on optical disks is fast and easy, and scanned information can be made available simultaneously to any number of users. Document scanning is also used to convert stored health record information into images that can be loaded onto new EHR systems.

Health Record Formats' Impact on HIM Functions

The format of health records affects how HIM professionals manage standard departmental functions. For example, in a paper-based facility deficiencies are identified by manually reviewing the paper health record. In the hybrid health record environment, adding an electronic process, such as electronic signatures, enables remote record completion. When a completely electronic health records system is implemented, deficiencies are identified automatically, and health records can be monitored for unsigned reports, unviewed results, and missing reports.

The transformation of HIM functions is not always easy. The path of change, especially in the hybrid record environment, has many different twists. There is no one right way to do things. The changes are not always efficient, nor are the outcomes perfect—in fact, at times, they may be downright difficult and ugly.

APPENDIX 6B discusses the transformation that occurs in HIM functions as the format of the health record moves from a paper-based state, through the hybrid transformation, and into the fully electronic health record.

Authentication of Health Record Entries

In the context of health records, **authentication** is the process of providing proof of the authorship of documentation in the health record, whether it is maintained in a paper or electronic format. Federal and state laws govern authentication of health records. Some states have no requirements, while others outline specific procedures for authentication, including acceptable methods and time frames. Many state laws apply exclusively to physicians' orders for drugs and services. Additionally, hospitals address authentication requirements for health records in medical staff rules and regulations, which provide minimum authentication requirements for documentation, including how it is authenticated.

Many hospitals produce health records in various formats as the organization transitions to an EHR; therefore, HIM professionals should have a good understanding of authentication requirements based on how health records are created. In the paper-based health record, written signatures are usually applied to handwritten documentation as it is created. Often signatures are illegible, and clinicians forget to date and time stamp entries. However, HIM professionals identify missing signatures when reviewing documentation for completeness.

As facilities implement EHRs, their health records become hybrid. The hybrid health record includes a combination of handwritten and electronic signatures. HIM departments using an EDMS to manage health records present an example of a hybrid state. An EDMS can be defined as interfaced and paper-based documents scanned into a document imaging system that has workflow functionality. Scanned paper-based documents and interfaced, transcribed documents can both be electronically authenticated with an electronic signature. The EDMS can trigger signature deficiencies in interfaced documents, or HIM professionals can assign a signature deficiency to scanned documents. An **electronic signature** is a unique personal identifier that is entered by the author of EHR documentation via electronic means. Benefits of the electronic signature include legibility and automatic dating and time stamping of entries.

Authentication in EHR systems is accomplished with electronic or digital signatures. Digital signatures use the same technology as automated credit card authentication systems. A **digital signature** is a digitized version of a handwritten signature. The author of the documentation signs his or her name on a pen pad, and the signature is automatically converted to a digital signature that is affixed to the electronic document (AHIMA e-HIM Workgroup 2009). Electronic authentication when documentation is completed within an application is the best practice because it saves time and all entries are legible, dated, and time stamped.

Each individual who has been authorized to document in the EHR uses a **unique personal identifier** in the form of a code or password. Some systems may use a combination of a unique logon ID and password as a means to validate the author of the documentation or a **biometric identifier**, such as a fingerprint or retinal scans.

Each unique personal identifier must be assigned exclusively to a specific clinician, and a master list of the electronic identifiers must be maintained in a secure environment. Electronic signatures are permitted under Medicare's Conditions of Participation for Hospitals (2006) regulations and accreditation standards. Some states outline requirements for the use of electronic signatures for authentication. States that do not address this issue may permit the use of electronic signatures with approval from fiscal intermediaries or state authorities (AHIMA e-HIM Workgroup 2009). Most states have enacted specific laws or regulations addressing electronic signatures, and HIM professionals should be familiar with their own state laws on electronic signatures.

Guidelines to Prevent Fraud and Ensure EHR Documentation Integrity

According to the National Health Care Anti-Fraud Association, healthcare fraud is defined as an "intentional deception or misrepresentation that the individual or entity makes knowing that the misrepresentation could result in some unauthorized benefit to the individual, or the entity, or to some other party." EHR users should not expect unintentional deception or misrepresentation to be viewed more gently by payers, evaluators, or litigators. However, one of the many changes HIPAA privacy legislation rendered is that the standard is now "when you knew or should have known" (OCR 2003, 17). This shifts burden significantly by including the concept that those submitting claims have a due diligence obligation to proactively identify and prevent fraud, as the burden now is that the deception or misrepresentation need not be known or intentional but should have been known. The Office of Inspector General Chief Council Lewis Morris testified to the Senate Finance Committee in 2009 that the United States spends more than $2 trillion on healthcare annually (HCPro 2009).

In addition, medical identity theft is one of the fastest-growing crimes in the United States. At least 3 percent of that spending—$68 billion—is lost to medical identity theft fraud each year (ProtectMyID 2011). In March 2011 the second annual Study on Medical Identity Theft released by the Ponemon Institute estimated that 1.5 million Americans are affected by medical identity theft. The average cost to resolve these cases is a staggering $20,663.00

There are four areas of concern regarding the EHR environment:

1. **Authorship integrity**: Borrowing record entries from another source or author and representing or displaying past as current documentation and (in some instances) misrepresenting or inflating the nature and intensity of services provided

2. **Auditing integrity**: Inadequate auditing functions that make it impossible to detect when an entry was modified or borrowed from another source and misrepresented as an original entry by an authorized user

3. **Documentation integrity**: Automated insertion of clinical data and visit documentation using templates or similar tools with predetermined documentation components with uncontrolled and uncertain clinical relevance

4. **Patient identification and demographic accuracy**: Automated demographic or registration entries generating erroneous patient identification, leading to patient safety and quality-of-care issues and enabling fraudulent activity involving patient identity theft or providing unjustified care for profit

Authorship Integrity

Authorship is the origin of recorded information that is attributed to a specific individual or entity (AHIMA e-HIM Workgroup 2009). EHRs must allow more than one party to add text to an entry while retaining and displaying the authorship of each entry. For example, a nurse or alternative user can begin a patient's encounter note, and later, the examining physician can add comments.

In systems that require a single authorization for visit notes, the entire note may be attributed to the physician, and entries or observations by alternative users may be edited or deleted before final physician authentication, despite the alternative users' authentication. Another example involves flowcharts allowing entries by multiple individuals over a period of time but requiring only one signature at the end of the encounter, causing the identities of caregivers who posted interim data to be lost.

In these situations, it may be impossible to verify the actual provider of care or the amount of work performed by each person providing services. When records are analyzed and clinical codes reported for billing, the claim may reflect the wrong provider and level or type of care. One method of healthcare fraud involves using unlicensed individuals to perform services, while submitting claims under the provider number of a legitimate provider. It is the user's duty to ensure that all documentation authorship is accurately recorded in all approved uses of the documentation tools available.

Auto-authentication or Systematic Authorship Misrepresentation

Progress notes are considered assertions of a person and are authenticated for legal admissibility in a court of law. Auto-authentication methods, which allow users to sign multiple documents at one time without opening the documents, do not require author review and therefore fall short of federal and state authentication requirements and place the organization at legal risk. Some providers choose not to enter their own progress notes electronically and instead use scribes or assistants to type entries into the system for subsequent authorization. Policies, procedures, and checks and balances must be in place to ensure that the physician or legally responsible individual reviews the health record entries and affixes an authorization compliant with existing law. Since health record documentation drives payment from health plans, inaccurate information may lead to perceived fraudulent activities.

Borrowing Data from Other Sources

Electronic tools make it easier to copy and paste documentation from one record to another or to pull information forward from a previous visit, someone else's records, or other sources, either intentionally or inadvertently. The ability to copy and paste entries leads to a record where a clinician may, upon signing the documentation, unwittingly swear to the accuracy and comprehensiveness of substantial amounts of duplicated, inapplicable, misleading, and erroneous information. Further, while helping to improve apparent timeliness and legibility of documentation, the inability to verify authors or authenticate services performed create additional adverse effects. Defaulting clinical information with previous existing documentation from other patient encounters facilitates billing at a higher level of service than was actually provided.

Because of industry and regulatory payment pressures, physicians may find it necessary to document each component of the history and physical or review of systems during a patient encounter for payment and quality measurement. Time constraints and patient care demands can sometimes make it difficult for clinicians to meet the evaluation and patient management documentation requirements, creating the temptation to copy and paste. Such shortcuts can result in erroneous records and elevate the potential for fraudulent activity unless clinicians carefully review each record. Difficulties resulting from these practices include the following:

- Inaccurate representation of authorship of documentation

- Duplication of inapplicable information (relevant to the original case but not true for current care)

- Incorporation of misleading or erroneous documentation due to loss of context that was available to users in the original source

- Inclusion of content created by others without their knowledge or consent

- Inability to accurately determine services and findings specific to a patient's encounter

- Inaccurate automated code generation associated with documentation

Auditing Integrity

If an EHR lacks adequate audit-trail functionality, there may be no way to determine if and when corrections or amendments were made to the documentation, by whom they were made, or the nature of the correction or amendment. In addition to the normal unintentional mistakes that occur in documentation, records may be altered to prevent the discovery of damaging information or to avoid legal action. Without an adequate auditing function, legitimate changes may be indistinguishable from illegitimate ones, and the latter may be accepted as fact and may be untraceable. Changes or deletions made outside of routine record use must be maintained in the EHR system. Any uncertainty as to the integrity of the record creates legal liability for the institution while protecting criminal activity.

The functionality of the EHR may also determine whether or not an original note or amendment includes the correct date and time. Some systems automatically assign the date that the entry was made, while others allow authorized users to revise the date of entry to the date of the visit or service. Any system must be able to identify the date the note or amendment originated and the service date that the note or amendment references. Otherwise, the date sequence may be impossible to follow, adversely affecting appropriate patient care and resulting in questionable supporting documentation for reported services. Some EHR systems allow more than one party to add text to the same entry; for example, when faculty physicians are required to cosign resident notes. If the EHR does not enable both providers to document and sign, it may be impossible to verify the actual provider of care or the amount of work performed by each. When records are analyzed and clinical codes are reported for billing, the claim may reflect the wrong provider or the incorrect level or type of care.

As stated before, auto-authentication falls short of federal and state authentication requirements and could place the organization at legal risk. Some providers use scribes or assistants to type entries into the system for subsequent authorization. In some situations, the physician or other provider gives his access codes to assistants to allow direct entry of the notes. The system recognizes the author as the physician or the other authorized provider of care instead of the assistant. Checks and balances must be in place to ensure that the physician or other legally responsible individual has reviewed the health record entries and authenticated them in compliance with existing law.

Documentation Integrity: Automated Insertion of Clinical Data

Documentation templates are sometimes employed to enter default common findings into health record documents. An example is the automatic generation of common negative findings within a review of systems for each body area or organ system. Template users (often physicians) should document pertinent positive results and delete incorrect autogenerated entries.

The primary reason templates are used is to save time. A physician not fully aware of the consequences of defaulting information in templates may fail to review all defaulted data for changes and leave incorrect information in the record. This can lead to an inappropriate clinical picture, and the accuracy of the entire documented entry may be questioned. Documentation can be especially suspect when default information is used as the basis for service justification or other payment concerns without evidence of clinical relevance.

EHR systems must allow limited automatic creation of information. In the hands of criminals, autogenerated documentation for health records can enable rapid and plausible claims to government and private health plans. Clinical coding professionals rely on documentation for code assignments used on health plans. If the documentation is not true, the codes do not accurately reflect the circumstances of the healthcare service even when the codes are completely consistent with the documentation in the record. The "dirty data" resulting from inappropriate use of these tools compromises patient care and data-mining capabilities.

Templates often provide clinical information by default and design. When used inappropriately, they may misrepresent a patient's condition and might not reflect changes in a condition. These tools may also include defaults such as "reviewed past, family, and social history" for frequent visits, which is often not indicated or performed each time. Unless the physician or other authorized provider removes the default documentation from the visit note, a higher level of service than is actually provided could be assigned.

All templates and autogenerated entries, such as laboratory results, have the potential to be problematic. Accordingly, management oversight is necessary. Appropriate care must be taken that the data captured and stored are accurate, complete, and associated with the correct patient record and encounter.

One beneficial feature of EHR systems is the autopopulation of discrete clinical data (such as laboratory results) in the appropriate data fields rather than requiring a physician or other authorized provider to document the results with a progress note. Anecdotal information indicates that data generated as close as possible to the point of care are the most accurate and least likely to be connected with healthcare fraud.

Patient Identification and Demographic Data

Some EHR systems include capabilities for additional efficiency in health service financial management transactions and billing processes. Demographic and insurance data may be defaulted for a patient's encounter. Based on a setting or type of service, the system can automatically assign a registration status or discharge disposition. Audit functions must be implemented to ensure that information is appropriate and legitimate, and errors can be tracked for correction and staff training purposes. Health plan or payer policies may include patient-care setting adjustments such as an office, hospital, or outpatient department for physician services. If a registration status is incorrectly assigned, the location of service and technical, professional, or global billing may be inappropriately reimbursed.

Patient identity theft is also an area of vulnerability for healthcare organizations. In the wrong hands, Medicare, Medicaid, and other health plan claims data, coupled with the ability to manufacture supporting documentation, creates the risk of false claims and criminal activity. Patient safety and quality-of-care issues arise when physician order entry system safeguards are insufficient to identify fraud and abuse or business agreements involving data management violate patient privacy or allow unscrupulous providers to provide care that is unnecessary or fails to meet community standards for quality.

The Red Flag Rule, a law the Federal Trade Commission (FTC) began to enforce in August 2009, requires certain businesses and organizations, including many doctors' offices, hospitals, and other healthcare providers, to develop a written program to spot the warning signs, or red flags, of identity theft. Every healthcare organization and practice must review its billing and payment procedures to determine whether it is covered by the Red Flag Rule. Providers who are covered must

- Identify the kinds of red flags that are relevant to their practice

- Explain the provider's process for detecting the red flags

- Describe how the provider will respond to red flags to prevent and mitigate identity theft

- Spell out how the provider will keep the program current

The FTC has provided some common examples, which include (Toporoff 2009)

- **Suspicious documents.** Has a new patient given you identification documents that look altered or forged? Is the photograph or physical description on the ID inconsistent with the patient's appearance? Did the patient give you other documentation inconsistent with what she has told you—for example, an inconsistent date of birth or a chronic medical condition not mentioned elsewhere? Under the Red Flag Rule, you may need to ask for additional information from that patient.

- **Suspicious personally identifying information.** If a patient gives you information that doesn't match what you've learned from other sources, it may be a red flag for identity theft. For example, if the patient gives you a home address, birth date, or Social Security number that doesn't match information on file or from the insurer, fraud could be afoot.

- **Suspicious activities.** Is mail repeatedly returned as undeliverable, even though the patient still shows up for appointments? Does a patient complain about receiving a bill for a service that he didn't get? Is there an inconsistency between a physical examination or medical history reported by the patient and the treatment records?

- **Notices from victims of identity theft, law enforcement authorities, insurers, or others suggesting possible identity theft.** Have you received word about identity theft from another source? Cooperation is key. Heed warnings from others that identity theft may be ongoing.

Corrections in Clinical Documentation

When erroneous entries are made in health records, written procedures should have provisions for how corrections are made. Educating clinicians who are authorized to document in the health record on the appropriate way to make corrections will promote consistency and standardization and maintain the integrity of the health record. Errors corrected in the paper-based record may be easier to identify visually than those corrected in electronic documentation systems. The following is the recommended process for correcting errors in paper-based records (Smith 2001):

1. The clinician making the correction should draw a single line in ink through the incorrect entry.

2. The clinician should then print the word "error" at the top of the entry.

3. The clinician should authenticate the error notation by signing or initialing the notation and noting the date and time. The signature should include the individual's credentials and title. The reason the change is needed should also be noted.

4. The correct information should then be added to the entry as a notation. Late entries should be labeled as such; that is, entries must never be antedated (assigned a date earlier than the current date).

Clinicians cannot use the same method for correcting erroneous electronic documentation. The practice of correcting transcribed reports has been for the clinician to dictate an addendum to the original report, especially if the report has been signed. However, when the transcribed report is interfaced into an EDMS, the clinician is able to edit the original report before applying an electronic signature. After the report is electronically signed, the text-editing feature should not be available for amending documentation. Organizational policy should consider mandating creation of an addendum rather than an amendment to a signed document.

A primary concern when making corrections to the EHR is the ripple effect of data passing to various data sets, systems, and warehouses in an electronic environment, which magnifies the risk of inaccuracies. When corrections are needed for electronic documentation, data capture methods should include a mechanism for correcting all the data sets to which information has been passed. Following are some best practices for correcting documents in an EHR:

1. Minimize the need for corrections by ensuring that documents are complete and accurate before electronic authentication occurs.

2. Determine whether data was received in the EHR through an interface from another documentation system.

3. Either edit or amend the original documentation and resend it through the interface to the EHR.

4. Add amendments to signed documentation, indicating the reason for the amendment.

5. The electronic system should identify authors of documentation and date and time stamp entries.

6. Redistribute corrections to recipients of the original/incorrect documentation.

7. Correct data in all electronic systems to ensure the integrity of data collected.

8. Limit the number of persons authorized to make amendments to a signed document.

9. If policy allows editing of signed documents, all versions of the documents must be available for legal purposes.

10. Signed documents in the EHR should never be permanently deleted from the system. Provide a link to the original version.

e-Discovery: Developing a Litigation Response Plan

This section was adapted from Kimberly Baldwin-Stried Reich's article "Developing a Litigation Response Plan," originally published in the October 2007 issue of the *Journal of American Health Information Management Association*. This topic is also discussed in chapter 3.

The e-discovery amendments to the Federal Rules of Civil Procedure (FRCP) (updated in 2006) and the Uniform Rules Relating to the Discovery of Electronically Stored Information (approved in August 2007 at the National Conference of Commissioners on Uniform State Laws) are creating new roles and responsibilities for legal counsel and HIM and IT professionals. Organizations must begin to consider how they will respond to e-discovery requests for information. The process by which electronic information is produced in response to threatened or impending litigation is changing, and those closely involved with it must be knowledgeable on the requirements for producing information.

Three concepts are important in developing a litigation response plan for e-discovery:

- An organization's duty to preserve documents in the face of threatened or pending litigation

- The legal hold

- The development of an organization's e-discovery response plan

New Requests, New Responsibilities

In general terms, *discovery* is the formal, pretrial legal process used by parties to a lawsuit to obtain information. Discovery helps ensure that neither party is subjected to surprises at trial. The scope of information that can be obtained through discovery is broad and is not limited to what will be used at trial. Federal courts and most state courts allow a party to discover any information relevant to the claim. Because of the broad nature of this standard, parties often disagree about what information must be exchanged and what is considered privileged. These disputes are resolved through court rulings on discovery motions.

In e-discovery, the court is alerted early in the litigation, and the district judge, magistrate judge, or special master may take an active role in addressing the handling of discovery of electronically stored information, when it is expected to occur.

While the FRCP amendments apply to civil cases brought before federal (district) courts, it is anticipated that these amendments, coupled with the Uniform Rules Relating to the Discovery of Electronically Stored Information, will define the standards for discovery and production of electronic information at the state and local court levels.

As a result, it is incumbent upon legal counsel and HIM and IT professionals to evaluate how their roles and responsibilities will change with regard to the discovery and production of electronically stored information.

E-discovery will be most effective when legal counsel has a good understanding of the rules, communicates and negotiates with opposing counsel and the court, and involves HIM and IT professionals in the process.

The Duty to Preserve

The basic principles regarding preservation of relevant electronically stored information are essentially the same as those governing the preservation of relevant paper-based business records. That is, at the moment when litigation is reasonably anticipated (known, threatened, or pending), the normal disposition and processing of information in either format should be suspended.

For example, some healthcare organizations make a copy of the paper-based record (usually the patient's health record) at the time litigation is known. The original is then given to risk management or legal counsel to secure in a locked file. Access to the original paper-based health record is then usually controlled or monitored to prevent unauthorized access or tampering.

The duty to preserve relevant electronically stored information also supersedes an organization's record retention and management policies that would normally result in the destruction of electronically stored information. The basic premise of common law doctrine is to avoid spoliation (intentional destruction, alteration, or concealment) of evidence for use at trial. The courts have inherent powers and rules that govern the imposition of sanctions for spoliation.

The Legal Hold

Once litigation can be reasonably anticipated, the organization should establish a legal (litigation) hold and take reasonable measures to identify and preserve all information relevant to the claim. A legal hold (also known as a preservation order) may or may not be issued by a court. An organization's key determination in establishing a legal hold is when litigation is "reasonably anticipated." For example, once an individual or organization is served with a complaint, subpoena, or subpoena duces tecum or receives notice of a government investigation, litigation can be reasonably anticipated. A legal hold should then be immediately established and reasonable measures taken to identify and preserve relevant information. The duty to preserve could arise well before an individual or organization is served with any of these documents or notices. Determining when the legal hold should be established is not a rote decision. When faced with potential litigation, the facts of the particular situation must be carefully weighed.

Organizations and their legal counsel may consider the following general factors prior to establishing a legal hold:

- The potential litigation risk to the organization (type, source, and credibility)

- The potential risk of information loss if a legal hold is not established

- Identification of all individuals identified as potential record custodians

- Assessment of the level of knowledge, sources, and location of information within the organization relevant to the potential claim

- Process by which the establishment of the legal hold will be communicated within the organization

- The time frame for reviewing the legal hold and when it can be lifted

The e-Discovery Litigation Response Team

The discovery of electronically stored information is not a simple, inexpensive, or straightforward process. The true costs to search, cull, and retrieve electronic information (including information contained in backup tapes and legacy systems) that may be relevant to a lawsuit could far outweigh the costs of providing photocopies of a patient's health records. Organizations must establish a plan and process to understand the true costs and burdens of producing electronic information.

Effective e-discovery administration requires a team of interdisciplinary professionals serving on a litigation response team. Legal counsel should oversee the e-discovery process and head the team. They will advise senior management and the governing board about any and all impending litigation, and they can define and delineate the measures the organization should take in the identification, preservation, search, retrieval, and production of responsive electronic and other potentially relevant information.

IT and HIM professionals should also be appointed to the team. They are best equipped to advise legal counsel about the forms, formats, methods, status, costs, location, and production burden of potentially responsive information. They also possess knowledge of the technical and administrative processes surrounding the use, management, storage, retention, and destruction of information within the organization.

An e-discovery plan should be prepared well in advance of litigation, and it should be tailored to the organization's needs as determined by its size, scope, and complexity. By becoming familiar with the FRCP, the Uniform Rules Relating to the Discovery of Electronically Stored Information, and state legislation involving electronic document production, legal counsel and HIM and IT professionals have the unique opportunity to work together to define and shape e-discovery processes for their organizations and states.

Disaster Planning

Another important aspect of health record documentation is planning for access to information during planned or unplanned computer systems down time or during a disaster. Hospitals are required to have backup plans to protect health information from damage and destruction. **Disaster recovery planning** is the technological aspect of business continuity planning. HIM professionals assist in designing disaster recovery plans that address documenting information in the health record during down time or a disaster.

A well-designed disaster-recovery plan should consider the following:

1. Daily backups and removal of electronic data/information to an offsite location for protection

2. Access to information needed to treat patients

3. Backup plan to collect and document health information

4. Protection of computer systems, data, and paper-based records from destruction

5. Protection against unauthorized use and disclosure

6. Safeguards to ensure integrity and confidentiality of information

7. Provision for orderly recovery of information

8. Periodic testing of disaster recovery plans before a disaster occurs

The Hurricane Katrina experience demonstrated not only that good contingency plans should include backing up patient data to other media but also that data need to be made accessible as soon as possible. Another lesson learned during Katrina was the importance of thorough planning for health information in disaster preparedness and response.

Disaster planning must account for manual processes to be used during down time, even when health information is electronic. HIM professionals play an important part in disaster planning by assuming leadership roles in ensuring that health records are safeguarded while the information is accessible.

Disaster recovery best practices include the following:

• Routinely reviewing emergency plans

• Regularly practicing and reviewing contingency plans

• Ensuring that employees are knowledgeable about and prepared to quickly implement plans

• Ensuring that hospital management has a serious dialogue about backup and recovery

• Routinely moving backup data to a remote location

• Routinely testing contingency plans

HIM professionals provide a unique perspective on disaster planning because they understand the workflow of the health record better than any other professional in the organization does, and they can identify strategies for making paper or electronic records available for patient care. HIM professionals should plan how to respond to different levels of disasters and how records will be created or maintained during this process. Additionally, they should plan how electronic databases will be made available during a disaster and how quickly information will be recovered.

In the aftermath of Hurricane Katrina in 2005, the VA initiated the development of the Health Data Repository to contain real-time copies of local clinical data. The

FIGURE 6.14. **Example of a decision tool**

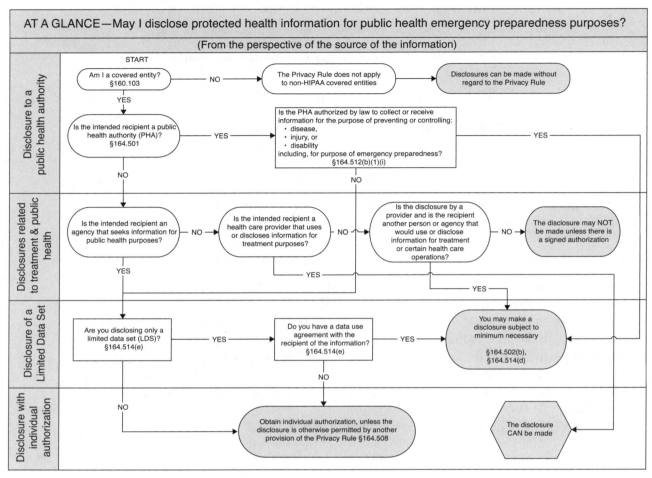

Source: OCR n.d.

Health Data Repository is a database that provides immediate national access to local data in the event of primary system failure or system unavailability. The repository is an effort to improve data accessibility and increase disaster preparedness. See **Figure 6.14** for a health information release decision tool from the Office for Civil Rights. This tool focuses on issues relevant to emergency preparedness and does not address other federal, state, or local confidentiality laws that may apply in specific circumstances. Although it does not discuss all the HIPAA Privacy Rule requirements for the uses and disclosures permitted, it can be used to guide development of a contingency plan for releasing protected health information in a disaster.

Summary

Adhering to a predetermined, published, standardized format for data entry can expedite the location of information within health records.. With a paper-based record, this is accomplished with well-designed forms that guide the entry of data elements. With an EHR, it is accomplished with a well-designed interface and edit prompts that guide data entry.

Healthcare organizations are in a transitional stage toward the EHR. Federal legislation plays an important role in the transition. However, SDOs and healthcare systems are responsible for realizing the EHR. There are 10 key components to the EHR that hospitals must work toward over the next five years. The VHA's EHR, VistA, is a microcosm of the NHIN and can be used for reference by healthcare organizations.

As facilities transition from paper-based health records to EHRs, hybrid health records use features of both formats. By standardizing the format and content of health records, providers can meet requirements for record completion and data quality and for storing information in a location that facilitates retrieval. The EHR also creates new challenges for data integrity and legal proceedings with which all HIM professionals need to be familiar.

References

Agency for Healthcare Research and Quality (AHRQ). 2011. Health Information Technology. http://healthit.ahrq.gov/portal/server.pt?open=514&objID=5554&mode=2&holderDisplayURL=http://wci-pubcontent/publish/communities/k_o/knowledge_library/key_topics/electronic_medical_record_systems/electronic_medical_record_systems.html.

AHIMA e-HIM Workgroup: Best Practices for Electronic Signature and Attestation. 2009. Electronic Signature, Attestation, and Authorship. *Journal of AHIMA* 80(11): expanded online edition.

Amatayakul, M. K. 2007. *Electronic Health Records: A Practical Guide for Professionals and Organizations*, 3rd ed. Chicago: AHIMA.

American Society of Testing Materials (ASTM). Standard E1384-07, 2007. Standard practice for content and structure of the electronic health record (EHR). West Conshohocken, PA: ASTM International.

Centers for Medicare and Medicaid Services (CMS). 2009. American Recovery and Reinvestment Act. http://www.cms.gov/Recovery/11_HealthIT.asp.

Cerrato, L., and Roberts, J. 2011. Health Information Technology Functions. In *Health Information Management Technology: An Applied Approach*, 3rd ed., edited by M. Johns. Chicago: AHIMA.

Centers for Medicare and Medicaid Services (CMS). 2006. Hospital Conditions of Participation: Patients' Rights. *Federal Register*. 71(236). http://www.edlawrc.com/CMS%20regs%20on%20restraint.pdf

Cote, R. A., D. J. Rothwell, J. L. Palotay, R. S. Becket, and L. Btochu. 1993. *The Systematized Nomenclature of Human and Veterinary Medicine – SNOMED International*. Lakefield, IL: College of American Pathologists.

Dick, R. S., E. B. Steen, and D. E. Detmer, eds. 1997. *The Computer-Based Patient Record: An Essential Technology for Health Care*, rev. ed. Washington, DC: National Academies Press.

EHR Collaborative. 2004. *EHR Functional Model*. www.ehrcollaborative.com.

Giannangelo, K. 2011. Healthcare Data Sets and Standards. In *Health Information Management Technology: An Applied Approach*, 3rd ed., edited by M. Johns. Chicago: AHIMA.

HCPro. 2009. OIG Official: Fighting Fraud is Critical to Healthcare Reform. *Healthcare Auditing Weekly*, April 28. http://www.hcpro.com/CCP-232146–1685/OIG-Official-Fighting-Fraud-is-Critical-to-Healthcare-Reform.html.

Health Insurance Portability and Accountability Act (HIPAA) of 1996. 1996. Public Law 104–191.

Health Level Seven (HL7). 2007. EHR Functional Model. http://www.hl7.org/ehr/downloads/index_2007.asp.

Healthcare Financial Management Association (HFMA). 2010. What to Consider When Purchasing an EHR System. http://www.hfma.org/Templates/InteriorMaster.aspx?id=20452.

*Healthcare Informatics.*2008. NAHIT Releases HIT Definitions. http://www.healthcare-informatics.com/ME2/dirmod.asp?sid=&nm=&type=news&mod=News&mid=9A02E3B96F2A415ABC72CB5F516B4C10&tier=3&nid=3672849E1D074C4ABD37D6C0B709F805.

Healthcare Information and Management Systems Society (HIMSS). 2010b. EMR Adoption Model. http://www.himssanalytics.org/stagesGraph.html.

Healthcare Information and Management Systems Society (HIMSS). 2010a. Clinical Decision Support Systems. Chicago: HIMSS.

Healthcare Information and Management Systems Society (HIMSS). 2009. HIMSS Analytics Database (derived from the Dorenfest IHDS+ Database). HIMSS Analytics Essentials of the US Hospital IT Market 2009.

Healthcare Information and Management Systems Society (HIMSS) EHR Association Membership Committee. 2006. HIMSS EHR Association Definitional Model and Application Process. http://www.himssehra.org/docs/EHRVA_application.pdf.

IBM. 1993. *Dictionary of Computing*, 10th ed. New York: McGraw-Hill.

Johns, M. 2011. Health Information Technology Functions. In *Health Information Management Technology: An Applied Approach*, 3rd ed., edited by M. Johns. Chicago: AHIMA.

LaTour, K., and S. Eichenwald Maki. 2010. *Health Information Management: Concepts, Principles, and Practice*, 3rd ed. Chicago: AHIMA.

National Alliance for Health Information Technology. 2008. Defining Key Health Information Technology Terms. http://www.hhs.gov/healthit/documents/m20080603/10_2_hit_terms.pdf.

National Committee on Vital and Health Statistics. 2011. Information for Health: A Strategy for Building the National Health Information Infrastructure. http://aspe.hhs.gov/sp/NHII/Documents/NHIIReport2001/report7.htm.

Office of Civil Rights (OCR). 2003. OCR Privacy Brief: Summary of the HIPAA Privacy Rule. http://www.hhs.gov/ocr/privacy/hipaa/understanding/summary/privacysummary.pdf.

Office of Civil Rights (OCR). n.d. Process Flow At-a-Glance. Washington, DC: Department of Health & Human Services. http://www.hhs.gov/ocr/privacy/hipaa/understanding/special/emergency/emergencyprepdisclose.pdf.

Office of the National Coordinator for Health Information Technology (ONC). 2010. National Health Information Network Exchange. http://healthit.hhs.gov/portal/server.pt?open=512&objID=1407&parentname=Community-Page&parentid=7&mode=2&in_hi_userid=10741&cached=true.

ProtectMyID. 2011. Medical Identity Theft: The Growing Cost of Indifference. http://blog.protectmyid.com/2011/03/16/medical-identity-theft-the-growing-cost-of-indifference.

Reich, Kimberly Baldwin-Stried. 2007. Developing a litigation response plan. *Journal of AHIMA*. 78(9): 76–78, 86.

Shortliffe, E., and J. Cimino. 2006. *Biomedical Informatics: Computer Applications in Health Care and Biomedicine*. New York: Springer Publishing.

Smith, C. M. 2001. Practice Brief: Documentation Requirements for the Acute Care Inpatient Record. *Journal of AHIMA* 72(3):56A–G.

Tegan, A., et al. 2005. The EHR's Impact on HIM Functions. *Journal of American Health Information Management Association* 76(5):56C–H.

Thompson, T. G., and D. J. Brailer. 2006. *The Decade of Health Information Technology: Delivering Consumer-Centric and Information-Rich Health Care Framework for Strategic Action*. Washington, DC: National Coordinator for Health Information Technology.

Toporoff, S. 2009. *The Red Flag Rule: What Health Care Providers Need to Know About Complying with New Requirements for Fighting Identity Theft*. Washington, DC: FTC.

US Department of Health and Human Services (HHS). 2010 Health Information Technology: Initial Set of Standards, Implementation Specifications, and Certification Criteria for Electronic Health Record Technology. Office of the National Coordinator for Health Information Technology (ONC), Department of Health and Human Services. http://edocket.access.gpo.gov/2010/pdf/2010-17210.pdf.

US Department of Veteran's Affairs Resource Center (US DVA). 2010. VistA: Description. http://www.virec.research.va.gov/DataSourcesName/VISTA/VistA.htm.

Walker, J. 2005. The Value of Health Care Information Exchange and Interoperability. *Health Affairs* Web exclusive: W5-10–W5-18.

Waller, D. 2006. How Veterans' Hospitals Became the Best in Health Care. *Time Magazine*. August 27. http://www.time.com/time/magazine/article/0,9171,1376238,00.html#ixzz0qlvp0Ghi.

Appendix 6A

Managing the Transition from Paper to EHRs

Background

The transition from a paper-based health record to an electronic health record (EHR) must be addressed and managed on many different and complex levels: administratively, financially, culturally, technologically, and institutionally. The EHR consists of many components that work together to create the foundation of the legal health record. These components may include software applications such as computerized physician order entry; integration with laboratory, radiology, and cardiology systems; an electronic document management system; or other solutions. The EHR journey is one that will evolve over many years, requiring many change-management dynamics that will challenge each of those involved with the transition process.

Given the complexities involved with the transition to an EHR environment, implementation has been slow yet steady, and many valuable lessons have emerged in recent years that are helping healthcare providers and organizations ease the transition to a workable, practical electronic record environment. A focus on patient safety, best practices, and return on investment, as well as ease of end-user adoption have driven healthcare organizations to adopt solutions that support workflow performance improvement versus those that simply automate existing process or system dysfunction.

In February 2009, President Obama signed the American Recovery and Reinvestment Act (ARRA) into law. Part of ARRA's goal is to encourage healthcare organizations to adopt EHRs through financial incentives. Because of the slowness of adoption, funding barriers, concurrent regulatory compliance timelines, competing technical priorities, strained human resources, and the lack of industry education, many healthcare providers are finding themselves maintaining a hybrid (combination of paper and electronic) health record as an alternative to full automation of the legal health record. It is widely recognized that a hybrid record state is not an ideal situation for any facility for any extended length of time. If an organization can avoid hybridization altogether, or minimize the effect of hybrid components, it will decrease the risk to patient safety and be more effective and cost-efficient. ARRA included the Health Information Technology for Economic and Clinical Health (HITECH) Act. HITECH is not meant to be the magic bullet for EHR implementation, so the hybrid record will continue to exist. Therefore, it is imperative for organizations to identify and address the challenges with the hybrid record and implement possible solutions to mitigate potential risks.

AHIMA. 2010. *Managing the Transition from Paper to EHRs.* Chicago: AHIMA.

This practice brief is intended to provide guidance and practical steps for managing the transition from paper to EHRs and for use and disclosure, authorship, and printing from paper to hybrid (paper and electronic) records and hybrid to electronic records.

Definition of the Legal Health Record

Organizations must define health record content and format in their policies. The health record comprises individually identifiable data, in any medium, that are collected, processed, stored, displayed, and used by healthcare professionals. The legal health record is generated at or for a healthcare organization as its business record and is the record that will be disclosed when required. It does not affect the discoverability of other information held by the organization. Healthcare organizations must designate the custodian of the legal health record. The custodian is responsible for the operational functions of the development and maintenance of the health record and may certify through affidavit or testimony the normal business practices used to create and maintain the record. Typically, this is the health information manager in collaboration with information technology professionals. HIM professionals oversee the operational functions related to collecting, protecting, and archiving the legal health record, whereas information technology staff members manage the technical infrastructure of the EHR.

The legal health record is the documentation of healthcare services provided to an individual during any aspect of healthcare delivery in any type of healthcare organization. It is consumer or patient centered. The legal health record contains individually identifiable data, stored on any medium, collected and directly used in documenting healthcare or health status.

Legal health records must meet accepted standards as defined by applicable Centers for Medicare and Medicaid Services (CMS) Conditions of Participation, federal regulations, state laws, and standards of accrediting agencies such as the Joint Commission, as well as the policies of the healthcare provider.[1]

Legal health records are records of care in any health-related setting used by healthcare professionals while providing patient care or for administrative, business, or payment purposes. Documentation that constitutes the legal health record may exist physically in separate and/or multiple paper-based or electronic systems.

Currently and into the near future, paper documents and various types of media containing patient health information will continue to exist. Documents that are produced outside a facility and are brought in for continuing care may be physical paper documents or exist on various types of media. This information may be technologically difficult to integrate into an EHR. If nothing else, access and readability, portability, and downtime backups all require some paper-based records.

Information that is both electronic and paper based is collected and/or directly used to document healthcare delivery or healthcare status and is the basis for research and planning functions in hospitals. A hybrid health record is a system with functional components that include any of the following:

- Both paper and electronic documents *without* a central electronic document management system where all patient information is maintained

- Manual and electronic processes to compile components of the medical record

- Multiple repositories (paper or electronic) of information that need to be accessed by the end user to compile the medical records for a single episode of care

Some examples of hybrid medical record scenarios are:

- Dictation, laboratory, and X-ray results are available electronically, whereas progress notes, ancillary care, provider information, graphic sheets, and doctors" orders are on paper.

- Patient health information may be maintained on various other media types such as film, video, or an imaging system.

- Patient information may be scanned images that are accessed in a separate part of the system versus being integrated together in a chronological packet of information defined as the legal health record.

- Hospital records are automated, but clinic records are on paper and processed and stored in the clinic, never becoming part of the core EHR.

Managing health information in this hybrid environment is challenging, particularly given the transition management requirements. It is also extremely costly to a facility because it requires duplicative efforts by staff to manage both paper and electronic documentation and the acts of compiling and retrieving information in a hybrid environment are labor-intensive and fraught with risk for errors. The costs of designing interfaces and integration in a partially electronic record system become increasingly expensive when written to manage only certain portions of the medical record. Increasingly, sites have learned lessons, and best practice is considered full adoption of an electronic document management system across the healthcare organization.

When creating the legal health record policy, healthcare organizations must evaluate accreditation standards and state and federal laws.

Legal and Accreditation Requirements

As organizations develop their vision and accompanying policies and procedures for the EHR, it is important to understand and address the many federal, state, accreditation, and other regulatory requirements that affect health information. Federal and state regulations are constantly changing and evolving, so it is crucial to keep up-to-date with these changes.

Federal

The HIPAA privacy rule requires that covered entities adhere to certain standards when using protected health information (PHI). It provides broad guidance insofar as defining to whom and under what circumstances information may or may not be requested, used, or disclosed.

The HIPAA security rule establishes the administrative, physical, and technical safeguards covered entities must implement to protect electronic PHI. ARRA and HITECH update the HIPAA rules and further establish privacy and security protections. The Confidentiality of Alcohol and Drug Abuse Patient Records 42CFR part 2 regulation establishes requirements for the use and disclosure of information maintained in connection with the performance of a drug abuse prevention function assisted directly or indirectly by the federal government.

The Privacy Act of 1974 grants people the right to find out what information has been collected about them, correct and amend that information, and exercise limited control over disclosure. The provisions of the Privacy Act apply to healthcare organizations operated by the federal government and record systems operated pursuant to a contract with the federal government. The Federal Rules of Evidence, Article VIII, outline the criteria necessary for health records to be acceptable as evidence in federal court.

State

Often states have laws or regulations that define the circumstances in which patient health information may be used, disclosed, and retained. Many states have special rules for access and disclosure of sexually transmitted disease, drug or alcohol abuse, or mental health information.

In addition to ensuring compliance with federal law, organizations must determine the laws and regulations within their states that affect EHRs in areas of electronic signature, access and disclosure of personal health information, and retention and destruction of information.

When federal and state laws exist, it is important that policies and procedures comply with both. When it is not possible for organizations to comply with both, the organization must comply with the more stringent law or regulation.

States also may have rules that relate to the use, disclosure, and retention of business records and/or materials that may be admitted into evidence. Organizations should examine and consider such rules when designing electronic or hybrid health information systems, policies, and procedures.

Accreditation

Many accreditation organizations such as the Joint Commission, American Osteopathic Association, CMS, and Accreditation Association for Ambulatory Health Care establish standards aimed at ensuring access to needed health information by authorized users and safeguards preventing access by unauthorized individuals. Organizations that are or wish to be accredited must look to these accreditation standards for guidance.

For example, the Joint Commission has posted prepublication editions of standards for hospitals and long-term care facilities on its Web site that state:

- Only authorized individuals make entries in the medical record

- Every medical record entry is dated, timed, and signed (TJC RC 01.01.01, CMS 482.24 (c)(1))

Managing the Transition

There are key differences to systems that are focused on being a clinical or patient-centric EHR and those that provide workflow and integration of a post-discharge document management. Both are important. The **TABLE 6A.1** illustrates some of the key differences between aspects of these systems. The first column focuses on managing a legal EHR. The second focuses on combining patient-centric clinical documentation solutions and electronic document management solutions.

TABLE 6A.1. Clinical/patient-centric systems versus workflow/integration systems

FUNCTIONS OF PATIENT-CENTRIC CLINICAL DOCUMENTATION SOLUTIONS	FUNCTIONS OF ELECTRONIC CONTENT MANAGEMENT AND ELECTRONIC DOCUMENT MANAGEMENT SOLUTIONS
Focuses on clinician workflow, including daily notes, transcribed documents, orders, and diagnostic results	Focuses on the legal health record in its entirety from preadmission to post-discharge documentation
Extremely dynamic, replacing temporary and working copies of documents with multiple versions of documents	Dynamic until point of completion, and then the record is considered sealed in a permanent state only to be altered through legal amendment and correction process
May be longitudinal in nature, potentially trending clinical results across multiple episodes of care	Typically episodic in nature, provides book-style chronological record for a single episode of care (i.e., outpatients within a single day, inpatients for an entire length of stay)
Requires separate repositories for data and scanned images	Incorporates paper documents through imaging (scanning), as well as alternate media and electronic feeds to capture the entire record through combination of computer output to laser disc (COLD) feeds and images
Provides input and results and, potentially, analytics around results within the components	Supports access, secure control, and workflow or work-routing functions for the entire record on an access, processing, maintenance, retrieval, and destruction basis

Managing the Change: Top 10 Paper/Hybrid/EHR Tenets

1. The EHR must be part of an organization's vision and strategic plan. As part of this plan, the organization should have a standard definition for the legal health record.

2. The organization must ensure that adequate leadership, consultation, staff training, equipment, policies and procedures, and funding or other resources are in place to support EHR development.

3. Organizations must establish a legal health record steering committee to guide the organization from a paper to an electronic environment. This group must be empowered to make proactive and constructive changes. Its members should include department managers from health information management; risk, quality, or compliance management; medical staff; nursing; ancillary departments; IT, and the privacy officer.

4. The legal health record steering committee must develop and publish policies and procedures for operating in the paper state, hybrid state, and electronic state and include long-term archive, purge, retention, and destruction guidelines.

5. HIM professionals must participate actively in the development and implementation of the EHR, given the significant operational management effects on workflow within HIM and their role as custodians of the legal health record.

6. There must be a formal process for approving EHR software and hardware to ensure that it can support the organization's operational needs adequately for the paper, hybrid, and electronic medical record.

7. There must be a formal process for managing paper, electronic, and hybrid forms, and system-generated records, including input, output, and versioning of document content and access.

8. There must be a formal process and written guidelines addressing access, confidentiality, security, print control, spoliation mitigation, disclosure, and e-discovery.

9. A complete record inventory of all existing storage and management of paper, hybrid, shadow (duplicate), and electronic records must be maintained by all healthcare organizations.

10. The facility must develop a policy for retention and destruction of medical records, regardless of whether paper, hybrid, or electronic medical records are used.

TABLE 6A.2 describes specific HIM functions, operational considerations, and suggested strategic guidelines for organizations to consider when planning the transition from a paper-based environment to a hybrid environment and then on to a fully electronic environment.

TABLE 6A.2. Strategic practice guidelines for traditional and emerging HIM operational functions

HIM OPERATIONAL FUNCTION	OPERATIONAL CONSIDERATIONS	STRATEGIC PRACTICE GUIDELINES
Transcription/Coding Staffing	In-house, home based, outsourced, or offshore	• Familiarize and synchronize transcription/coding staff with your organization's strategic plan • Become knowledgeable about system integration capabilities, limitations, and opportunities of both source and interfacing information systems • Ensure availability and implementation of quality control features and reporting capabilities of all source and interfacing systems • Ensure compliance with any and all privacy, confidentiality, and security laws (e.g., state, federal, or organization specific) • Ensure organization has planned its off-site EHR content carefully before implementing any off-site coding or transcription functions (e.g., have major clinical documentation needed by coders, such as physician progress notes, available online to coders before implementing off-site coding) • Consider bidirectional interfacing for edits, changes, and other source document integrity • Consider electronic signature authentication; encourage online signature

TABLE 6A.2. (continued)

HIM OPERATIONAL FUNCTION	OPERATIONAL CONSIDERATIONS	STRATEGIC PRACTICE GUIDELINES
Transcription Delivery Media	Fax, tape, disc or CD, paper, electronic (e.g., batch mode, uploading, integrity maintenance)	• Standardize delivery media to minimize paper and/or duplicate delivery modalities • Ensure device availability (e.g., remote access) and notification to recipients of delivered electronic documents • Ensure proper privacy and security controls are in place regardless of media
Electronic Signature	Transcription and other critical EHR documentation	• Review and consider e-signature processing capabilities, limitations, opportunities (see practice brief: Electronic Signature, Attestation, and Authorship) • Consider versioning control and replacement of temporary versus permanent (after review and authentication) document storage • Understand clearly the minimal operational workflow requirements for processing e-signatures when working with information systems and vendor representatives
Release of Information (ROI)	Customer service when ROI function is off-site or remote; electronic transfers rather than paper printing	• Consider expansion of HIM responsibilities for ROI functions into decentralized areas, including off-site clinics, if not already responsible • Consider how to continue to meet standards and laws if ROI function is decentralized (e.g., disclosure laws with respect to ETOH, HIV, and mental health; have HIM continue to handle all requests for amendments coming through ROI) • Consider whether HIM will continue to maintain oversight or be a subject matter resource to those managing ROI; consider centralization of ROI and other printing and access functions for greater confidentiality, compliance, audit control, and cost efficiencies • Ensure EHR plans incorporate ROI workflow capabilities both on-site and remotely (e.g., disclosure tracking and auditing capabilities) • Consider electronic rules and alerts on ROI requirements to allow for expanded delegation of ROI operational capabilities and responsibilities

TABLE 6A.2. (continued)

HIM OPERATIONAL FUNCTION	OPERATIONAL CONSIDERATIONS	STRATEGIC PRACTICE GUIDELINES
Record Processing	Completion, abstracting, assembly, indexing	• Establish business rules for online EHR viewing that are based on an individual's role and completion status of online document (e.g., ROI only sees complete online records) • Ensure EHR system capabilities to monitor and track record completion (e.g., online alerts to individual clinicians, aggregated management screens and reports for HIM) • Manage record completion business processes, regardless of where organization is along the EHR transition continuum • Transfer and/or retrain staff members for other operational areas (e.g., assemblers become preppers and scanners where imaging has been deployed) as the need to print and assemble paper-based records diminishes • Develop standardized assembly order based on user needs for printed EHRs (e.g., different EHR views may necessitate different assembly orders [lawyers, patients, etc.]) • Work with EHR vendor toward use of expert rules for automated abstracting, where possible • Ensure productivity standards are in place for all record-processing functions • Determine which information will be back loaded into the EHR system • Ensure that the workflow and work routing support COLD electronic document/results feed is used to reduce dependency on manual scanning of documents
Data Management	Data quality and integrity	• Ensure backlogs are eliminated before any EHR implementation • Ensure periodic spot-checks are made to ensure data integrity within the medical record • Ensure daily reconciliation of all interfaces for exported and imported feeds to ensure integrity of the medical record • Ensure processing standards (availability standards) are maintained as immediately as possible seven days a week 24 hours a day via adequate processing, staffing, and backups • Develop and review a data dictionary

TABLE 6A.2. (continued)

HIM OPERATIONAL FUNCTION	OPERATIONAL CONSIDERATIONS	STRATEGIC PRACTICE GUIDELINES
File Room	Define the file room in terms of where files are stored and whether scanned images are used (are files paper, electronic, both?) Need to consider staffing support for retrieval of older records for length of retention; records are used most heavily the first three years after discharge	• Conduct an assessment to determine where along the EHR transition continuum your organization's current and planned state of the file room is or will be: – Paper-based health record – Shadow health record – Hybrid health record – Complete EHR • Consider logistically what kinds of HIM policies, processes, procedures, and management practices are needed as the file room transforms from a physical environment to a virtual operation: – Elimination of shadow records – Shelving and hard-copy paper folders or files stored in a fixed location accessed and managed by staff – Electronic records contained on a server managed by information technology business rules for access, retrieval, retention, etc. • Consider which file room operations may need to shift to ensure acceptable productivity levels (e.g., timeliness, accessibility, completeness) in a hybrid file room environment (e.g., combination of hard-copy records, scanned records, and data repository records): – List of functions – Hours of operation – After-hours access and backup – Staffing needs – Record control – Filing and indexing – Retention, purging, and archiving – Other
Dynamic Data Handling	Alerts, flow data, e-mails, e-logs, and practice protocols	• Determine whether dynamic data will be considered part of the legal medical record • Ensure proper security measures are taken to protect your PHI if dynamic data are being maintained at a remote community health information network location • Determine whether online alerts and associated audit information should be included as part of the legal EHR

TABLE 6A.2. (continued)

HIM OPERATIONAL FUNCTION	OPERATIONAL CONSIDERATIONS	STRATEGIC PRACTICE GUIDELINES
Data Integration Issues	System merges, conversion issues, and multiple EHR systems in a given environment	• Ensure appropriate quality control mechanisms are in place to ensure data integrity (e.g., enterprise-wide master patient index encounters or episodes as part of the overall IT conversion process) for multifacility and/or multidepartmental EHR system integrations • Ensure HIM plays a strong role in all quality control planning and implementation activities (e.g., audit reporting and monitoring)
Retention/Destruction Issues	State and federal mandates, legal counsel recommendations, and system limitations and needs; e-discovery policies	• Conduct a compliance review to ensure current policies are up-to-date with all state and federal laws on retention and destruction • Ensure that your retention and destruction policies include the components of the legal medical record that are stored in nonpaper-based media (e.g., remote and local servers, tapes, film, fiche) if the legal medical record is defined as being in a hybrid environment • Ensure that EHR systems have the ability to retain and destroy health information in accordance with your facility's legal medical record definition (e.g., fetal monitor data)
Definitions/Glossary of Terms	Varying definitions of original, legal, complete, or hard-copy record; business rules	• Define what a complete medical record is in a paper-based versus EHR environment (e.g., transcribed outpatient clinic notes)

Transition of HIM Professional Responsibilities

In collaboration with the information technology professionals, HIM professionals will serve as the custodians of patient health information, regardless of the media on which health information is maintained (e.g., film, video, paper, electronic, or other media).

- HIM professionals will establish policies, procedures, systems, and safeguards to ensure that patient health information is documented, maintained, and disclosed in accordance with all health information laws, regulations, and standards.

- HIM professionals will maintain a matrix of sources for various reports or types of information that constitute the hybrid health record. (See **APPENDIX 6A.1**, Legal Source Legend.)

- HIM professionals should evaluate the adequacy and validity of authorizations and requests for patient health information, making sure that the sources used are from the legal source as designated by the organization.

- HIM professionals will participate actively in the periodic reassessment of policies and procedures for accessing and disclosing information in the hybrid and electronic environments.

- HIM professionals will ensure standardization and ongoing maintenance of all forms (paper based) or templates (electronic).

- HIM professionals will play a key role in ensuring the functionality of EHR systems with respect to the practice of HIM and its support of other business functions of the organization.

Evolving Roles for HIM Professionals in the Electronic Environment

The 2010 AHIMA practice brief "e-HIM Practice Transformation" identified several additional roles for the HIM professional. Building on that resource, HIM roles should be reviewed and updated when planning the transition from a paper-based environment to a hybrid or completely electronic environment.

Guidelines for Access and Disclosure

Access and Disclosure Overview

It is important to understand exactly what access and disclosure means as it relates to sensitive information—electronic and paper. The National Institute of Standards and Technology (NIST) set forth guidelines for the federal government. The following concepts will be helpful to understand in your planning efforts.

Confidentiality

Confidentiality of information refers to authorizing disclosure to authorized users for authorized purposes and accessed in an authorized manner. As defined by NIST:

"Preserving authorized restrictions on information access and disclosure, including means for protecting personal privacy and proprietary information..." [44 U.S.C., Sec. 3542]

A loss of confidentiality is the unauthorized disclosure of information.[2]

Integrity

Integrity of information refers to maintaining safeguards to prevent alteration or modification of that data by unauthorized users.

"Guarding against improper information modification or destruction, and includes ensuring information non-repudiation and authenticity..." [44 U.S.C., Sec. 3542]

A loss of integrity is the unauthorized modification or destruction of information.[3]

Availability

Availability refers to making information available to authorized users.

"Ensuring timely and reliable access to and use of information..." [44 U.S.C., Sec. 3542]

A loss of availability is the disruption of access to or use of information or an information system.[4]

Organizations that successfully implement an EHR will have a shared vision with measurable outcomes. Relative to access and disclosure, the EHR vision and, to the extent possible, the hybrid health record should:

- Be protected by a rigorous information security structure consistent with laws and regulations, standards of practice, and available technology

- Support the organization's ability to perform electronic security audits

- Allow the organization to authorize or limit access based on user, record, document, and data element

- Provide access to all relevant information from a patient's hybrid record when needed for use in patient care, regardless of storage medium

- Provide for retrieval of information on a timely basis without compromising the data or the patient's confidentiality

- Bring together information contained in multiple systems, applications, or other media so complete information can be retrieved from a single point of access, where feasible

- Facilitate effective retrieval, display, reporting, and dissemination of data and information individually, comparatively, and collectively

- Minimize the need for printing while facilitating the delivery of efficient and effective healthcare

- Facilitate printing or copying of concise and easy-to-use documents that support continuity of care, patient requests, subpoenas, accreditation, legal requirements, and other business needs

- Facilitate electronic requests and disclosures of personal health information to authorized external users

- Give patients the opportunity to see, copy, and amend the information contained in their designated record set

- Support electronic tracking of disclosures that can be made available to the patient

- Support a personal health record that may be used for care decisions

- Support not only the delivery of patient care, decision support, and performance improvement but also the performance of all HIM and other required business functions

Practical Discussion for Managing Access and Disclosure

Access and Retrieval

Healthcare organizations must document where the components of their hybrid records are stored so they can access, use, and disclose the information as necessary, regardless of the information's location or the media on which it is maintained. To accomplish this task, organizations must define and describe the location of information contained in the legal health record and the designated record set. (See **APPENDIX 6A.1**.) AHIMA's practice briefs "Defining and Disclosing the Designated Record Set and the Legal Health Record" and "Update: Guidelines for Defining the Legal Health Record for Disclosure Purposes assist organizations with these two topics.

The location of components of the legal medical record and designated record set may need to be cross-referenced to alert users of the health record to which information exists across both the paper-based record and EHR, particularly as new or revised computer systems are implemented or updated. In addition, organizations will need to consider reviewing and updating their policies and procedures on access, disclosure, and printing for both the legal medical record and designated record set at least annually. Consideration also should be given to information stored on legacy systems that use technology that is old or no longer supported and how this information will be retrieved as the EHR evolves.

Organizations will need to consider the access afforded to hybrid health records by affiliates and business associates and formalize these decisions in their policies. Although it may be expedient to provide affiliates and business associates with access, organizations must consider carefully such access or disclosure in the context of the HIPAA privacy rule's "minimum necessary" standard.

Patient Access

During the transition to an EHR, information available to the patient electronically may be a subset of the patient's designated record set. In such cases, the EHR should indicate where the primary or complete information resides and how it can be accessed.

Because EHRs will contain many abbreviations and words with which patients may be unfamiliar, organizations will find it advisable to provide patients with links to abbreviation lists, references, medical dictionaries, and information about diseases and illnesses. They also will want to provide patients with information about how to contact their physicians should they have questions.

As the organization allows patients access to their EHRs, they should determine if the selected portions or the entire content of the EHR will be accessible to the patient and how it will be accessible. In addition, organizations will want to discuss disposition of clinician-to-clinician and patient-to-provider e-mail messages and text messages as it pertains to the hybrid health record. Any organization contemplating e-mail communications should review AHIMA's practice brief "Provider-Patient E-mail Security."

In an ambulatory care situation, patients may document various types of clinical information. For example, diabetic patients may track their blood sugar levels over time. Organizations should consider allowing patients to access and record such information electronically. Organizations should determine whether such information will be part of the legal medical record and designated record set, to whom access will be granted, and under what circumstances.

Referral Provider Access

Organizations that allow referral providers access to their EHRs should determine which information will be accessible. Steps should be taken to ensure this is a view-only access. It should be tested at each upgrade to ensure the view-only status continues. In addition, organizations should determine if referral providers will be allowed to print a copy of the EHR.

Potentially, referral providers could ask for access for their patient care team because of the workflow of the provider and the nurse preparing the chart for them to see the patient. Organizations will need to determine if they are willing to extend this access and if the tools are in place to audit such access.

Outside Reviewer Access

Payers, accreditation reviewers, and other external reviewers requiring access to review the medical record need access to both the hybrid chart and the electronic chart, whether on-site or off-site. Organizations must develop policies and procedures governing system access by external reviewers (e.g., for purposes such as auditing and accreditation). These could include creating queues that can be populated with requested charts, individual log-ins, and timed expiration date for access. This procedure would allow view-only access. Access to the electronic record is more efficient than printing and mailing to the reviewer, but all steps must be maintained to ensure that the protected heath information is secure.

Dissemination and Disclosure

In a hybrid environment, it is important that organizations develop and implement policies and procedures that describe the circumstances in which electronic documents may be duplicated. This determination is important because:

- The electronic copy likely will contain the most current information.

- Duplicating documents prevents the organization from optimizing its return on investment. The organization will be spending money on printers, toner, paper, CDs, USBs, and other media, as well as retention and destruction. These resources could be applied better toward making sure that there are adequate points of access to the electronic information wherever needed.

- Users may be inclined to make notes on the printed copies, further complicating operational management of these documents, since these notated copies would need to be retained as part of the legal health record. This potentially could create a data management issue because of the paper record and the electronic record containing disparate information.

- It is difficult to manage and secure duplicated copies.

- Once users are given permission to print, it is difficult to remove this permission.

In particular, organizations must address the handling and disposition of interim reports, weighing the risk to the organization of the performance of the following options:

- Maintaining *all* interim results reports within the health record

- Maintaining interim results reports only when the final results differ

Maintaining all interim results reports provides the greatest measure of security for the organization but causes a high volume of duplicate reports within the health record, particularly in a paper-based environment. This duplication also can lead to confusion regarding which report to use, especially for future access and disclosure.

The hybrid health record also should reflect who received disclosed information and whether it was paper based or electronic. As organizations work toward tracking disclosures electronically, they must interface disparate systems components to capture and track the required details of the disclosures (i.e., who, where, and what). The accounting should be available for review by the patient when it is requested.

Guidelines for Authorship and Printing of the Health Record

As the healthcare organization transitions from the paper-based record to the EHR, authorship and printing policies must be put in place. Identifying individuals who have rights for authorship will ensure the integrity of the health record. Printing policies need to be identified to ensure users are reviewing the most up-to-date information in the EHR. The following guidelines should be considered when developing the authorship and printing policies:

- The organization must have a multidisciplinary steering committee to develop and express the vision, strategic plan, and policies and procedures for the hybrid environment.

- With regard to policy issues about authorship, the HIM committee should:

  o Designate which individuals are authorized to make entries (author) in the hybrid record across all predesignated legal media

  o Identify documents and authors requiring cosignatures across all media such as medical students, residents, physician assistants, and nurse practitioners

  o Identify who is authorized to make changes when someone has discovered a nonclinical error such as wrong title of template, wrong patient, or wrong attending assigned

  o Establish the appropriate cosignature (e.g., name, credentials, date/time stamp)

  o Determine the method to capture patient-originated data, as approved

  o Establish guidelines about automated tools such as copy and paste, copy forward, and "blown-in" data elements

  o Identify and help the organization procure and implement software that supports the organization's authorship guidelines, including date/time stamp of entries and modifications

- The HIM department and the HIM committee should address policy issues regarding printing, including:

  o Designating the electronic components of the legal health record for which printing will occur and requiring authorized users to access clinical information in the EHR rather than keeping paper copies. (Refer to AHIMA's practice brief Update: Guidelines for Defining the Legal Health Record for Disclosure Purposes.) Organizational policy must address and regulate the keeping of and referring to shadow records.

- o Identifying the date when an electronic report will no longer be routinely printed and available only through the EHR (See Appendix 6A.1, "Legal Source Legend.") For example:
  - □ Transcribed reports (discharge summaries, operative notes)
  - □ Diagnostic reports (laboratory, radiology, cardiology, pathology)
- o Developing methods to ensure all components of the hybrid medical record are compiled when providing a copy of the medical record
- o Developing methods to ensure STAT printing queues for customer service and patient transfers between facilities
- o Overriding print queues to meet turnaround time requirements or customer needs
- o Mass printing requests (RAC, PERM, MIC, ZPICs, etc.) queued to meet system efficiency and response time
- o Developing an online data pushed to patients or legal guardians via direct EHR access or PHR access or CDs
- o Ensuring that CDs and other electronic media copies contain the correct patient information, are labeled correctly, and are formatted for easy access
- o Ensuring that procedures exist for producing paper or electronic copies of the EHR for external reviewers, including RAC, MIC, PERM, or ZPIC in a format that optimizes:
  - □ Review of documentation by a reviewer not familiar with your organization's medical record;
  - □ Presentation of key information first, such as discharge summary, history and physical examination, coding summary, etc.;
  - □ Ensuring attestation or coding summary is included and is one of the initial documents in the printout or CD;
  - □ All documents being accounted for in the copies;
  - □ All like documents being formatted in either reverse chronological or chronological order so that the medical record tells the story of the care provided;
  - □ The medical record being complete, including all reports dictated and signed.
- o Identifying the date(s) on which the following will be or is eliminated:
  - □ Routine printing of reports by ancillary departments and nursing units
  - □ Concurrent filing of in-house reports into facility patient records
  - □ Discharge report filing
- o Availability or nonavailability of online transcribed reports before verification and attestation (please refer to AHIMA's practice brief on Electronic Signature, Attestation, and Authorship)

o Determining the method to be used to indicate any online changes to a signed EHR document to ensure clear visibility of any changes for users

o Identifying those few roles allowed to print from the EHR and how this will be tracked for accounting of disclosure

o Determining a formal process for review and approval of all new requests for access and printing for accounting of disclosure

o Designating where copies of an EHR may be printed in the organization and methods to be used for copy disposal

o Labeling reports printed by authorized users to include a prominent watermark or label with the following information:

  □ "Confidential medical information"

    – Instructions for use such as:

    – "Do not file or scan in patient's medical record"

    – "Document any clinically pertinent information in the medical record"

    – "Do not remove report from facility"

    – "Discard report in designated disposal area"

  □ For all unauthenticated reports, indication that the report has not been reviewed for accuracy or authenticated

o When information is no longer printed, users are notified by one of the following methods:

  □ Medical record folder or tabs in paper-based record alert users that additional medical information is in the EHR with similar cross-references in the EHR, where feasible.

  □ The EHR has an online reference listing of all available reports and dates of availability (see **Appendix 6A.1**, "Legal Source Legend").

  □ When remote access to the EHR is allowed, a determination should be made if the ability to print information from the EHR will be allowed.

  □ Auditing of printing through the development of audit trails and associated processes to identify and monitor users who have printed reports or screen-printed patient information

o Disclosure of information, subpoenas and audits

  □ Requests for disclosure of information, subpoenas, and audits requiring printing from all designated sources of the legal health record that may be in a hybrid environment, in addition to photocopying the paper medical record or downloading onto disks or CDs

  □ In a hybrid environment, it may be difficult and confusing to tell the story of the patient's care when it resides in both paper and electronic media. When releasing information, consideration should be given to printing out the electronic record and combining the electronic record and paper record into a closed chart order before releasing so that the continuity of care can be reflected. Recommend documenting on a cover sheet that pages that are copied from paper may not be in numerical order as printed from the EHR so that the component of the patient's stay that is documented on paper can be integrated into the printout of the electronic record, eliminating confusion. The story of the patient's care is integral to all users of the record being released.

☐ For on-site audits and regulatory reviews requiring printing reports or allowing auditors to have online access to EHRs, development of viewing stations for on-site requesters and staff training to support them is needed.

☐ When possible, create a review queue for auditors who are reviewing the record; the records available in the queue are only the ones requested for the audit. The auditor does not have the ability to search the system.

Conclusion

Managing the transition from paper-based records to EHRs is a complex process intensified by the multitude of systems, functionality, and rapid technology advances. No single standard approach exists for solving the transitional process concerns, and each healthcare organization must determine the steps and policies that are needed as they evolve into using a fully functioning EHR. Many healthcare organizations have some degree of hybridization that coincides with the implementation plan. There are many decisions to consider when determining steps and guidelines for managing the transition process from paper to hybrid records and hybrid to electronic records. To ensure accurate and timely business records, healthcare organizations need to define the legal health record and ensure that the quality and integrity of the health record remains intact during the transition process.

Notes

1. AHIMA e-HIM Work Group on the Legal Health Record. "Update: Guidelines for Defining the Legal Health Record for Disclosure Purposes." *Journal of AHIMA* 76, no. 8 (Sept.2005): 64A–G. Available in the AHIMA Body of Knowledge at www .ahima.org.

2. National Institute of Standards and Technology. "Standards for Security Categorization of Federal Information and Information Systems." FIPS Pub 199. February 2004. Available online at http://csrc.nist.gov/publications/fips/fips199/ FIPS-PUB-199-final.pdf.

3. Ibid.

4. Ibid

References

AHIMA. "e-HIM Practice Transformation (Updated)." *Journal of AHIMA* 81, no. 8 (Aug. 2010): 52–55. Available online in the AHIMA Body of Knowledge at www.ahima.org.

AHIMA e-HIM Workgroup: Best Practices for Electronic Signature and Attestation. "Electronic Signature, Attestation, and Authorship (Updated)." *Journal of AHIMA* 80, no. 11 (Nov.–Dec. 2009): 62–69. Available online in the AHIMA Body of Knowledge at www.ahima.org

AHIMA e-HIM Work Group on the Legal Health Record. "Update: Guidelines for Defining the Legal Health Record for Disclosure Purposes." *Journal of AHIMA* 76, no. 8 (Sept. 2005): 64A–G. Available online in the AHIMA Body of Knowledge at www.ahima.org.

Amatayakul, Margret, et al. "Definition of the Health Record for Legal Purposes (AHIMA Practice Brief)." *Journal of AHIMA* 72, no. 9 (Sept. 2001): 88A–H. Available online in the AHIMA Body of Knowledge at www.ahima.org.

Burrington-Brown, Jill, and Gwen Hughes. "AHIMA Practice Brief: Provider-Patient E-mail Security." Updated June 2003. Available online in the AHIMA Body of Knowledge at www.ahima.org.

Department of Health and Human Services. "Breach Notification for Unsecured Protected Health Information; Interim Final Rule." *Federal Register* 74, no. 162 (Aug. 24, 2009). Available online at http://edocket.access.gpo.gov/2009/pdf/E9-20169.pdf.

Department of Health and Human Services. "Health Insurance Reform: Security Standards, Final Rule." 45 CFR, subtitle A, subchapter C, parts 160 and 164, *Federal Register* 68, no. 34 (Feb. 20, 2003). Available online at http://aspe.hhs.gov/admnsimp/final/fr03-8334.pdf.

Department of Health and Human Services. "Standards for Privacy of Individually Identifiable Health Information; Final Rule." 45 CFR, subtitle A, subchapter C, parts 160 and 162. *Federal Register* 67, no. 157 (Aug. 14, 2002). Available online at www.hhs.gov/ocr/privacy/hipaa/administrative/privacyrule/privruletxt.txt.

Department of the Treasury, et al. "Identity Theft Red Flags and Address Discrepancies under the Fair and Accurate Credit Transactions Act of 2003." *Federal Register* 72, no. 217 (Nov. 9, 2007). Available online at www.ftc.gov/os/fedreg/2007/november/071109redflags.pdf.

Federal Rules of Civil Procedure—Rule 26. Available online at http://judiciary.house.gov/hearings/printers/111th/civil2009.pdf

Federal Rules of Evidence, article VIII, rule 803. Available online at http://judiciary.house.gov/hearings/printers/111th/evid2009.pdf.

Hughes, Gwen. "Defining the Designated Record Set (AHIMA Practice Brief)." *Journal of AHIMA* 74, no. 1 (2003): 64A–D. Available online in the AHIMA Body of Knowledge at www.ahima.org.

National Institute of Standards and Technology. "Guideline for Identifying an Information System as a National Security System." Special Publication 800-59. August 2003. Available online at http://csrc.nist.gov/publications/nistpubs/800-59/SP800-59.pdf.

The Joint Commission. Standard Record of Care, Treatment and Services (RC). Available online at www.jcrinc.com/Joint-Commission-Requirements/Hospitals/#RC

The Privacy Act of 1974. Section 5 U.S.C. §552a. Available online at www.justice.gov/opcl/privstat.htm.

Public Health Service, Department of Health and Human Services. "Confidentiality of Alcohol and Drug Abuse Patient Records." *Code of Federal Regulations*, 2000. 42 CFR, chapter 1, part 2. Available online at www.access.gpo.gov/nara/cfr/waisidx_00/42cfr2_00.html.

Prepared by

This practice brief was updated by the following AHIMA e-HIM workgroup:
Cris Berry, RHIA
Susan Dolack, MHIM, RHIA
Denise Dunyak
Darice M. Grzybowski, MA, RHIA, FAHIMA

Karl Koob, MS, RHIA
Cindy Loragner
Cindy Rupe
Diana Warner, MS, RHIA, CHPS

Acknowledgments

Kathy Arner, LPN, RHIT, CCS, CPC, MCS, CPMA
Roberta Baranda, RHIA, CHP
Donna Barnard, RHIA
June Bronnert, RHIA, CCS, CCS-P
Jill Clark, RHIA
Karen Czirr, RHIA, CHP
Emily Macko, RHIA
Nicole Miller, RHIA
Edith Okenquist, RHIT, CCS, CCS-P
Catherine Ptak, MS, RHIA
Melinda Teel, RHIA, CCS
Lou Ann Wiedemann, MS, RHIA, CPEHR
Henryetta Wynne, RHIT

Prepared by (original)

This practice brief was developed by the following AHIMA e-HIM workgroup:
Cris Berry, RHIA
Jill Burrington-Brown, MS, RHIA
Cindy Doyon, RHIA
Linda Frank, MBA, RHIA
Aviva Halpert, RHIA
Susan Helbig, MA, RHIA
Gwen Hughes, RHIA, CHP
Julie King, RHIA
Karl Koob, MS, RHIA
Carole Okamoto, MBA, RHIA, CPHQ
Tracy Peabody, RHIA
Carol Ann Quinsey, RHIA (staff)
Mary Reeves, RHIA
Clarice Smith, RHIA
Melanie Thomas, RHIT
Lydia Washington, MS, RHIA
Ann Zeisset, RHIT, CCS, CCS-P (staff)
Lin Zhang, RHIA, CHP

Appendix 6A.1

Legal Source Legend

Health information may be stored in a variety of paper-based and electronic systems during the transition to an electronic health record (EHR). Regardless of the originating or generating source of content in the EHR, all components, results, and documentation need to be unified within a single system as a complete episodic legal health record for purposes of review and printed output. A useful tool for planning and managing the transition is a grid or matrix that describes where and how to find specific document types that constitute the hybrid health record. The grid can be used as a planning tool to ensure each major document type is addressed during the document's transition from paper to electronic media. It is important to maintain the grid in real time so that users will be able to see the paper-to-electronic status of all documents. Over time, the grid will serve as a monitoring tool and as a dynamic source that can be used to help define the legal status of each document (for example, the point at which an electronic document stored in a system replaces its former paper document as the legal document).

Depending on the complexity and type of organization (academic, healthcare, community, research, physician office, etc.), this grid may be expanded to include additional columns. Such additional columns may list more specific information or include super groups or classes for enhanced clarity and usability. For example, for designation of a document class, organizations may opt to use their paper-based chart tabs, forms inventory or catalog, or even the items listed in their designated record set (nonfinancial or non-health-plan plan components).

As a tool, the grid should be published and updated wherever it will be most accessible and helpful for users of the hybrid record. Possible locations for publication may include an internal organization's Web page, policies and procedures, or even in the EHR itself. Maintenance, responsibility, and frequency of updates should be considered when deciding where to publish the grid for interested parties.

Hybrid Health Record Legal Source Legend

REPORT/DOCUMENT TYPES	MEDIA TYPE (P)APER/ (E)LEC- TRONIC	SOURCE SYSTEM APPLICATION (NONPAPER)	CURRENTLY PRINTED	CURRENTLY SCANNED	DATE STORED ELECTRONICALLY	STOP PRINTING START DATE
Admission History and Physical	P/E	System 1 (e.g., laboratory system)			1/1/2002	1/1/2003
Attending Admission Notes	P					
Physician Orders	E					
Inpatient Progress Notes	P					
Discharge Summary	E	System 2 (e.g., transcription system)			1/1/2002	4/1/2002
Inpatient Transfer Notes	E	System 1			1/1/2002	
Outpatient Progress Notes	P					
Clinical Laboratory Results (Preliminary/Interim)	E	System 2			1/1/1999	1/1/1999
Clinical Laboratory Results (Final)	E	System 2			1/1/1999	1/1/2000
Radiology Reports	E	System 3 (e.g., radiology system)			7/1/2003	
Care Flow Sheets	E	System 1			6/1/2003	
Medication Records	E	System 1			7/1/2003	
Clinical Consult Reports	E	System 1			1/1/2002	
Preoperative, Preprocedure Notes	P					

(continued)

REPORT/DOCUMENT TYPES	MEDIA TYPE (P)APER/ (E)LEC- TRONIC	SOURCE SYSTEM APPLICATION (NONPAPER)	CURRENTLY PRINTED	CURRENTLY SCANNED	DATE STORED ELECTRONICALLY	STOP PRINTING START DATE
Pathology Reports	E	System 2			1/1/1999	1/1/2000
Organ or Tissue Donation or Transplants	P					
Patient Problem List (Summary List)	E	System 1			8/1/2003	
Urgent Care and Emergency Records	P					
Consents*	E	System 4 (e.g., docu- ment imaging system)			TBD	
Advance Directive						
Correspondence*	E	System 4			TBD	
Preoperative Anesthetic Assess- ments and Plans	P					
Intraoperative Documentation	P					
Postoperative Documentation	P					
Brief Postoperative Notes	P					
Surgical Operative Reports	E	System 1			1/1/2002	

*Scanned electronic documents.

e-HIM Practice Transformation

The migration to electronic health records (EHRs) will change the design and operations of traditional HIM departments. HIM professionals will be tasked with new responsibilities that require clinical leadership, management skills, and IT knowledge. Roles will continue to evolve, and opportunities await HIM professionals who evaluate and upgrade their expertise to keep pace with changing practice.

This practice brief outlines how health IT will change information management and how HIM professionals and their departments can prepare for this transformation.

The Industry Impact

Federal and state laws are constantly changing the healthcare landscape, including the use of technology. Most recently, the American Recovery and Reinvestment Act created new regulations for EHR use and incentives for EHR adoption.

Technologies such as portals are enabling individual, longitudinal health records that can be accessed by consumers, care providers, HIM professionals, and others as appropriate. Consumers can access their medical information online to maintain personal health records. They can schedule appointments, register, pay bills, and authorize disclosure of their personal health information to employers and schools through facility kiosks or via the healthcare organization's secured Web site.

In addition, technologies related to telemedicine and e-visits enhance the way physicians offer consultation services to one another and care to their patients, further affecting the way information is exchanged and maintained.

These changes add complexity to the management of health information. In this transition to e-HIM, HIM professionals will serve a broad range of roles planning, organizing, and managing clinical content, integrity, accessibility, use, and protection.

They will be called on to identify work process improvements and implementation techniques and redefine information management practices. They will work at the convergence of people, processes, regulations, organizational structure, standards, and system design. Given this magnitude of upheaval, change management and expectation management will be critical to the successful creation of the emerging digital HIM department.

From Paper to Hybrid to Electronic

The transformation to e-HIM encompasses three states:

- The traditional state of the paper health record

- A transitional, hybrid state featuring both paper and electronic records

- The future state of the fully electronic record

AHIMA. 2010. e-HIM practice transformation. *Journal of AHIMA* 81(8):52–55.

HIM professionals must assume a leadership role in transforming all HIM functions to e-HIM. They must analyze and visualize documented and undocumented intradepartmental and interdepartmental information management functions to understand the current and future state of the HIM department, while ensuring that HIM best practices and standards such as privacy, the legal health record, and information integrity are consistently maintained.

HIM functions that will be transformed include:

- Analysis
- Abstracting
- Assembly
- Vital records
- Coding
- Data reporting
- Data quality and integrity
- Denial management
- Document identification
- Documentation training
- Forms design
- Chart completion
- MPI maintenance
- Release of information
- Chargemaster maintenance
- Revenue cycle management

New functions will also emerge as the organization's EHR evolves, such as document management (scanning), application coordination, clinical application training, clinical vocabulary management, information privacy, and process improvement.

To support this transformation, HIM professionals will require new skills as well as training opportunities to continually upgrade their skills. They must be comfortable with changing technology and able to adapt to a changing environment as systems are upgraded, replaced, and optimized.

Critical thinking and decision-making skills are valuable as staff transition to more unique and complex workflows in both hybrid and electronic systems. HIM professionals must gain a thorough knowledge of the workflows in the electronic system in order to follow the flow of the medical record. To ensure the legality of the EHR and the downstream effects of information practices, workflows must focus on quality with attention to record completeness, timeliness, and authenticity, which are important factors for data integrity, validity, and reliability. Familiarity with paper workflows will still be needed to support those processes that remain in paper during the transition.

The ability to work independently and troubleshoot IT issues is also necessary to remain productive in remote locations as facilities transition HIM functions off site. Newer roles that are created to support the transformation also require skills in information management and information technology.

HIM professionals will need to be leaders in change management for their organizations, both prior to and during the three states of the transformation process. They will also need to drive continual process improvement as the EHR evolves. HIM professionals thus must understand the changing demands of federal regulations and organizational requirements, strive to achieve professional designations of EHR adoption, and support organizational attempts to attract providers and professionals with EHR systems that support improved clinical and administrative workflows.

Envisioning e-HIM Practice

Envisioning the future of e-HIM can be a daunting task; however, it does not have to be complex. A good envisioning approach will help HIM professionals think about the future and ready them for the most significant transition in HIM history.

An envisioning process should include research, evaluating common situations that staff encounter and how the workflow may change in the electronic environment, and a review of the current and future state of HIM departments. HIM professionals should read about other organizations' transformations and talk with colleagues to determine current HIM practices and how they are transformed into electronic practices.

The envisioning process should also include visits to other sites that have transitioned to hybrid or fully electronic processes. Before visiting other sites, HIM professionals should discuss their practices, asking pertinent questions to frame the visit.

HIM leaders should understand change management principles in order to transition their departments to the EHR. It is critical for HIM professionals to be knowledgeable about the current momentum of EHR development (e.g., functionality), technology (e.g., peripheral devices and interfaces used to ensure all information is in the EHR), and industry initiatives within the organization and the industry (e.g., ARRA, new EHR functionality requirements, HIE, access to records) and their effects on HIM practice.

The HIM director should plan the department's intentional transition to e-HIM. The first step in accomplishing this is to define the current state of the department, including an analysis of all critical processes. The next step is to define the desired future state. Once the current and future states are defined, the HIM director should compare and contrast these to create a road map to move the department to e-HIM.

Envisioning a future state should begin now. Proper preparation for a change takes a minimum of six months and includes assessing the gaps between the current workflows and expected future workflows, identifying what new functions will be added, and determining how to plan the transition from paper to electronic. This transition takes a minimum of six months to ensure all workflows and downstream effects are evaluated.

Even after the organization makes the leap to a hybrid or electronic record, the HIM department's vision for its future state requires ongoing fine tuning for continued readiness as practice evolves.

Planning for Change

The first step in change management is defining the current state within the HIM department. This includes defining all major processes and the number of staff associated with each one, identifying current staff strengths and skills, job descriptions, job requirements, and qualifications.

Understanding staffing needs will assist in assessing how to manage the HIM department in the interim. For example, if the assessment indicates there are currently more employees in record operations than will be required in the future, the HIM director may choose to freeze openings to avoid future layoffs. In addition, if the extent of resources required for upcoming changes is significant in one particular area, adjustments to major projects and services can be made in advance.

The next step is defining the desired future state. The HIM director should plan for the optimal environment, although revisions may occur as the plan progresses toward realization. The future state should be defined to the best of the HIM professional's knowledge.

Directors and managers can rely on other facilities that have already made the change to e-HIM. They should visit other facilities of similar size and business model to gain a better understanding of the processes associated with such a change and identify lessons learned. Directors should include staff and managers in site visits and ensure an opportunity to talk to managers, staff, and support staff.

Once the current and future states are defined, the HIM director should compare and contrast the current and future states to identify the gaps that exist. For example, if the director expects that a new scanning process will replace the filing process, some questions to ask are:

- What other work do the file clerks perform (e.g., are they entering information into a computer system before filing a document, sorting loose sheets, assigning medical record numbers)?

- How many staff currently performs this function?

- How many full-time employees are anticipated to maintain the file room once scanning has been implemented?

Some current staff may not be able to make the leap to the new e-HIM technical requirements. To address this concern, the gap analysis should include both a quantitative and qualitative assessment of the staffing requirements for the department. For example, to build upon the scanning process above, the HIM director may identify that quantitatively five additional staff will be required for the implementation phase.

Some additional questions to ask include:

- What is the skill set of the workforce?

- Will the current skill set enable staff to perform job functions in the new role?

- Will the new role require the ability to answer phones, release information, prepare and scan documents, perform scanning quality control, and answer questions about EHR functionality?

- Where will additional training be needed?

- Which current staff can both adapt to new roles and be fully functional?

- How will the new staff be selected?

It will be vital for HIM professionals to secure a senior manager as a change sponsor for the transition from HIM to e-HIM. This position may be a vice president or a C-level position. Since staff will be affected by the e-HIM transition, a discussion of the need for HIM transformation should occur with the human resources vice president in order to gain his or her support and move forward with budget and personnel concerns. The team supporting the e-HIM transformation should include the HIM vice president and the financial and human resources representatives for HIM.

HR must be consulted when job requirements change and skills are re-assessed. Some questions they must consider include:

- Will the department keep staff on for the new roles?

- Will staff require financial increases due to new functions?

- Will staff be laid off due to a decrease in staffing needs?

Buy-in from upper management is essential in order to ensure funding for transformational changes like an EHR implementation.

Organizations should also fully educate HIM employees on the e-HIM transition and prepare them for the change. At a minimum, all clerical staff should be made aware that clerical tasks are diminishing and that new skills are necessary for continued employment. Clerical staff should be encouraged to seek education to further their career options.

Defining the Virtual HIM Department

Not only will EHR technology change HIM roles, it also will change how and where HIM professionals work. Because EHRs offer electronic access to medical record documentation, traditional HIM functions, such as coding, transcription, record completion, release of information, and auditing will be transformed into new virtual workflows. These may exist between buildings, towns, or the facility and the employee's home. For example, an auditor may no longer need to travel to a hospital to complete a review when the EHR documents can be viewed online with authorized access.

Transitioning an HIM department to this virtual environment offers many operational and financial advantages. However, it does not mean the HIM department itself will disappear.

The HIM department will remain present with job roles such as document imaging and customer support. For example, while the auditor, coder, or release of information clerk may be able to access records electronically, on-site staff will still be needed to assist with scanning documents into the system and supporting facility staff, patients, and physicians who have record questions.

New roles also will be prominent, such as project managers, EHR system managers, and workflow and data analysts. Privacy coordinators, different from privacy officers, will act as directors, creating policy, implementing programs, and directing the goals.

Facility leaders must carefully assess how the e-HIM transition will affect staff, understanding that not all staff may desire or have the ability to work remotely. The successful remote employee is disciplined, self-motivated, and able to work alone with little social interaction. Remote staffing adds human resource complexities. For instance, the facility will need to decide if a remote employee has the option to work on-site periodically or to change to on-site status.

Every HIM function performed to support the paper health record today will be re-engineered. This will challenge HIM directors and managers to not only manage new workflow processes, but to do so remotely. Therefore, in order to ensure success, healthcare executives will need to be actively engaged in and support their HIM teams in accomplishing this virtual transformation.

Future Roles of HIM Professionals

According to the Bureau of Labor Statistics 2010–2011 *Occupational Handbook* "employment of medical and health services managers is expected to grow 16 percent from 2008 to 2018, faster than the average for all occupations." In addition, only 38 percent of medical and health service managers work in hospitals. Nineteen percent of these positions indicate opportunities in physician offices or nursing or residential care facilities. Additional opportunities are available in home health, government facilities, outpatient facilities, insurance payer groups, or community healthcare facilities.

New roles may include business change manager, EHR system manager, IT training specialist, business process engineer, clinical vocabulary manager, workflow and data analyst, consumer advocate, clinical alerts and reminders manager, clinical research coordinator, privacy coordinator, enterprise application specialist, and many more.

Federal funding is accelerating the entry of health IT specialists into the workforce. Section 3016 of the Health Information Technology for Economic and Clinical Health (HITECH) Act authorizes the creation of programs that will offer training designed to create a skilled workforce of health IT professionals. These professionals are expected to help implement EHRs and train providers on their use, primarily through the Health IT Regional Extension Centers.

Under this authority the Office of the National Coordinator for Health Information Technology has awarded $120 million in funding toward health IT education through four initiatives:

- Community college training programs to be completed in six months or less

- Development of educational materials to support those programs

- University-based certificates and advanced IT programs

- Development of a set of health IT competency exams

Roles are identified on the Community College Consortia to Educate Health Information Technology Professionals in Health Care Program Web site at http://healthit.hhs.gov. In addition, HIM professionals can view an illustration of these REC resources and the HIM skill set at www.ahima.org/advocacy/arraresources.

HIM professionals are a key participant in the current skilled healthcare workforce. As an established discipline with four academic pathways and more than 250 accredited HIM programs, AHIMA's members are ideally suited for many of ONC's defined roles.

HIM professionals will need to continuously upgrade their skills and expertise to keep pace and be successful in the new e-HIM practice. Healthcare executives, ever mindful of the need to empower and advance their workforce, should place a high priority on empowering HIM professionals as key leaders in EHR implementation and management.

References

AHIMA e-HIM Task Force. "A Vision of the e-HIM Future: A Report from the AHIMA e-HIM Task Force." Available online in the AHIMA Body of Knowledge at www.ahima.org.

Bloomrosen, Meryl. "e-HIM: From Vision to Reality." *Journal of AHIMA* 76, no. 9 (Oct. 2005): 36–41.

Health and Human Services. "HITECH Programs." Available online at http://healthit.hhs.gov.

Kohn, Deborah. "Technologies Support Transition to Virtual HIM Department." 2008 AHIMA Convention Proceedings, October 2008. Available online in the AHIMA Body of Knowledge at www.ahima.org.

Sheridan, Patty Thierry, Michele D'Ambrosio, and Kerry Heinecke. "Visioning e-HIM: A Process for Imagining—and Anticipating—HIM's Future." *Journal of AHIMA* 76, no. 5 (May 2005): 24–28.

Appendixes

Two additional appendixes are included in this book and in the online version of this brief, available in the AHIMA Body of Knowledge at www.ahima.org:

- **APPENDIX 6B.1**: Sample Job Description Format
- **APPENDIX 6B.2**: Sample Job Titles, Functions, and Skill Sets

Appendix 6B.1

Sample Job Description Format

Department Name:	Cost Center:
Status/Pay Grade:	Effective Date:
Job Title: Health Data Analyst/Health System Specialist	Reports to:
Hire Date:	Annual Review Date:

Position Summary/General Purpose: Provide expertise to acquire, manage, manipulate, and analyze data and report results

Position Requirements/Qualifications:

Licensure/Certification/Registration: RHIA, RHIT, CHDA certification preferred

Education: Bachelor's degree in health information management, healthcare informatics, computer science, statistics, or related field

Experience: Prior healthcare experience required; previous health data analyst experience preferred.

Degree of Supervision: Employee must be able to work independently, effectively, and efficiently on their own. This position has no direct reports.

Physical Requirements: Employee must be able to perform the essential functions of this job. This position includes a requirement to walk, climb stairs, balance, and sit. Lifting is limited to health information charts and is not expected to exceed 25 pounds. Vision requirements include the ability to read paper and electronic health records.

Responsibilities:

Daily Operations

- Identify problematic data areas and conduct research to determine best course of action

- Analyze and problem solve issues with legacy, current, and planned systems as they relate to the integration and management of patient data (e.g., review for accuracy in record merge, unmerge processes)

- Analyze reports of data duplicates or other errors to provide ongoing appropriate interdepartmental communication and monthly or daily data reports (e.g., related to the EMPI)

- Monitor metadata for process improvement opportunities (e.g., monitoring orders for successful CPOE implementation)

- Identify, analyze, and interpret trends or patterns in complex data sets

- Monitor data dictionary statistics

Data Capture

- In collaboration with others, develop and maintain databases and data systems necessary for projects and department functions

- Acquire and abstract primary or secondary data from existing internal or external data sources

- In collaboration with others, develop and implement data collection systems and other strategies that optimize statistical efficiency and data quality

- Enter data either manually or using scanning technology when needed or required

Data Reporting

- In collaboration with others, interpret data and develop recommendations based on findings

- Develop graphs, reports, and presentations of project results, trending, data mining

- Perform basic statistical analyses for projects and reports

- Create and present quality dashboards

- Generate routine and/or ad-hoc reports

Knowledge/Skills

- Technical expertise regarding data models and database design development; understanding of XML and SQL

- Proficient in MS Word, Excel, Access, and PowerPoint

- Experience using SAS, SPSS, or other statistical package to analyze large data sets

- Programming skills; adept at queries and report writing

- Knowledge of statistics, at least to the degree necessary in order to communicate easily with statisticians

- Experience in data-mining techniques and procedures and knowing when their use is appropriate

- Ability to present complex information in an understandable and compelling manner

- Knowledge of coding classification systems

Appendix 6B.2

Sample Job Titles, Functions, and Skill Sets

The sample descriptions of new HIM roles below come from an informal survey conducted among members of AHIMA's HIM Practice Transformation e-HIM Workgroup in January 2005 and Electronic Health Records Practice Council in 2010. These are just a few of the positions held in the e-HIM world across the US today that are filled by experienced HIM professionals and new graduates. This list should not be considered comprehensive. In addition, individual organizations have template job description formats that make it difficult to develop a standardized job description for every position.

Appendix 6B.1 includes a sample job description format so that readers can identify how a job description may be developed.

Note: In terms of experience, the workgroup chose not to include references to years of experience or previous management experience required. These specificities should be developed at an organizational level.

In addition, some titles are staff positions and others reflect management positions. Reporting structures are organization specific and are not listed in these job titles for that reason.

Title: Clinical Health Analyst

Job Purpose: Depending on the organization's titles, clinical analysts can either coordinate and manage specific clinical applications such as online documentation tool development (e.g., electronic forms, clinical screens) or serve as the interpreter between clinical staff and IT technical programmer/analysts in the development of the EHR or clinical report development. Clinical analysts ensure that the product being developed meets the needs of clinical staff and that tools enhance or improve workflow. Depending on their role, clinical analysts can report to IT, HIM, or an individual clinical department (e.g., laboratory, pharmacy).

Key Job Functions:

- Format, design, and build relevant content into online forms, mapping data collection and documentation to clinical workflows

- Lead discussions on clinical and functional design with multidisciplinary teams, interpreting user needs into relevant electronic tools

- Provide key knowledge on implementation of standardized, streamlined clinical content

- Design clinical content for software applications across all care processes (including documentation, ordering, alerting and notification actions, and reporting needs)

- Develop and document current and future state processes and knowledge structures using careful listening skills and advanced capability to ask questions to arrive at root processes

- Develop detailed content design documents
- Facilitate validation sessions with clinical staff
- Develop and publish supporting documentation

Skills and Experience:

- Excellent written and verbal communication skills including ability to understand and interpret clinical needs and transform IT technical tools to meet these needs
- Solid ability to use Microsoft Office, including Word, Excel, PowerPoint, Visio, and Project and ability to do Internet searches
- Experience with EHRs
- HIM education and experience with healthcare operations, including a basic understanding of different departments and their role in healthcare delivery

Applicable AHIMA Credentials:

- CHDA
- RHIT
- RHIA

Title: Clinical Applications Coordinator

Job Purpose: Primary functions include hands-on development and maintenance of clinical EHR applications. Clinical application coordinators ensure that the product being integrated meets the needs of clinical staff through workflow analysis. Depending on their role, clinical application coordinators can report to IT, HIM, or clinical department (e.g., laboratory or pharmacy).

Key Job Functions:

- Implement and support multiservice software packages
- Manage the customization of site parameters
- Address integration issues with other software packages
- Review site parameters and local tables with each service for accuracy and completeness
- Coordinate implementation of new software products that cover these functions
- Analyze and evaluate processes related to information flow
- Provide training to all services on current software applications and new features

- Ensure training is scheduled for new users

- Work with IT and clinical staff to develop processes to address access to historical information, manual documentation tools, and remediation for EHR downtime events

- Partner with HIM to coordinate efforts to correct errors that occur in the electronic record (e.g., incorrect ordering physician chosen at the point of care)

- Test and troubleshoot problems within the applications

- Test and troubleshoot new codes, upgrades, and fixes

Skills and Experience:

- Excellent written and verbal communication skills, including ability to understand and interpret clinical needs and transform IT technical tools to meet these needs

- Solid ability to use Microsoft Office, including Word, Excel, PowerPoint, Visio, and Project and ability to do Internet searches

- Experience with the EHR

- HIM education and experience with healthcare operations, including a basic understanding of different departments and their role in healthcare delivery

Applicable AHIMA Credentials:

- RHIA

Title: Clinical Project Manager/Senior Project Manager

Job Purpose: The clinical project manager provides overall leadership for all phases of the implementation including, but not limited to, budget management, outlining project risks and contingency planning, project timeline development, timeline management, development and management of tracking tools, and overall communication for successful implementation of the project.

Key Job Functions:

- Manage the scope of work, objectives, and other project management activities of assigned projects

- Manage the project team

- Delegate individual tasks assigned to team members

- Finalize project budget and scope of work

- Act as primary project contact with sponsor to ensure appropriate communication channels are maintained and reporting schedules adhered to

- Manage project budget to meet financial and company goals (realization targets); identify and develop change orders

- Develop project plans, schedules, and other scope definition documents for assigned projects as outlined in the project operations database

- Maintain project management information and tracking systems

- Coordinate and evaluate the probability and impact of risks

- Develop plans for minimizing risk impact on project objectives

- Implement improvement processes for assigned projects

Skills and Experience:

- Strong project management skills

- Previous healthcare and information management experience required

- Demonstrated strong leadership and management skills

- Excellent verbal and written communication skills

- Excellent interpersonal and organizational skills and attention to detail

- Computer literacy, including proficiency in word processing, spreadsheet, and data management software programs

Applicable AHIMA Credentials:

- RHIA

Title: Clinical Research Associate

Job Purpose: The clinical research associate plans, organizes, and coordinates clinical studies and institutional review board activities. This position assists in the development of clinical study protocols, informed consents, case report forms, and other documents. The clinical research associate provides monitoring of clinical research projects by ensuring regulatory compliance and adherence to good clinical practices, standard operating procedures, and study protocols.

Key Job Functions:

- Monitor activities at clinical study sites to ensure adherence to good clinical practices, standard operating procedures, and study protocols

- Assist in the development of clinical study protocols

- Review regulatory documents as required and prepare site visit reports

- Manage multiple projects

- Manage the location and retention of clinical research-related documentation

- Understand release of information guidelines pertaining to research records

- Work both independently and in team environments

- Participate in the study development and start-up process, including reviewing protocols and designing or reviewing study follow-up

- Prepare informed consent forms

- Develop study documents

- Organize and present at investigator meetings

- Work with management on monitoring strategy

- Develop project-specific clinical research associate training

- Participate in clinical training programs and maintain awareness of developments in the field of clinical research

Skills and Experience:

- Sound knowledge of medical terminology and clinical monitoring process

- Trained in good clinical practice guidelines

- Excellent written and verbal skills

- Previous healthcare experience required

- Excellent interpersonal and organizational skills, attention to detail

- Computer literacy, including proficiency in word processing, spreadsheet, and data management software programs

Applicable AHIMA Credentials:

- CHDA

- RHIA

- RHIT

Title: Clinical Vocabulary Manager/ Terminology Asset Manager

Job Purpose: The clinical vocabulary manager/terminology asset manager leads organizational efforts for the appropriate application of classification, nomenclature, and other standardized vocabularies to ensure consistent codes and data for reimbursement, EHR documentation, comparative reporting, and statistical classification of morbidity and mortality.

Key Job Functions:

- Create, maintain, and implement terminologies, validation files, and maps for a variety of use cases in the EHR

- Perform ongoing review of the auto and manual encoder systems for terminology and classification systems, including methods and processes; implement recommendations for improving and optimizing the encoding process

- Ensure quality (accuracy, consistency, relevancy) and productivity of clinical classification processes and applications

- Develop and deliver education sessions for coding staff relative to coding and classification systems; coordinate coding staff clinical education with clinical experts for anatomy, physiology, pharmacology, clinical assessment and procedure at and drug/biologic interventions

- Educate data analysts in coding and classification systems

- Recommend and lead development of application of appropriate classification and terminology systems for clinical documentation, including but not limited to problem list vocabularies/pick lists/favorites, nursing clinical terminologies/languages, and standardized documentation tools (e.g., point and click/templates, etc.), ensuring that documentation is complete, accurate, and compliant and reflects appropriate E&M levels/rules

- Understand and communicate/educate others on the strengths and weaknesses of all classification and nomenclatures including best use

- Assist in the analysis of the enterprise's classification and grouping system assignment trends and use data from classification and grouping systems to assist in decision making

- Proactively monitor standards requirements and technology development in the field of clinical terminologies and medical vocabularies (e.g., computer-assisted coding)

- Recommend the most appropriate classification or terminology systems to meet all required information reporting needs

- Possess expertise in clinical terminology, medical vocabulary, and classification systems and skill in mining, deriving, or engineering clinical ontologies

Skills and Experience:

- Advanced knowledge of the appropriate application of ICD-9-CM, SNOMED CT, CPT, and ICD-10

- Previous experience with ICD-9-CM and at least one other classification or nomenclature

- Ability to lead coding staff in application of ICD-9-CM and CPT code sets

- Knowledge of resources for other classification and nomenclatures

- Auditing experience

Applicable AHIMA Credentials:

- RHIA
- RHIT
- CCS
- CCS-P
- CHDA

Title: Enterprise Applications Specialist

Job Purpose: Primary functions include hands-on development and maintenance of enterprise EHR applications. Enterprise applications specialists show an optimal blend of HIM and IT domains with the use of increasingly complex documentation systems and data repositories. They ensure that the product being integrated meets the needs of the enterprise staff (e.g., physicians, clinicians, and HIM personnel) through workflow analysis. Depending on their role, enterprise applications specialists can report to IT, HIM, or a clinical department (e.g., laboratory or pharmacy).

Key Job Functions:

- Facilitate the identification, creation, implementation, and maintenance of enterprise policies and procedures related to the EHR

- Serve as a clinical information liaison to facilitate communication between clinical caregivers and technical implementation teams

- Serve as EHR consultant to the enterprise

- Coordinate and assemble appropriate personnel for task force assignments related to EHR projects and issues

- Coordinate activities related to the integrity of the enterprise master patient index file

- Provide development guidance and coordination to ensure clinical data generated and stored in disparate clinical systems are made available in the enterprise EHR when appropriate

- Work cooperatively with the administrative director of HIM and other applicable enterprise entities to ensure policies and procedures meet or exceed existing legal and regulatory requirements as related to the EHR and accepted medical record standards of practice

- Work cooperatively with privacy and security officer to ensure compliance with all existing and emerging requirements related to privacy and confidentiality of health information

Skills and Experience:

- Possess knowledge of existing and emerging federal and state requirements related to privacy and security of health information

- Possess knowledge of existing EHR policies and procedures associated with the collection and distribution of clinical data via the repository

- Maintain current knowledge of applicable federal and state EHR-related laws and accreditation standards; monitor and communicate changes to ensure organizational adaptation and compliance

- Manage multiple projects simultaneously

- Possess advanced knowledge of EHR systems

- Possess knowledge of federal and state requirements for record retention

- Ability to manage, maintain, and retrieve legacy system information

Applicable AHIMA Credentials:

- RHIA

- CHPS

Title: Health Information Services Department Technician

Note: This title has historically been an entry level position. Previous education was limited to a high school diploma or GED. In order to prepare for e-HIM the workgroup determined that education, skills, and knowledge for this particular title must be expanded upon in order to recruit and retain qualified staff.

Job Purpose: The health information services department technician provides quality services to all customers (e.g., patients, physicians, and employees), which requires assistance from the health information services department. Services might include physician support, release of information, audit support, document imaging, or scanning and other technical functions.

Key Job Functions:

- Possess knowledge of hospital and departmental policies and procedures

- Possess knowledge of EHR functions to guide users in note amendments, corrections, and retractions

- Ensure release of information is completed according to policy

- Retrieve electronic medical records for internal and external requests as appropriate (e.g., release of information, audits, review)

- Process and compile statistics for delinquency

- Process and monitor bill hold reports

- Process documentation deficiencies

- Abstract records

- Manage interfaces, reviewing reject reports and correcting errors

- Merge duplicate medical record numbers

- Prepare, scan, verify, and index paper documents into the EHR

- Provide technical and administrative assistance for other health information services functions

Skills and Experience:

- Excellent communication skills

- Strong computer skills

- Ability to organize work priorities and meet specific objectives under time constraints

- Ability to manage multiple tasks simultaneously

- Good problem-solving skills and attention to detail

- Ability to be a team player in a team-oriented environment

- Previous healthcare experience or credential required

Preferred AHIMA credential:

- RHIT

Title: Optical Imaging Manager/Coordinator

Job Purpose: The optical imaging manager/coordinator coordinates all activities and staff in a records center, including the scanning process management of on-site or archived off-site historic records (e.g., paper, DVDs, microfilm, etc.), movement of paper records with internal couriers or contracted paper warehouse, and pulling/filing paper records in a hybrid environment.

Key Job Functions:

- Assist in the implementation of new scanning systems including equipment and workflow processes

- Interface with users about timely collection of paper documents

- Ensure rapid turnaround times to optimize the usability of the EHR

- Manage all staff including schedules, training, recruitment, and adherence to work and organization standards

- Develop and monitor quality and productivity measures for all work

- Ensure proper maintenance of all equipment and troubleshoot for the records operations, including scanners, copiers, printers, and fax machines

- Coordinate with forms coordinator to ensure documents reflect scanning needs, including format, bar codes, and shading, to optimize workflow and legibility

- Coordinate with HIM director/manager regarding best placement (hierarchy, index, etc.) of documents in the EHR

- Ensure quality control of documents and determine post-scanning retention of paper to optimize legibility

- Train users and provide follow-up training when required

- Monitor workflow

- Function as a liaison between health informatics and information services departments

- Lead and maintain the change control process and maintain the change records

- Post changes to computerized or manual records, release documents, and notify affected departments

- Confer with others as directed to prepare documents and change requests and with document originators to resolve discrepancies and make required changes to the documentation

- Manage and maintain active, obsolete, and computerized files that support the documentation system

- Test upgrades on test and live systems and determine go/no-go status

Skills and Experience:

- Advanced knowledge of/experience with the EHR

- HIM experience

- Experience with workflow design

- Experience with paper record systems

- Basic understanding of Microsoft Office tools

- Good communication skills

Applicable AHIMA credentials:

- RHIT

Title: Enterprise Content Record Manager

Other titles: Records and Information Manager (RIM), Senior RIM or ECRM Supervisor

Job Purpose: The enterprise content record manager manages, controls, and directs active business records systems and centers, including records organization, inactive records systems, centers and maintenance, correspondence control, reports and directives control, and records retention.

Key Job Functions:

- Provide reference services to all departments and levels of personnel and process incoming information

- Sort, classify, and verify coded material for integration into systems

- Create and maintain logs, computerized indexes, and databases to provide accurate status and retrieval information

- Plan, develop, and implement appropriate methods for creating, receiving, retrieving, retaining, storing, and disposing of records and other information, regardless of media and in compliance with all applicable laws and regulations

- Develop, implement, and document effective guidelines and processes for all aspects of records workflow, regardless of media, that is compliant with facility, state, and federal records management standards, rules, and regulations

- Work to ensure compliance and coordination activities, including transfer of permanent records and creation of inventories

- Administer records management processes, including identification and classification of all records, establishing file structures and naming conventions according to established guidelines

- Manage, control, and direct production, quality assurance, and records

- Identify the custodian as listed in the records retention schedules

- Ensure proper disposal of nonessential copies of records

- Configure and monitor information storage so access to records is limited to appropriate individuals

- Document and publish office procedures as they relate to assurance of business continuity

- Provide user training relating to records management process to employees

- Act as a resource for other units for questions related to records and information management

Skills and Experience:

- Knowledge of facility, state, and federal records management standards, rules, and regulations.

- Advanced communication skills

- Advanced organization skills

- Strong computer skills and proficient in Microsoft Office applications (Word, Excel, Access, and Outlook)

- Ability to train staff

- Ability to make independent decisions based on knowledge of policies and procedures

- Knowledge of and experience with paper record systems and electronic health records

Applicable AHIMA Credentials:

- RHIT

- RHIA

HITECH Continuing Education e-HIM Opportunities

The HITECH Act mandated that the Office of the National Coordinator for Health Information Technology create the Community College Consortia. The purpose of the Community College Consortia is to help higher education institutions establish or expand health IT education programs. These academic programs may be offered through traditional on-campus instruction, distance learning modalities, or a combination of both.

Training is designed to be completed within six months or less. The programs will be flexibly implemented to provide each trainee with skills and competencies that he or she does not already possess. Training at all consortia member colleges is expected to begin by September 30, 2010. The anticipated training capacity of the consortia as a whole is expected to be least 10,500 students annually.

- Practice workflow and information management redesign specialist

- Clinician/practitioner consultant

- Implementation support specialist

- Implementation manager

- Technical/software support staff

- Trainer

For a list of community colleges participating in the program, visit http://healthit.hhs.gov/portal/server.pt?open=512&objID=1804&mode=2.

Chapter 7

Best Practices in Health Record Documentation

Ruthann Russo, PhD, MPH, RHIT

Learning Objectives

- Explain the concept and importance of clinical documentation improvement and identify the seven criteria for high-quality clinical documentation.

- Define evidence-based medicine and evidence-based clinical documentation

- Identify documentation that meets the seven criteria for high-quality clinical documentation and documentation that does not meet the criteria

- Describe the background and functions of a clinical documentation specialist

- Explain the physician query process and the difference between a concurrent query and a retrospective query

- Describe how clinical documentation improvement functions are likely to change once hospitals have made the full transition to an electronic health record

- Explain the role of clinical documentation in the coding process

- Describe the process of clinical documentation analysis and assessment

- Describe the type of data reports that can be used in the clinical documentation analysis process

- Explain the purpose of health record analysis and the differences between quantitative and qualitative analysis

- Discuss the importance of ongoing record review and data quality management

Key Terms

Case-mix index (CMI)

Clinical documentation

Clinical documentation specialist

Complication and/or comorbidity (CC)

Concurrent query

Data collection

Deficiency system

Electronic document management system (EDMS)

Encoder

Evidence-based documentation

Evidence-based medicine

Health data repository

Health record analysis

Medical record delinquency rate

Medicare quality indicators

MedPAR data

Ongoing record review

Precise clinical documentation

Principal diagnosis

Quality

Qualitative analysis

Retrospective query

Secondary diagnosis

Severity of illness (SOI)

Seven criteria for high-quality clinical documentation

Introduction

Best practices in health record documentation involve activities that ensure the highest-quality data and information. Although the terms *data* and *information* are often used interchangeably, they actually represent two different things. *Data* is defined as individual facts, statistics, or items, such as a patient's weight, height, or lab results. When data are processed or organized, it becomes *information*. For example, when a physician processes a patient's symptoms, lab values, and radiology results, the diagnosis is the information that results. In most disciplines, the information that comes from data processing is the final result. However, in healthcare, the information can then be turned back into another form of data. In the example, we begin with lab and radiology data, which is processed into diagnostic information and then translated into a more refined form of data through the process of coding. For example, a culture and sensitivity value of >100,000 colonies of bacteria is data that can be transformed through the integration of this data element along with other data elements, such as fever, chills, and lower back pain, into a diagnosis of urinary tract infection, which is information. This information can then be translated by a coder into ICD-9-CM code 599.0 which another form of data—coded data.

This chapter explores the health information management (HIM) functions that ensure that all three of these levels of data and information are created and maintained at the highest possible levels of quality. First, we discuss the assurance of high-quality clinical documentation. This is generally obtained through a clinical documentation improvement (CDI) program staffed by clinical documentation specialists. The ultimate purpose of a CDI program is to ensure that physicians provide the most complete, clear, reliable, timely, legible, and precise documentation (information) consistent with the clinical findings (data) in the medical record. A CDI program includes review of patient records while the patient is still in the hospital to concurrently identify any opportunity for improvement in clinical documentation. With the transition to the electronic health record (EHR), some of the documentation reviews now being performed by clinical documentation specialists are likely to be replaced by clinical decision-support systems, alerts, and other automated clinical messaging.

Second, the evidence-based theory of high-quality clinical documentation is reviewed. The standards for high-quality clinical documentation are that clinical documentation be complete, clear, consistent, reliable, timely, legible, and precise. The seven criteria are described, and examples are provided of documentation that meet and do not meet the criteria. The role of the clinical documentation specialists is explained, and the physician query process is described.

Third, quantitative analysis, which involves reviewing the health record for completeness, is described. Quantitative analysis is based on the regulatory, accrediting, licensing, and reimbursement requirements that apply to the hospital. The same requirements apply whether the patient record is paper-based or electronic. However, the methodologies for review may vary.

The Importance of Clinical Documentation

Clinical documentation is any manual or electronic notation (or recording) made by a physician or other healthcare clinician related to a patient's medical condition or treatment. Clinical documentation is the primary means clinicians use to communicate their opinions about a patient's condition(s) and decisions about how to treat the patient. Since coding professionals use clinical documentation to determine which codes to assign to a patient's record, clinical documentation is the basis for ICD-9-CM and CPT coding. In this section, the definition of high-quality clinical documentation is described. In addition, we discuss who is usually responsible for the review of clinical documentation to ensure that it meets the high-quality criteria.

Evidence-based Documentation: The Theory of High-Quality Clinical Documentation

Because clinical documentation in patient health records is highly regulated, the theory must begin with regulatory and legal requirements. Medicare Conditions of Participation require all healthcare providers to maintain patient health records and dictates certain content. In addition, the Department of Health and Human Services' (HHS) Office of the Inspector General (OIG) guidance recommends the following minimum compliance for health record documentation:

1. The health record should be complete and legible.

2. Past and present diagnoses should be accessible in the health record.

3. Appropriate health risk factors should be identified.

4. If not documented, the rationale for ordering diagnostic and ancillary services should be easily inferred by an independent reviewer.

5. The patient's progress and response to any changes in treatment and any revision in diagnoses should be documented.

6. Documentation of each patient encounter should include the reason for the encounter along with any relevant history, physician examination findings, prior diagnostic test results, assessments, clinical impressions, diagnoses, plan of care, date of service, and legible identity of the observer (AMA n.d.).

Government, regulatory, and accreditation resources for health record content are shown in **TABLE 7.1**.

Evidence-based medicine (EBM) means practicing medicine using only the best scientific data available. Just as in medical practice, physicians should only be practicing clinical documentation using the best scientific data available. If physicians are trained in the seven criteria for high-quality clinical documentation (described in the next

TABLE 7.1. Resources for clinical documentation in health records

RESOURCE	INTERNET ADDRESS
Medicare Conditions of Participation	http://www.access.gpo.gov/nara/cfr/waisidx_01/42cfr482_01.html
The Joint Commission	http://www.jcaho.org/search_frm.html
PRO Directory	http://www.hcfa.gov/quality/5b5.htm
Official Guidelines for Coding and Reporting (CDC)	http://www.cdc.gov/nchs/data/icdguide.pdf
OIG—3rd Party Billing Guidance (p.7—fn.48–51)	http://oig.hhs.gov/fraud/docs/complianceguidance/thirdparty.pdf

section), the quality of their clinical documentation will improve (Russo and Fitzgerald 2008). If physicians and clinicians practice using the seven criteria, they are practicing **evidence-based documentation**.

Seven Criteria for High-Quality Clinical Documentation

The seven criteria for high-**quality** clinical documentation require that all entries in the patient record be:

1. Legible

2. Reliable

3. Precise

4. Complete

5. Consistent

6. Clear

7. Timely

The first six criteria are focused on the step during which records are being reviewed or screened through EHR criteria because corrections can be made or documentation added after the initial documentation occurred, if necessary. The last criteria, timeliness, cannot be corrected after the fact. Once an entry is late, it remains late. A description and an example for each of the seven criteria for high-quality clinical documentation follow (Russo and Fitzgerald 2008; Russo 2007). The initial definition provided for each criterion is taken from the 6th edition of the *Oxford English Dictionary*. Following the dictionary definition is a description of how the criteria can be applied to patient health record documentation. Examples of documentation that meet and do not meet the criteria are also included after each definition, with the exceptions of legibility and timeliness.

Legible: Clear Enough to Be Read and Easily Deciphered

The inability to read a record entry is usually due to the fact that the physician's handwriting is indecipherable. Legibility is a clinical documentation requirement by every regulatory body and law that addresses health record content. The most recent nod to the importance of legibility came when Health Insurance Portability and Accountability Act gave patients the right to ask for clarification of illegible information in their records. Illegible handwriting is usually the result of a rushed or careless documentation practice. As we evolve toward an EHR, handwriting becomes less of an issue. However, rushed or careless use of an EHR carries other risks that may require the definition of legibility to be amended for these purposes.

Reliable: Trustworthy, Safe, Yielding the Same Result When Repeated

These criteria relates to treatment provided to the patient and whether the physician's documentation supports that treatment. For example, assume that a physician orders a blood transfusion for a patient who has an upper gastrointestinal bleed and severely low hemoglobin and hematocrit levels. The physician's diagnosis for the patient is a bleeding gastric ulcer. The physician's diagnosis of a bleeding gastric ulcer does not appear to be reliable based on the treatment given, as blood transfusion is not an accepted treatment for a gastric ulcer. If the physician documents bleeding gastric ulcer with acute blood loss anemia (if clinically indicated), based on the treatment given, this is a reliable diagnosis.

Example: Documentation That Does Not Meet Criteria for Reliability

A patient is admitted with shortness of breath and chest pain. The patient is treated with Lasix, oxygen, and theophylline. The physician's final documented diagnosis for the patient is acute exacerbation of chronic obstructive pulmonary disease (COPD).

Example: Documentation That Meets Criteria for Reliability

The patient was given Lasix to treat an acute and chronic congestive heart failure (CHF). The physician amends the final progress note to reflect the final diagnosis: acute exacerbation of chronic bronchitis and COPD and acute and chronic CHF. In this case, the patient had bronchitis with the COPD and so the initial documentation did not meet criteria for both reliability and precision.

Precise: Accurate, Exact, Strictly Defined

Detail, if available and clinically appropriate, is an important component of every patient's health record. The more detailed the physician's documentation, the more representative and accurate the clinical documentation in the patient's record is likely to be.

Example: Documentation That Does Not Meet Criteria for Precision

A patient is admitted with chest pain, shortness of breath, fever, and cough. Chest X-ray shows aspiration pneumonia. The physician's final documented diagnosis for the patient is pneumonia.

Example: Documentation That Meets Criteria for Precision

The physician reviews the chest X-ray and documents the patient's final diagnosis in the discharge summary as aspiration pneumonia.

Complete: Has the Maximum Content; Thorough

This means that the physician has fully addressed all concerns in the patient record. Completeness also includes the appropriate authentication by the physician or clinician, which generally includes a signature and a date. Diagnostic documentation concerns apply to anything from the patient's initial complaint (did the physician provide a working and final diagnosis?) to ordering of tests (did the physician document the reason for the tests?) to abnormal diagnostic test results (did the physician document the clinical significance of any abnormal diagnostic test?)

Example: Documentation That Does Not Meet Criteria for Completeness

The physician orders comprehensive blood chemistries. The tests show low sodium levels, low magnesium levels, and low potassium levels. The physician does not document diagnoses to represent any of these abnormal results, nor does he document that the results are clinically insignificant.

Example: Documentation That Meets Criteria for Completeness

The physician documents the following in the patient's progress notes on the day after the test results were received:

> *Na 131 Mg 1.3 K+ 3.1; Patient dehydrated. Potassium within normal limits. Patient given CAD and hypertensive medication.*

The physician should not document a diagnosis if the clinical evidence did not support it. However, if the abnormal test results do not support a diagnosis, the physician should document "abnormal test results are clinically insignificant."

Consistent: Not Contradictory

Clinical documentation about a patient that contradicts itself from one progress note to the next or among entries from different physicians is a documentation deficiency. The overall rule is that when another physician's documentation conflicts with the attending physician's documentation, and the attending is unavailable to state otherwise, the attending physician's documentation takes precedence. However, if the attending physician has provided documentation that appears to contradict itself, she must clarify and add an addendum to the discharge summary or a final progress note.

Example: Documentation That Does Not Meet Criteria for Consistency

A patient is admitted by her primary care physician with vertigo and confusion. The primary care physician documents the patient's preliminary diagnosis as transient ischemic attack (TIA) and asks for a neurology consult. The neurologist examines the patient and documents the diagnosis in his final consultation as cerebrovascular accident (CVA). The attending physician provides no further documentation regarding the patient's diagnosis. (In this case, the attending physician's diagnosis and the neurologist's diagnosis are inconsistent).

Example: Documentation That Meets Criteria for Consistency

The attending physician is asked to re-review the neurologist's consultation. The attending physician adds a final progress note to the patient's record that states the final diagnosis is CVA.

Clear: Unambiguous, Intelligible; Not Vague

Vagueness and ambiguity exist when the clinical documentation does not fully describe what is wrong with the patient. This may result in the documentation of symptoms without etiology or possible etiology. For example, if a patient presents with a symptom such as chest pain and the physician provides no other insight in his documentation, it would be considered vague. If there is no clinical evidence for any diagnosis, then the appropriate documentation would be "chest pain etiology undetermined."

Example: Documentation That Does Not Meet Criteria for Clarity

A patient presents with syncope. The physician orders a CT scan and MRI of the brain, an EKG, and blood tests, all of which are within normal limits. The physician's final diagnosis on discharge is syncope.

Example: Documentation That Meets Criteria for Clarity

In the previous example, the following documentation would meet criteria for clarity if these clinical indicators were present:

1. Syncope, etiology undetermined

2. Syncope, possible bradycardia

3. Syncope, probable TIA

Timely: At the Time of Service

Timeliness of clinical documentation is essential for the best treatment of the patient. The EHR can help with timeliness, but the clinician's input is still necessary. In addition to daily progress-note entries and timely discharge summaries, physicians also need to be timely with diagnoses that are present on admission. Hospitals need to report when a diagnosis was present on admission as evidence that the condition did not develop in the hospital. Present on admission documentation impacts research, reimbursement, quality indicators, and planning.

TABLE 7.2 provides a summary of criteria for high-quality clinical documentation with representative examples.

TABLE 7.2. Criteria for high-quality clinical documentation

CRITERIA	EXAMPLE/DESCRIPTION
Legibility	Required under all government and regulatory agencies
Completeness	Abnormal test results without documentation for clinical significance (Joint Commission requirement)
Clarity	Vague or ambiguous documentation, especially in the case of a symptom principal diagnosis (chest pain vs. gastroesophageal reflux disease [GERD] or syncope vs. dehydration)
Consistency	Disagreement between two or more treating physicians without obvious resolution of the conflicting documentation upon discharge
Precision	Nonspecific diagnosis documented, more specific diagnosis appears to be supported (anemia vs. acute or chronic blood loss anemia)
Reliability	Treatment provided without documentation of condition being treated (Lasix, no CHF documented; potassium chloride administered, no hypokalemia documented)

The Clinical Documentation Specialist

The review of acute care hospital clinical documentation is usually performed while the patient is still in the hospital or concurrently with the care of the patient. Reviewing the record concurrently ensures that the improved documentation will also have a positive impact on the patient's care. The individual who is chiefly responsible for reviewing the patient's record to determine whether it meets the criteria for high-quality clinical documentation is the **clinical documentation specialist**. Clinical documentation specialists must have strong skills in the following four areas: (1) healthcare regulations, including reimbursement and documentation requirements; (2) clinical knowledge with training in the pathology of disease processes; (3) ability to read and analyze all information in a patient's health record; and (4) communication with physicians and other clinicians. Ideally, clinical documentation specialists should be credentialed in either a clinical or health information discipline, or both. **FIGURE 7.1** is a sample job description for a clinical documentation specialist.

FIGURE 7.1. Sample clinical documentation specialist job description

Anytime Hospital Anywhere USA		
Job Title: Clinical Documentation Specialist	**Job Description Approval:**	
Department: Health Information	Human Resources	Date
Job Code: X0092	Department Head	Date

GENERAL SUMMARY:

Specific Job Duties

1. Reviews inpatient health records as directed on admission and throughout hospitalization. Analyzes clinical status of patient, current treatment plan, and past medical history and identifies when clinical documentation does not meet any of the seven criteria for high quality.

2. Communicates with attending physician either verbally or through written queries to ask the physician to provide documentation remedying the deficiency.

3. Works closely with coding staff to ensure that documentation of discharged diagnosis(es) is a complete reflection of the patient's clinical status and care.

4. Demonstrates basic knowledge about standards of coding and applies this knowledge to ongoing evaluation of health record documentation.

5. Consistently meets established productivity targets for record review.

6. Designs and implements, in collaboration with physician leadership, specific tools to support improvement of physician clinical documentation.

7. Develops and implements plans for formal and informal education of physician, nursing, and other clinical staff.

8. Identifies strategies for sustained work process changes that facilitate high-quality clinical documentation.

9. Maintains good rapport and cooperative relationships. Approaches conflict in a constructive manner. Helps identify problems, offers solutions, and participates in their resolution.

10. Maintains the confidentiality of information acquired pertaining to patients, physicians, associates, and visitors to Anywhere Hospital. Discusses patient and hospital information only among appropriate personnel in appropriately private places.

11. Behaves in accordance with the mission, vision, and values of Anywhere Hospital.

When a clinical documentation specialist identifies documentation in the patient's record that does not meet one or more of the criteria for high-quality clinical documentation, he will ask the physician to clarify the documentation. This is called a physician query. The physician query can be spoken or written. If the query is spoken, the clinical documentation specialist must document the reason for the query (that is, which of the seven criteria the documentation did not meet). Queries are usually performed during the patient's stay. However, when the patient is discharged before the query can be resolved, the query can be resolved retrospectively. Retrospective queries are usually the responsibility of the coding staff. Definitions for both types of queries follow.

Concurrent Query

A **concurrent query** is a question posed to the documenting physician during the patient's hospital stay to obtain additional, clarifying documentation to improve both the quality of documentation in the patient's record and the treatment of the patient.

Retrospective Query

A **retrospective query** is a question posed to the documenting or attending physician after the patient has been discharged to obtain additional, clarifying documentation to improve the specificity and completeness of the data used to assign diagnosis and procedure codes in the patient's health record. The AHIMA Standards of Ethical Coding (2008a) state:

> Coding professionals should query provider (physician or other qualified healthcare practitioner) for clarification and additional documentation prior to code assignment when there is conflicting, incomplete, or ambiguous information in the health record regarding a significant reportable condition or procedure or other reportable data element dependent on health record documentation (e.g., present on admission indicator).

FIGURE 7.2 is an example of a retrospective query form

An organization must create a query policy and procedure that should be part of the overall clinical documentation policies and procedures. To ensure that the policy and procedure are complete, the organization should seek input from all relevant functions, including, but not limited to, health information management, the medical staff, quality improvement, compliance, legal and risk management, and case management. Input from each of these areas is likely to ensure a complete policy that is consistent with other practices of the organization.

The organization's clinical documentation procedure should include, at a minimum, the following sections: (1) When will queries be performed? (concurrently versus retrospectively) (2) Who will perform queries? (3) Who will respond to queries? (4) What is the specific criteria for when a query should be performed? In addition, the procedure should address how a query should be asked. For example, will the query be written or spoken, or are both forms acceptable? If a spoken query is performed, how will it be documented?

FIGURE 7.3 is an example of a query policy showing both concurrent and retrospective query policies and procedures.

FIGURE 7.2. Example of a retrospective query form

Physician Query to Clarify Documentation
General Hospital

Dear Dr: _____

RE: Patient health record # _____   Discharge date: _____

After a review of this record to ensure that the clinical documentation contained in inpatient records at General Hospital is as complete and precise as possible for coding and reporting purposes, we have identified a need for additional, clarifying information and possible additional documentation in this patient's record.

Location of documentation supporting this query:

☐ H&P ☐ PN of _____   ☐ Consult ☐ Lab ☐ X-ray ☐ Op report ☐ C&S ☐ ER ☐ Order

☐ Other test result: _____   ☐ Anesthesiology report   ☐ Nurse's note of _____

☐ Nutrition note of : _____   ☐ Other: _____

Other clinical indicators supporting the query:

Description of information requiring clarification:

Can you please add clarifying documentation in the form of an addendum progress note to this patient's record? Thank you.

Query generated by: _____   Date: _____

Query communicated to physician by: _____   Date: _____

CDI and the EHR

The EHR poses significant challenges for the CDI process as it exists in most hospitals today. As discussed in chapter 6, most hospitals today have a hybrid record, or one that contains both electronic and paper-based documents. In some of these organizations, queries may be performed electronically. There may be a messaging system for physicians to receive queries either through secure e-mail or through the EHR program. In other organizations, the query may be performed on paper and then scanned and filed as a permanent part of the patient record. In others, the query may be filed in its paper format in the patient's record.

As we transition to more refined EHR systems over the course of the next 5 to 10 years, the role of the clinical documentation specialist and the query as we now know it will

FIGURE 7.3. Sample query policy

Sample Physician Query Procedure

Purpose

To provide a standardized policy regarding querying of physician staff regarding documentation clarification for inpatients at the ABC Hospital that meets corporate compliance guidelines.

Scope

This policy applies to all ABC Hospital inpatients.

Responsibility

It is the responsibility of all clinical documentation specialists (CDSs), health information management (HIM), and medical staff to implement this policy. It is the responsibility of the chief of service, director of case management, and director of HIM to ensure compliance to this policy.

The physician (MD) will be queried when an opportunity to improve the quality of documentation in the inpatient record is noted; queries may be made concurrently by CDSs or retrospectively by HIM in-patient coders or auditing staff. Queries should be supported by clinical evidence in the patient's record. A query is never to be generated to misrepresent a patient's diagnosis or condition.

Concurrent queries—CDSs will query the patient's MD if opportunities to improve documentation are noted during concurrent review of the patient's record. Queries will be written on the facility's concurrent query form or may be made verbally if the MD is on the patient care unit at the time of the query.

MDs will be queried by CDSs for:

1. Specificity in documentation

2. Evaluation of lab data/radiology and other reports, such as pathology, as to the significance of any abnormalities or findings (and the name of the suspected/treated condition)

3. Agreement and documentation of diagnoses documented by other members of the health care team (e.g., nutrition, substance abuse team [if not completed by the MD member of the team], wound care team)

4. Co-signature of nurse practitioner and physician assistant notes to be used for APR-DRG (all patient refined diagnosis-related group) assignment and coding

5. Differential diagnoses ruled in/out by discharge

6. Conditions/procedure names that do not use approved hospital abbreviations

7. Clarification if there are conflicts of diagnoses between consultant and the attending MD

MDs (attending or resident) shall review and respond to queries within 24 hours whenever possible.

1. If the MD agrees with the query, he or she is to document the applicable condition/procedure the next time he or she documents in the progress notes.

2. If the MD does not agree with the query (i.e., there is no clinical significance for an abnormal lab test), he or she is to check off on the sticky note "disagree with the query."

Retrospective queries—HIM coders will query the patient's MD if opportunities to improve documentation are noted during retrospective review of the patient's record. Queries of the attending MD after discharge should be made only when there is sufficient supporting documentation within the body of the health record to warrant a query. Questions about documentation in the record may arise during the coding process or as a result of a special audit.

The MD will be queried in the following situations:

1. Documentation is inconsistent and/or ambiguous, unclear, incomplete, or unspecified or general in nature (AHIMA Standards of Ethical Coding and Compliance Guidance for Third Party Billing Companies, 1999)

2. Principal diagnosis (reason for admission, after study) is not clearly identified

3. Significant case manager queries not answered prior to discharge (e.g., those that would affect severity level)

FIGURE 7.3. (continued)

4. Abnormal diagnostic test results indicate the possible addition of a secondary diagnosis or increased specificity of an already documented condition

5. Lack of clarity as to whether a condition has been ruled out

6. Patient is receiving treatment for a condition that has not been documented

7. Significance of abnormal operative/procedural/pathologic findings are not documented

8. Predetermined and agreed upon (with medical staff) clinical criteria are met

9. Agreement and documentation of diagnoses documented by other members of the health care team (e.g., nutrition, substance abuse team (if not completed by the MD member of the team), wound care team)

Query format

The physician query form will be used for all queries, including patient identification, reason for query, directions as to how to provide the requested documentation clarification, and contact information of the person executing the query. If there are multiple questions for one case, the MD is to be alerted that there is more than one query requiring a response.

1. In completing the reason for query on the MD query form, the coder will use open-ended questions and allow the MD to render and document his or her clinical interpretation of the diagnosis, condition, procedure, etc. based on the facts of the case. Closed-ended yes/no or leading questions will be avoided.

2. Exceptions to the open-ended query, when it is appropriate to query for a specific diagnosis, include the following:

   a. Positive lab or radiology findings clinically supporting the diagnosis (Coding Clinic, 2nd quarter 1998)

   b. Medication is prescribed that supports the specific diagnosis (Coding Clinic, 1st quarter 1993 and 2nd quarter 1998)

3. MDs (attending or resident) are to respond to retrospective queries within 5 business days (or on the same day for special audits).

4. If they agree with the query, they are to document on a late-entry documentation note form (see attached). All entries must be signed and dated for the date the current entry is made.

5. If they disagree with the query, they are to indicate their reasons on the MD query form and return the form to HIM.

The late-entry documentation note form shall be documented by the MD and, if applicable scanned into the hospital's imaging system, if the MD documents additional information.

---

change forever. Ideally, the clinical decision support system should be front loaded with query logic that will not permit a physician to provide any documentation in the patient's record unless it meets all of the criteria for high-quality clinical documentation. For example, if a patient has abnormal lab tests, the system should automatically query the physician about the abnormal test results and require her to either document that the abnormal tests are not clinically significant or document the condition that the abnormal tests represent. Literally hundreds of different types of automated queries can be created for the EHR.

Clinical decision-support systems that contain these kinds of criteria are just beginning to be created and tested. It is probably impossible to predict every scenario in which clinical documentation might not meet the quality criteria at this point. Clinical documentation specialists will likely continue in the same roles for the next few years. Then, they will transition into roles where they provide an audit function, identifying query opportunities that the EHR has missed. Each time a clinical documentation specialist identifies an opportunity manually, however, it will be recorded and eventually added into the EHR system. At some point, the clinical documentation query function will be 90 to 95 percent automated. An audit role, as well as education and training for the clinical documentation specialist, will likely always exist. But, like coders, their job duties will be upgraded to an audit, instructor, and analytical function as opposed to merely a reviewer function.

Translating Clinical Documentation into Coded Data

Coding is the act of translating physician clinical documentation into diagnostic and procedural coded data. It is essentially another language, one that allows the patient's diagnostic, treatment, and response information to be aggregated into a uniform data set. This efficient aggregation of millions of pages of clinical documentation enables the analysis of health record information for research, planning, billing, and patient-care purposes. Without the coding professional applying a specific set of specialized skills and expertise to arrive at the coded data set for each patient, this analysis would not be possible. The coding professional needs high-quality clinical documentation to create quality data. Like the artist whose sculpture will be better if it is created with high-quality clay, so the coding professional's data product will be of higher accuracy and quality if created from superior clinical documentation.

How a Coding Professional Views an Inpatient Health Record

Within about 48 hours of a patient's discharge from the hospital, his health record is in the hands of a hospital coding professional. The coding professional is definitely the first, and may be the only, person ever to read the complete health record from front to back, and this may be the first time all of the record is (or should be) in one place. It is the coding professional's job to methodically review all of the information in the record so the clinical documentation can be translated into the language of coding. The next few paragraphs describe the steps a typical coding professional is likely to take in reviewing a patient health record for coding purposes. The exact order of review may vary by coding professional or by the way a record, especially an EHR, is compiled. The coding professional begins the review with the first page of the record, which is commonly known as the *face sheet* or the *admission and discharge form*. The face sheet is a summary that contains primarily demographic information. A coding professional may take note of the patient's age and the admission and discharge dates, which are also on the form, and then quickly calculate how long the patient was in the hospital by subtracting the admission date from the discharge date. These two pieces of information give the coding professional a basic idea of the complexity of the record. For example, the record of an 89-year-old patient in the hospital for nine days would be more complex to review and code than the record of a 29-year-old who was in and out of the hospital within two days. Of course, another simple and obvious clue to the record's complexity is its size. Usually, the thicker the record or, in the case of a hybrid record or EHR, the more screen entries, the more complex the case was. The physician documents the patient's diagnoses and procedures on the face-sheet page or screen of the patient's record. This documentation may be fairly sketchy, but it gives the coding professional some initial clues about what was going on with the patient.

The next form in the patient's record is usually the discharge summary, if it was completed by the physician immediately after discharge. The discharge summary, which should provide a complete overview of the patient's entire stay, is generally the last document completed for the patient's record. The next document that appears in the record, the history and physical, is the first document completed during the patient's stay. As coding professionals read the complete history and physical, they look for key pieces of information, such as symptoms upon admission, medications that the patient was taking, and chronic conditions. The attending physician's "impression and plan," which usually appears at the end of the history and physical, helps the coding professional piece together the patient's diagnoses.

The next section of the patient's record for review contains the progress notes. For a coding professional, the progress notes are the essence of the patient's record. Reading and deciphering the progress notes, which in most hospitals are still handwritten, can be challenging. The notes represent what was going on in the physician's mind at that point in time. There is something about the candidness of the progress notes that cannot be captured in a dictated and transcribed formal report. The difference between the discharge summary and the day-by-day description of treatment activities and the patient's reactions to treatment is like the difference between watching the news on television and watching the events happen in person.

Consultation reports are typically the next set of documents for review. Consultation reports are particularly important to coding professionals. When coding professionals review the consultation report, they try to determine whether the attending physician and the consultant agreed on the patient's diagnosis. If not, the coding professional may need to contact the attending physician to clarify the patient's diagnosis. If one physician documents that the patient had a stroke and another physician documents that the same patient had a TIA, the coding professional needs a tiebreaker; and the attending or primary physician breaks the tie in every case. When a documentation discrepancy between the attending and another treating physician occurs, the coding professional generates a retrospective query to the attending physician to clarify the patient's diagnosis and resolve the conflicting documentation in the patient's record.

Diagnostic test results are the next piece of data reviewed by coding professionals. Diagnostic test results present some of the biggest challenges for hospital coding professionals. Abnormal test results without a physician verification of a diagnosis or documentation as to whether the test result is clinically-significant prompts the coding professional to query the physician. If the physician documents the diagnosis, the coding professional can translate that documentation into a code. If the physician does not document the diagnosis, the coding professional cannot assume that the patient has a diagnosis based solely on abnormal test results. **FIGURES 7.4** and **7.5** illustrate the required documentation from the physician that a coding professional needs to use clinical information such as abnormal lab results, orders, or medication administration records for coding purposes.

If a patient has surgery during her hospital stay, the next documents in the record for review are the surgical reports, which include a preoperative or preanesthesia assessment completed by the anesthesiologist; a formal operative report completed by the surgeon; a postoperative assessment completed by the anesthesiologist; and,

FIGURE 7.4. Required documentation for coding abnormal laboratory tests

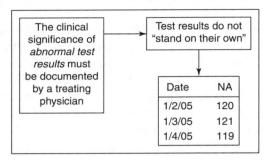

if any tissue was removed during the surgery, a pathology report completed by the hospital pathologist. Coding professionals read the surgical report very closely to determine exactly what surgeries were performed that need to be coded. In addition, anesthesiologists often document patient conditions that might not be documented by other physicians who are treating the patient. This is particularly true of chronic respiratory conditions or heart murmurs that may be significant for the anesthesiologist to monitor while the patient is under anesthesia. Any information documented by the anesthesiologist that conflicts with that of the attending physician may require a query to the attending physician.

Physician orders are the next part of the patient record. Coding professionals check to make sure that they have been able to assign a diagnostic code to the reason for every order placed. For example, if the physician places an order on a record for Lasix, a drug used to treat CHF, but there is no documentation for CHF on the record, this may trigger a question from the coding professional to the physician to clarify the diagnosis.

Nurses' graphic records appear after physician orders in the patient record. One of the common items coding professionals look for here is the patient's temperature. If a nurse charted a high temperature and the patient was treated with antibiotics or analgesics, coding professionals want to make sure there is a corresponding diagnosis documented by the physician for this activity. Coding professionals are always looking to close the loop and make sure that the activities in the record match the diagnoses. Closing the loop means that the codes present an accurate picture of what actually happened to the patient during the stay.

FIGURE 7.5. Required documentation for coding from physician order

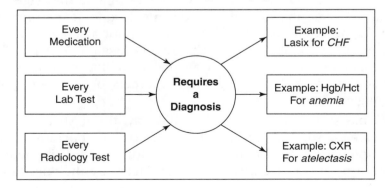

Finally, medication administration records appear in the record. Many coding professionals first review the medication administration forms. By looking at these forms, coding professionals can quickly get an idea of what is wrong with the patient. The medications or intravenous (IV) fluids that were administered to the patient during the stay provide good evidence of what happened. So, a coding professional may begin with a hypothesis, such as the patient received antibiotics, Lasix, and potassium in her IV fluids, therefore, the patient probably had an infection (treated with antibiotics), CHF (treated with Lasix), and low potassium, also known as hypokalemia (treated with potassium supplements). Next, the coding professional begins at the front of the record, looking for evidence to support the hypothesis. Of course, coding professionals identify other information while wading through the record, but using the medication administration forms to formulate a hypothesis can be quite reliable.

The Relationship Between Clinical Documentation and Coding

The coding professional's job includes

1. Reviewing all clinical documentation in the patient's record

2. Separating out clinical information that has been documented with high-quality criteria by the physician into diagnoses for coding purposes

3. Applying rules for whose documentation counts for coding purposes

4. Incorporating only diagnoses and procedures that should be coded under official coding guidelines

5. Arriving at the correct code number to represent the diagnosis or procedure (CMS and NCHS 2007)

6. Asking the physician about any gaps in documentation that may represent a diagnosis that is clinically relevant but not sufficiently documented. The preferred methodology for physician querying is concurrent, while the patient is still in the hospital, as illustrated in **FIGURE 7.6**. However, when a query cannot be performed concurrently because of a short length of stay or because the physician does not respond, the coding professional is charged with asking the physician to clarify any documentation that does not meet high-quality clinical documentation criteria (AHIMA 2008b).

FIGURE 7.6. Methodology for querying physicians

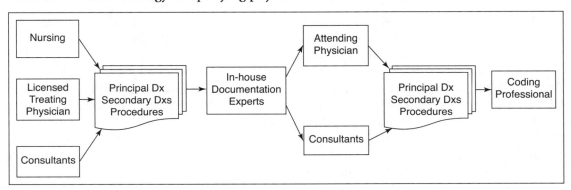

Basic Coding Guidelines

All codes are assigned using the official ICD-9-CM coding manuals. These manuals contain directions for assigning codes. For cases in which a coding professional encounters an issue that is not addressed in the manual, the Centers for Medicare and Medicaid Services (CMS) and the National Center for Health Statistics (NCHS), two departments within the HHS, have created the *ICD-9-CM Official Guidelines for Coding and Reporting* (CMS and NCHS 2007).

The guidelines for ICD-9-CM were developed and approved by the American Hospital Association (AHA), the American Health Information Management Association (AHIMA), CMS, and NCHS (CMS and NCHS 2007). The first paragraph of the guidelines contains the following sentence: "A joint effort between the attending physician and coder is essential to achieve complete and accurate documentation, code assignment, and reporting of diagnoses and procedures." This statement emphasizes the importance of high-quality clinical documentation and the role of the coding professional in ensuring that the final coded data is consistent with the documentation in the patient's record. Detailed information can be obtained from the guidelines, but the two most important and basic definitions are for the assignment of a patient's principal diagnosis and for the secondary diagnoses in the inpatient setting. The definitions are as follows:

> **Principal diagnosis:** Every inpatient is assigned one principal ICD-9-CM diagnostic code. The principal diagnosis is the condition that is determined, after study, to have caused the admission of the patient to the acute care setting and is documented by a licensed, treating physician.

> **Secondary diagnosis:** Every inpatient is assigned one ICD-9-CM diagnostic code for each secondary diagnosis. Secondary diagnoses include any diagnosis that is documented by a licensed, treating physician and is either clinically evaluated, treated, or tested during the stay or responsible for increasing the length of stay or use of resources (CMS and NCHS 2007).

Another way to view the patient's principal and secondary diagnoses is illustrated in **TABLE 7.3**. This table shows the differences between acute and chronic conditions as well as the importance of precision and completeness in all clinical documentation for diagnoses.

Example of Coding for a Myocardial Infarction (Heart Attack)

The following example provides some insight into the detail involved in coding a patient's diagnosis. A coding professional needs to be adept at reading the entire health record. The individual must then be able to translate the material, through his or her expertise and a series of filters, provided by the encoder, into the representative codes. An **encoder** is a computer program that assists the coder in assigning ICD-9-CM or CPT codes to the documentation in the patient's health record. **TABLE 7.4** presents a list that includes all the different codes available for patients who are admitted to the hospital with a current, acute myocardial infarction (MI) or heart attack. There are additional codes for patients who had the MI prior to hospital admission, or in situations where the physician has not documented exactly when the heart attack

TABLE 7.3. Clinical documentation characteristics

IMPORTANT CONSIDERATIONS	DOCUMENT....	EXAMPLES: IF PRESENT OR *SUSPECTED*, DOCUMENT....
Patient's principal diagnosis	Detail, precision	*"Aspiration"* pneumonia *"Acute"* renal failure Cerebral *"infarct"*
Chronic coexisting diagnoses	Everything under consideration	COPD CHF Seizure disorder Pulmonary fibrosis
Acute coexisting diagnoses	Everything being evaluated or treated	Malnutrition Respiratory failure Dehydration
Abnormal diagnostic tests	The clinical significance of	Hyponatremia Mitral regurgitation Atrial fibrillation
Symptoms	The etiology or "suspected etiology"	Instead of chest pain—Possible GERD or angina due to CAD Instead of syncope—Arrhythmia

occurred.

Each code designates very specific information. The digits to the left of the decimal represent the main condition (for example, MI or heart attack). The digits to the right are based on the specific location and timing of the patient's heart attack. Examples in **TABLE 7.4** using the fifth digit, 1, show that the MI occurred during the current admission. Other fifth digits are available to identify that an MI occurred during a prior admission (410.02) or during neither the current nor a prior admission (410.00). In particular, the use of 0 or 2 as the fifth digit would be a red flag to identify that the physician's clinical documentation does not meet the criteria for high-quality clinical documentation. The coding professional, especially in the inpatient setting, should always be able to deter-

TABLE 7.4. Examples of the use of the fifth digit for coding

CODE	CONDITION
410.01	[MI/heart attack] of the anteriolateral wall
410.11	[MI/heart attack] of other anterior wall (i.e., anterioapical or anteroseptal wall)
410.21	[MI/heart attack] of the inferolateral wall
410.31	[MI/heart attack] of the interoposterior wall
410.41	[MI/heart attack] of other interior wall (i.e., diaphragmatic wall)
410.51	[MI/heart attack] of other lateral wall (i.e., basal-lateral, high lateral)
410.61	[MI/heart attack] of the true posterior wall
410.71	[MI/heart attack] of the subendocardium (also nontransmural infarct)
410.81	[MI/heart attack] of other specified sites (i.e., atrium, papillary muscle)
410.91	[MI/heart attack] of unspecified site of heart

mine, based on the physician's documentation, whether an MI occurred during the current or a prior admission (CMS and NCHS 2007).

The details used in codes in the ICD-9-CM coding book are generally intended to facilitate medical research. For example, certain areas of the heart affected by heart attacks may respond better to certain drugs or interventions than others. However, if coding professionals grouped all patients' heart attacks together under one general code, there would be no way of comparing large databases of patients with heart attacks as researchers do today.

Insurance companies and Medicare also use the detailed ICD-9-CM coding to determine whether the information is sufficient for them to pay the bill. Certain insurance companies and Medicare may reject codes that are unspecified. For example, the heart attack code 410.90 represents "heart attack of unspecified site of the heart, unspecified as to episode of care." If this code is submitted on a patient's bill, it could be a red flag for an insurance company, and the bill could be rejected unless the provider submits more detailed codes. The insurance company's perspective is that if the hospital treated the patient for a heart attack, it should know if it was a current, acute attack (a fifth digit of 1 instead of 0), and should probably know where in the heart muscle the blood flow was stopped.

Clinical Documentation Analysis and Assessment

An assessment is a snapshot in time that gives the CDI review team or CDI specialists a starting point for their activities. Unless the review team is familiar with the organization's documentation and the data produced from it, it cannot determine whether its efforts to improve clinical documentation have been successful. Reviewing actual documentation and data prior to investing in a CDI program prevents the CDI review team from acting on assumptions. For example, the management team may believe that there is a quality problem with clinical documentation based on discussions, a drop in case mix, and a few documentation problems identified in patient records during the coding process. In this case, the organization should perform an objective analysis of data and documentation for two reasons. First, an analysis will determine whether the perceived problem exists. Second, the analysis, if performed according to the recommendations in this chapter, will provide a valid baseline for measuring the impact of any CDI efforts.

If the organization already has a CDI program in place, it can use the information in this chapter to validate its current baseline. The information can also be used to determine whether current analyses include all of the necessary components. If not, this chapter can be used to include some new baseline analytics in the process. Finally, if a program is currently in place that focuses only on inpatient documentation, this information can be used to analyze outpatient or long-term care data and create a baseline for those care areas. In every case, it is important to include analyses of data and documentation.

Data Review

Every healthcare organization produces significant amounts of data on an ongoing basis. As noted in the introduction to this book, these data are used for everything from reimbursement and quality indicators to research and planning. A management team that knows, understands, and uses the data produced by its organization is more likely to make better decisions than a team that is not datacentered (Drucker 1999). The use of data for decision making is most imperative when the decisions involve a new or established CDI program.

What Data Matter?

Two types of data should be considered in the CDI process. The first is the data the organization produces. The second is the data that others produce about the organization. An organization produces data from coding, data collected for Medicare quality indicators, and other specialized data collected for the organization's mortality and morbidity review (MMR) or other internal clinical committees or groups. The following terms and their definitions will be helpful in understanding how clinical documentation is reflected in data about a hospital:

Case-mix index (CMI)—CMI is the average relative weight for all inpatients in a hospital. CMI reflects the expected intensity of resources needed to care for patients.

Complication and/or comorbidity (CC)—CCs are secondary diagnoses that, if documented on a patient record, are likely to increase the intensity of services needed to care for the patient.

Diagnosis-related groups (DRGs)—DRGs are a way to group ICD-9-CM coded data from an inpatient stay into categories that are similar clinically and in the intensity of services they are likely to require. Each DRG is assigned a relative weight based on the intensity of services patients in that DRG are likely to require. The DRG is the larger category that includes refined groupings such as the Medicare Severity DRGs (MS-DRGs) and all patient refined (APR) DRGs.

Medicare Quality Indicators—These are criteria determined by Medicare that, if present in a patient's record, are likely to result in higher quality of care than if they are not present. Examples of Medicare Quality Indicators include smoking cessation counseling and aspirin given to patients with acute MI within minutes of their admission to the emergency department.

Severity of illness—Severity of illness (SOI) is a system of classifying inpatient cases into categories that are likely to be similar in severity using demographic and clinical information. Several SOI DRG systems are available. The two most common systems are the MS-DRGs, which group patients into three different levels of severity, and the 3M APR-DRGs, which group patients into four different levels of SOI. In both systems, the higher the level, the higher the severity of illness for patients assigned to it.

An organization collects a significant amount of data that must be prioritized if it is to focus its efforts and obtain maximum benefit from this data review. General guidelines are included in this chapter, but data vary for each organization. One of the first questions to ask is what level of aggregation to look at. Many organizations want to begin at a high level and drill down to the details if a problem or unexpected finding is discovered. For coded data, one of the highest levels of aggregation is by DRG. The organization may also want to consider reviewing data by severity level or by the presence or absence of

TABLE 7.5. Hospital severity levels from the APR grouper based on service type

SERVICE	MINOR (LEVEL 1)	MODERATE (LEVEL 2)	MAJOR (LEVEL 3)	EXTREME (LEVEL 4)
Internal medicine	40%	32%	25%	3%
Cardiology	35%	35%	28%	2%
Neurology	30%	40%	27%	3%
General surgery	28%	42%	25%	5%
Orthopedic surgery	45%	40%	14%	1%

CC codes. One of the most detailed levels of data is found at the diagnosis or procedure code level. Table 4.1 shows hospital severity levels from the APR grouper broken out by service type. This shows another way to drill into high-level data. The review begins with data by severity. Within each severity level, the type of service is specified. This type of data review can help determine whether there may be specific problems in certain clinical departments. In **TABLE 7.5**, the orthopedic service shows 45 percent of patients with severity level 1 and only 14 percent of patients with severity level 3. These two numbers show that orthopedic patients have lower severity levels than patients in all other services. There may be a reason to expect that orthopedic patients are less severely ill than those in all other services. If not, this data finding is a red flag that orthopedic services may have a more significant problem with documentation practices than other services.

Data that others produce about the organization affect patient perception, accreditation status, and reimbursement. These data include Medicare quality indicators, The Joint Commission's Quality Check, data from private quality organizations like HealthGrades, and data from state-specific quality programs like the Medisgroup data abstracting used by such states as Colorado and Pennsylvania (PHCCCC 2006). An adaptation of data produced by HealthGrades for patients to review appears in **FIGURE 7.7**.

For the diagnosis or procedure analyzed, hospitals with one star are providing care below the quality expected, those with three stars are providing care at the level of quality expected, and those with five stars are providing better quality care than expected. If an organization has a one- or three-star rating that it believes should be a five-star rating, documentation may be the reason. Analysis at this level will also allow comparison of ratings by service, because HealthGrades provides ratings by diagnosis and by procedure.

Using Criteria to Screen the Data

Everything is relative, and a valid comparison is needed for the data. Following are three sources of comparative data:

1. National normative data

2. Regulatory guidance

3. The organization's own benchmarks

FIGURE 7.7. Example of a hospital quality rating by HealthGrades

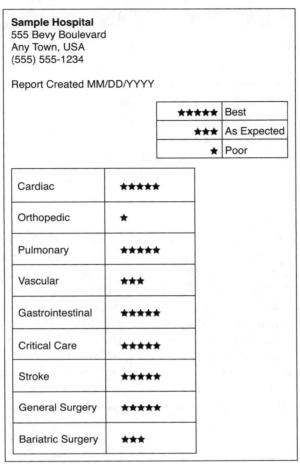

Source: Adapted from HealthGrades 2011.

National normative data can be used, but it is much more relevant to use data from hospitals that are similar in size, teaching status, and geographic status. Some organizations have their own information staff who are able to obtain detailed levels of data. Data can also be purchased for reasonable rates from organizations such as the American Hospital Directory (AHD). Other sources of data may include the regulatory guidance provided by the OIG, Medicare, quality improvement organizations (QIOs), and other government agencies. For example, on some occasions local QIOs have published CC rates or certain DRG pair proportions that raise a red flag for the review team. Finally, the organization's own benchmarks can be used to screen data (so long as this is consistent with legal and regulatory requirements). Ideally, an organization will develop its own set of criteria based on the three sources.

Deciding What Data to Review

Once the CDI review team has decided what criteria to use, it needs to determine what data to review. Ultimately, this determination is driven by two things: the

TABLE 7.6. Discharges for a 300-bed hospital Over a 12-month period

DIAGNOSIS	MEDICARE	OTHER PAYERS
Chest pain	53	436
Syncope	50	166
Angina	70	250
Back pain	43	128
Vertigo	26	223
Epistaxis	12	61
Shortness of breath	11	90
Musculoskeletal pain	10	36

criteria used to screen the data for decision making and the purpose of the review. For example, what is the team trying to get out of the data review? For high-quality clinical documentation, one criterion is completeness. One way to apply the criteria to aggregate-level data is to identify patient records with vague principal diagnoses. While these may be valid from a high-level data perspective, a vague or symptomatic principal diagnosis can be a red flag. **TABLE 7.6** illustrates this type of data. Medicare is separated out from other payers since the age difference may affect the data. The table represents discharges for a 300-bed hospital over the course of a year. The hospital in this case was concerned about the high numbers of chest pain and vertigo cases. At a minimum, this type of data analysis can provide the organization with enough information that it will know it should further explore the issue of clinical documentation quality.

Recommended Data to Review

This section presents a list of recommended data to review. It is important, however, to ensure that the data review reflects the organization. This list is intended as a general guide only. Each organization should create a data review that will accomplish its specific objectives.

It is important that the CDI review team understand which services admit the most patients to the hospital. It is particularly important to review the data by service if the service is assigned by an indicator other than the major diagnostic category (MDC). Then, discharges by service should be compared with discharges by MDC. Lack of agreement between the two may point to a problem with clinical documentation. For example, when cardiologists admit a significant number of patients with chest pain to the hospital, discharges by MDC may show a lower number of cardiac admissions than discharges by service. This difference could represent a problem with precision in documenting a principal diagnosis.

Example: Discharges by Service and by Major Diagnostic Category

TABLE 7.7 is an example of data about the organization that can be obtained from the AHD (2008). These data are derived from **MedPAR data**, so they are usually more than a year old. They are a starting point for analysis, but ultimately, more

TABLE 7.7. Examples of data that can be obtained from the American Hospital Directory

	MEDICARE INPATIENTS	AVERAGE LENGTH OF STAY	AVERAGE CHARGES	AVERAGE COST	MEDICARE CMI
Burns	28	12.11	$78,359	$21,436	2.6269
Cardiology	1,925	4.79	$22,065	$6,314	1.0917
Cardiovascular surgery	1,667	6.13	$88,352	$19,704	3.7755
Gynecology	92	3.49	$21,137	$5,505	1.1344
Medicine	3,304	4.23	$18,367	$5,159	0.8810
Neurology	977	4.56	$22,068	$6,098	1.0861
Neurosurgery	108	8.85	$67,128	$17,910	2.9322
Oncology	290	6.80	$26,945	$7,545	1.4957
Orthopedics	1,766	5.25	$31,757	$8,135	1.7000
Psychiatry	601	11.82	$21,155	$8,180	0.6840
Pulmonology	1,322	7.54	$51,775	$13,428	2.5170
Surgery	1,018	8.43	$52,132	$13,687	2.3922
Surgery for malignancy	74	4.70	$30,470	$8,019	1.6887
Urology	812	4.85	$25,879	$8,107	1.2416
Vascular surgery	394	6.37	$42,201	$11,444	2.0163
TOTAL	14,387	5.79	$36,259	$9,451	1.6964

Source: Adapted from AHD 2008.

recent data provided by the organization's internal information or finance staff will be wanted. MedPAR data are publicly available, de-identified data from Medicare inpatient billing files.

TABLE 7.7 can also be used to identify and analyze the following data.

Discharges by DRG

Most organizations review data by DRG on a regular basis as part of their case-mix analysis. For clinical documentation purposes, actual DRG data should be reviewed against the organization's expectations. For example, an organization may believe that there have been no (or very few) inpatient admissions for chest pain since it opened a chest pain clinic. If an analysis of DRG-level data reveals several cases in the chest pain DRG, this is a red flag for documentation.

Case-Mix Index

Most organizations review CMI over time, both overall and by specialty. For clinical documentation analysis purposes, an unexpected change in CMI could signal a possible problem with clinical documentation. For example, if the CMI for orthopedic surgery has dropped for the past six months with no change in admitting physicians or types

TABLE 7.8. Example of Complication and comorbidity (CC) capture rates—combined and by specialty

CC CAPTURE RATE	MEDICARE	OTHER PAYERS	MEDICARE PEER NORMS
All medicine specialties	68%	50%	81%
All surgical specialties	77%	39%	72%
General medicine	70%	50%	80%
Cardiology	79%	46%	93%
General surgery	68%	43%	78%
Orthopedic surgery	59%	28%	69%

of surgery performed, the orthopedic surgeons may not be completely documenting all diagnoses in their patients' records.

Complication and Major Complication Rates

Changes in rates, or rates that are not consistent with an organization's expectations or normative data, may indicate a problem with clinical documentation quality. **TABLE 7.8** is an example of a report that shows overall CC capture rate by all medicine and all surgical specialties together and then by each specialty. The comparison with peer norms for Medicare cases is helpful in determining whether rates appear to be lower or higher than an organization's norms. Any inconsistency provides support for further clinical documentation review and analysis.

Table 7.8 can also be used to identify and analyze the data described in the following paragraphs.

Severity Levels (MS-DRGs and APR DRGs)

If the CDI review team has access to the MS-DRG and the APR-DRG grouper, it is helpful to look at the organization's severity levels for each. While MS-DRGs are used for Medicare reimbursement, the APR-DRG grouper is used for quality indicators for HealthGrades' analysis and, in many states, for Medicaid reimbursement. Changes in rates or inconsistency with expectations or normative data may indicate a problem with clinical documentation quality.

Medical Quality Indicators

Because Medicare quality indicators are important for both reimbursement (pay for performance) and accreditation (The Joint Commission uses many of the same measures), the organization must be familiar with its outcomes data. **TABLE 7.9** contains a summary of the Medicare quality indicators for a hospital for current, reported indicators (CMS 2008). In this example, a hospital may identify that documentation of influenza and pneumococcal vaccination status may be an issue for physicians.

Table 7.9 can also be used to identify and analyze the data in the following paragraphs.

TABLE 7.9. **Example of summary of Medicare quality indicators**

CONDITION	NUMBER OF PATIENTS	HOSPITAL SCORE	NATIONAL AVERAGE	90TH PERCENTILE	STATE AVERAGE
Appropriate initial antibiotic selection	140	89%	87%	97%	88%
Blood cultures performed in the emergency department before initial antibiotic received in hospital	237	86%	90%	100%	90%
Influenza vaccination status	65	97%	75%	99%	79%
Initial antibiotic(s) administered within 6 hours after arrival	190	93%	93%	100%	93%
Oxygenation assessment	344	99%	99%	100%	100%
Pneumococcal vaccination status	310	95%	78%	97%	85%
Smoking cessation advice/ counseling	91	100%	85%	100%	93%

Secondary Diagnoses

The numbers of secondary diagnoses for inpatient cases can provide some insight into the level of detail of documentation available to the coding staff for code assignment. If this measure is used for CDI, the review team will want to make sure its members are familiar with the coding guidelines at the hospital and understand any possible limitations. The team may also want to delete one-day stays from the data since they can skew overall averages. **Table 7.10** further breaks down the data by using severity levels to stratify numbers of secondary diagnoses. This table reveals that the numbers of secondary diagnoses for this hospital for all cases are less than those for peer hospitals. It points in particular to a possible significant problem with surgery cases since the peer norms figure is 6.5 secondary diagnoses on average, while the hospital has only 5.6 secondary diagnoses for surgery cases. Secondary diagnoses can also be stratified by service and physician for more detail.

TABLE 7.10. **Comparison of secondary diagnoses**

SECONDARY DIAGNOSIS CATEGORY	NUMBER	PEER NORMS
All inpatient cases	5.3	6.8
Medicine cases	5.6	7.2
Surgical cases	4.2	6.6
Severity level 1 cases	2.6	2.8
Severity level 2 cases	5.3	5.5
Severity level 3 cases	8.6	9.0
Severity level 4 cases	11.8	12.0

Quantitative Analysis

Health record analysis is the review of patient records to ensure the quality and completeness of clinical documentation. Health record analysis is generally performed after the patient is discharged. The review does not entail an evaluation of the clinical care provided to the patient. However, quality improvement and accreditation organizations depend on health record documentation for evidence that appropriate and effective care is being provided to patients. And, as we have already discussed, the quality of clinical documentation significantly affects the coding and billing processes that lead to reimbursement for provided services.

Traditional health record analysis is made up of two separate but related processes: quantitative analysis and qualitative analysis. **Quantitative analysis** is a review of the health record to determine its completeness and accuracy. Examples of quantitative analysis include ensuring that procedure reports are dictated and filed into the patient record in a timely manner and that progress notes are recorded daily and contain the time, date, and signature of the author. **Qualitative analysis** is a review of the health record to ensure the quality of clinical documentation.

In hospitals that use traditional, paper-based health record systems, HIM department personnel are responsible for ensuring receipt of the health records of discharged, transferred, and deceased patients (Coffman-Kadish 2002). (See **Figure 7.8**.) HIM personnel compare records received with discharge lists or logs to ensure that all records are accounted for from each unit or department. Depending on the hospital's health record policies, HIM personnel may reassemble the contents of the record in a specific order for storage. However, most hospitals have replaced the reassembly of records with the best practice of maintaining the record in reverse chronological order. Assembling the record after discharge is not necessary in facilities that use an **electronic document management system (EDMS)** or EHR system.

FIGURE 7.8. Steps in the flow of paper-based health records after discharge

1. Records of discharged patients arrive or are delivered to HIM department.

2. Receipt of records is verified by comparing discharge lists to actual charts received.

3. Folder corresponding to records is pulled.

4. Record is assembled according to prescribed format, ensuring that all pages belong to the correct patient and that forms are in the correct date order.

5. Deficiencies such as missing signatures, reports needing completion, and so on are assigned to the responsible provider.

6. Diagnoses and procedures are coded.

7. Record is held for final completion by providers either in the incomplete chart area or some other filing area.

8. Charts are rechecked after the providers have done their work to ensure that all have been completed.

9. The complete record is filed in the permanent filing area.

Source: Reynolds and Bowman 2010, 206.

Facilities using an EDMS to organize hybrid health records require a format that facilitates easy retrieval of interfaced and scanned documents. The ideal scanning process would automatically organize documents within the health record through the use of bar codes and tables that are designed to define document location.

The purpose of quantitative analysis is to assess the completeness and accuracy of patient health records. Quantitative evaluations are based on the regulatory, accrediting, licensing, and reimbursement requirements that apply to the hospital, all of which are discussed in chapters 5 and 8. Therefore, the timing and extent of quantitative health record analysis depend on policies developed by individual organizations. Both paper-based and computer-based records are subject to quantitative review. This chapter describes the manual involved in quantitative and qualitative record review. In a fully implemented EHR, the system itself would be programmed to identify deficiencies and alert the individual responsible for the completion of deficiencies. In the future, the health information professional's responsibility for completeness of records will entail a higher-level auditing function. Because this change may be as much as ten years into the future, we will focus on manual health record analysis.

Although most quantitative health record analysis is performed retrospectively, concurrent inpatient record analysis is possible. Concurrent analysis is more costly to the organization because it requires more time to perform. However, it positively affects patient care and safety when findings are corrected immediately. Another benefit of concurrent quantitative analysis is that content or authentication issues can be addressed before the patient has been discharged, which enhances the timeliness of documentation and the quality of the record. In addition, it is an effective way to ensure that documentation is completed when services are performed.

Deficiencies may be auto-assigned by the EDMS or HIM personnel in the hybrid environment. The EDMS can be configured to present deficiencies in a queue for HIM personnel to review for completeness. HIM personnel assign the deficiency to the appropriate physician for completion. Deficiency types may include missing reports, electronic documents that need editing, scanned documents that need annotating, or missing electronic signatures. After documents are electronically signed, no additional review is required by HIM personnel.

In the EHR, interfacing missing items automatically updates the deficiency from "missing" to "signed." Ideally, electronic systems auto-assign deficiencies based on record completion criteria established by the organization. For example, when the history and physical examination are incomplete or not documented within the established time frame, the system autogenerates a deficiency for the attending physician to complete the required documentation.

During record analysis, missing or incomplete information is identified, and the reviewer can attempt to find the missing documentation. If missing documentation cannot be located, HIM personnel can issue deficiency notifications to the appropriate caregivers.

Deficiency systems may be paper based, computer based, or electronic. A deficiency system is designed to track and report elements of documentation missing from health records. Paper-based deficiency systems use a checklist to indicate missing reports, signatures, consents, and other documentation. (See **Figure 7.9** for an example of a paper-based deficiency slip.) Computer-based deficiency systems provide logs for reporting and tracking health record deficiencies. Deficiencies created in an electronic system are automatically placed in the physician's inbox or work queue. The oldest deficiencies are listed first, but the physician can use the EDMS's sort feature to prioritize deficiencies processing.

FIGURE 7.9. Sample paper-based deficiency slip

Physician/Practitioner's Name: _____
Health Record Number: _____
Patient's Name: _____
Discharge Date: _____
Analyzed by: _____
Date: _____

Signatures Required	Dictation Required	Missing Reports
_____ History	_____ History	_____ History
_____ Physical	_____ Physical	_____ Physical
_____ Consultation	_____ Consultation	_____ Consultation
_____ Operative Report	_____ Operative Report	_____ Operative Report
_____ Discharge Summary	_____ Discharge Summary	_____ Discharge Summary
		_____ Radiology Report
		_____ Pathology Report
Other	Other	_____ Progress Notes
_____ _____	_____ _____	Other
_____ _____	_____ _____	_____ _____
_____ _____	_____ _____	_____ _____
		_____ _____

Most HIM personnel periodically remind physicians to complete their patients' records for past admissions. The value of temporarily identifying deficiencies is that it allows the aggregation of information that can be used for performance improvement and credentialing functions. It plays a role in enforcing medical staff bylaws and hospital policies and thus the accreditation measurement of standards compliance through average health record delinquency rate metrics. Hospitals using an EHR usually achieve single-digit delinquency rates for incomplete records.

Accreditation standards require hospitals to track the number of delinquent health records. The Joint Commission (2006) requires hospitals to monitor the **medical record delinquency rate** at least quarterly. Delinquency statistics data are used during Joint Commission accreditation surveys to show past evidence of compliance with record completion standards. The delinquency rate is calculated by dividing the monthly average number of discharges by the monthly average number of delinquent records.

Qualitative Analysis

The primary goal of qualitative analysis is to ensure that the clinical documentation in the patient's health record meets the criteria for high-quality clinical documentation. As discussed earlier in the chapter, concurrent qualitative analysis is a responsibility of the clinical documentation function. As a result, the terms *qualitative analysis* and *clinical documentation analysis* mean essentially the same thing. Retrospective qualitative analysis is usually performed in the HIM department by coding professionals. To achieve the best outcomes, there should be close collaboration between the clinical documentation specialists and the coding professionals responsible for analyzing the same patient records. For example, a clinical documentation specialist may generate a physician query on the patient record. If the patient is discharged before the physician responds to the query, the coder should be made aware of the clinical documentation specialist's query. The coder can determine when a query has been asked and not answered if an incomplete query form is on the patient's record or an electronic query has not been completed.

Hospitals may establish a reporting structure such as a health records committee or performance improvement manager to receive the results of qualitative analysis. The designated group or person addresses any problems that are identified and implements actions to improve the quality of the health record documentation.

Ongoing Record Review

Ongoing record review is a continuous health record quality review process. Clinical and/or HIM professionals review the records of current inpatients or outpatients to ensure that health records are complete and accurate and that the facility's clinical documentation practices meet relevant accreditation standards, state licensing laws, and federal regulatory requirements. Ongoing record reviews also address quality and patient safety initiatives by improving documentation practices. The Joint Commission (2006) requires review of health records at the point of care. For example, tracking, trending, and reporting data collected about national patient safety goals such as prohibited abbreviations or legibility can produce changes within the organization.

HIM professionals should take the lead to make the review process happen. Providing an automated **data collection** and reporting tool for clinical and HIM departments improves the timeliness of decision making. Hospitals may purchase vendor software or collaborate with their internal information services departments to implement electronic data collection tools. The abilities to customize data collection and provide feedback allow HIM professionals to easily focus on problem-prone areas, implement action plans, and measure progress. Policies and procedures should address the functions of the ongoing record review program and should include the responsibilities of the healthcare staff and other clinical disciplines. The result should be a meaningful ongoing record review plan designed to meet the needs of the organization (Lewis and Reinicke 2005).

See **FIGURES 7.10** and **7.11** for examples of ongoing records review checklists. A sample of an electronic ongoing record review is illustrated in **FIGURE 7.12**.

FIGURE 7.10. Example of an open record review checklist: Initial assessments

Information/Indicator	Record Number	Record Number	Record Number	Record Number	Record Number	Record Number	Record Number
	004303	193847					
1. Nursing unit	11B	12B					
2. Admission date	04/06/20xx	04/06/20xx					
3. Primary physician	Jones	Smith					
4. Was the history and physical report available within 24 hours of the admission?	**No**	Yes					
5. Does the history and physical report include information of the patient's the past history, examination of heart, lungs, and mental status and other body systems related to the condition for which the patient was admitted?	Yes	Yes					
6. Is the nursing initial assessment complete and free of blanks?	Yes	Yes					
7. Was the nursing initial assessment completed within 24 hours of the admission?	Yes	Yes					
8. Was a functional status screen completed when warranted by the patient's condition?	Yes	Yes					
9. Was a nutritional status screen completed when warranted by the patient's condition?	Yes	Yes					
10. Was the need to plan for discharge or transfer determined?	Yes	Yes					
11. Was the patient's level of pain assessed?	Yes	Yes					
12. Did the patient sign the consent to treatment?	Yes	Yes					
13. Was it determined whether the patient had an advance directive?	**No**	Yes					
Comments							

Actions Needed	Who	When Due
Supply missing report of history and physical.	Dr. Jones	04/08/200x

FIGURE 7.11. Example of a closed record review checklist: Discharge summary

Information/Indicator	Record Number 000011	Record Number 000026	Record Number 001000	Record Number 000090	Record Number 000087	Record Number 000560	Record Number 000777
1. Nursing unit	10A	12B	10A	10A	10A	12B	10A
2. Primary physician	Smith	Green	Jones	Smith	Black	White	Jones
3. Discharge date	04/04/20xx	04/04/20xx	04/04/20xx	04/04/20xx	04/04/20xx	04/04/20xx	04/04/20xx
4. Was the discharge summary in the record within 30 days of discharge?	Yes	Yes	Yes	Yes	Yes	Yes	Yes
5. Does the discharge summary include the reason for the patient's hospitalization?	Yes	Yes	Yes	Yes	Yes	Yes	Yes
6. Does the discharge summary include documentation of significant findings?	Yes	Yes	Yes	Yes	Yes	Yes	Yes
7. Does the discharge summary include documentation of all of the procedures performed and the other care, treatment, and services provided?	Yes	Yes	Yes	Yes	Yes	Yes	Yes
8. Does the discharge summary include documentation of the patient's condition at discharge?	Yes	Yes	Yes	**No**	Yes	Yes	Yes
9. Does the discharge summary include documentation of the patient aftercare instructions?	Yes	Yes	Yes	Yes	Yes	Yes	Yes
10. Is the discharge summary readable, complete, and free of blanks?	Yes	Yes	Yes	Yes	Yes	Yes	Yes
11. Is the discharge summary free of abbreviations from the prohibited list?	**No**	Yes	Yes	Yes	Yes	Yes	Yes
12. Is the discharge summary signed and dated by the author or otherwise authenticated?	Yes	Yes	Yes	Yes	Yes	Yes	Yes
Comments	Trend						

Actions Needed	Who	When Due
Send Dr. Smith another reminder about the use of prohibited abbreviations from the JCAHO list, specifically SO4.	Tilly	Today
Ask Dr. Smith to add specific information about the patient's condition at discharge.	Dr. Smith	04/10/200x

FIGURE 7.12. Sample electronic open health records review form

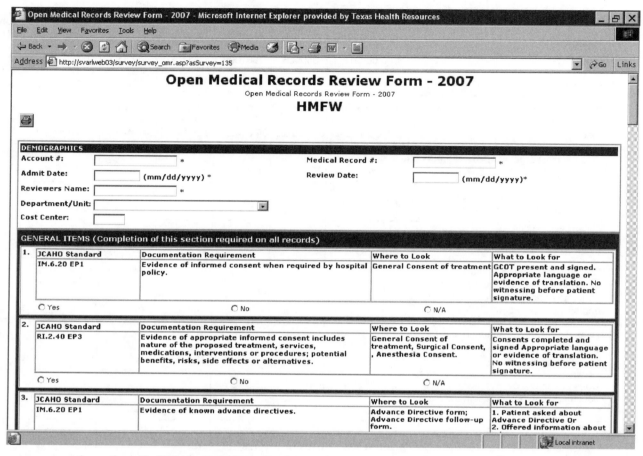

Source: Texas Health Resources 2007.

Summary

High-quality clinical documentation is necessary for every healthcare organization. To achieve high-quality clinical documentation on a national level, healthcare providers must use a standardized set of guidelines and definitions. In this chapter, we reviewed a theory of high-quality clinical documentation supported by evidence-based research.

Coding is the act of translating physician clinical documentation into diagnostic and procedural coded data. It is essentially another language—a language that allows the diagnostic, treatment, and response information of the patient to be aggregated into a uniform data set. This efficient aggregation of millions of pages of clinical documentation enables the analysis of health record information for research, planning, billing, and patient-care purposes. High-quality clinical documentation is needed to produce high-quality coded data.

It may be helpful for clinical documentation professionals and other clinicians to understand how a coding professional views a health record. Documentation professionals can use this understanding to guide their review and query process. It is also helpful for documentation professionals to understand the complexity of both the ICD-9-CM coding system and the official coding guidelines. The level of detail required by the coding system is one reason such detail is needed in clinical documentation.

HIM professionals' role in healthcare settings has advanced from ensuring compliance with documentation requirements to developing and implementing best practices and processes that help support clinical staff to create accurate documentation and complete it in a timely manner. During the process of health record analysis, HIM professionals identify deficiencies in health records that range from authentication to missing documentation. Organizations use data documented in the health record to improve quality of care and patient safety.

References

AHIMA. 2008a. Standards of Ethical Coding. http://library.ahima.org/xpedio/groups/public/documents/ahima/bok2_001166.hcsp?dDocName=bok2_001166.

AHIMA. 2008b. Managing an Effective Query Process. *Journal of AHIMA* 79(10):83–88.

American Hospital Directory (AHD). 2008. *American Hospital Directory.* http://www.ahd.com.

American Medical Association (AMA). n.d. Physician Compliance: Federal fraud enforcement—physician compliance planning. http://www.ama-assn.org/ama/pub/physician-resources/legal-topics/regulatory-compliance-topics/health-care-fraud-abuse/federal-fraud-enforcement-physician-compliance/compliance-planning/physician-compliance.page.

Centers for Medicare and Medicaid Services (CMS). 2008. Public Quality Indicator and Resident Reports. http://www.cms.hhs.gov/MDSPubQIandResRep.

Centers for Medicare and Medicaid Services (CMS) and the National Center for Health Statistics (NCHS). 2007. *ICD-9-CM Coding Book.* Washington, DC: Government Printing Office.

Coffman-Kadish, N. 2002. Health Record Analysis. In *Health Information Management: Principles and Organization for Health Information Services,* 5th ed., edited by M. Skurka. San Francisco: Jossey-Bass.

Drucker, P. 1999. Knowledge Worker Productivity: The Biggest Challenge. *California Management Review* 41(2):83–94.

HealthGrades. 2011. Hospital Quality Report. http://www.healthgrades.com/consumer/index.cfm?fuseaction=modnw&modtype=content&modact=SHOP_HospQual_Example.

The Joint Commission. 2006. *2010 Accreditation Process Guide for Hospitals*; Oakbrook Terrace, IL: The Joint Commission.

Lewis, S., and S. Reinicke. 2005. To Review or Not to Review: Finding the Solution for Ongoing Record Review. Proceedings of the AHIMA 77th National Convention and Exhibit. San Diego, CA.

Pennsylvania Health Care Cost Containment Council (PHCCC). 2006. Cardiac Surgery in Pennsylvania 2005–2006. http://www.phc4.org/reports/cabg/06/docs/cabg2006keyfindings.pdf.

Reynolds, R. B., and E. D. Bowman. 2010. Paper-based and Hybrid Health Records. Chapter 8 in *Health Information Management: Concepts, Principles, and Practice,* 3rd ed., edited by K. LaTour and S. Eichenwald Maki. Chicago: AHIMA.

Russo, R. 2007. Improving Self-Efficacy and Organizational Performance: Identifying the Differences That May Exist from Educational Interventions Crafted to Utilize Two Versus All Four Self-Efficacy Constructs. Dissertation. Cypress, CA: Touro University International.

Russo, R., and S. Fitzgerald. 2008. Physician Clinical Documentation: Implications for Healthcare Quality and Cost. Academy of Management Annual Meeting. Anaheim, CA.

Texas Health Resources. 2007. *Open Medical Records Review Form.* Arlington, TX: Texas Health Resources.

PART III

Organization and Management
of the Health Record

Chapter 8

Federal and State Requirements and Accreditation Guidelines

Ruthann Russo, PhD, JD, MPH, RHIT

Learning Objectives

- List and explain accreditation and licensure requirements that apply to acute care health records

- Differentiate a statute from a regulation

- List and explain the documentation standards in the Medicare Conditions of Participation for Hospitals

- Explain the purpose of Centers for Medicare and Medicaid Services (CMS) quality measures and provide examples

- Identify the five elements of a healthcare corporate compliance program

- Explain the purpose of the Office of the Inspector General's (OIG) compliance guidance and annual work plan

- List the functions of the Office of the National Coordinator for Health Information Technology (ONCHIT)

- Describe the basic hospital licensure process

- Clarify the concept of deemed status

- Identify the difference between regulatory standards and accreditation standards

- Describe The Joint Commission's accreditation process

- Define The Joint Commission's sentinel event policy

- Explain the purpose of tracer methodology

- Briefly describe the American Osteopathic Association's (AOA) Healthcare Facilities Accreditation Process (HFAP)

- Describe the purpose of developing health record policies and procedures and explain the difference between a policy and a procedure

Key Terms

Accreditation

Accreditation organizations

American Osteopathic Association (AOA)

Board certification

Centers for Medicare and Medicaid Services (CMS)

CMS quality measures

Code of Federal Regulations (CFR)

Compliance guidance

Conditions of Participation (COP) for Hospitals

Credentialing

Deemed status

Federal Register

Healthcare Facilities Accreditation Program (HFAP)

Health Information Technology for Economic and Clinical Health (HITECH) Act

Health Insurance Portability and Accountability Act (HIPAA)

Individual-based system tracer activity

Individual tracer activity

The Joint Commission

Licensure

Medical staff bylaws, rules, and regulations

National Committee for Quality Assurance (NCQA)

Office of the Inspector General (OIG)

Office of the National Coordinator for Health Information Technology (ONCHIT)

ORYX

Periodic performance review (PPR)

Policy

Priority focus area (PFA)

Priority focus process (PFP)

Procedure

Protected health information (PHI)

Recovery audit contractor (RAC)

Regulation

Sentinel event

Statute

Tracer methodology

Unannounced survey

Introduction

Chapters 1 through 7 addressed accreditation, regulation, and licensure standards as they apply to health record content and maintenance. This chapter examines in detail federal and state requirements and accreditation guidelines for acute care hospitals. Requirements may include laws, administrative regulations, and guidance. Federal regulations applicable to acute care hospitals in the United States are managed by the Department of Health and Human Services (HHS). Within HHS, the **Centers for Medicare and Medicaid Services (CMS)** manages all regulations that apply to reimbursement for care provided to Medicare and Medicaid recipients. Licensure refers to state laws that govern the operation of healthcare providers, and accreditation refers to voluntary standards of accrediting agencies such as The Joint Commission.

Mandatory federal and state requirements for acute care hospitals will be addressed first, followed by voluntary accreditation guidelines. Finally, hospital-specific policies and procedures are discussed. Although accreditation is voluntary for acute care hospitals, most hospitals today elect to be accredited by The Joint Commission. Federal requirements for acute care hospitals include three levels: laws, regulations, and guidelines. Each level is addressed separately.

Many federal laws apply to healthcare providers. This chapter addresses those laws that apply to acute care hospitals and have specific relevance for health information professionals. Examples include the **Health Insurance Portability and Accountability Act (HIPAA)** and the **Health Information Technology for Economic and Clinical Health (HITECH)** Act.

Federal regulations are also addressed. Medicare is the federal government–sponsored health plan, and Medicaid is the health plan cosponsored by the federal and state governments. Together, Medicare and Medicaid are the largest single health insurer in the United States, accounting for about 37 percent of payments to healthcare providers (HHS 2008). Hospitals that provide services to Medicare or Medicaid recipients must meet the regulations administered by the CMS.

Health information management (HIM) professionals need to be familiar with the **compliance guidance** for hospitals published by the **Office of the Inspector General (OIG)**, addressed in the section on healthcare compliance. Although the OIG's guidance is not mandatory, most hospitals follow it closely to avoid fines, penalties, and possible exclusion from the Medicare program.

States require every hospital operating within their borders to maintain a current and valid license to provide healthcare services to patients. Each state has its own licensing laws, but most contain similar provisions. State licensure is addressed generally, and examples of some state licensing statutes are provided. State compliance programs are also addressed.

Most hospitals in the United States are accredited by either The Joint Commission or the **American Osteopathic Association (AOA)**. Accreditation, by these organizations is voluntary, but most hospitals seek accreditation because it can be used as evidence to patients of the quality and safety of care provided. Accreditation standards for hospitals are addressed generally, and standards for health record content and maintenance are addressed in detail.

Hospital internal policies and procedures are also addressed. Regulation, licensing, and accreditation standards all require hospital-specific policies and procedures to be developed and updated in certain areas. Each hospital's location, services, and organizational structure are unique. Therefore, each hospital must design and follow its own operating policies and procedures to ensure that its services and health records fulfill all of the applicable standards and regulations. Regulatory and accreditation agencies rely heavily on the information documented in health records to determine whether patient-care standards are being met.

Federal and State Requirements

The mandatory rules that apply to hospitals and other healthcare organizations come from several different sources:

- Federal statutes and regulations, which apply throughout the United States

- State statutes and regulations, which apply only within individual states

- County and municipal ordinances and codes, which apply only to local communities

A **statute** is a piece of legislation written and approved by a state or federal legislature and then signed into law by the state's governor or the president. HIPAA is an example of a federal statute.

A **regulation** is a rule established by an administrative agency of government. Regulations have the same effect as legislation. Failure to abide by regulations or statutes results in fines and/or disciplinary action.

Acute care hospitals must meet additional requirements, such as the following:

- State licensure requirements

- State public health regulations

- County and municipal building safety codes

- Legal doctrines of medical liability based on judicial decisions

- HITECH Act provisions of the American Recovery and Reinvestment Act of 2009 (ARRA)

- Occupational Safety and Health Administration (OSHA) guidelines

FIGURE 8.1 illustrates the steps involved in creating a regulation and a statute. While both are mandatory and carry the same legal effect, regulations are generally less

FIGURE 8.1. Creating federal regulations and statutes

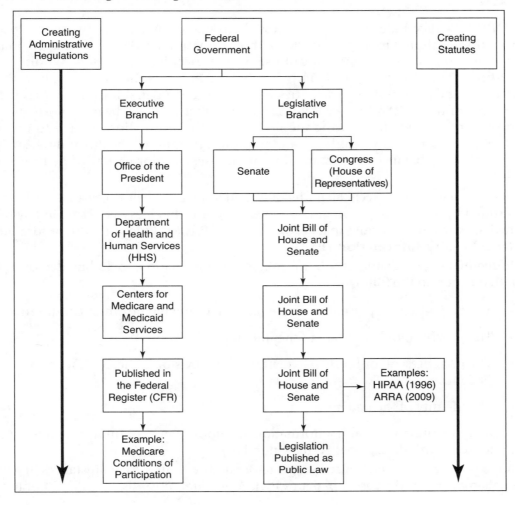

cumbersome to enact because they do not require a majority vote of Congress and the Senate. Healthcare providers must abide by both federal and state laws. However, when a state law and federal law regarding the same topic differ, the healthcare provider must apply the stricter of the two laws. For example, if a federal law requires maintaining documentation for seven years and the state law requires ten years, then the healthcare provider must maintain documentation for ten years—the stricter of the two requirements.

State and federal regulations, national accreditation standards, and clinical practice standards are created, updated, and changed frequently. Therefore, HIM professionals must routinely review the sources of regulations and standards. Although this chapter cannot describe all of the requirements that acute care records must fulfill, it will provide a starting point for health record policy and procedure development.

Federal Healthcare Statutes

Many federal statutes apply to acute care hospitals. In this section, we will address three statutes that have significant implications for acute care hospitals and HIM professionals: HIPAA, the HITECH Act, and the federal patient safety legislation.

HIPAA

The HIPAA Privacy Rule standards address the use and disclosure of patients' health information—referred to as protected health information (PHI)—as well as standards for patients to understand and control use of their health information. Within HHS, the Office for Civil Rights (OCR) implements and enforces the Privacy Rule with respect to voluntary compliance activities and civil money penalties (HHS 2011c). The major goal of the HIPAA Privacy Rule is to ensure that patients' health information is properly protected while allowing the flow of health information needed to provide and promote high-quality healthcare and to protect the public's health and well-being. The rule strikes a balance that permits important uses of information while protecting patient privacy.

The Privacy Rule protects all individually identifiable health information held or transmitted by a hospital (or other covered entity) or its business associate, in any form or media, whether electronic, paper, or oral. The Privacy Rule calls this information **protected health information (PHI).**

Individually identifiable health information is information, including demographic data, that relates to the following:

- The patient's past, present or future physical or mental health or condition

- The provision of healthcare to the individual

- The past, present, or future payment for the provision of health care to the patient

- The identity of the patient

Individually identifiable health information includes many common identifiers (e.g., name, address, birth date, Social Security number).

A major purpose of the Privacy Rule is to define and limit the circumstances in which hospitals may use or disclose a patient's PHI. A hospital must disclose PHI in only two situations: (a) to individuals (or their personal representatives) when they request access to their PHI and (b) to HHS when it is undertaking a compliance investigation or a review or enforcement action.

Permitted Uses and Disclosures

A hospital is permitted, but not required, to use and disclose PHI, without an individual's authorization for the following purposes or situations: (1) to the patient; (2) for treatment, payment, and healthcare operations; (3) to give patients opportunity to agree or object; (4) incident to an otherwise permitted use and disclosure; (5) for public interest and benefit activities; and (6) as part of a limited data set for the purposes of research, public health, or health care operations. Each of these permitted uses are described in the following paragraphs. (HHS 2011c).

1. **To the patient.** A hospital may disclose PHI to the patient who is the subject of the information.

2. **Treatment, payment, healthcare operations.** A hospital may use and disclose PHI for its own treatment, payment, and healthcare operations activities. Treatment is the provision, coordination, or management of healthcare and related services for a patient by one or more healthcare providers, including consultation between providers regarding a patient and referral of a patient by one provider to another. Payment encompasses a health plan's activities to obtain premiums, determine or fulfill responsibilities for coverage and provision of benefits, and furnish or obtain reimbursement for healthcare delivered to a patient and a healthcare provider's activities to obtain payment or be reimbursed for the provision of healthcare to a patient. Healthcare operations are any of the following activities: (a) quality assessment and improvement activities, including case management and care coordination; (b) competency assurance activities, including provider or health plan performance evaluation, **credentialing**, and accreditation; (c) conduct or arrangements for medical reviews, audits, or legal services, including fraud and abuse detection and compliance programs; (d) specified insurance functions, such as underwriting, risk rating, and reinsuring risk; (e) business planning, development, management, and administration; and (f) business management and general administrative activities of the entity.

3. **Uses and disclosures with opportunity to agree or object.** Informal permission may be obtained by asking the patient outright or in circumstances that clearly give the patient the opportunity to agree, acquiesce, or object. If the patient is incapacitated, in an emergency situation, or not available, the hospital may make such uses and disclosures if, in the exercise of their professional judgment, the use or disclosure is determined to be in the best interests of the patient.

   Facility directories. Maintaining a directory of patient contact information is a common practice in hospitals. Hospitals may rely on a patient's informal permission to list in its facility directory the patient's name, general condition, religious affiliation, and location in the provider's facility. The provider may then disclose the patient's condition and location in the facility to anyone asking for the patient by name and may also disclose religious affiliation to clergy. Members of the clergy are not required to ask for the patient by name when inquiring about patient religious affiliation.

For notification and other purposes. A hospital may rely on a patient's informal permission to disclose to the patient's family, relatives, or friends, or to other persons whom the patient identifies, PHI directly relevant to that person's involvement in the patient's care or payment for care. This provision, for example, allows a pharmacist to dispense filled prescriptions to a person acting on behalf of the patient.

4. **Incidental use and disclosure.** The Privacy Rule does not require that every risk of an incidental use or disclosure of PHI be eliminated. A use or disclosure of this information that occurs as a result of, or as "incident to," an otherwise permitted use or disclosure is permitted as long as the covered entity has adopted reasonable safeguards as required by the Privacy Rule, and the information being shared was limited to the "minimum necessary," as required by the Privacy Rule.

5. **Public interest and benefit activities.** The Privacy Rule permits use and disclosure of PHI without a patient's authorization or permission for 12 national priority purposes (see **FIGURE 8.2**). These 12 purposes are:

Required by law. Hospitals may use and disclose PHI without individual authorization as required by law (including by statute, regulation, or court orders).

Public health activities. Hospitals may disclose PHI to (1) public health authorities authorized by law to collect or receive such information to prevent or control disease, injury, or disability and to public health or other government authorities authorized to receive reports of child abuse and neglect; (2) entities subject to Food and Drug Administration (FDA) regulation regarding FDA-regulated products or activities for purposes such as adverse event reporting, tracking of products, product recalls, and post-marketing surveillance; (3) individuals who may have contracted or been exposed to a communicable disease when notification is authorized by law; and (4) employers, regarding employees, when requested by employers, for information concerning a work-related illness or injury or workplace-related medical surveillance, because such information is needed by the employer to comply with OSHA, the Mine Safety and Health Administration, or similar state law.

Victims of abuse, neglect, or domestic violence. In certain circumstances, hospitals may disclose PHI to appropriate government authorities regarding victims of abuse, neglect, or domestic violence.

Health oversight activities. Hospitals may disclose PHI to health oversight agencies (as defined in the rule) for purposes of legally authorized health oversight activities, such as audits and investigations necessary for oversight of the healthcare system and government benefit programs.

Judicial and administrative proceedings. Hospitals may disclose PHI in a judicial or administrative proceeding if the request for the information is through an order from a court or administrative tribunal. Such information may also be disclosed in response to a subpoena or other lawful process if certain assurances regarding notice to the individual or a protective order are provided.

Law enforcement purposes. Hospitals may disclose PHI to law enforcement officials for law enforcement purposes under the following six circumstances, and subject to specified conditions: (1) as required by law (including court orders, court-ordered warrants, subpoenas), and administrative requests; (2) to identify or locate a suspect, fugitive, material witness, or missing person; (3) in response to a law enforcement official's request for information about a victim or suspected victim of a crime; (4) to alert law enforcement of a person's death, if the covered entity suspects that criminal activity caused the death; (5) when a covered entity believes PHI is evidence of a crime that occurred on its premises; and (6) by a covered healthcare provider in a medical emergency not occurring on its premises, when necessary to inform law enforcement about the commission and nature of a crime, the location of the crime or crime victims, and the perpetrator of the crime.

Decedents. Hospitals may disclose PHI to funeral directors as needed, and to coroners or medical examiners to identify a deceased person, determine the cause of death, and perform other functions authorized by law.

Cadaveric organ, eye, or tissue donation. Hospitals may use or disclose PHI to facilitate the donation and transplantation of cadaveric organs, eyes, and tissue.

Research. Research is any systematic investigation designed to develop or contribute to generalizable knowledge. The Privacy Rule permits a hospital to use and disclose PHI for research purposes without an individual's authorization, provided the covered entity obtains certain specified waivers.

Serious threat to health or safety. Hospitals may disclose PHI that they believe is necessary to prevent or lessen a serious and imminent threat to a person or the public, when such disclosure is made to someone they believe can prevent or lessen the threat (including the target of the threat).

Essential government functions. An authorization is not required to use or disclose PHI for certain essential government functions.

Workers' compensation. Hospitals may disclose PHI as authorized by, and to comply with, workers' compensation laws and other similar programs providing benefits for work-related injuries or illnesses.

6. **Limited data set.** A limited data set is PHI from which certain specified direct identifiers of individuals and their relatives, household members, and employers have been removed. A limited data set may be used and disclosed for research, healthcare operations, and public health purposes, provided the recipient enters into a data use agreement promising specified safeguards for the PHI within the limited data set.

Figure 8.2 lists the 12 national priority purposes that permit the use and disclosure of PHI without a patient's authorization or permission.

FIGURE 8.2. **Disclosure of PHI permitted without a patient's authorization**

1. Required by law	7. Decedents
2. Public health activities	8. Cadaveric organ, eye, or tissue donation
3. Victims of abuse, neglect, or domestic violence	9. Research
4. Health oversight activities	10. Serious threat to health or safety
5. Judicial and administrative proceedings	11. Essential government functions
6. Law enforcement purposes	12. Workers' compensation

HITECH Act

The HITECH Act gives HHS the authority to promulgate regulations and guidance to support the development of an interoperable, private, and secure nationwide health information technology (IT) infrastructure. The **Office of the National Coordinator for Health Information Technology (ONCHIT)** is responsible for administering the HITECH Act. The functions of the ONCHIT are

- Promoting development of a nationwide health IT infrastructure that allows for electronic use and exchange of information that
  - Ensures secure and protected patient health information
  - Improves healthcare quality
  - Reduces healthcare costs
  - Informs medical decisions at the time/place of care
  - Includes meaningful public input on infrastructure development
  - Improves coordination of care and information among hospitals, labs, physicians, and the like.
  - Improves public health activities and facilitates early identification of and rapid response to public health emergencies
  - Facilitates health and clinical research
  - Promotes early detection, prevention, and management of chronic diseases
  - Promotes a more effective marketplace
  - Improves efforts to reduce health disparities
- Providing leadership in the development, recognition, and implementation of standards and the certification of Health IT products
- Coordinating health IT policy
- Overseeing strategic planning for Health IT adoption and health information exchange
- Establishing governance for the Nationwide Health Information Network

The overriding goal of the HITECH Act is to improve the quality of patient care while simultaneously decreasing healthcare costs. The specific objective of the HITECH Act is to ensure that healthcare providers have

- Accurate and complete information about patient's health to provide the best possible care
- The ability to better coordinate care
- A way to securely share information with patients and their family caregivers over the Internet, which allows patients and their families to be more proactive about their healthcare

- Information to help doctors diagnose health problems sooner, reduce medical errors, and provide safer care at lower costs

The HITECH Act addresses five primary areas:

1. **Standards and Certification**
   a. Standards and certification criteria for electronic health records (EHRs) assure eligible professionals and hospitals that the systems they adopt are capable of performing the required functions
   b. Certification programs provide a defined process to ensure that EHR technologies meet the adopted standards, certification criteria, and other technical requirements to achieve meaningful use of those records in systems.

2. **Meaningful Use**

   ARRA authorizes CMS to provide reimbursement incentives for eligible professionals and hospitals who succeed in becoming "meaningful users" of certified EHR technology.

3. **Privacy and Security**
   a. Modifications to the HIPAA Privacy, Security, and Enforcement Rules under the HITECH Act give patients the right to receive their medical information electronically and set new limits on the use of PHI.
   b. The HITECH Breach Notification Interim Final Rule includes guidance specifying encryption and destruction as the technologies and methodologies that render PHI unusable, unreadable, or indecipherable to unauthorized individuals.
   c. The Substance Abuse Confidentiality Regulations FAQs serve as a resource for practitioners in the field, as they apply the Substance Abuse Confidentiality Regulations to health information exchange activities but do not provide legal advice to its user.

4. **Electronic Eligibility and Enrollment**

5. **Electronic Prescriptions for Controlled Substances**

The regulations will also permit pharmacies to receive, dispense, and archive these electronic prescriptions.

Federal Patient Safety Legislation

In July 2004, the US Senate passed the Patient Safety and Quality Improvement Act, which was signed into law on July 29 of that year. This legislation creates a confidential and voluntary system for reporting medical errors. The overall goal of the national reporting system is to improve patient safety and reduce the number of medical errors nationwide. In addition, the Patient Safety Act

- Encourages the development of patient safety organizations (PSOs)—organizations that can work with clinicians and healthcare organizations to identify, analyze, and reduce the risks and hazards associated with patient care. PSOs are organizations to which hospitals, doctors, and other healthcare providers may voluntarily report information about patient safety events on a privileged and confidential basis.

- Fosters a culture of safety by establishing strong federal confidentiality and privilege protections for information assembled and developed by provider organizations, physicians, and other clinicians for deliberations and analyses regarding quality and safety.

- Accelerates the speed with which solutions can be identified for the risks and hazards associated with patient care by facilitating the aggregation of a sufficient number of events in a protected legal environment (HHS 2011b).

Eight patient safety activities are carried out by, or on behalf of, a PSO or a healthcare provider (HHS 2011b).

1. Efforts to improve patient safety and the quality of healthcare delivery

2. The collection and analysis of patient safety work product (PSWP)

3. The development and dissemination of information regarding patient safety, such as recommendations, protocols, or information regarding best practices

4. The utilization of PSWP for the purposes of encouraging a culture of safety as well as providing feedback and assistance to effectively minimize patient risk

5. The maintenance of procedures to preserve confidentiality with respect to PSWP

6. The provision of appropriate security measures with respect to PSWP

7. The utilization of qualified staff

8. Activities related to the operation of a patient safety evaluation system and to the provision of feedback to participants in a patient safety evaluation system

CMS Regulations

In 1965, amendments to the Social Security Act of 1935 established the Medicare and Medicaid programs. Federal healthcare programs were originally administered by the US Department of Health, Education, and Welfare (now HHS).The Health Care Financing Administration (HCFA, now CMS), was established in 1977 to coordinate Medicare and Medicaid benefits on the federal level. Medicare provides health insurance to individuals 65 years of age and older, certain individuals with end-stage renal disease, disabled individuals, and individuals who have collected Social Security or disability for at least 24 months (Medicare 2011). Medicare benefits are divided into four parts known as Medicare A, B, C, and D. Medicare Part A is hospital insurance that helps cover inpatient care in hospitals and skilled nursing facility, hospice, and home health care. Part B helps cover medically necessary services such as doctors' services, outpatient care, home health services, and other medical services. Part B also covers some preventive services. Part C is also known as a Medicare Advantage Plan. Part C plans are offered by private companies approved by Medicare that provide all of a patient's Part A and Part B coverage. Medicare Part D provides coverage for prescription drugs.

Medicaid provides health insurance predominantly to individuals with limited financial means and most children under the age of 18 who have no other health insurance. In the case of Medicaid, each state determines eligibility for residents of that state. Together, the Medicare and Medicaid health insurance programs cover 37 percent of Americans (HHS 2008). The health records of Medicare beneficiaries are subject to federal Medicare regulations and policies. Likewise, the records of Medicaid beneficiaries must fulfill the requirements of state medical assistance programs. Like other third-party payers, state Medicaid agencies and Medicare fiscal intermediaries may request information from patient records to support reimbursement of claims. More details about Medicaid eligibility and administration are provided in the following section on state requirements.

Medicare Conditions of Participation

Hospitals supply services to Medicare beneficiaries under contractual arrangements with HHS. To qualify for Medicare participation, hospitals must meet Medicare **Conditions of Participation (COP) for Hospitals** (2010). To treat Medicare patients and receive payment for those services, healthcare providers must comply with the COP for hospitals. Providers in other specialty areas, such as long-term care or ambulatory healthcare services, are required to follow the COP that apply specifically to them.

The Medicare COP for Hospitals are published under title 42, part 482, of the **Code of Federal Regulations (CFR)**. The CFR is updated whenever statutes or regulations are added or changed. Final changes and updates and proposed changes and updates are also published in the *Federal Register*, a daily publication of the US Government Printing Office. Up-to-date information is also available in other print and online resources provided by the Government Printing Office. HIM professionals are advised to check the *Federal Register* for the most current version of the Medicare COP for Hospitals, available online at www.gpoaccess.gov/fr.

Section 482.24 of the Medicare COP (2010) lists the requirements for medical record services in a hospital. **Figure 8.3** lists current COP for health record services for acute care hospitals.

Medicare COP (2010) section 482.13 requires hospitals to protect the personal and medical rights of patients. This section of the regulation lists the patients' rights provisions of the Medicare program. It also requires hospitals to provide a notice of rights to patients or their legal representatives, as follows:

1. A notice of the rights of patients must be provided to patients or their legal representatives, and the notice should be furnished in advance of providing or discontinuing services whenever possible.

2. The notice must describe the facility's procedures for receiving and resolving patients' grievances.

FIGURE 8.3. Current Medicare Conditions of Participation for acute care hospitals

---

§482.24 Condition of participation: Medical record services.

The hospital must have a medical record service that has administrative responsibility for medical records. A medical record must be maintained for every individual evaluated or treated in the hospital.

a. **Standard:** Organization and staffing. The organization of the medical record service must be appropriate to the scope and complexity of the services performed. The hospital must employ adequate personnel to ensure prompt completion, filing, and retrieval of records.

b. **Standard:** Form and retention of record. The hospital must maintain a medical record for each inpatient and outpatient. Medical records must be accurately written, promptly completed, properly filed and retained, and accessible. The hospital must use a system of author identification and record maintenance that ensures the integrity of the authentication and protects the security of all record entries.

   1. Medical records must be retained in their original or legally reproduced form for a period of at least 5 years.

   2. The hospital must have a system of coding and indexing medical records. The system must allow for timely retrieval by diagnosis and procedure, in order to support medical care evaluation studies.

   3. The hospital must have a procedure for ensuring the confidentiality of patient records. Information from or copies of records may be released only to authorized individuals, and the hospital must ensure that unauthorized individuals cannot gain access to or alter patient records. Original medical records must be released by the hospital only in accordance with federal or state laws, court orders, or subpoenas.

c. **Standard:** Content of record. The medical record must contain information to justify admission and continued hospitalization, support the diagnosis, and describe the patient's progress and response to medications and services.

   1. All patient medical record entries must be legible, complete, dated, timed, and authenticated in written or electronic form by the person responsible for providing or evaluating the service provided, consistent with hospital policies and procedures.

      i. All orders, including verbal orders, must be dated, timed, and authenticated promptly by the ordering practitioner, except as noted in paragraph (c)(1)(ii) of this section.

      ii. For the 5-year period following January 26, 2007, all orders, including verbal orders, must be dated, timed, and authenticated by the ordering practitioner or another practitioner who is responsible for the care of the patient as specified under § 482.12(c) and authorized to write orders by hospital policy in accordance with state law.

      iii. All verbal orders must be authenticated based upon federal and state law. If there is no state law that designates a specific timeframe for the authentication of verbal orders, verbal orders must be authenticated within 48 hours.

   2. All records must document the following, as appropriate:

      i. Evidence of

         A. A medical history and physical examination completed and documented no more than 30 days before or 24 hours after admission or registration, but prior to surgery or a procedure requiring anesthesia services. The medical history and physical examination must be placed in the patient's medical record within 24 hours after admission or registration, but prior to surgery or a procedure requiring anesthesia services.

         B. An updated examination of the patient, including any changes in the patient's condition, when the medical history and physical examination are completed within 30 days before admission or registration. Documentation of the updated examination must be placed in the patient's medical record within 24 hours after admission or registration, but prior to surgery or a procedure requiring anesthesia services.

      ii. Admitting diagnosis.

      iii. Results of all consultative evaluations of the patient and appropriate findings by clinical and other staff involved in the care of the patient.

      iv. Documentation of complications, hospital-acquired infections, and unfavorable reactions to drugs and anesthesia.

FIGURE 8.3. (Continued)

> v. Properly executed informed consent forms for procedures and treatments specified by the medical staff, or by federal or state law if applicable, to require written patient consent.
>
> vi. All practitioners' orders, nursing notes, reports of treatment, medication records, radiology and laboratory reports, and vital signs and other information necessary to monitor the patient's condition.
>
> vii. Discharge summary with outcome of hospitalization, disposition of case, and provisions for follow-up care.
>
> viii. Final diagnosis with completion of medical records within 30 days following discharge.

Source: CMS 2010.

3. The patient's rights notice must include the following provisions (42 CFR Section 482.13):

    a. The patient's right to participate in the development and implementation of his care plan

    b. The patient's right to accept or refuse treatment

    c. The patient's right to formulate advance directives and expect caregivers to follow those directives

    d. The patient's right to have a family member or personal representative as well as her personal physician notified promptly of her hospital admission

    e. The patient's right to personal privacy and safety

    f. The patient's right to be free from all forms of abuse and harassment

    g. The patient's right to the confidentiality of his clinical records

    h. The patient's right to access her clinical records within a reasonable time frame

    i. The patient's right to be free from restraints of any form (physical or chemical) that are not medically necessary and established by a physician's order (specifically, to be free of restraints applied as a means of coercion, discipline, convenience, or retaliation by staff)

The hospital should ask patients or their representatives to sign acknowledgment forms to document the fact that information about patient's rights was provided.

Several other sections of the Medicare COP for hospitals (2010) also include documentation requirements. These sections can be summarized as follows:

- *Section 482.22, Medical Staff:* The hospital must have a system for documenting the family's (or legal representative's) permission to perform an autopsy on a patient who died while under the hospital's care.

- *Section 482.23, Nursing Services:* (1) A registered nurse must supervise and ensure the documentation, development, and maintenance of a care plan for every patient. (2) All orders for drugs and biologicals must be made in writing and signed by the physician responsible for the patient's care. (3) Telephone and verbal orders must be accepted only by personnel authorized by medical staff rules, consistent with applicable state and federal regulations. (4) Telephone and verbal orders must be signed, dated, and timed by the prescribing practitioner within 48 hours. (5) The hospital must have a procedure in place for reporting transfusion reactions, adverse drug reactions, and medication errors.

- *Section 482.26, Radiology Services:* (1) The radiologist responsible for interpreting diagnostic images must authenticate the reports of her findings. (2) The hospital must maintain records of radiology procedures, consultations, and interpretations for at least five years.

- *Section 482.27, Laboratory Services:* The hospital must have a system in place for notifying patients who may have been exposed to infectious diseases through contaminated blood transfusions.

- *Section 482.43, Discharge Planning:* (1) Hospital personnel must complete a discharge evaluation for every patient who is likely to require posthospital services. (2) The discharge evaluation and plan must be completed in time to avoid unnecessary delays in arranging posthospital services. (3) The discharge plan must be documented in the patient's health record.

- *Section 482.51, Surgical Services:* (1) A complete history and physical must be documented in the patient's health record before surgery begins, except in emergencies. (2) A fully executed consent form must be placed in the patient's health record before surgery begins, except in emergencies. (3) The operating room register must be complete and up to date. (4) An operative report that describes surgical techniques, surgical findings, and any tissues removed or altered must be written or dictated and authenticated by the surgeon immediately following surgery.

- *Section 482.52, Anesthesia Services:* (1) A preanesthesia patient evaluation must be performed and documented no more than 48 hours before surgery. (2) An intraoperative record must be maintained while the procedure is in progress. (3) For inpatients, a postanesthesia follow-up report must be written within 48 hours after surgery. (4) For outpatients, a postanesthesia evaluation must be performed and documented according to medical staff policy.

- *Section 482, Nuclear Medicine Services:* (1) The practitioner approved by the medical staff to interpret the results of diagnostic procedures that use nuclear materials must sign and date the reports of her interpretation of the findings. (2) The hospital must maintain records of nuclear medicine procedures, consultations, and interpretations for at least five years.

Medicare Compliance Surveys

For a healthcare organization to participate in and receive payment from Medicare or Medicaid, it must meet the eligibility requirements for program participation, including a certification of compliance with the COP, or standards, set forth in federal regulations. Certification of hospital compliance with the COP is accomplished through observations, interviews, and document/record reviews. The survey process focuses on a hospital's performance of patient-focused and organizational functions and processes. The hospital survey is used to assess compliance with federal health, safety, and quality standards that will ensure that the beneficiary receives safe, quality care and services.

This certification is based on a survey conducted by a state agency on behalf of CMS. However, if a national accrediting organization, such as The Joint Commission, has and enforces standards that meet or exceed Medicare requirements, CMS may grant the accrediting organization deeming authority and deem each accredited healthcare organization as meeting Medicare and Medicaid certification requirements. The healthcare organization would then have deemed status and would not be subject to Medicare's routine survey and certification process (Joint Commission 2010).

Hospitals accredited through The Joint Commission's Hospital Accreditation Program or the AOA's **Healthcare Facilities Accreditation Program (HFAP)** may participate in Medicare because the accrediting agency has been granted deemed status by the Medicare program. **Deemed status** means accrediting bodies such as The Joint Commission or AOA can survey facilities for compliance with the Medicare COP in place of of the government.

Seeking deemed status through accreditation is an option, not a requirement. Organizations seeking Medicare approval may choose to be surveyed either by an accrediting body, such as The Joint Commission or the AOA, or by a state agency on behalf of CMS. All surveys for Medicare certification are unannounced, whether they are performed by a state agency, The Joint Commission, or another CMS-approved accrediting body.

Medicare/Medicaid certification programs are conducted by state licensure agencies working under contract with CMS. Hospitals must undergo Medicare and Medicaid certification surveys annually if they do not qualify for deemed status. Such facilities may have chosen not to participate in one of the accreditation programs, or they may have lost their accreditation temporarily because of compliance deficiencies.

CMS Quality Measures

HHS first introduced CMS quality measures in 2001 as the department's commitment to ensure quality healthcare for all Americans through published consumer information. Since then, CMS has joined forces with The Joint Commission and the National Quality Forum (NQF) to create validated clinical measures for hospital inpatient cases. Since 2003, these three organizations have combined their data collection efforts to create a common set of measures published as the *Specifications Manual for National Hospital Inpatient Quality Measures.*

Quality measures help measure or quantify healthcare processes, outcomes, patient perceptions, and organizational structure and systems. These measures are associated with high-quality healthcare and effective, safe, efficient, patient-centered, equitable, and timely care (CMS 2011a). Publicly reporting these measures increases the transparency of hospital care, provides useful information for consumers choosing care, and helps hospitals maintain quality. Hospitals currently report the following measures to CMS (Hospital Quality Initiative 2009):

Heart Attack (acute myocardial infarction)

- Aspirin at arrival

- Aspirin prescribed at discharge

- Angiotensin-converting enzyme (ACE) inhibitor or angiotensin II receptor blocker for left ventricular systolic dysfunction

- Beta blocker at arrival

- Beta blocker prescribed at discharge

- Fibrinolytic (thrombolytic) agent received within 30 minutes of hospital arrival

- Timing of receipt of primary percutaneous coronary intervention

- Adult smoking cessation advice/counseling

Heart Failure

- Left ventricular function assessment
- ACE inhibitor or angiotensin II receptor blocker for left ventricular systolic dysfunction
- Discharge instructions
- Adult smoking cessation advice/counseling

Pneumonia

- Timing of receipt of initial antibiotic following hospital arrival
- Pneumococcal vaccination status
- Blood culture performed before first antibiotic is received in the hospital
- Adult smoking cessation advice/counseling
- Appropriate initial antibiotic selection
- Influenza vaccination status

Surgical Care Improvement Project

- Prophylactic antibiotic received within one hour prior to surgical incision
- Prophylactic antibiotics discontinued within 24 hours after surgery end time
- Venous thromboembolism prophylaxis ordered for surgery patients
- Venous thromboembolism prophylaxis within 24 hours before or after surgery
- Prophylactic antibiotic selection for surgical patients
- Cardiac surgery patients with controlled 6 a.m. postoperative serum glucose
- Surgery patients with appropriate hair removal

Mortality Measures

- Acute myocardial infarction 30-day mortality (Medicare patients)
- Heart failure 30-day mortality (Medicare patients)
- Pneumonia 30-day mortality (Medicare patients)

Patients' Experience of Care

- Hospital Patient Perspectives on Care Survey (HCAHPS) patient survey

Patient Safety Indicators

- Death among surgical patients with treatable serious complications
- Iatrogenic pneumothorax, adult
- Postoperative wound dehiscence

FIGURE 8.4. Example of a hospital comparison report for coronary artery bypass graft surgical procedure

Process Measure	Hoboken University Medical Center	New York Downtown Hospital	NYU Hospital Center
Surgery patients who were taking heart drugs called beta blockers before coming to the hospital and who were kept on the beta blockers during the period just before and after their surgery	78%	97%	99%
Surgery patients who were given an antibiotic at the right time (within one hour before surgery) to help prevent infection	99%	100%	99%
Surgery patients who were given the right kind of antibiotic to help prevent infection	97%	96%	98%
Surgery patients whose preventive antibiotics were stopped at the right time (within 24 hours after surgery)	93%	98%	98%
Heart surgery patients whose blood sugar (blood glucose) is kept under good control in the days right after surgery	Not available	Not available	97%
Surgery patients needing hair removed from the surgical area before surgery, who had hair removed using a safe method (electric clippers or hair removal cream, not a razor)	100%	100%	100%
Surgery patients whose urinary catheters were removed on the first or second day after surgery	84%	88%	94%
Surgery patients whose doctors ordered treatments to prevent blood clots after certain types of surgeries	89%	96%	100%
Patients who received treatment at the right time (within 24 hours before or after their surgery) to help prevent blood clots after certain types of surgery	85%	94%	98%

Source: HHS 2011a.

- Accidental puncture or laceration

- Inpatient quality indicator measures

- Abdominal aortic aneurysm mortality rate (with or without volume)

- Hip fracture mortality rate

- Mortality for selected medical conditions (composite)

- Mortality for selected surgical procedures (composite)

- Complication/patient safety for selected indicators

CMS created the Hospital Compare website (www.hospitalcompare.gov) as a tool patients can use to analyze hospitals' outcomes and to help patients and their families make better-informed choices about where to receive care. See **FIGURE 8.4** for an example of a report patients can generate from the Hospital Compare website that analyzes outcomes for coronary artery bypass graft surgery.

Patient Satisfaction as a Quality Measure

CMS recently added patient satisfaction as a measure of quality of care provided in the hospital setting. CMS worked with the Agency for Healthcare Research and Quality (AHRQ) to develop the standardized HCAHPS. The hospital patient perspectives data

FIGURE 8.5. Example of a HCAHPS hospital patient satisfaction survey

During this hospital stay, how often did doctors treat you with courtesy and respect?

During this hospital stay, how often did doctors listen carefully to you?

During this hospital stay, how often did doctors explain things in a way you could understand?

During this hospital stay, how often were your room and bathroom cleaned?

During this hospital stay, how often was the area around your room quiet at night?

Before giving you any new medicine, how often did hospital staff tell you what the medicine was for?

Before giving you any new medicine, how often did hospital staff describe possible side effects in a way you could understand?

During this hospital stay, did you get information in writing about what symptoms or health problems to look out for after you left the hospital?

Would you recommend this hospital to your friends and family?

Source: HCAHPS 2011.

are published to help consumers make more informed hospital choices and to create incentives for hospitals to improve quality of care. See **FIGURE 8.5** for sample hospital patient satisfaction questions from the HCAHPS survey and **FIGURE 8.6** for an example of a comparison of patient satisfaction measures from three different hospitals that can be generated from the Hospital Compare website.

FIGURE 8.6. A sample hospital compare report for coronary artery bypass graft patient satisfaction

Patient Satisfaction Measure	Hoboken University Medical Center	New York Downtown Hospital	NYU Hospital Center
Patients who reported that their nurses always communicated well	71%	54%	71%
Patients who reported that their doctors always communicated well	81%	64%	75%
Patients who reported that they always received help as soon as they wanted	59%	44%	54%
Patients who reported that their pain was always well controlled	67%	50%	65%
Patients who reported that staff always explained a medicine before giving it to them	51%	48%	58%
Patients who reported that their room and bathroom were always clean	61%	56%	61%
Patients who reported that the area around their room was always quiet at night	48%	34%	44%
Patients at each hospital who reported that they were given information about what to do during their recovery at home	80%	75%	79%
Patients who gave their hospital a rating of 9 or 10 on a scale from 0 (lowest) to 10 (highest)	58%	35%	62%
Patients who reported that they would definitely recommend the hospital	64%	42%	71%

Source: HHS 2011a.

Healthcare Corporate Compliance

Healthcare corporate compliance requires that all healthcare providers abide by the laws and regulations governing them and the guidelines of the organizations by which they choose to be accredited. Compliance further requires organizations and their employees to act ethically. Often, the first document produced as part of a healthcare provider's corporate compliance program is the standards of conduct by which all employees are expected to abide.

Five components of a compliance plan are

1. Standards of conduct and policies and procedures

2. Compliance plan development and validation

3. Education and training of nonmedical and medical staff

4. Monitoring of high-risk activities

5. Auditing of high-risk activities

FIGURE 8.7 illustrates the dynamic and interrelated nature of these five components of a compliance program.

The primary difference between monitoring and auditing is that monitoring is less formal and is performed regularly (daily, weekly, or monthly) by internal employees, while auditing is more formal and is performed less frequently (annually or quarterly) by an external professional services firm.

Hospital compliance is overseen by the OIG, which publishes *Compliance Guidance for Hospitals* in 1998 and updates the document on a regular basis. Special areas of OIG concern include (OIG 1998):

FIGURE 8.7. Components of a corporate compliance program as described in the OIG's Compliance Guidance

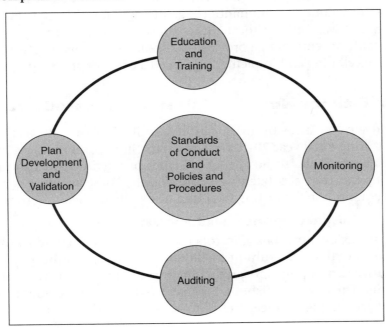

- The billing of items or services not actually rendered

- The provision of medically unnecessary services

- Upcoding

- Diagnosis-related group (DRG) creep

- Outpatient services rendered in connection with inpatient stays

- Physician and resident requirements for teaching hospitals

- Duplicate billing

- False cost reports

Several of the areas of concern either directly affect the HIM function or are managed by the HIM department in a hospital. These include upcoding and DRG creep (which is defined as the practice of billing using a DRG code that provides a higher payment rate than the DRG code that accurately reflects the service furnished to the patient) (OIG 1998).

In addition to its *Compliance Guidance for Hospitals,* OIG publishes a Compliance Work Plan each year, which highlights the specific activities on which their compliance investigations will focus that year. Because some of the target activities may be directly managed by or affect the HIM department, HIM professionals must be familiar with the current OIG Compliance Work Plan.

Office of the Inspector General

In the late 1990s the OIG began to promote voluntary compliance programs for the healthcare industry. It issued guidelines to help healthcare entities develop effective internal controls that promote adherence to applicable federal and state laws and the program requirements of federal, state, and private health plans. The OIG believes the adoption and implementation of voluntary compliance programs significantly advances the prevention of fraud, abuse, and waste in healthcare. It issued sample compliance programs for multiple types of healthcare entities that provide details on specific elements each entity should consider when developing and implementing an effective compliance program.

OIG's Work Plan for Hospitals 2011: HIM-Related Activities

Following are five of the areas of investigation identified by the OIG as targets for acute care hospitals during fiscal year 2011. Each has some impact on the HIM professional in a hospital. This list provides some idea of the types of activities that can present risk for hospitals if not performed accurately and compliantly. These activities generally involve coding documentation or abstracting data from the patient's health record.

Reliability of hospital-reported quality measure data
The OIG will review hospitals' controls for ensuring the accuracy of data related to quality of care that they submit to CMS for Medicare reimbursement. The Social Security Act, requires hospitals to report quality measures for a set of 10 indicators. The law establishes a 2 percent reduction in payments to hospitals that do not report quality measures to CMS. The OIG determines whether

hospitals have implemented sufficient controls to ensure that their quality measurement data are valid.

Hospital readmissions

The OIG will review Medicare claims to determine trends in the number of hospital readmission cases. CMS implemented an edit in 2004 by which it would reject subsequent claims on behalf of beneficiaries who were readmitted to the same hospital on the same day. If a same-day readmission occurs for symptoms related to or for evaluation or management of the prior stay's medical condition, the hospital is entitled to only one DRG payment and should combine the original and subsequent stays into a single claim. Providers are permitted to override the edit in certain situations. The OIG tests the effectiveness of the edit and determines the extent of oversight of readmission cases.

Hospital admissions with conditions coded "present on admission"

The OIG will review Medicare claims to determine which types of facilities most frequently transfer patients with certain diagnoses that were coded as being present on admission (POA). Acute care hospitals are required to report POA diagnoses on their Medicare claims. For certain diagnoses specified by CMS, hospitals receive a lower payment if the specified diagnoses were acquired in the hospital. The OIG will also determine whether specific providers transferred a high number of patients to hospitals with POA diagnoses.

Early implementation of Medicare's policy for hospital-acquired conditions

The OIG will review the early implementation of CMS's hospital-acquired conditions (HACs) policy. CMS implemented the HAC policy, which prevents additional payment under Medicare's hospital inpatient prospective payment system for certain conditions or complications determined to be reasonably preventable. The OIG reviews Medicare claims data to identify the number of beneficiary stays associated with HACs and determine their impact on reimbursement.

Hospital inpatient outlier payments

The OIG will review hospital inpatient outlier payments. Medicare typically reimburses hospitals for inpatient services based on a predetermined per-discharge amount, regardless of the actual costs incurred. The Social Security Act allows Medicare to pay hospitals supplemental, or outlier, payments for patients incurring extraordinarily high costs. In 2009, outlier payments represented about 5 percent of total Medicare inpatient payments.

Recovery Audit Contractors

The purpose of the Recovery Audit Contractors (RAC) Program is to reduce improper Medicare payments and prevent future improper payments by identifying improper payments made on claims of healthcare services provided to Medicare beneficiaries. Improper payments may be overpayments or underpayments. Overpayments can occur when healthcare providers submit claims that do not meet Medicare's coding or medical necessity policies. Underpayments can occur when healthcare providers submit claims for a simple procedure but the medical record reveals that a more complicated procedure was actually performed.

In March 2008, the RAC demonstration program ended with more than $1.03 billion recovered from improper payments. Approximately 96 percent of the improper payments were overpayments collected from providers, and the remaining 4 percent were underpayments paid to providers. Most of the overpayments (85 percent) were collected from inpatient hospital providers, 6 percent were collected from inpatient rehabilitation facilities, and 4 percent were collected from outpatient hospital providers.

With regards to the RAC process, CMS recommends that providers (CMS 2011b)

- Identify where improper payments have been persistent by reviewing the RAC websites to identify any patterns of denied claims within their own practice or facility

- Implement procedures to promptly respond to RAC requests for medical records

- File an appeal before the 120-day deadline for any cases where the provider disagrees with the RAC's findings

- Keep track of denied claims and correct these previous errors

- Determine what corrective actions need to be taken to ensure compliance with Medicare's requirements and to avoid submitting incorrect claims in the future

Federal Requirements for Special Health Record Protection

The confidentiality of all patient-identifiable health information must be protected, but several types of health-related information are particularly sensitive. The inappropriate disclosure of information related to substance abuse treatment or psychiatric care can have devastating consequences for patients and their families. Information about a patient's HIV status or sexually transmitted illness can lead to discrimination in employment and housing. Concerns related to the release of genetic information and the potential for discrimination based on genetic profiles are relatively new. Several federal regulations supplement state laws and voluntary accreditation standards to provide special protection to particularly sensitive health information.

Records of HIV/AIDS Diagnosis and Treatment

The illness caused by HIV (AIDS) has been a worldwide public health concern for more than two decades. In response to the AIDS epidemic in the United States, most state legislatures have enacted laws that require HIV/AIDS reporting. Because individuals infected with HIV often face discrimination in housing, employment, and healthcare services, many state regulations also specifically address confidentiality issues related to HIV testing and AIDS treatment.

HIV Testing

HIV testing has become a common practice. Many individuals at risk for contracting HIV voluntarily choose to be tested. However, individuals may also be compelled by court order to undergo involuntary testing. In addition, many states have enacted statutes that require specific groups of individuals to undergo routine HIV testing, most commonly healthcare workers.

Most HIV testing in the United States is performed on a voluntary basis. Some states have even developed anonymous HIV testing programs to encourage individuals at risk of infection to be tested without identifying themselves by name. In addition, many individuals undergo routine voluntary testing when they donate blood, plasma, semen, and other human tissue to blood and tissue banks. HIV testing has become a routine element in prenatal care, and infants are usually tested shortly after birth when their mothers are known or suspected to be HIV-positive.

Involuntary HIV testing, however, may be required for specific groups of individuals by state statute or for individuals by court order. Where they exist, state regulations mandating HIV testing apply to specific groups whose infection would present the greatest potential threat to public health. Examples of such groups include convicted sex offenders and prison inmates entering or leaving correctional facilities (McWay 2009).

Some states require mandatory testing of specific groups of employees, while others permit only voluntary employee-testing programs. Other states prohibit mandatory employee testing or allow it only under specific circumstances, that is, when health status affects the employees' ability to perform their jobs safely. Healthcare workers who perform invasive procedures are one example.

Court orders for mandatory HIV testing of individuals differ from state to state. Specific risks may be identified, such as that the individual is likely to be infected with HIV or that the individual's HIV status presents a serious threat to the health of other people.

Discrimination based on disability status is prohibited by law in some states as well as by the federal Americans with Disabilities Act of 1990. The collection of information about an employee's HIV status is a serious issue. The federal regulations in this area also apply to applicants for employment. Hospitals and other healthcare facilities must consult legal counsel before establishing policies and procedures related to human resources issues.

Confidentiality Issues Related to HIV/AIDS

In general, state regulations developed to protect the identity of HIV-positive individuals address confidentiality practices in three areas: consent for testing, general information on testing, and reporting of test results. Individuals must sign a formal informed consent before testing. Most states also require healthcare providers to provide information about HIV testing and AIDS to patients before they perform the test. The provider's method of communicating test results to patients is also covered in many states' HIV-testing regulations (McWay 2009).

Virtually every state requires providers to report cases of positive HIV results to the state's public health department. Some counties and municipalities may also require reporting. In general, reporting involves the identification of the infected individual. Therefore, the communication of public health reports containing HIV/AIDS information should be accomplished through a confidential medium, specifically, not via telephone, e-mail, or facsimile transmission (Carpenter 1999).

AHIMA has recommended the following procedures for managing health information related to HIV infection and AIDS (Carpenter 1999):

- HIV employee-screening programs should protect the confidentiality of test results.
- Specific, written informed consent should be obtained from the individual or the individual's legal representative before voluntary testing.

- When state regulations permit the mandatory testing of patients after healthcare workers have been exposed to blood or bodily fluids, the need for testing should be discussed with the patient or his legal representative before testing.

- Counseling provided before or after testing should be performed by a qualified healthcare professional.

- The records of HIV-positive patients should not be subject to special handling procedures because special procedures are more likely to draw attention than routine security measures. In states where special handling is required for the records of HIV-positive individuals or HIV test results, the records should be identified with an obscure code or symbol to avoid inadvertent release of HIV-related information.

- Facilities should implement and monitor compliance with clear policies and procedures on the disclosure of health information related to HIV/AIDS. Policies should dictate that HIV/AIDS information must be used only for diagnosis, treatment, and patient care management. Other disclosures, including disclosures for billing and claims purposes, must be allowed only with the patient's written consent and should be limited to the minimum amount needed for the authorized purpose. Authorized disclosures of HIV/AIDS information should include a notice that redisclosure is prohibited except when required by law.

- HIV/AIDS-related information should only be discussed via telephone in emergencies.

- Clinical coding should be based only on the diagnoses verified in patient records and not on the basis of laboratory results alone.

- Information related to the HIV-positive status of healthcare workers, including information on any restrictions to their practice, should be protected according to all applicable state and federal regulations. Such information should only be disclosed to patients on the advice of legal counsel.

Genetic Information Nondiscrimination Act (GINA)

The Genetic Information Nondiscrimination Act (GINA), which prohibits US insurance companies and employers from discriminating on the basis of information derived from genetic tests, was signed into law in May 2008. GINA protects Americans from discrimination based on information derived from genetic tests. It forbids insurance companies from discriminating through reduced coverage or pricing and prohibits employers from making adverse employment decisions based on a person's genetic code. In addition, insurers and employers are not allowed under the law to request or demand a genetic test (GINA 2008).

In 2003, the Human Genome Project identified all of the approximately 20,000 to 25,000 genes in human DNA. The US Department of Energy (DOE) and the National Institutes of Health (NIH) jointly sponsored the effort, which was one of the largest scientific projects ever undertaken. Its research identified the function of every human gene. This information promises to revolutionize the future of medicine. The DOE promotes scientific and technological innovation, and the NIH supports medical research.

Genetic information can be used to predict an individual's risk of eventually contracting many types of illness, including diabetes, heart disease, cancer, and even mental health disorders such as alcoholism and schizophrenia. For this reason, the potential for using genetic information as the basis of discrimination against individuals cannot be ignored.

HIPAA also addresses the issue of health insurance discrimination based on genetic information. The act specifically prohibits healthcare insurance plans from basing coverage decisions and premiums on genetic information alone. Several states, including Missouri, California, Arizona, Maryland, and Wisconsin, have enacted similar health insurance and genetic testing regulations (McWay 2009).

Definition of "Genetic Information"

Genetic information includes information about an individual's genetic tests, the genetic tests of an individual's family members, and the manifestation of a disease or disorder in an individual's family members (that is, family medical history). Family medical history is included in the definition of genetic information because it is often used to determine the individual's risk of developing a disease, disorder, or condition in the future. Genetic information also includes an individual's request for, or receipt of, genetic services; the participation in clinical research that includes genetic services by the individual or a family member of the individual; the genetic information of a fetus carried by an individual or by a pregnant woman who is a family member of the individual; and the genetic information of any embryo legally held by the individual or family member using an assisted reproductive technology (EEOC 2011).

Under Title II of GINA, it is illegal to discriminate against employees or applicants because of genetic information. Title II of GINA prohibits the use of genetic information in making employment decisions; restricts employers and other entities covered by Title II (employment agencies, labor organizations, and joint labor-management training and apprenticeship programs—referred to as "covered entities") from requesting, requiring, or purchasing genetic information; and strictly limits the disclosure of genetic information.

State Requirements

Licensure

All states require that hospitals and other healthcare facilities within their border be licensed by the state. **Licensure** is the mandatory process whereby state governments grant individual facilities permission to operate within a specific geopolitical area and provide a specific range of healthcare services. Licensure is also mandatory for individual healthcare providers such as physicians and nurses. Licensing of individual healthcare providers is addressed in chapter 13.

The state agency charged with administering hospital licensure is usually the department of health. According to Cassidy (2011, 721):

> Although licensure requirements vary, healthcare facilities must meet certain basic criteria determined by state regulatory agencies. These standards address concerns such as adequacy of staffing, physical aspects of the facility (equipment, buildings), and services provided, including the maintenance of health records. Most licensing agencies perform reviews annually.

Typical hospital licensure standards address minimum operating requirements in the areas of operational procedures, staffing, and environmental safety. Some states require hospitals to maintain additional licenses for specific services, such as laboratory, radiology, renal dialysis, and substance abuse treatment. Most states have separate licensure requirements for pharmacies.

Documentation within health records is an important source of information in licensure surveys. States conduct annual surveys to determine the hospital's continued compliance with licensure standards. Surveys are often unannounced and generally focus on clinical services and the environment of care. The health record is the source document requested during these surveys, along with hospital policies and procedures, to validate compliance with licensure requirements. In addition, state surveyors conduct reviews in response to specific complaints from consumers. State surveys are also used to validate compliance with Medicaid regulations. **FIGURE 8.8** contains the portion of state

FIGURE 8.8. Massachusetts state licensure requirements for health records

130.370: Retention of Records

(A) In accordance with M.G.L. c. 111, § 70 a hospital shall maintain records of the diagnosis and treatment of patients under its care for a minimum of 20 years after the discharge or the final treatment of the patient to whom the record relates. Medical records may be handwritten, printed, typed or in electronic digital format, or converted to electronic digital format or an alternative archival method. Handwritten, printed or typed medical records that have been converted to electronic digital format or an alternative archival format may be destroyed before the expiration of the 20 year retention period. The manner of destruction must ensure the confidentiality of patient information. For purposes of 105 CMR 130.370, medical records in electronic digital format shall have the same force and effect as the original records from which they were made. A hospital shall include with the patient's medical record all trip records submitted by Emergency Medical Technicians on each ambulance run in accordance with 105 CMR 170.345(C). A hospital shall maintain the unprotected exposure forms in compliance with the requirements of 105 CMR 172.002(C).

(B) For the purpose of 105 CMR 130.370, a hospital shall not be required to consider the following as part of the medical record subject to the retention requirements in M.G.L. c. 111, § 70: radiological films, scans, other image records, raw psychological testing data, electronic fetal monitoring tracings, electroencephalograph, electrocardiography tracings and the like, provided that any signed narrative reports, interpretations or, sample tracings that are generated to report the results of such tests and procedures shall be maintained as part of the record. Such records as described in 105 CMR 130.370(B) shall be retained for a period of at least five years following the date of service. The purpose of 105 CMR 130.370 is to establish a minimum retention period and does not preclude hospitals from maintaining records for a longer period of time.

(C) Medical records retained by the hospital in accordance with 130.370(A) or (B) shall be made available for inspection and copying upon written request of the patient or his or her authorized representative. The hospital may charge a reasonable fee for copying, not to exceed the rate of copying expenses as specified in M.G.L. c. 111, § 70.

(D) A hospital shall maintain and use patient records in a manner that protects the confidentiality of the information contained therein. Printed copies of electronically stored records shall be destroyed in a manner that ensures the confidentiality of patient information.

(E) A hospital shall make all patient records available promptly to any agent of the Department.

(F) At the expiration of 20 years after the discharge or the final treatment of the patient to whom a retained medical record relates, a hospital may destroy the medical record. The manner of destruction must ensure the confidentiality of patient information. At least 30 days prior to the proposed date of destruction of a medical record(s), a hospital shall provide written notification to the Department, generally indicating the type of records to be destroyed and the dates of service which exceed the applicable retention period, in a manner specified by the Department, of the hospital's intent to destroy medical record(s) that exceed the 20 year retention period. A hospital may, but is not required to, notify a patient before destroying the patient's medical record pursuant to 105 CMR 130.370.

(G) A hospital shall provide written notice to a patient of the patient's right to inspect and to receive a copy of the patient's medical records and the hospital's medical record retention policy, as specified in M.G.L. c. 111, § 70.

Source: Massachusetts Department of Public Health 2010.

licensure requirements that addresses health records for the state of Massachusetts. The entire set of regulations for the state of Massachusetts is quite voluminous at 114 total pages (Massachusetts Department of Public Health 2010).

Medicaid Eligibility and Administration

States are required to include certain types of individuals or eligibility groups under their Medicaid plans, and they may include others. States' eligibility groups include categorically needy, medically needy, and special groups. Following are brief descriptions of some of the key eligibility groups included under states' plans.

Categorically Needy:

- Families who meet states' Aid to Families with Dependent Children eligibility requirements in effect on July 16, 1996

- Pregnant women and children younger than 6 years whose family income is at or below 133 percent of the federal poverty level

- Children aged 6 to 19 years with family income up to 100 percent of the federal poverty level

- Caretakers (relatives or legal guardians who take care of children younger than 18 years [or 19 if still in high school])

- Supplemental Security Income (SSI) recipients (or, in certain states, aged, blind, and disabled people who meet requirements that are more restrictive than those of the SSI program)

- Individuals and couples who are living in medical institutions and who have monthly income up to 300 percent of the SSI income standard (federal benefit rate).

Medically Needy:

The medically needy have too much money (and in some cases, resources such as savings) to be eligible as categorically needy. If a state has a medically needy program, it must include pregnant women through a 60-day postpartum period, children younger than 18 years, certain newborns for one year, and certain protected blind persons. At the state's option, they may also provide Medicaid to (CMS 2005):

- Children younger than 21, 20, or 19 years, or children younger than 19 years who are full-time students; if a state doesn't want to cover all of these children, it can limit eligibility to reasonable groups of these children

- Caretaker relatives (relatives or legal guardians who live with and take care of children)

- Aged persons (65 years and older)

- Blind persons (blindness is determined using the SSI program standards or state standards)

FIGURE 8.9. Services that must be provided to economically needy Medicaid recipients in all states

- Inpatient hospital (excluding inpatient services in institutions for mental disease)

- Outpatient hospital including federally qualified health centers and, if permitted under state law, rural health clinic and other ambulatory services provided by a rural health clinic that are otherwise included under states' plans

- Other laboratory and X-ray

- Certified pediatric and family nurse practitioners (when licensed to practice under state law)

- Nursing facility services for beneficiaries age 21 years and older

- Early and periodic screening, diagnosis, and treatment for children younger than 21 years

- Family planning services and supplies

- Physicians' services

- Medical and surgical services of a dentist

- Home health services for beneficiaries who are entitled to nursing facility services under the state's Medicaid plan

- Intermittent or part-time nursing services provided by a home health agency or by a registered nurse when there is no home health agency in the area

- Home health aides

- Medical supplies and appliances for use in the home

- Nurse midwife services

- Pregnancy-related services and service for other conditions that might complicate pregnancy

- 60 days postpartum pregnancy-related services

Source: CMS 2005.

- Disabled persons (disability is determined using the SSI program standards or state standards).

- Persons who would be eligible if not enrolled in a health maintenance organization.

FIGURE 8.9 lists those services that must be provided to economically needy Medicaid recipients.

Medicaid Compliance Programs

In addition to being in compliance with federal requirements, acute care hospitals must also be in compliance with state Medicaid requirements. Many states have enacted laws that require all healthcare providers to have a compliance program in place. For example, Title 18 of the Codes, Rules, and Regulations of the state of New York says, "To be eligible to receive medical assistance payments for care, services, or supplies, or to be eligible to submit claims for care, services, or supplies for or on behalf of another person, [healthcare providers] shall adopt and implement effective compliance programs...." (New York State 2011).

New York State has also published examples of best practices in healthcare compliance. One of these examples, Training and Education for Compliance, is illustrated in **FIGURE 8.10**.

FIGURE 8.10. New York State healthcare compliance best practices example

---

Training and Education

1. Use electronic training and education system that tracks mandatory compliance education of employees via an electronic system that is: customized to the organization, sends an individualized email to employees to announce upcoming required and elective training, and tracks each employee's required compliance training and educational needs.

2. Results of online compliance education quiz scores are analyzed and tracked to identify areas of weakness for both the education program and those being trained. Additional training and education is provided if needed. Results of the online post test quizzes are used to identify risk areas and assess the need for internal monitoring and auditing.

3. Compliance training of the various organizational constituencies is specialized. For example, general staff compliance training need not include the same level of detail on billing and coding issues that should be included for those engaged in the billing functions.

4. The compliance training and educational materials delivered to staff were uniquely developed and tailored to the educational backgrounds of all the employees.

5. Clients/patients receive information on how to identify Medicaid fraud and examples of Medicaid fraud, and compliance-related issues are provided. Home care clients are encouraged to contact the provider's office to report any concerns regarding care provided and inconsistencies with service dates and time.

6. Issuance of a brochure to consumers, partners, and vendors that highlights the provider's quality initiatives and commitment to performance and quality improvement. The brochure includes a "contact us" section, which identifies contact names and numbers of the compliance staff.

Source: State of New York Office of the Medicaid Inspector General 2011.

Accreditation Requirements for Acute Care Hospitals

Acute care facilities must fulfill the various regulatory requirements of federal, local, and state governments, but most also choose to participate in one or more voluntary accreditation programs. One benefit of accreditation is enhancement of the hospital's public reputation for providing high-quality clinical services. In some cases, accreditation also satisfies eligibility requirements for hospitals participating in programs that affect their financial status, such as Medicare and Medicaid. In addition, many state licensure agencies base their licensure requirements for hospitals on Joint Commission standards.

Accreditation is a systematic quality review process that evaluates the healthcare facility's performance against preestablished, written criteria, or standards. Healthcare organizations voluntarily seek accreditation from a variety of private, not-for-profit accreditation organizations. Different types of healthcare organizations and services are accredited by different accreditation organizations.

Either The Joint Commission or the AOA's Healthcare Facilities Accreditation Program accredits most acute care hospitals. Psychiatric and rehabilitation specialty hospitals and hospital departments devoted to psychiatric and rehabilitation services may also be accredited through the Commission on Accreditation of Rehabilitation Facilities. Managed-care programs that provide acute care services may be accredited through the **National Committee for Quality Assurance (NSQA)**. Ambulatory surgery centers and outpatient diagnostic imaging and radiation oncology treatment facilities may be accredited through the Accreditation Association for Ambulatory Health Care.

See chapters 9 through 13 for information about The Joint Commission regulations pertaining to the ambulatory, long-term care, hospice and home care, and behavioral healthcare settings.

The Joint Commission

The Joint Commission is a not-for-profit, standards-setting organization whose primary mission is "to continuously improve health care for the public, in collaboration with other stakeholders, by evaluating health care organizations and inspiring them to excel in providing safe and effective care of the highest quality and value" (Joint Commission 2011a). Currently, it accredits more than 4,250 general, children's, long-term acute, psychiatric, rehabilitation, and surgical specialty hospitals, and 358 critical access hospitals, through a separate accreditation program. Approximately 88 percent of the nation's hospitals are accredited by The Joint Commission.

The Joint Commission currently provides the following accreditation programs:

- Ambulatory Care Accreditation Program

- Behavioral Health Care Accreditation Program

- Critical Access Hospital Accreditation Program

- Home Health Care Accreditation Program

- Hospital Accreditation Program

- Laboratory Services Accreditation Program

- Long Term Care Accreditation Program

- Office-Based Surgery Accreditation Program

- Office-Based Surgery Accreditation Program

The Joint Commission uses a **periodic performance review** (PPR) designed to promote continuous standards compliance. The PPR was created to help hospitals shift from a mentality of survey preparation to one of continuous improvement. The Joint Commission hopes to transfer the focus from getting a score on an exam to using standards to achieve and maintain excellent performance. Hospitals can fulfill the PPR requirement in the following ways with options for either a limited PPR survey or a full-length PPR survey under PPR Options 2 and 3 (Joint Commission 2010):

- The full PPR, in which hospitals assess themselves against the applicable standards and elements of performance (EPs) and submit their assessment electronically. This option has the greatest benefits for hospitals, including educational benefits for physicians and staff and time and technology efficiencies.

- Option 1, in which hospitals assess themselves against the standards and EPs that apply to them and attest to their assessment without submitting their data to The Joint Commission.

- Option 2, in which hospitals can request and undergo either a limited on-site visit from The Joint Commission or a full-length announced or unannounced PPR survey and then participate in an optional follow-up call with Joint Commission staff.

- Option 3, in which hospitals can request and undergo either a limited on-site visit from The Joint Commission or a full-length announced or unannounced

PPR survey and then participate in an optional follow-up call with Joint Commission staff. All findings from the on-site visit are communicated verbally, and no written report is provided to the hospital or transmitted to The Joint Commission (Joint Commission 2010).

To earn and maintain accreditation, a hospital must undergo an on-site Joint Commission survey. The Joint Commission accreditation process focuses on systems critical to the safety and quality of patient care, treatment, and services. Hospital surveys are unannounced. An organization can have an **unannounced survey** 18 to 36 months after its last full survey. Surveys are conducted by a Joint Commission survey team that can include physicians, nurses, life safety code specialists, and hospital administrators. The Joint Commission evaluates an organization's performance of functions and processes aimed at continuously improving patient outcomes, as evidenced in the hospital or healthcare system's PPR. The assessment is accomplished through an evaluation of the organization's compliance with the applicable standards, based on

- Documents provided by the healthcare facility
- A tracing of the care delivered to patients
- Verbal and written information provided to The Joint Commission
- On-site observations and interviews by surveyors

The *Accreditation Compliance Guide* contains compliance assessments for the following functional areas in the hospital or healthcare system (Joint Commission 2010):

- Emergency management
- Environment of care
- Human resources
- Infection prevention and control
- Information management
- Leadership
- Life safety
- Medication management
- Medical staff
- National patient safety goals
- Nursing
- Performance improvement
- Provisions of care, treatment, and services
- Record of care, treatment, and services
- Rights and responsibilities of the individual
- Transplant safety
- Waived testing

Health record functions are included in two of these areas: information management and record of care, treatment, and services. The information management section contains compliance assessments for EHR technology, destruction of records, hospital policies on acceptable abbreviations and terminology, accessibility of records, and accuracy of record content validated through an audit or review process (Joint Commission 2010).

The record of care, treatment, and services section contains compliance assessments for hospital policies (and compliance with such policies) for defining complete components of the record; a unique patient identifier; documentation to support the patient's care, treatment, and course of care; policies on standard formats for documentation, date, time, and authentication of records; and a timeliness policy. In addition, The Joint Commission defines demographic and clinical content in the section on record of care (Joint Commission 2010).

Priority Focus Process

The priority focus process is an important component of the survey process because it guides the surveyor(s) in planning and conducting on-site surveys. The Joint Commission defines the **priority focus process (PFP)** as focusing survey activities on the organization-specific issues that are most relevant to safety and quality of care. Internal and external data about the organization are integrated to identify clinical service groups and priority focus areas for each hospital. The Joint Commission provides the hospital with information about its top clinical service groups and priority focus areas on its secure extranet site.

Priority focus areas (PFAs) include the processes, systems, and structures that have the most substantial effect on patient-care services. The Joint Commission designates information management as one of 14 PFAs vital to successful operation in hospitals (Joint Commission 2007, ACC-19).

The Joint Commission uses the tracer methodology for on-site surveys. The **tracer methodology** incorporates the use of the PFP, follows the experience of care through the organization's entire healthcare process, and allows the surveyor to identify performance issues. Surveyors may perform two different types of tracers: individual tracer activity or individual-based system tracer activity. **Individual tracer activity** permits the evaluation of the care experience of a specific patient while he is in the hospital. This method analyzes a hospital's system of providing care, treatment, and services used as the framework for assessing standards of compliance. The **individual-based system tracer activity** explores a specific system or process across the organization. The surveyor evaluates the integration of related processes, coordination, and communication among disciplines and departments during the individual-based system tracer. Data use, infection control, and medical management are key components evaluated during the individual-based system tracer activity.

Hospital staff will be involved in the tracer methodology process. The surveyor will ask staff to provide a list of active patients that will include the patient's name, current location, and diagnosis. The surveyor will interview physicians and hospital staff involved in the care of the patient as she proceeds through the hospital visiting areas where service was provided.

Each performance area has an overview that provides background information. Additionally, each performance area includes the following:

- The *standard*, which defines the performance expectations and/or structures or process that must be in place

- The *rationale for the standard*, which provides additional text describing the purpose of the standard

- The *elements of performance* (EPs), which detail specific performance expectations and/or structures or processes that must be in place

The Joint Commission has six accreditation decision categories. They are (Joint Commission 2010):

- Accredited: The organization is in compliance with all standards.

- Provisional Accreditation: The organization fails to successfully address all requirements for improvement within 45 or 60 days of the on-site survey.

- Conditional Accreditation: The organization fails to resolve the requirements of a Provisional Accreditation status or is in substantial noncompliance with standards.

- Preliminary Denial of Accreditation: There is justification to deny accreditation to the organization as evidenced by an immediate threat to health or safety for patients or the public, or failure to resolve the requirements of a Conditional Accreditation.

- Denial of Accreditation: The organization has been denied accreditation. All review and appeal opportunities have been exhausted.

- Preliminary Accreditation: The organization demonstrates compliance with selected standards in the surveys conducted under the Early Survey Policy.

Joint Commission Sentinel Event Policy

The Joint Commission reviews healthcare organizational activities in response to sentinel events to support its mission to continuously improve the safety and quality of healthcare provided to the community. The Joint Commission requires accredited hospitals and other healthcare facilities to implement systems for identifying and addressing sentinel events.

- A **sentinel event** is an unexpected occurrence involving death, serious physical or psychological injury, or the risk thereof. Serious injury specifically includes loss of limb or function. The phrase "or the risk thereof" includes any process variation for which a recurrence would carry a significant chance of a serious adverse outcome.

- Such events are called "sentinel" because they signal the need for immediate investigation and response.

- The terms *"sentinel event"* and *"error"* are not synonymous; not all sentinel events occur because of an error, and not all errors result in sentinel events (Joint Commission 2011a).

FIGURE 8.11. Examples of reviewable and nonreviewable sentinel events

There is no one-size-fits-all approach to developing and using problem lists, but rather multiple approaches to be considered. This sample policy is intended to provide guidance for organizations developing problem list policy. Organizations must take national standards and organizational operation into account when developing problem list policy.

SAMPLE PROBLEM LIST POLICY

Policy Statement:

Patients receiving continuing care in the acute and ambulatory setting are required to have a problem list as part of the medical record. The problem list is intended to promote continuity of care over time and among providers for the patient.

PURPOSE

The purpose of this policy is to provide guidance on initiating and maintaining the patient problem list. When used properly and consistently, the problem list serves as a valuable tool in patient care management. The problem list compiles all past and current patient problems, including social, psychological, and medical problems, in one location. At a glance, providers can determine which problems are active or resolved and formulate treatment plans accordingly. Additionally, the problem list serves as a communication tool and aids in the evaluation and treatment decision when the patient is referred to a specialty physician for care.

DEFINITIONS

Active patient: a patient who has had a visit to any [Facility Name] location within the previous three years.

Problem list: a list of illnesses, injuries, and other factors that affect the health of an individual patient, usually identifying the time of occurrence or identification and resolution. The electronic summary of the patient's medical information includes at least the following:

- Items from organization-defined national standards

- Known significant medical diagnoses and conditions

- Known significant operative and invasive procedures affecting current health

- Known adverse and allergic reactions

Healthcare provider: a physician, nurse practitioner, nurse midwife, physician assistant, or other licensed individual authorized to write patient care orders.

Significant medical diagnosis/condition: any nontransient problem that is significant enough to be relevant to the health of the patient going forward, including significant signs or symptoms that are undiagnosed (i.e., chronic abdominal pain) as well as diagnoses that are confirmed and relevant to future care.

Significant operative and invasive procedures: any operative or invasive procedure that is significant enough to be relevant to the health of the patient going forward.

PROCEDURE

1. All clinic patients will have a problem list initiated and maintained by the third visit. For inpatients treated for chronic or critical conditions, problems are entered into the problem list upon discharge.

2. All providers should review the problem list, add problems, and enter updates as appropriate.

3. Primary care providers have ultimate responsibility for maintaining an accurate problem list.

4. To maintain usefulness of the problem list, problems will be entered in a timely manner. (Organizations should consider further defining time specifications.)

5. Only approved staff will enter problems. Medical directors will identify approved staff within their clinic/department.

6. All problems will be listed as active until a licensed independent practitioner changes the problem to "resolved."

7. If copy/paste functionality is utilized, the entry must be edited to ensure documentation integrity.

FIGURE 8.11. (Continued)

8. Problems will include

   o Items from organization-defined national standards

   o Known significant medical diagnoses and conditions

   o Known significant operative and invasive procedures affecting current health

   o Known adverse and allergic reactions

9. All entries, when possible, will utilize a standard vocabulary to ensure classification of data for rules, alerts, and potential reporting. HIM professionals and clinical users will determine whether a classification or vocabulary system should be used for the entries on the problem list.

10. If directed by a specialty, approved by the HIM committee, and resources are allocated, HIM coders or routine automated entry will be allowed to enter designated problems onto the problem list.

11. Development of system-level problem folders requires approval by the HIM committee.

12. Abbreviations will be avoided in the problem list to ensure clear communication among all disciplines.

13. The HIM committee must approve all rules, alerts, and system-generated problems at least one month before implementation. System-generated problems will be updated with resolved status by the requesting provider group.

14. The problem list is considered a permanent part of the medical record and is included in the designated record set.

REFERENCES

[Include any references used to develop problem list policy]

RELATED POLICIES

1103.00 Medical Record Documentation

REVIEW/REVISION DATES

[Provide original and revised dates for problem list policy]

APPROVAL GROUPS

[Outline groups that have approved problem list policy]

Source: AHIMA 2011.

The sentinel event policy has four goals:

1. To have a positive impact in improving patient care, treatment, and services and preventing sentinel events

2. To focus the attention of a hospital that has experienced a sentinel event on understanding the factors that contributed to the event (such as underlying causes, latent conditions and active failures in defense systems, or organizational culture) and changing the hospital's culture, systems, and processes to reduce the probability of such an event in the future

3. To increase the general knowledge about sentinel events, their contributing factors, and strategies for prevention

4. To maintain the confidence of the public and accredited hospitals in the accreditation process (Joint Commission 2011c).

Each hospital is encouraged, but not required, to report to The Joint Commission any event that meets the criteria for reviewable sentinel events. (See Figure 8.11 for examples of reviewable and nonreviewable sentinel events.) The Joint Commission may become aware of a sentinel event by some other means, such as communication from a patient, a family member, an employee of the hospital, or a surveyor, or through the media. Although self-reporting a sentinel event is not required and the expected response, time frames, and review procedures are the same, whether the hospital voluntarily reports the event or The Joint Commission becomes aware of the event by some other means, self-reporting has several advantages (Joint Commission 2011c):

- Reporting the event enables the lessons learned from the event to be added to The Joint Commission's Sentinel Event Database, thereby contributing to the general knowledge about sentinel events and to the reduction of risk for such events in many other hospitals.

- Early reporting provides an opportunity for consultation with Joint Commission staff during the development of the root-cause analysis and action plan.

- The hospital's acknowledged collaboration with The Joint Commission to understand how the event happened and how to prevent it from happening again strengthens the message to the public that the hospital is doing everything possible to ensure that such an event will not happen again.

Joint Commission National Patient Safety Goals

The Joint Commission measures hospital performance against a set of goals designed to complement its longstanding patient safety standards. Annually, the National Patient Safety Goals process undergoes a review and update, and some goals become standards and are replaced by new, more pressing quality issues. The purpose of these goals is to promote specific improvements in patient safety.

The HIM role in patient safety is one of direct leadership, and opportunities for providing critical support exist in many areas. Many HIM professionals are directly involved in clinical quality issues and outcomes through quality management programs. Organizations use the health record to support and validate patient safety goals. Evidence of compliance with these goals is often found in the documentation within the record. For example, to demonstrate compliance with medication reconciliation, organizations use the health record to document reconciliation between nursing units, such as a patient being transferred from the intensive care unit (ICU) to a general medical floor. The ICU lists medications, their dosages, and their timing, and the general medical floor uses a specific form developed by the organization to validate this information. If this form is not located within the health record during the hospital survey, the organization could not demonstrate compliance with this patient safety goal. Others affect quality through improved medical record documentation, accurate coding, and index integrity (Hjort 2005).

Most patient safety goals focus on system-wide solutions. The 2007 National Patient Safety Goals that affect accredited hospitals include the following:

Goal 1: Improve the accuracy of patient identification

Goal 2: Improve the effectiveness of communication among caregivers

Goal 3: Improve the safety of using medications

Goal 7: Reduce the risk of healthcare-associated infections

Goal 8: Accurately and completely reconcile medications across the continuum of care

Goal 9: Reduce the risk of patient harm resulting from falls

Goal 13: Encourage patients' active involvement in their own care as a patient safety strategy

Goal 15: Identify safety risks inherent in the organization's patient population

Joint Commission ORYX

The Joint Commission's **ORYX** initiative integrates outcomes and other performance measure data into the accreditation process. ORYX measurement requirements are intended to support Joint Commission–accredited organizations in their quality improvement efforts. Performance measures are essential to the credibility of evaluation activity for healthcare organizations. Data collected or submitted to The Joint Commission are reviewed during the on-site survey.

On July 1, 2002, accredited hospitals began collecting data on standardized—or core—performance measures. In September 2004, The Joint Commission and CMS began working together to align measures common to both organizations. These standardized common measures, called National Hospital Quality Measures, are integral to improving the quality of care provided to hospital patients and bringing value to stakeholders by focusing on the actual results of care. Measure alignment benefits hospitals by making it easier and less costly to collect and report data because the same data set can be used to satisfy both CMS and Joint Commission requirements.

In 2004, National Hospital Quality Measures and other core measure data were integrated into the PFP The Joint Commission uses to help focus on-site survey evaluation activities. These data are also incorporated into The Joint Commission's Strategic Surveillance System (S3), a tool available exclusively to Joint Commission–accredited hospitals and designed to help accredited hospitals identify potential areas of risk and opportunities for improvement, and are publicly reported on The Joint Commission website. The public availability of performance measure data permits users to compare hospital performance at the state and national levels.

Hospitals are required to collect and transmit data to The Joint Commission for a minimum of four core measure sets or a combination of applicable core measure sets and noncore measures. The measure sets currently available for selection are (Joint Commission 2011b):

- Acute myocardial infarction (AMI)
- Heart failure (HF)
- Pneumonia (PN)
- Perinatal care (PR)
- Hospital-based inpatient psychiatric services (HBIPS)
- Children's asthma care (CAC)
- Surgical care improvement project (SCIP)

- Hospital outpatient measures (HOP)

- Venous thromboembolism (VTE)

- Stroke (STK)

The data collection process for these ORYX measures is the same as that for CMS quality measures. One of the main differences between CMS Quality Measures and ORYX is that CMS measures only apply to CMS beneficiaries, while ORYX applies to all patients treated in the hospital setting, regardless of the age or insurance coverage. One example of an ORYX measure that CMS does not collect is the children's asthma care measure.

American Osteopathic Association

The AOA is a professional membership association that represents more than 56,000 osteopathic physicians in practice in the United States. The AOA is also the primary certification agency for osteopathic physicians and the accreditation agency for all osteopathic medical colleges and many osteopathic healthcare facilities (AOA 2007).

The practice of osteopathic medicine began at the end of the nineteenth century. Osteopathy is a therapeutic approach to the practice of medicine that uses all the usual forms of medical therapy and diagnosis, including drugs and surgery. However, it places greater emphasis on the influence of the relationship between the organs and the musculoskeletal system than traditional medical science does. Osteopathic physicians diagnose and correct structural problems using manipulation techniques similar to those employed by doctors of chiropractic. The difference is that osteopaths attempt to address structural problems within the body through physical manipulation, while chiropractors are not considered medical physicians, and their practices are limited to spinal manipulation and other skeletal "adjustments.")

The AOA first initiated its hospital accreditation program in 1945 to ensure the quality of residency training programs for doctors of osteopathy. Today, the association's Healthcare Facilities Accreditation Program (HFAP) accredits a number of healthcare facilities and services, including laboratories, ambulatory care clinics, ambulatory surgery centers, behavioral health and substance abuse treatment facilities, physical rehabilitation facilities, acute care hospitals, and critical access hospitals.

Healthcare facilities that have been accredited by the AOA earn deemed status from CMS. CMS extended the AOA HFAP deemed status effective through September 25, 2009. Like hospitals accredited by The Joint Commission, AOA-accredited hospitals are not required to undergo yearly Medicare certification surveys; however, as stated previously, a sample of approximately 10 percent of accredited osteopathic hospitals undergo Medicare validation surveys each year (Shaw et al. 2010). State licensure agencies conduct Medicare certification surveys under contracts with CMS. CMS has also granted the AOA accreditation program deeming authority for hospital laboratory services under the Clinical Laboratory Improvements Act of 1988.

Healthcare Facilities Accreditation Program Documentation Standards

The HFAP's acute care accreditation standards relate closely to the Medicare COP for Hospitals (AOA 2007). The AOA's documentation standards are very similar to Joint Commission standards, except in the area of osteopathic medical practice. According to the HFAP's standards, osteopathic physicians are required to perform musculoskeletal examinations in addition to traditional physical examinations shortly before or after a patient's admission to the hospital unless the patient's condition contraindicates such an examination. One standard specifically requires osteopathic physicians to document the results of such examinations in the patient's health record or to document the reason an osteopathic examination was not performed. Failure to meet this standard is one of the most common deficiencies cited during the survey process (AOA 2004).

The HFAP standards in which deficiencies most commonly occur are the following (AOA 2008):

- **Legible and complete:** Orders and progress notes not timed; orders not authenticated within required timeframes; entries not legible

- **Consultations:** Reason for consultation not indicated; level of involvement not indicated

Healthcare Facilities Accreditation Program Survey and Accreditation Processes

Similar to Joint Commission–accredited hospitals, hospitals requesting initial accreditation or renewed accreditation from the AOA initiate the process by submitting an application. The HFAP application requests the same types of information The Joint Commission's application requires. Likewise, the HFAP conducts on-site surveys at accredited hospitals at least once every three years, and accreditation decisions are based on compliance with the HFAP standards and participation requirements (AOA 2004).

Internal Hospital Policies and Procedures

Every hospital must develop, implement, and enforce policies and procedures to ensure the quality of clinical care and the safety of patients, visitors, and staff. **Policies** are general written guidelines that dictate behavior or direct and constrain decision making within the organization. **Procedures** provide detailed written instructions on how functions and processes are implemented. Procedures should explicitly fulfill the stipulations of general policies.

Hospitals generally model their internal policies and procedures after applicable state and federal regulations, legal guidelines, accreditation standards, clinical practice standards, and voluntary industry standards. However, internal policies must also reflect the facility's own service goals and standards of care. Some organizations choose to develop internal policies and procedures that are stricter than state, federal, or accreditation guidelines. For example, a hospital may develop a policy that defines a delinquent record as any record with outstanding deficiencies seven days after discharge, while the state guideline is 30 days after discharge. This type of policy is acceptable; however, the hospital should be aware that during the accreditation survey, it will be held accountable for meeting its own internal policy and not the less restrictive state requirement.

Policies should use clear language and follow a consistent format. In addition, every policy, procedure, and revision should be dated to ensure effective version control.

Policies and procedures should be reviewed on a regular basis and communicated to employees and the medical staff during initial employee and provider orientation.

Employees and caregivers may also be required to review and sign acknowledgments of particularly important policies at regular intervals. Examples might include patient confidentiality and health record access and security policies. Many healthcare organizations post policies and procedures on their internal information networks to make them easy for employees to access.

Policies and procedures may apply across the hospital's departments or pertain specifically to one group of employees or one functional department. Hospital policies and procedures can be grouped into the following general categories:

- Administration, including HIM

- Medical staff

- Nursing services

- Human resources

- Safety

- Environment of care

HIM Policies and Procedures

HIM professionals work with representatives of the hospital's clinical departments to develop health record policies and procedures. Like other hospital policies, health record policies must comply with applicable state and federal regulations, accreditation standards, and clinical standards. Policies and procedures must fulfill the specific legal requirements that apply to the facility. **FIGURE 8.12** provides a sample policy and procedure template.

FIGURE 8.12. HIM Policy and Procedure on Legibility of Handwritten Entries in Patient Health Records

---

POLICY STATEMENT:

Medical record entries shall be documented in a manner that meets the requirements of the legal and regulatory agencies with jurisdiction over the Hospital and the Joint Commission accrediting standards. The health record shall be free from inadvertent or intentional alterations and potential for such altering. There shall be no change or deletion whatsoever of recorded data in the medical record. All members of the Hospital who are authorized to document within the medical record shall provide clear and legible documentation of the patient's condition according to all guidelines.

PROCEDURE:

CORRECTIONS AND ALTERATIONS

- Corrections shall be done in a manner that does not obliterate the original entry. **Use of white-out is not permitted.** No erasure or eradication is permitted. If an error has been made, a single line shall be drawn through the error, labeled as an error, the correction made, dated and initialed.

- Pages of medical records shall not be removed, torn out or cut. Any actions which may be construed as tampering with the record must be avoided. All entries are to be made in permanent black ink (preferred) or blue ink.

FIGURE 8.12. (Continued)

GENERAL ENTRIES

- Entries in the medical record shall be continuous with no blank pages, lines or spaces. A line shall be drawn to the end of the page when an entry does not fill the page.

- Entries shall be made in permanent black ink (preferred) or blue ink. Using other colors is discouraged. Pencil may not be used.

- Entries shall be documented as close to the time of the actual event as feasible. Entries shall be dated, timed and signed at the time the entry is written. Signatures shall include initials or titles indicating professional credentials. Each entry shall be individually authenticated.

- The attending physician for each patient shall be responsible for the preparations and completion of the medical record. However, he/she can countersign history and physical examinations written by a member of the House Staff. He/she does not have to countersign progress notes, treatment orders or other entries written by House Staff appointees (per Medical Staff Bylaws).

- Symbols and abbreviations may be used if the Medical Records Committee approves them. Only abbreviations that are approved and listed on the Medical Records website will be used. Abbreviations on the "Dangerous Abbreviations" List are not to be used.

- All entries must be in chronological order.

- The patient's name must appear on both sides of every page in the record. The addressograph should be used.

- All entries shall be promptly recorded to reflect the accuracy of the patient's condition.

LEGIBILITY

- All entries into the medical record shall be written legibly.

- Handwriting, including signatures, must be legible.

LATE ENTRIES AND ADDENDA

- Late entries and addenda shall be entered in chronological order according to the time and date of the late entries or addenda. Notes shall be labeled as late entries or addenda.

- Attending physicians shall be notified of patient requests to amend records. After discussion with the attending physician regarding the amendment, patients may add a letter of amendment to the record.

FIGURE 8.13 lists the policies and procedures commonly maintained by hospital HIM departments.

Medical Staff Bylaws, Rules, and Regulations

Medical staff bylaws, rules, and regulations govern the conduct of the independent healthcare professionals who provide patient care services in acute care facilities. Bylaws are similar to policies in that they describe general guidelines. Rules and regulations, like procedures, describe the specific activities to be performed to carry out the bylaws. The bylaws describe the structure of the medical staff and its membership qualifications, rights, and responsibilities.

Rules and regulations are generally easier to amend and therefore should be used to communicate elements that are likely to change frequently. Medical staff rules and regulations establish the medical staff's specific responsibilities for patient care and health record documentation.

FIGURE 8.13. HIM policy and procedures on legibility of handwritten entries in patient health records

The following list provides an example of the types of policy and procedures that may be included in a manual for health information services. The titles and content of the policy and procedures may vary by facility or corporation. Some of the policy and procedures are listed more than once for cross-referencing purposes.

Abbreviations
Access to Automated/Computerized Records
Access to Records (Release of Information) by
    Resident and by Staff
Admission/Discharge Register
Admission Procedures
    Facility Procedures–Establishing/Closing the
      Record
    Preparing the Medical Record
    Preparing the Master Patient Index Card
    Readmission–Continued Use of Previous
      Record
    Readmission–New Record
Amendment of Clinical Records
Audit Schedule
Audit and Monitoring System
    Audit/Monitoring Schedule
    Admission/Readmission Audit
    Concurrent Audit
    Discharge Audit
    Specialized Audits (examples)
    Change in Condition
    MDS
    Nursing Assistant Flow Sheet
    Psychotropic Drug Documentation
    Pressure Sore
    Restrictive Device/Restraint
    Therapy
Certification, Medicare
Chart Removal and Chart Locator Log
Clinical Records, Definition of Records,
    and Record Service
General Policies
    Access to Records
    Automation of Records (See also
      Computerization)
    Availability
    Change in Ownership
    Completion and Correction of Records
    Confidentiality
    Definition of the Legal Record,
      Coding from home
    Indexes
    Ownership of Records

Permanent and Capable of Being
    Photocopied
Retention
Storage of Records
Subpoena
Unit Record
Willful Falsification/Willful Omission
Closing the Record
Coding and Indexing, Disease Index
Committee Minutes Guidelines
Computerization and Security of Automated
    Data/Records
Confidentiality (See Release of Information)
Consulting Services for Clinical Records and Plan
    of Service
Content, Record *(the list provided is not all-
    inclusive and should be tailored to the
    facility/corporation)*
    General
    Advanced Directives
    Transfer Form/Discharge Plan of Care
    Discharge against Medical Advice
    Physician Consultant Reports
    Medicare Certification/Recertification
    Physician Orders/Telephone Orders
    Physician Services Guidelines and Progress
      Notes
    Physician History and Physical Exam
    Discharge Summary
    Interdisciplinary Progress Notes
Copying/Release of Records—General
Correcting Clinical Records
Data Collection/Monitoring
Definition of Clinical Records/Health Information
    Service
Delinquent Physician Visit
Denial Letters, Medicare
Destruction of Records, Log
Disaster Planning for Health Information
Discharge Procedures
    Assembly of Discharge Record
    Chart Order on Discharge

FIGURE 8.13. (Continued)

Completing and Filing Master Patient
    Index Card
Discharge Chart Audit
Notification of Deficiencies
Incomplete Record File
Closure of Incomplete Clinical Record
Preparation of the Record, Imaging of
    Records, Quality Review
Emergency Disaster Evacuation
Establishing/Closing Record
Falsification of Records, Willful
Fax/Facsimile, Faxing
Filing Order, Discharge (Chart Order)
Filing Order, In-house (Chart Order)
Filing System
Filing System, Unit Record
Forms Management
Forms, Release of Information
Forms, Subpoena
Guide to Location of Items in the Health
    Information Department
Guidelines, Committee Minutes
Incomplete Record File
Indexes
    Disease Index and Forms for Indexing
    Master Patient Index
    Release of Information Index/Log
In-service Training Minutes/Record
Job Descriptions
    Health Information Coordinator
    Health Unit Coordinator
    Other Health Information Staff (if
        applicable)
Late Entries
Lost Record—Reconstruction
Master Patient Index
Medicare Documentation
    Certification and Recertification
    Medicare Denial Procedure and Letter
    Medicare Log
Numbering System
Ombudsman, Review/Access to Records
Omission, Willful
Order of Filing, Discharge
Order of Filing, In-house
Organizational Chart for Health Information
    Department
Orientation/Training of Health Information
    Department

Outguides
Physician Visit Schedule, Letters, and
    Monitoring
Physician Visits, Delinquent Visit Follow-up
Quality Assurance
    Health Information Participation
    QA Studies and Reporting
Readmission—Continued Use of Previous
    Record
Readmission—New Record
Recertification or Certification (Medicare)
Reconstruction of Lost Record
Refusal of Treatment
Release of Information
    Confidentiality
    Confidentiality Statement by Staff
    Copying/Release of Records—General
    Faxing Medical Information
    Procedure for Release—Sample Letters
        and Authorizations
    Redisclosure of Clinical Information
    Resident Access to Records
    Retrieval of Records (sign-out system)
    Subpoena
    Uses and Disclosures of Protected Health
        Information, Uses and Disclosures of
        Deidentified Documentation, Business-
        Associated Contracts, Audit Trails
    Witnessing Legal Documents
Requesting Information
    From Hospitals and Other Healthcare Providers
    Request for Information Form
Retention of Records and Destruction after
    Retention Period
    Example Statement for Destruction
    Retention Guidelines
Retrieval of Records
Security of Automated Data/Electronic Medical
    Records
    General Procedures
    Back-up Procedures
    Passwords
Sign-out Logs
Storage of Records
Telephone Orders
Thinning
    In-house Records
    Maintaining Overflow Record
Unit Record System

Medical Records Committee

Medical staff bylaws prescribe the duties and functions of the medical records committee. Usually the committee consists of physician members, the president or designee, a nursing service representative, the director of health information services, and others as required to accomplish the duties and responsibilities of the committee at the request of the chairperson. Another committee, as defined by medical staff bylaws, may perform the functions of the medical records committee.

Duties of the medical records committee include the following:

- Evaluating medical records using criteria developed and approved by the medical board to assess whether records describe the conditions and progress of the patients, the therapies provided, and the results thereof

- Evaluating and making recommendations to the medical board regarding form and format of the medical records

- Monitoring the promptness, adequacy, pertinence, and completeness of medical records

- Referring identified deficiencies to the appropriate department or committee for review

- Reviewing the number of incomplete charts for each practitioner and referring information to the medical board as appropriate

- Preparing reports as requested by the medical board, a division's quality review officer/committee, or the credentials committee for use during the reappointment and renewal of clinical privileges

Interface Between Joint Commission Standards and Hospital Policy and Procedure Development

The Joint Commission's standards for information management and record of care contain many provisions that defer to the hospital to set the specifics for meeting the standard through development and compliance with internal policies and procedures. Examples of Joint Commission record of care standards that defer to internal hospital policies and procedures include the following (Joint Commission 2010):

1. Does the hospital implement its policy requiring timely entry of information into the patient's medical record? (RC.01.03.01 #3)

2. Does the hospital define the types of entries in the medical record made by nonindependent practitioners that require countersigning, in accordance with law and regulation? (RC.01.02.01 #2)

3. Does the hospital identify in writing the staff who are authorized to receive and record verbal orders, in accordance with law and regulation? (RC.02.03.07 #1)

Summary

Acute care hospitals are regulated through a complex and constantly changing system of mandatory and voluntary standards promulgated by federal government agencies, state government departments of health, and accrediting organizations. Regulations vary at the federal and state levels, and Medicare and Medicaid have their own COP based on the healthcare setting. Although several accreditation programs are available for hospitals, The Joint Commission brings together these disparate regulations to provide a launching point for most healthcare facilities. For each of these mandatory and voluntary standards, it is usually the health rerecord and the documentation contained therein that hospitals use to demonstrate compliance. The HIM professional is a key member of the organization team that addresses the ongoing compliance efforts. Hospital internal policies and procedures are essential not only for internal operations efficiencies and quality purposes, but also to meeting ongoing PPR requirements of The Joint Commission.

References

American Health Information Management Association (AHIMA). n.d. Healthcare Compliance. http://www.ahima.org/resources/compliance.aspx.

American Osteopathic Association (AOA). 2008. HFAP Most Commonly Occurring Deficiencies 2008. http://www.hfap.org/pdf/hfap_most_commonly_occurring_deficiencies_2008.pdf-wi.

American Osteopathic Association (AOA). 2007. *Accreditation Requirements for Healthcare Facilities, 2004-2005.* Chicago: AOA.

American Osteopathic Association (AOA). 2004. About the Healthcare Facilities Accreditation Program. http://do-online.osteotech.org.

Carpenter, J. 1999. Practice Brief: Managing Health Information Relating to Infection with the Human Immunodeficiency Virus. *Journal of American Health Information Management Association* 70(5): Suppl.

Cassidy, B. 2011. "Healthcare Delivery Systems." In *Health Information Management Technology: An Applied Approach,* 3rd ed., edited by M. Johns. Chicago: AHIMA.

Centers for Medicare and Medicaid Services (CMS). 2011a. Quality Measures: Overview. https://www.cms.gov/qualitymeasures.

Centers for Medicare and Medicaid Services (CMS). 2011b. Recovery Audit Program: Overview. https://www.cms.gov/recovery-audit-program/.

Centers for Medicare and Medicaid Services (CMS). 2005. Medicaid at a Glance. http://www.cms.gov/MedicaidDataSourcesGenInfo/downloads/maag2005.pdf.

Centers for Medicare and Medicaid Services (CMS). 2010. Medicare and Medicaid Programs; Hospital conditions of participation: Final rule. 42 CFR Part 482. *Federal Register* 71(236): 71377–71428. http://edocket.access.gpo.gov/cfr_2010/octqtr/pdf/42cfr482.24.pdf.

Commonwealth of Massachusetts. 2010. 105 CMR-130.370: Retention of Records. http://www.lawlib.state.ma.us/source/mass/cmr/cmrtext/105CMR130.pdf.

Department of Health and Human Services (HHS). 2011. Summary of the HIPAA Privacy Rule. http://www.hhs.gov/ocr/privacy/hipaa/understanding/summary/privacysummary.pdf.

Department of Health and Human Services (HHS). 2008. http://aspe.hhs.gov/health/Reports/05/uninsured-cps/index.htm#Insurance.

Department of Health and Human Services (HHS). 2005. Medicaid At-a-Glance 2005: A Medicaid Information Source. Publication No. CMS-11024-05. https://www.cms.gov/MedicaidDataSourcesGenInfo/downloads/maag2005.pdf.

Department of Health and Human Services (HHS). n.d. Hospital Compare. http://www.hospitalcompare.hhs.gov/.

Equal Opportunity Employment Commission. (EEOC). 2011. Genetic Information Discrimination. http://www.eeoc.gov/laws/types/genetic.cfm.

Genetic Information Nondiscrimination Act (GINA). 2008. Public Law 110-233, 122 STST. 881. http://www.ornl.gov/sci/techresources/Human_Genome/publicat/GINAMay2008.pdf.

Human Genome Project (HGP). 2004. Human Genome Project. http://www.ornl.gov/sci/techresources/Human_Genome/project/about.shtml.

Hjort, B. 2005. Practice Brief: The HIM Role in Patient Safety and Quality of Care. *Journal of American Health Information Management Association* 76 (1): 56A–G.

Hospital Care Quality Information from the Consumer Perspective (HCAHPS). 2011. HCAHPS Survey. http://www.hcahpsonline.org/Files/HCAHPS%20V6%200%20Appendix%20A%20-%20HCAHPS%20Mail%20Survey%20Materials%20(English)%202-16-2011.pdf.

Hospital Quality Initiative. 2009. Fiscal Year 2009 Quality Measure Reporting for 2010 Payment Update. https://www.cms.gov/HospitalQualityInits/downloads/HospitalRHQDAPU200808.pdf.

The Joint Commission. 2007. Joint Commission International Accreditation Standards for Hospitals 3rd Edition: Standards Only. http://www.google.com/url?sa=t&rct=j&q=&esrc=s&source=web&cd=1&ved=0CCUQFjAA&url=http%3A%2F%2Fjointcommissioninternational.org%2Fcommon%2Fpdfs%2Fjcia%2FStandards_Only-Hosp_3rd_ed.pdf&ei=gbmNT4uRPIWatwekks3GCw&usg=AFQjCNEXFYcMlbGAUKPBna9ISdMlYcL5Fg&sig2=dbNaxsVcA55ahJkLU9lTRg.

The Joint Commission. 2011a. About The Joint Commission. http://www.jointcommission.org/about_us/about_the_joint_commission_main.aspx.

The Joint Commission, 2011b. Sentinel Events. http://www.jointcommission.org/assets/1/6/2011_CAMH_SE.pdf.

The Joint Commission. 2010. *Accreditation Guide.* Oakbrook Terrace, IL: Joint Commission. www.jointcommission.org/AccreditationPrograms/Hospitals/AccreditationProcess/PPR_QA.htm.

Massachusetts Department of Public Health. 2010. 130.370: Retention of Records. 105 CMR—568.2. http://www.mass.gov/Eeohhs2/docs/dph/regs/105cmr130.pdf.

McWay, D. 2009. *Legal and Ethical Aspects of Health Information Management.* Clifton Park, NY: Delmar Learning.

New York State. 2011. Codes, Rules and Regulations. Title 18. http://www.omig.ny.gov/data/images/stories/provider_compliance/adopted_regulations_521.pdf.

Office of Inspector General (OIG). 2011. Work Plan Fiscal Year 2011. http://oig.hhs.gov/publications/workplan/2011/FY11_WorkPlan-All.pdf.

Office of Inspector General (OIG). 1998. *OIG Compliance Guidance for Hospitals.* http://oig.hhs.gov/authorities/docs/cpghosp.pdf.

ORYX. 2011. Facts About ORYX for Hospitals. http://www.jointcommission.org/assets/1/18/ORYX_for_Hospitals_1_25_11.pdf.

Agency for Healthcare Research and Quality (AHRQ). 2011. Patient Safety Organizations. http://www.pso
.ahrq.gov/index.html.

Shaw, P., et al. 2010. *Quality and Performance Improvement in Healthcare: A Tool for Programmed Learning,*
4th ed. Chicago: AHIMA.

State of New York Office of the Medicaid Inspector General. 2011. Bureau of Compliance Best Practices in
Compliance by Provider Type. http://www.omig.ny.gov/data/images/stories/compliance/best_practices_
list_7_8_f_%2011_2_%203.pdf.

Chapter 9

Health Records in Ambulatory Care

Susan Rossiter, RHIA

Learning Objectives

- Describe the role of the federal government in regulating ambulatory care providers

- Explain the role of state governments in regulating ambulatory care providers

- Identify at least four reasons an ambulatory care provider would seek out voluntary accreditation

- Evaluate the different accreditation agencies for ambulatory care

- Describe The Joint Commission's accreditation methodology for ambulatory care, including elements of performance and sentinel events

- Describe the emerging documentation requirements for each type of accreditation

- Compare the differences in acute care and ambulatory care documentation

- Describe the challenges of obtaining informed consent in a large multispecialty setting

- Explain the unique difference in the internal policies for a multisite ambulatory healthcare organization

- Outline the internal health information management policies that professionals should address to meet current regulation challenges

Key Terms

Accreditation

Accreditation Association for Ambulatory Health Care (AAAHC)

Accreditation Commission for Healthcare (ACHC)

American Association for Accreditation of Ambulatory Surgery Facilities (AAAASF)

American College of Radiology (ACR)

CARF

Clinical Laboratory Improvement Amendments (CLIA)

Closing practice policy

College of American Pathologists (CAP)

Commission on Cancer (CoC)

Community Health Accreditation Program (CHAP)

Deemed status

Elements of performance (EP)

Failed/missed appointment policy

General consent

Hand-off communication

Informed consent

The Joint Commission

Medication list

National Committee for Quality
Assurance (NCQA)

Outstanding record policy

Problem list

Sentinel event

Shadow chart policy

Summary list

Telephone encounter

Introduction

Ambulatory care is preventive or corrective healthcare services provided on a nonresident basis in a provider's office, clinic setting, or hospital outpatient setting. Ambulatory care services can be divided into hospital based and independent, or non–hospital based. Hospital-based ambulatory services generally include emergency departments, ambulatory surgery, and outpatient diagnostic and therapeutic services. General descriptions and record content for hospital-based ambulatory services were addressed in chapter 5. There are many types of non–hospital-based outpatient services. A description of these services is provided in chapter 13. The current chapter focuses on the regulatory and accrediting agencies for ambulatory care and health record content.

First we address the organizations that create health record standards for ambulatory care. These include the federal government, state governments, The Joint Commission, and other accrediting organizations. Medicare Conditions of Participation (COP) for ambulatory services are reviewed. Some examples of state legislation are provided; however, an health information management (HIM) professional will need to be familiar with the laws in the state where his healthcare organization is located. The Joint Commission accreditation standards for ambulatory care are addressed generally. However, the information in these standards is quite detailed. Again, HIM professionals need to familiarize themselves with the standards that apply to their organization. Finally, other accrediting organizations for ambulatory care services are described.

Second, health record content for non–hospital-based ambulatory services is addressed. The content included and the HIM professional's responsibilities for maintaining that content are addressed. References are made to the electronic health record (EHR), and some examples of computerized forms are provided. For an in-depth look at the EHR, refer to chapter 6.

Finally, regulation and policy topics such as informed consent and closing a practice are addressed.

Governmental Regulation of Ambulatory Care

Healthcare provider entities must comply with certain federal regulations to receive reimbursement under Medicare and Medicaid. Additionally, each state has specific rules that must be met to qualify for licensing.

Federal Government: CMS

To treat Medicare or Medicaid patients, healthcare providers must demonstrate that they meet the Medicare COP. The COP standards for ambulatory surgery centers (ASCs) are included in chapter IV, Part 416 of the Code of Federal Regulations (CFR). Although ASCs are only one example of ambulatory or outpatient care, these guidelines provide an example of federal government regulation requirements in this area. **Figure 9.1** contains the health record requirements for an ASC.

State Governments

Any provider of ambulatory care services must be licensed by the state where the facility is located. In addition, the provider must abide by all laws and regulations for that state's department of health. Because laws and regulations vary by state, an HIM professional must be familiar with all state regulations and laws that apply to the type of providing setting where she is employed. **Figure 9.2** lists the medical record state-specific regulations for an ASC in Illinois.

FIGURE 9.1. **Medicare Conditions of Participation for medical records for ambulatory surgery centers**

TITLE 42—PUBLIC HEALTH

CHAPTER IV—CENTERS FOR MEDICARE
& MEDICAID SERVICES,
DEPARTMENT OF HEALTH AND
HUMAN SERVICES

PART 416_AMBULATORY SURGICAL SERVICES—Table of Contents

Subpart C_Specific Conditions for Coverage

Sec. 416.47 Condition for coverage—Medical records.

The ASC must maintain complete, comprehensive, and accurate medical records to ensure adequate patient care.

    a. Standard: Organization. The ASC must develop and maintain a system for the proper collection, storage, and use of patient records.

    b. Standard: Form and content of record. The ASC must maintain a medical record for each patient. Every record must be accurate, legible, and promptly completed. Medical records must include at least the following:

        1. Patient identification.

        2. Significant medical history and results of physical examination.

        3. Pre-operative diagnostic studies (entered before surgery), if performed.

        4. Findings and techniques of the operation, including a pathologist's report on all tissues removed during surgery, except those exempted by the governing body.

        5. Any allergies and abnormal drug reactions.

        6. Entries related to anesthesia administration.

        7. Documentation of properly executed informed patient consent.

        8. Discharge diagnosis.

Source: 42 CFR 416.47, 728

FIGURE 9.2. Illinois regulations for medical records in an ambulatory surgery center

---

TITLE 77: PUBLIC HEALTH

CHAPTER I: DEPARTMENT OF PUBLIC HEALTH

SUBCHAPTER b: HOSPITAL AND AMBULATORY CARE FACILITIES

PART 205 AMBULATORY SURGICAL TREATMENT CENTER LICENSING REQUIREMENTS

SECTION 205.610 CLINICAL RECORDS

Section 205.610 Clinical Records

Accurate and complete clinical records shall be maintained for each patient and all entries in the clinical record shall be made at the time the surgical procedure is performed and when care, treatment, medications, or other medical services are given. The record shall include, but not be limited to, the following:

    a. patient identification.

    b. admitting information including patient history, physical examination findings, diagnosis or need for medical services.

    c. pre-counseling notes.

    d. signed informed consent.

    e. confirmation of pregnancy (when abortion is performed).

    f. signed physician orders.

    g. laboratory test reports, pathologist's report of tissue, and radiologist's report of x-rays.

    h. anesthesia record.

    i. operative record.

    j. medication and medical treatments.

    k. recovery room progress notes.

    l. physician and nurses' progress notes.

    m. condition at time of discharge.

    n. patient instructions.

    o. post-counseling notes.

Source: Illinois General Assembly 1973.

Ambulatory Care Accreditation Standards

Accreditation is defined as recognition by an external entity of achievement of predefined standards of excellence. The ambulatory care environment is changing rapidly. New technology, prospective payment systems, compliance requirements, an increasing shift in patient volume, competition in the marketplace, and continuous updates in patient quality of care are some of the ongoing pressures. Many regulatory agencies, payers, and managed-care contractors require accreditation for reimbursement, certification, licensure, and participation agreement.

Because ambulatory care is becoming so common and so diversified, the numbers and types of accrediting bodies have grown since 2000. In addition, the services that are accredited by existing agencies, such as The Joint Commission, have expanded. This section describes the organizations that provide accreditation for entire ambulatory care centers or specific services within a center. The Joint Commission remains the largest and most diversified accrediting body. However, many other organizations have grown to meet the increased demand for accreditation in ambulatory care.

Advantages of Accreditation

Ambulatory care organizations benefit from being accredited. Probably the most significant benefit is recognition from the federal government as having **deemed status**. As we discussed earlier, for a healthcare organization to participate in and receive payment from the Medicare or Medicaid programs, it must be certified as complying with the COP, or standards, set forth in federal regulations. This certification is based on a survey conducted by a state agency on behalf of the Centers for Medicare and Medicaid Services (CMS). However, if national accrediting organizations, such as The Joint Commission or the American Association for Accreditation of Ambulatory Surgery Facilities (AAAASF), have and enforce standards that meet the federal COP, CMS may grant the accrediting organization deeming authority and deem each accredited healthcare organization as meeting the Medicare and Medicaid certification requirements. As a result, the healthcare organization would have deemed status and would not be subject to the Medicare survey and certification process. Not every accrediting organization has deemed status.

Deemed status options are available for Joint Commission–accredited ASCs, clinical laboratories, home health agencies, hospice organizations, and hospitals, and the AAAASF.

In addition to deemed status, recognition from an accrediting association provides the following advantages:

- Enhances community confidence by visibly demonstrating the organization's commitment to improving the quality of patient care and makes a strong statement to the community about the organization's efforts to provide the highest-quality services possible

- Provides a report card or benchmark of quality for the organization's performance standards, including performance improvement concepts

- Assists in performance improvement efforts, enabling the organization to perform a variety of activities to raise the quality of care to the highest possible level

- Assists in the recruitment of professional staff

- Provides an education tool and ongoing educational support

- Helps the organization meet certain regulatory agency certification and state licensure requirements

- Helps the organization meet the eligibility prerequisites or requirements for insurance reimbursement and expedites payment by insurers and other third parties, ensures participation in managed-care plans, facilitates bidding on contracts, and increases financing capabilities because lenders may require accreditation as a condition of financing

In addition, accreditation enhances risk management efforts and may improve access to and reduce the cost of liability insurance coverage.

The Joint Commission

The Joint Commission established the Ambulatory Care Accreditation program in 1975 to encourage quality patient care in all types of freestanding ambulatory care facilities. These centers may not be owned or operated by a hospital. See **FIGURE 9.3** for a list of the types of ambulatory centers that are certified by The Joint Commission.

In 2007, The Joint Commission made available for the first time a separate manual of accreditation standards for ASCs. Until that time, ambulatory care standards were combined into one manual for all ambulatory care settings. The *Accreditation Manual for Ambulatory Care Organizations* (Joint Commission 2008a) provides an in-depth review of required standards for all other freestanding ambulatory care organizations. A condensed version of the standards pertaining specifically to information management in a freestanding ambulatory surgical center follows.

Refer to the most current Joint Commission manual. Standards and elements of performance (EPs) are updated periodically.

FIGURE 9.3. Types of freestanding and specialty ambulatory healthcare centers certified by The Joint Commission

Freestanding Ambulatory Centers	Specialty Care Providers
• Ambulatory surgery centers	• Birthing centers
• Community health centers	• Cardiac catheterization centers
• Correctional facilities health centers	• Dental clinics
• Group medical practices	• Dialysis centers
• Indian health clinics	• Endoscopy centers
• Military clinics	• Imaging centers
• Mobile services	• Infusion therapy services
• Multispecialty group practices	• Laser centers
• Occupational health centers	• Lithotripsy services
• Office-based surgery offices	• Magnetic resonance imaging (MRI) centers
• Physicians' offices	• Ophthalmology practices
• Student health services	• Oral and maxillofacial surgery centers
	• Pain management centers
	• Plastic surgery centers
	• Podiatric clinics
	• Radiation/oncology clinics
	• Rehabilitation centers
	• Sleep centers
	• Urgent/emergency care centers
	• Women's health centers

Elements of Performance

Elements of Performance (EPs) are The Joint Commission's specific performance expectations and/or structures or processes that must be in place for an organization to provide safe, high-quality care, treatment, and services. Knowledge of EPs pertaining directly to the health record and documentation in the record are critical for HIM professionals working in an accredited facility. This includes compliance with the following federal and state laws and regulations:

- Health Insurance Portability and Accountability Act (HIPAA)
- State medical board regulations
- State and local health department regulations

In addition to having written policies, organizations must

- Implement the policy
- Ensure the policy and any updates have been communicated to all staff members
- Monitor the policy (such as by doing an organization-wide HIPAA audit)
- Stay abreast of developments in technology to continually improve privacy and confidentiality
- Preserve the privacy and confidentiality of data and information identified as sensitive
- Inform individuals with identifiable health data and information that is maintained or collected about how their information will be used or disclosed
- Remove personal identifiers, to the extent possible, for uses and disclosures of health information consistent with maintaining the usefulness of the information
- Protect health information by ensuring that it is used for the purposes identified or as required by law or regulation and not redisclosed without patient permission

The Joint Commission requires that healthcare provider entities have written policies addressing information security and data integrity consistent with law or regulation. Sample HIM policies might include the following:

- A policy to allow staff access to the HIM department on a need-to-know basis (for example, HIM staff and physicians)
- A visitor log and policy
- A policy on transporting medical records to and from the clinic
- A chain-of-custody policy to ensure that the medical record is never in the patient's hands without a member of the organization present

The requirement concerning implementation and monitoring of any written policy also applies.

Developing and implementing controls to safeguard data and information, including the patient record, against loss, destruction, and tampering include the following:

- Policies indicating when the removal of records is permitted

- Protection against unauthorized intrusion, corruption, or damage

- Minimization of risk of falsification of data and information

- Guidelines for preventing the loss and destruction of records

- Guidelines for destroying copies of records

- Protection of records in a manner that minimizes the possibility of damage from fire and water

- Policies and procedures, including plans for electronic information systems, that address data integrity, authentication, nonrepudiation, encryption as warranted, and auditability as appropriate to the system and types of information (such as patient information and billing information)

Electronic medical record systems requirements include backing up electronic medical record systems. Contingency plans must be in place for interruptions of service due to system failures. The plan must be tested periodically as defined by the organization. See **FIGURE 9.4** for EPs related to the following:

IM.6.10: Requirements for patient-specific information

IM.6.30: Documentation for operative and high-risk procedures

IM.6.40: Summary list(s) for patients with continuing ambulatory care needs

IM.6.50: Process for authenticating verbal or telephone orders

Access to relevant information from a patient must be available as needed for use in patient services. To accomplish this, the organization must do the following:

- Have a process for tracking all components of the medical record

- Use a system to assemble required information or make available a summary or information relative to the patient services provided

Use of these comprehensive documentation requirements helps ambulatory healthcare organizations improve patient outcomes, healthcare documentation, patient safety, and performance in patient services.

Ambulatory Care and Office-Based Surgery National Patient Safety Goals

In 2006, The Joint Commission announced patient safety standards that apply specifically to ambulatory care facilities. New requirements for **hand-off communication** of patient information between caregivers and improvement in the safety of medication received special attention. The primary objective of a handoff is to provide accurate information about a patient's care, treatment, services, current condition, and any recent or anticipated changes. The information communicated during a

FIGURE 9.4. The Joint Commission elements of performance

IM.6.10: Requirements for patient-specific information

- Only authorized users make entries in the medical record.

- The organization defines which entries made by nonindependent practitioners require countersigning consistent with law or regulation.

- Standardized formats are used for documenting all services provided to patients.

- Medical record entries are dated, the author identified, and when necessary according to law or regulation, authenticated by written signature, electronic signature, computer key, or rubber stamp. Use of a computer key or rubber stamp requires the author to sign a statement that he or she alone uses the key or stamp.

- The author authenticates the following per above requirements:
    1. History and physical (H&P)
    2. Operative reports
    3. Consultations
    4. Diagnostic and therapeutic procedures
    5. Follow-up or discharge orders

- The medical record contains sufficient information to identify the patient, support the diagnosis/condition, justify the services, document the course and results of services, and promote continuity of care among providers.

- Policy on timely entry of information into the patient's medical record

- Definition of what is a complete record and time frame to complete the record

- Medical records are reviewed on an ongoing basis.

- Review of the record is based on organization-defined indicators that address the presence, timeliness, readability, quality, consistency, clarity, accuracy, completeness, and authentication of data and information contained within the record.

- The retention time of medical record information is determined by the organization based on law or regulation and its use for patient services; legal, research, operational purposes; and educational activities.

- Original medical records are not released unless responding to laws or regulations, court orders, or subpoenas.

- Medical records of patients who have received urgent or immediate services contain (1) time and means of arrival, (2) whether the patient left against medical advice, and (3) conclusions at termination of treatment, including final disposition and instructions for follow-up services.

- A copy of the record is available to the practitioner or medical organization providing follow-up care, treatment, and services.

- Documentation and findings of assessments

- Conclusions or impressions drawn from the H&P exam

- Diagnosis, diagnostic impression, or conditions

- Diagnostic and therapeutic orders

- Diagnostic and therapeutic procedures, tests, and results

- Operative and other invasive procedures

- Progress notes made by authorized individuals, including the date, staff person, and service provided

- Reassessments and plan of care revisions

- Consultation reports

- Allergies to food and medications

- Medications ordered or prescribed

- Dosages of medications administered (including the strength, dose, and rate of administration), administration devices used, access site or route, known drug allergies, patient's response to medication, and adverse drug reactions

- Relevant diagnoses/conditions established during the course of services

FIGURE 9.4. (continued)

- Demographic information: patient's name, gender, address, phone number, date of birth, height, weight, phone number of a legally authorized representative, legal status of patient receiving behavioral health services, patient's language and communication needs

- Evidence of known advance directives when indicated, evidence of informed consent, referrals or communications made to external or internal care providers and community agencies

- Treatment summaries and other pertinent documents to promote continuity of care

- Documentation of clinical research interventions that is distinct from entries related to regular patient care

- Records of communication with patient regarding services (such as telephone calls or e-mail)

- Patient-generated information (such as information entered into the record over the Internet or via previsit computer systems)

- When appropriate, summaries of treatment and other documents provided by the organization are forwarded to other care providers.

- Discharge diagnosis

IM.6.30: Documentation for operative and high-risk procedures

- Provisional diagnosis recorded prior to the operative or other high-risk procedure

- Written or dictated reports are recorded immediately after the procedure. The written report must include the name of the licensed independent practitioner and assistants, procedure(s) performed and description of the procedure(s), finding(s), estimated blood loss, specimen(s) removed, and postoperative diagnosis.

- A progress note written immediately after the procedure can take the place of the full report being recorded immediately. However, the full report must be recorded within a specified time frame defined by the organization.

- The completed procedure report is authenticated by the practitioner and made available in the medical record as soon as possible.

- Postoperative documentation records the patient's vital signs and level of consciousness, medications (including intravenous fluids), blood and blood components administered, unusual events or complications (including blood transfusion reactions), and the management of those events.

  o Postoperative documentation records the patient's discharge from the postsedation or postanesthesia care area by the responsible licensed independent practitioner or according to discharge criteria.

  o Use of approved discharge criteria to determine the patient's readiness for discharge is documented in the medical record.

  o Postoperative documentation records the name of the licensed independent practitioner responsible for discharge.

  o For Medicare-certified ambulatory centers, the results of preoperative diagnostic studies before surgery, if performed, must be documented.

IM.6.40: Summary list(s) for patients with continuing ambulatory care needs

- The summary list must be initiated by the third visit and maintained thereafter.

- The summary list must contain known significant medical diagnoses and conditions and operative and invasive procedures.

- Known adverse and allergic drug reactions

- Known long-term medications, including current medications, over-the counter drugs, and herbal preparations

- The summary list must be quickly and easily available for healthcare professionals to access needed information.

IM.6.50: Process for authenticating verbal or telephone orders

- Qualified personnel are identified per law and regulation.

- Verbal or telephone orders are dated and identify the names of the individuals who gave, received, and implemented the orders.

- Authenticated within the specified time frame, if required by law or regulation

- Verification of the complete verbal or telephone order when reporting critical test results by having the person receiving the order record and "read back" the complete order or test result.

Source: Joint Commission 2008a.

handoff must be accurate to meet patient safety goals. Types of patient handoffs include nursing shift changes; physicians transferring complete responsibility for a patient; physicians transferring on-call responsibility; temporary responsibility for staff leaving the unit for a short time; an anesthesiologist reporting to a postanesthesia recovery room nurse; nursing and physician handoff from the emergency department to inpatient units; transfers to different hospitals, nursing homes, and home health care; and critical laboratory and radiology results being sent to physician offices (Joint Commission 2008a).

> **Standard 2E**: Implement a standardized approach to hand off communications, including an opportunity to ask and respond to questions.

> **Standard 3D**: Label all medications, medication containers, or other solutions on and off the sterile field in perioperative and other procedural settings.

Sentinel Event Policy

The Joint Commission (2008b) describes a **sentinel event** as "an unexpected occurrence involving death or serious physical or psychological injury or the risk thereof." Specifically, it includes "loss of limb or function." Sentinel events are immediate in nature. Accreditation standards include having an organization-specific sentinel event policy. Examples of a reportable event for an ambulatory care organization include

- Operating on the wrong side of the patient's body

- Leaving a foreign body such as a sponge in a patient after surgery

- A patient fall resulting in death

- Medication errors that cause paralysis, coma, or other permanent loss of function

The Joint Commission's Improving Organization Performance indicators are closely tied to the management of sentinel events and outcome of services provided.

Accreditation Association for Ambulatory Health Care

The **Accreditation Association for Ambulatory Health Care (AAAHC)** is a nonprofit organization incorporated in 1979. AAAHC (2008) states that it is the "leader in developing standards to advance and promote patient safety, quality and value for ambulatory health care through peer-based accreditation processes, education and research." AAAHC has a fundamental commitment to high-quality healthcare. The association is dedicated to educating providers in quality assurance and accreditation standards and procedures. It has conducted thousands of accreditation surveys of all types of ambulatory care organizations, including ambulatory surgical facilities, college and university health centers, single and multispecialty group practices, and health networks. The association currently accredits more than 3,700 organizations nationwide.

AAAHC's Core Standards include the following:

- Rights of patients

- Governance

- Administration

- Quality of care provided

- Quality management and improvement

- Clinical records and health information

- Facilities and environment

In the AAAHC's accreditation process, the following questions are asked regarding "clinical records and health information" (2008):

- Does the organization have an organized system for collecting, processing, maintaining, and storing patient records?

- Are the presence or absence of allergies and untoward reactions toward drugs and other materials recorded in a uniform location in patient charts?

- Are patient records transferred to the new healthcare professional when a patient is transferred?

AAAHC requires that the following data be recorded for each patient visit (AAAHC 2008):

- Patient identification

- Date, department (if appropriate), and provider's name and profession (for example, physical therapist, registered nurse)

- Chief complaint or purpose of visit

- Significant medical history and results of physical examination

- Preoperative diagnostic studies (entered before surgery), if performed

- Clinical findings

- Diagnosis or medical impression

- Findings/techniques of operation including pathology report on all tissues removed during surgery, except those exempted by GB

- Any allergies and abnormal drug reactions

- Entries related to anesthesia administration

- Documentation of properly executed informed patient consent

- Discharge diagnosis

- Therapies administered

- Disposition, recommendations, and instructions given to the patient

- Signature or initials of the practitioner

- When the initials of the practitioner are used, the record must also contain key listing initials and a corresponding full signature

American Association for Accreditation of Ambulatory Surgery Facilities

The **American Association for Accreditation of Ambulatory Surgery Facilities, Inc. (AAAASF)** is an accreditation program that certifies to the medical community and the public that a surgical facility meets nationally recognized standards. The accreditation program is operated by physicians who set and evaluate the standards under the direction of a board of directors. AAAASF strives for the highest standards of excellence for its accredited facilities by regularly revising and updating its requirements for patient safety and quality of care (AAAASF 2010b).

Mission

To accomplish its mission, AAAASF has set the following goals (AAAASF 2010a):

- To provide the medical community and the public with a means of standardizing and improving the quality of medical and surgical care in the ambulatory environment

- To encourage the highest level of competence for medical and surgical care of patients in the ambulatory setting

- To provide a forum for the discussion of new concepts in ambulatory surgery care and a repository of information that can be disseminated to the public and medical community

- To encourage constant improvement in the quality of care provided to patients in the ambulatory surgery setting

- To provide a means of measuring medical and surgical competence and ethical conduct by providing an external source for the evaluation of professional credentialing, patient safety, and quality of care

Medical Record Content Standards

The following are examples of the medical record content standards for ASCs seeking accreditation by the AAAASF (2010b):

- The medical record includes responses to questions about current medications, previous illness, current and chronic illness, previous surgery, bleeding tendencies.

- Treating physicians or appropriate consultants are contacted as to the advisability of office surgery when the history and physical examination so warrant.

- Appropriate laboratory procedures are performed where indicated and are entered in the chart before surgery.

- An **informed consent** is routinely obtained that specifically authorizes the surgeon, by name, to perform surgery and names or describes the operative procedure.

- Expectations, alternatives, risks, and complications are discussed with the patient and documented.

- The informed consent form provides consent for administration of anesthesia or sedatives under the direction of the surgeon, certified registered nurse anesthetist, or anesthesiologist.

- Printed or written copies of laboratory, pathology, X-ray, consultation, and treating physician reports are kept in the medical record.

- All laboratory results must be reviewed by the registered nurse or surgeon. All abnormal results must be reviewed and initialed by the surgeon. All other reports, such as pathology and medical clearance reports, are reviewed and initialed by the surgeon.

- Vital signs are recorded during surgery.

- All medications given to a patient are recorded by date, time, and dosage.

- Type and volume of all intravenously and subcutaneously administered fluids given pre operatively, intra operatively, and post operatively are recorded.

- Post operative vital signs are recorded at suitable intervals until the patient is discharged from the facility.

- There is an operative report that includes operative technique, unusual findings, and unanticipated sequelae.

- Post operative progress notes are recorded.

- All medical records include a discharge diagnosis.

American College of Radiology

The American College of Radiology (ACR) is the most widely recognized diagnostic medical imaging accrediting body, with nearly 16,000 accredited facilities in the United States (ACR 2007). Accreditation is an outward sign that a facility is set up to provide quality patient care. The accreditation process evaluates a practice's quality assurance activities, personnel, and equipment. It includes self-assessment by the facility and an independent audit by experts. Using ACR guidelines and technical standards, the accreditation process measures the facility's personnel qualifications, facility policies and procedures; equipment specifications; quality assurance activities; patient safety; and, ultimately, the quality of patient care.

ACR (2007) accreditation requires that the physicians supervising and interpreting medical imaging meet stringent education and training standards. ACR accreditation also requires that the imaging equipment be surveyed regularly by qualified medical physicists to ensure that it is functioning properly and that the technologists administering the tests are appropriately certified (ACR 2007).

All facilities providing mammography must be certified by the Food and Drug Administrationn (FDA). To be certified, a facility must be accredited. The FDA has designated the ACR as an accrediting body for mammography. In addition, after January 2010, any organization providing magnetic resonance imaging (MRI), computed tomography, positron emission tomography, and nuclear medicine procedures must be accredited.

Documentation requirements for accreditation are specific to the type of imaging. The following excerpt is from the ACR's accreditation requirements for breast MRI and details the documentation and health record requirements (ACR 2010):

The interpreting physician must prepare a written report containing the results of each examination in addition to the following information:

- Name of the patient and an additional patient identifier

- Date of the examination

- Name of the interpreting physician

- An overall final assessment

This written report, signed by the interpreting physician, must be provided to the patient's healthcare provider within 30 days of the examination date. If the assessment is "suspicious abnormality" or "highly suggestive of malignancy" reasonable attempts must be made to communicate this to the healthcare provider (or designee) as soon as possible. The ACR recommends that this communication be no more than 3 business days.

CARF

Founded in 1966 as the Commission on Accreditation of Rehabilitation Facilities, **CARF** International is an independent, nonprofit accrediting agency for health and human services in the following areas:

- Aging services

- Behavioral health

- Opioid treatment programs

- Business and services management networks

- Child and youth services

- Employment and community services

- Vision rehabilitation

- Medical rehabilitation

- Durable medical equipment, prosthetics, orthotics, and supplies

CARF currently accredits close to 47,000 programs and services at more than 20,000 locations on five continents. More than 8.3 million persons of all ages are served annually by more than 6,000 CARF-accredited providers. CARF accreditation requirements for rehabilitation facilities are addressed in chapter 5.

CARF recommendations about record documentation and management are as follows (CARF 2005):

- Never alter your records. Any corrections to records should be initialed and dated.

- Record all clinical findings and observations. This includes consultations; assessments; treatment plans; the nature of other health problems, if any; and the clinical reasoning process, treatments, and responses to treatments.

- Document all instructions and procedures with the person served. In addition, document that any risks were discussed with the person served or someone authorized to make a decision on behalf of the person served.

- Document all missed appointments, any nonadherence to directed treatment, and any treatment refusals by the person served.

- Keep a written record of all telephone conversations regarding the person served, especially information about symptoms.

- Print or clearly write all instructions for the person served.

- Do not release records of the person served without first obtaining his or her written permission unless required by a court order or other legal requirement.

- Keep your closed files secured and protected in storage or somewhere easily accessible for at least the length of time required by law.

- Make sure your records reflect the high quality of care you provide to the persons served.

Accreditation Commission for Healthcare

The **Accreditation Commission for Healthcare (ACHC)** provides accreditation to the following types of healthcare providers (including providers of medical supplies and technology):

- Specialty pharmacy

- Women's post–breast surgery filter services

- Medical supply providers services

- Complex rehabilitation and assistive technology suppliers

ACHC's core competencies, which reflect its accreditation philosophy, include the following (ACHC 2010):

- To develop comprehensive and relevant healthcare accreditation standards and programs

- To provide impartial third-party peer reviews in the evaluation of patient care services

- To use a systematic approach for chart review and data analysis

- To employ best-practice education and quality suggestions from certified and qualified surveyors for business operations and evidence-based healthcare

- To provide data analysis and evaluation for organization improvement

The ACHC accreditation process requires that patient record review be conducted by all disciplines involved in the patient's care. An adequate sampling of open and closed records is selected to determine completeness of documentation. Minimally, the patient assessment, intake, and referral will be reviewed during the survey process.

Community Health Accreditation Program

The **Community Health Accreditation Program, Inc. (CHAP)** is an independent, non-profit accrediting body. Created in 1965 as a joint venture between the American Public Health Association (APHA) and the National League for Nursing (NLN), it was the first accrediting body for community-based healthcare organizations in the United States (CHAP 2010). In 2001, it became an independent, nonprofit corporation. CHAP was granted deeming authority by CMS in 1992 for home health and in 1999 for hospice. This means that CHAP has regulatory authorization to survey agencies providing home health and hospice services and determine whether they meet the Medicare COPs. In 2006, CMS granted CHAP full deeming authority for home medical equipment. Review of patient medical record content is part of the CHAP accreditation process. Once an organization applies for accreditation, it is provided with access to the web-based self-study materials. HIM professionals who work in an organization seeking CHAP accreditation should obtain access to any requirements for health record review prior to the organization's completion of the self-study.

College of American Pathologists

The **College of American Pathologists' (CAP)** Laboratory Accreditation Program is required by CMS for laboratory providers. CMS regulates all laboratory testing performed on humans in the United States through the **Clinical Laboratory Improvement Amendments (CLIA)**. CLIA covers approximately 200,000 laboratory entities. The objective of the program is to ensure quality laboratory testing.

CAP also provides a voluntary accreditation process designed to complement CLIA. Known as CAP 15189, the program is intended to (CAP 2010):

- Improve patient care

- Strengthen the deployment of quality standards

- Reduce errors and risk

- Control costs

General requirements for supporting clinical documentation are included in the CAP accreditation standards.

Commission on Cancer

The Commission on Cancer (CoC) Accreditation Program encourages hospitals, treatment centers, and other facilities to improve their quality of patient care through various cancer-related programs. These programs focus on prevention, early diagnosis, pretreatment evaluation, staging, optimal treatment, rehabilitation, surveillance for recurrent disease, support services, and end-of-life care. The availability of a full range of medical services, along with a multidisciplinary team approach to patient care at accredited cancer programs, has resulted in approximately 80 percent of all newly diagnosed cancer patients being treated in CoC-accredited cancer programs.

Recognizing that cancer is a complex group of diseases, the CoC Cancer Program Standards promote consultation among surgeons, medical and radiation oncologists, diagnostic radiologists, pathologists, and other cancer specialists. This multidisciplinary cooperation improves patient care.

Five elements are key to the success of a CoC-accredited cancer program (CoC 2010):

1. The clinical services provide state-of-the-art pretreatment evaluation, staging, treatment, and clinical follow-up for cancer patients seen at the facility for primary, secondary, tertiary, or quaternary care.

2. The cancer committee leads the program through setting goals, monitoring activity, evaluating patient outcomes, and improving care.

3. The cancer conferences provide a forum for patient consultation and contribute to physician education.

4. The quality improvement program is the mechanism for evaluating and improving patient outcomes.

5. The cancer registry and database are the basis for monitoring the quality of care.

Patient health records are reviewed as part of the accreditation process to support clinical care, cancer registry operations, early detection, and patient education.

National Committee for Quality Assurance

Although the **National Committee for Quality Assurance (NCQA)** is primarily an accrediting body for health insurance plans, it is included in this chapter because its accreditation is branching out to include managed care and wellness programs that are both providers and payers. Purchasers, patients, policy makers, and health plans consider NCQA accreditation to be the gold standard for evaluating healthcare quality and value. NCQA regularly revises and improves its standards to reflect the evolving needs of stakeholders. NCQA currently accredits the following types of programs (NCQA 2007):

- Health plan accreditation
- Wellness and health promotion
- Managed behavioral healthcare organizations
- New health plans
- Disease management

Ambulatory Care Health Record Content and Formats

Accurate and timely documentation is critical in every ambulatory organization, no matter the size or scope of patient care. The health record is a compilation of identifying information about the patient and pertinent facts about his or her current health status and medical history. Provided by the healthcare professionals who participate in the patient's care, the information in the health record is used in planning and managing care, evaluating its adequacy and appropriateness, substantiating reimbursement claims, and protecting the legal interests of the patient and her healthcare providers. Moreover, the health record is a tool for communication among the patient's providers along the continuum of care. Finally, it is used for education, research, public health, and organizational activities such as performance improvement, risk management, and strategic planning.

For documentation in the paper-based and hybrid ambulatory health record to be meaningful, the information must be arranged in a predefined format. This requirement is especially important when multiple providers use the same record. The health record can be arranged according to one of three formats: source-oriented, problem-oriented, or integrated system (see chapter 6).

The advantages and disadvantages of each format must be weighed against the needs of the providers using the health record. For example, because it was developed to enhance comprehensive patient care, the problem-oriented record system is especially appropriate for health maintenance organizations and neighborhood health centers, where a team of professionals offers total patient care. Different practitioners can easily identify existing conditions and current treatments and adjust their own treatment strategies accordingly. In an urgent-care setting, however, an integrated record system may be more suitable. Urgent-care patients usually present for treatment of a single acute problem and then return to their primary care physician for follow-up care. Of course, the record formats can be combined. The only requirement is that the resulting record contains sufficient information to identify the patient and to support the diagnosis and plan of treatment for each episode of care. Providing discharge instructions to the patient and hand-off information to his other healthcare providers is critical to the patient's continuity of care.

Certain basic components are required in every record of ambulatory care. These include the following:

- Registration record, which documents demographic data about the patient

- Problem list, which summarizes all of the medical and surgical problems that have long-term clinical significance for the patient's care, including allergies

- Medication list, which contains pertinent information about the medications the patient is taking

- Patient history questionnaire, which asks the patient for information about current and past medical conditions

- Medical history, which documents the provider's findings on the patient's health status

- Physical examination report, which contains the provider's findings on examination of the patient

- Immunization and injection records, which chronicle the patient's vaccinations

- Progress notes, which provide a chronological summary of the patient's illness and treatment at each encounter

- Physician orders, which document the physician's instructions to other parties involved in providing the patient's care

The following items are recommended:

- Patient instructions, which document the instructions the provider gave the patient regarding follow-up care

- Failed/missed appointment form, which documents patient noncompliance with recommendations for follow-up appointments with the provider

- Flow sheets, which can be used to document treatment between patient visits

- Telephone contact records, which document telephone communications between the patient and his or her healthcare providers

Registration Record

The registration record documents the basic demographic data collected before or during the initial patient visit. This information is maintained and updated on subsequent visits, as needed.

Individual facilities must determine what additional data they need to collect for the purpose of performing various internal activities such as research, utilization management, planning, and marketing. For example, an analysis of basic demographic data might provide answers to questions about the need to hire additional staff or to open facilities in different locations. The goals and objectives of an ambulatory care facility also play a role in determining what data should be collected. For example, facilities featuring family-centered care may collect basic demographic data on all of the patient's family members. In general, the following data elements are collected and maintained for every patient:

- Surname, first name, and middle name or initial

- Unique identifying number

- Residence address and telephone

- Date of birth

- Gender

- Marital status

- Race or ethnic origin

- Social Security number

- Medicare, Medicaid, or insurance group number

- Insurance company, address, and name of subscriber

- Guarantor, if applicable

- Name of insured

- Patient relationship to insured

- Employer

- Occupation

- Business address and telephone

- Name, address, and telephone of nearest relative, friend, or guardian or emergency contact

- Any other emergency contact

- Primary-care physician

- Referring physician's name and address, if applicable

In many clinics, registration information is maintained on the clinic's practice management or billing software. A copy is printed and placed in the patient's record. This copy may contain only limited data elements. A new registration record may be printed and placed in the patient's record whenever the registration information changes.

For greater efficiency, an identifying number unique to each patient should be assigned. The use of the patient's Social Security number as an identifier is not recommended due to the potential for identity theft and regulations governing the use of Social Security numbers.

Problem/Summary List

According to the *Accreditation Manual for Ambulatory Surgical Centers* (Joint Commission 2008a), for each patient who receives continuing ambulatory services, a list of known significant diagnoses, conditions, procedures, and drug allergies must be included in the health record by the third visit.

The **problem list** (sometimes called the **summary list**) is a valuable tool in patient care management and should always be visible and easy to read. A single page summarizes the major medical and surgical problems that have long-term clinical significance for the patient, including social and psychiatric problems, along with the dates of onset and resolution for each problem. The healthcare provider can use the problem list to determine at a glance which problems are active or resolved and can adjust treatment plans accordingly. As a communication tool, the problem list helps specialty physicians make evaluation and treatment decisions about the patients referred to them for care; having this information often eliminates the need to duplicate costly tests. Each provider documents her care of the patient on the same list, thereby creating a comprehensive overview of the patient's medical status. For consistency and clarity, facilities should develop guidelines for recording several key elements in the problem list, including problems, dates of onset, active versus inactive status, and resolution dates.

Significant problems include chronic and acute conditions that affect patient management. For example, both hypercholesterolemia and status post-cholecystectomy would be included on the problem list. Although the cholecystectomy occurred in the past, knowledge of this major surgical event could prove valuable in future clinical evaluations. Abnormal signs and symptoms that have the potential to become significant problems also are recorded, but short-term illnesses that were resolved quickly and ruled-out conditions are not. Including ruled-out conditions would defeat the list's purpose, which is to provide a quick reference to the patient's confirmed conditions and their management status. The problem list also records allergies, social situations that may have a significant impact on clinical management (for example, the fact that the patient lives alone or has a history of child abuse), and risk factors (smoking, alcohol and drug usage, and personal and family history of conditions such as cancer, diabetes, or heart disease). Every clinician involved in a patient's care should have information on these factors. NCQA requires notation on the use of cigarettes, alcohol, and substances for all patients older than 14 years of age. Frequently, this information is included on the problem list.

The date of onset for each problem should be documented. Guidelines should specify which date should be used—the date the patient reported first noting the condition or the date the provider confirmed the condition. Consistency in documentation is important for interpretation and use in evaluation. Each problem should be labeled as active or inactive so that clinicians can determine treatment priorities quickly and develop a treatment plan. Resolved or inactive problems may still be relevant to management of the patient. When its cause is confirmed, the symptom is not erased. but rather linked to the new diagnosis. The resolution date is important as an indicator of problems that have been resolved and as a means for monitoring recurrences.

Medication List

The **medication list** is an ongoing record of the medications a patient has received in the past and those he is currently taking. Key data elements include

- Names of medications

- Dosages and amounts dispensed

- Dispensing instructions (with signature)

- Prescription dates and discontinued dates

- Problem numbers for which each medication was prescribed

Organizations may decide to omit medications prescribed for a single, short-term course of therapy, such as an antibiotic prescribed for an infection. In pediatric patients, however, even short-term medications should be included. Many pediatric illnesses (for example, otitis media) are recurrent in nature, so the physician needs a record that shows which medications were effective in past episodes of the illness.

Dates of medication refills often are charted on the medication list. The list is an acceptable location for documenting patient allergies. However, this information should be documented in a single, specific location of the chart to ensure its completeness and consistency. The patient's current medications and allergies should be verified during each visit, and the chart should be updated appropriately.

When consistent, accurate, and properly updated, the medication list serves multiple purposes, including alerting the physician to drug sensitivities and allergies. When used in conjunction with the problem list, the medication list can help clarify the reason a patient is taking a particular medication (Benson, Van Osdol, and Townes 1988, 197). For patients who are taking several medications or seeing several practitioners, the medication list helps providers evaluate and adjust the drug regimen appropriately by taking into account potential incompatibilities or interactions.

Medication reconciliation is the comparison of a patient's current medications to the medication list from the patient's prior visit. Failure to complete this comparison can lead to medication errors when the patient has been prescribed medications by providers that she may have seen since her last visit.

Patient History Questionnaire

The patient history questionnaire is structured to prompt the patient to provide certain items of information, including the presence or absence of significant conditions that may represent potential medical problems. Responses to specific questions not only provide information but also serve as starting points for the clinician to gather additional historical data. The patient should be asked to complete a new history questionnaire at periodic intervals (approximately every five years). Placing an updated patient questionnaire in the health record makes it possible to have a complete, current history in one place and frees providers from having to read through multiple progress notes.

Medical History

A comprehensive medical history should be obtained periodically from the patient or his representative. Frequency depends on the patient's age and health status. Often the initial medical history is obtained by questioning patients in detail about their health history. Clinicians may use short history forms to supplement and expand the information provided on the patient's general health history questionnaire. Updates to the history often are included in the progress note made during the patient visit (Cofer 1994).

A complete medical history establishes the foundation for comprehensive care by documenting current complaints and symptoms in addition to past medical, personal, and family history. It should include pertinent aspects of basic physiological systems as well. The medical histories obtained by specialists such as gynecologists and gastroenterologists are comprehensive for the particular organ system involved.

Cofer (1994) suggests including the following information in a complete medical history. Note that the second element, present illness, may not be included in a primary-care ambulatory record when the patient presents for preventive care or health maintenance.

- **Chief complaint or reason for visit**: Nature and duration of the symptoms that caused the patient to seek medical attention as stated in the patient's own words

- **Present illness**: Detailed chronological description of the development of the patient's illness, from the appearance of the first symptom to the present situation

- **Past medical history**: A summary of childhood and adult illnesses and conditions, such as infectious diseases, pregnancies, allergies and drug sensitivities, accidents, operations, hospitalizations, and current medications

- **Social or personal history**: Marital status; dietary, sleep, and exercise patterns; use of coffee, tobacco, alcohol, and other drugs; occupation; home environment; daily routine; and so on

- **Family history**: Diseases among relatives in which heredity or contact may play a role, such as allergies, cancer, and infections: psychiatric, metabolic, endocrine, cardiovascular, and renal diseases; health status or cause of and age at death for immediate relatives

The medical history is a record of subjective statements made by the patient. The physical examination is a record of the physician's assessment of the patient's current health status. Information on all of the major organ systems should be documented in the physical examination report:

- **Review of systems**: A systemic inventory designed to uncover current or past subjective symptoms

- **Immunization and injection records**: A list of immunizations or injections of medication, including the date(s) of administration; information on the manufacturer and lot number, drug, dosage, and route of administration; signature of the person administering the vaccine; and a consent form for the vaccination

Progress Notes

Progress notes summarize the patient's status and treatment at each encounter. Progress notes may be structured or narrative, but to be useful to other reviewers of the health record, they must be legible (if paper based) and uniform. The best example of a structured progress note is the SOAP format (also addressed in chapter 6), commonly used with the problem-oriented medical record. In this format, the note itself is divided into four parts, each identified by a letter from the SOAP acronym:

Subjective: Patient's complaints and comments

Objective: Physical findings and laboratory data

Assessment: Diagnosis and impression

Plan: Medication, therapy, referral, consultation, and patient education

The SOAP format helps the clinician structure her decision making to match the problems identified on the problem list. The patient's complaints, diagnoses, and treatments can be viewed at a glance. Under S, the reason for the visit as stated by the patient is commonly recorded in quotes. For O, medical facts established during physical examinations and diagnostic workups are recorded. Under A, documentation of a diagnosis or status of an identified problem is written. Under P, the practitioner records the patient's individualized treatment plan. Every progress note need not contain documentation for every part of the SOAP acronym, but using this format can help professionals ensure that their medical documentation is complete.

Physician Orders

Physician orders are the instructions the physician gives to other parties to provide specific medications, services, diagnostic tests, or treatments to a particular patient. Given the nature of ambulatory care, patients frequently have to visit another site for the orders to be carried out. For example, they must go to the pharmacy to have prescriptions filled or the laboratory to have blood drawn for testing. Orders for medication are written on prescription forms and presented to the pharmacy. Orders for diagnostic tests are written on requisition or referral forms that the patient may or may not receive. To comply with accreditation standards requiring that information on all studies, tests, and treatments be entered into the patient's health record at each visit, physician orders often are documented in the progress note. The orders must be written legibly and accompanied by the date and the physician's signature. Standing orders, which the medical staff or an individual practitioner has established as routine care for a specific diagnosis or procedure, are commonly given to recovery room staff in ambulatory surgery facilities. Usually, standing orders are preprinted on a single sheet of paper and, like other physician orders, must be signed, dated, and filed in the individual patient's health record.

Patient Instructions

Unlike the hospital setting, where a healthcare team headed by a physician is responsible for all patient care, the ambulatory setting leaves aftercare in the patient's hands. Therefore, it is essential that the patient be given clear, concise instructions. The Joint Commission's *Accreditation Manual for Ambulatory Surgical Centers* (2008a) requires that disposition of and recommendations and instructions to the patient are recorded in the health record, including all handoffs provided for continuity of care. It is standard practice to ask for evidence regarding follow-up care, calls, or visits and specified timing of follow-up appointments. Ideally, instructions to the patient should be communicated verbally and in writing, with a copy of the written instructions filed in the health record. When a group or individual other than the patient has assumed responsibility for the patient's aftercare, the record should indicate that the instructions were given to that group or individual. The healthcare professional should sign the record to indicate that he issued the verbal instructions, and the person receiving the instructions should sign the record to verify that understanding. Moreover, patient comments or questions should be documented, along with the healthcare professional's responses. Documentation of patient education during office visits may be accomplished by using forms that prompt the person providing instruction to cover important information.

Missed Appointment Forms

In the ambulatory care setting, patients assume responsibility for much of their own healthcare. For example, they have their prescriptions filled and take their medications as prescribed, follow a prescribed diet, report to the laboratory to have diagnostic tests performed, or schedule follow-up appointments as their physicians advise. By documenting when the patient fails to keep such appointments, the practitioner can protect the organization in case of litigation by demonstrating compliance with clinical practice standards and offering evidence of the quality of care provided. It is important that the provider review the reason the patient was scheduled for an office visit and determine whether the patient should be contacted to reschedule. Attempts to contact the patient and the advice given should be documented.

Flow sheets can be an effective way to display information about the patient's treatment from episode to episode. Another useful application for flow sheets is to document the healthcare maintenance provided to the patient (such as health maintenance forms). Used in this manner, flow sheets serve to remind providers when tests or exams are due for the patients they serve.

Telephone Encounters

From a risk management perspective as well as a patient-care perspective, documentation of any advice (instructions, prescriptions, orders, medication changes, and such) or patient follow-up communicated by a **telephone encounter** is critical. Documentation should include the date and time of the call, the caller's name and telephone number, the patient's name and identifying information, the reason for the call, the date and time of the response (or attempts to return the call), the response given, and the signature of the person returning the call. Because messages may be relayed among several people, a standard telephone encounter form should be used to document all information regarding phone calls with every patient.

Regulation and Policy

In some states, regulations covering hospitals differ from those governing ambulatory care organizations. Independent physician office practices may fall under the guidance of the medical board for physicians' offices, not under the regulation for hospitals. The state of Texas is an example. Ambulatory organizations must decide which rule applies to them and coordinate their internal policies accordingly. For example, a large multispecialty group practice would have different copying fees for release of medical records than would hospitals. See **FIGURE 9.5** for an example of board rules concerning documentation and maintenance of the medical record. Note that the physician is required to keep a copy of any information obtained from another healthcare provider as part of the medical record. Another notation should be made concerning the fact that HIPAA regulations preempt state law provisions that are "contrary" to a provision or requirement of HIPAA (DHHS 2006).

Due to the multiple appointment sites in large, multisite, ambulatory care organizations, HIM professionals face unique documentation challenges for new and existing patients. Often, these organizations have a large, campus-type setting where clinics are established in numerous buildings. Very large centers can include as many as 50 different clinical specialties within the same physicians' practice group. At times, a patient may have several visits scheduled at different clinics (such as internal medicine first and then dermatology) on the same day. Without a centralized record-tracking system in place, one clinic may think another clinic has completed the required documentation for a patient. Physicians, fearing records may be unavailable when needed, may keep shadow charts of patient information or hold on to the original medical records.

Chart management of underdocumented and overdue records is essential. Usually, multisite facilities have a unit record with a centralized HIM department. As many as 1,500 records may be needed for clinic visits on any one day. Location and movement of medical records in these circumstances is challenging, and an electronic record tracking system is vital. Following are some of the different internal HIM policies needed to manage these challenges.

General Consent

The **general consent** for treatment policy is a challenge to large multispecialty physicians' practices due to patients' multiple points of entry. For systems that have transitioned to the EHR, this is not a concern. One clinic may assume that another clinic has already had a patient sign the informed consent. Options for managing this challenge include the following:

- Having each patient sign a new consent upon each visit
- Establishing a monitoring system that alerts clinics when consent is needed

FIGURE 9.5. **Example of board rules on medical records documentation**

Chapter 165. Medical Records

§§165.1-165.6

§165.1. Medical Records.

(a) Contents of Medical Record. Each licensed physician of the board shall maintain an adequate medical record for each patient that is complete, contemporaneous and legible. For purposes of this section, an "adequate medical record" should meet the following standards:

  (1) The documentation of each patient encounter should include:

    (A) reason for the encounter and relevant history, physical examination findings and prior diagnostic test results;

    (B) an assessment, clinical impression, or diagnosis;

    (C) plan for care (including discharge plan if appropriate); and

    (D) the date and legible identity of the observer.

  (2) Past and present diagnoses should be accessible to the treating and/or consulting physician.

  (3) The rationale for and results of diagnostic and other ancillary services should be included in the medical record.

  (4) The patient's progress, including response to treatment, change in diagnosis, and patient's non-compliance should be documented.

  (5) Relevant risk factors should be identified.

  (6) The written plan for care should include when appropriate:

    (A) treatments and medications (prescriptions and samples) specifying amount, frequency, number of refills, and dosage;

    (B) any referrals and consultations;

    (C) patient/family education; and

    (D) specific instructions for follow up.

  (7) any written consents for treatment or surgery requested from the patient/family by the physician.

  (8) Billing codes, including CPT and ICD-9-CM codes, reported on health insurance claim forms or billing statements should be supported by the documentation in the medical record.

  (9) Any amendment, supplementation, change, or correction in a medical record not made contemporaneously with the act or observation shall be noted by indicating the time and date of the amendment, supplementation, change, or correction, and clearly indicating that there has been an amendment, supplementation, change, or correction.

  (10) Salient records received from another physician or health care provider involved in the care or treatment of the patient shall be maintained as part of the patient's medical records.

  (11) The board acknowledges that the nature and amount of physician work and documentation varies by type of services, place of service and the patient's status. Paragraphs (1) – (11) of this subsection may be modified to account for these variable circumstances in providing medical care.

(b) Maintenance of Medical Records.

  (1) A licensed physician shall maintain adequate medical records of a patient for a minimum of seven years from the anniversary date of the date of last treatment by the physician.

  (2) If a patient was younger than 18 years of age when last treated by the physician, the medical records of the patient shall be maintained by the physician until the patient reaches age 21 or for seven years from the date of last treatment, whichever is longer.

FIGURE 9.5. (continued)

---

(3) A physician may destroy medical records that relate to any civil, criminal or administrative proceeding only if the physician knows the proceeding has been finally resolved.

(4) Physicians shall retain medical records for such longer length of time than that imposed herein when mandated by other federal or state statute or regulation.

(5) Physicians may transfer ownership of records to another licensed physician or group of physicians only if the physician provides notice consistent with §165.5 of this chapter (relating to Transfer and Disposal of Medical Records) and the physician who assumes ownership of the records maintains the records consistent with this chapter.

(6) Medical records may be owned by a physician's employer, to include group practices, professional associations, and non-profit health organizations, provided records are maintained by these entities consistent with this chapter.

(7) Destruction of medical records shall be done in a manner that ensures continued confidentiality.

Source Note: The provisions of this §165.1 adopted to be effective December 29, 1997, 22 TexReg 12490; amended to be effective September 14, 2003, 28 TexReg 7703; amended to be effective March 4, 2004, 29 TexReg 1946; amended to be effective September 28, 2006, 31 TexReg 8090; amended to be effective January 20, 2009, 34 TexReg 337; amended to be effective September 19, 2010, 35 TexReg 8350

Source: Texas Medical Board 2010

Patients often respond negatively to the first option. The perception is that the organization should know when the consent has been signed. The second choice presents an economic challenge due to the high cost associated with the staff time required to monitor and audit for compliance.

Physicians New to Practice

The new-to-practice policy should outline how physicians coming into a practice handle their medical records from a prior practice. The policy should direct the physician to review information in patient records from her previous practice and place copies of those records in new records at the new practice. Often, physicians want to place an original, prior record into the medical record at the new location. When an original record is incorporated into a new medical record in this manner, it becomes a part of the medical record at the new practice and should not be removed, even if the physician decides to leave the new practice.

Missed Appointments

The organization should have a **failed/missed appointment policy** that tracks appointments that are canceled or missed. The policy should state the required documentation of information concerning the missed appointment.

Closing Practice

A **closing practice policy** directs an organization to send letters to patients of physicians who are closing their practice at a facility. Information should include options for patients to either continue receiving care from another physician at the facility or to receive copies of their medical records if they decide to transfer to another practice. The specific actions that must be taken when a physician or other healthcare practitioner closes a practice are outlined in the state laws for the state where the practice is located. HIM professionals and healthcare practitioners should be familiar with these laws.

Shadow Charts

A **shadow chart policy** should require that all original information and medical reports be kept in the medical record located in the HIM department. Physicians should be discouraged from keeping copies of records or reports in a shadow chart in their offices. Incorporating and reconciling shadow charts from a physician's practice places an economic burden on the healthcare facility and the HIM department.

Outstanding Records

An **outstanding record policy** should detail the time frame in which a medical record can be kept in the clinic or physician's office. The recommended time is no longer than 48 hours.

Chart Delivery

A chart-delivery policy should detail the day and time of delivery for records of patients with regularly scheduled appointments. Because such appointments are scheduled ahead of time, the HIM department and the clinic can plan for delivery of these records at a time that is convenient for all. Typically, records are delivered the day before the appointment.

Risk Management and Liability

Risk management efforts are designed to minimize the facility's potential risks and, when an incident occurs, its losses. A comprehensive risk management program incorporates the identification, analysis, evaluation, and elimination or reduction of potential liability by addressing the following issues:

- **Liability insurance**: Ambulatory care facilities must secure adequate liability insurance. Liability for patient or employee injury applies to both physicians and nonphysicians who provide medical care to patients as well as to healthcare facilities with responsibility for supervising the actions of the medical staff.

- **Credentialing and licensure**: Ambulatory care facilities must obtain state licensure and adopt a method to properly renew and ensure their licensure status. Specific policies and procedures should address credential verification and monitor compliance with continuing education requirements for all licensed and credentialed personnel.

- **Equipment**: Maintenance and quality-control policies should be developed to ensure that all equipment is functional, operated properly, and checked on a regular basis and that appropriate parts and supplies are available.

Summary

The percentage of care provided in ambulatory care settings continues to grow. In addition, the different types of ambulatory care settings are growing. Additional ambulatory care settings are addressed in chapter 13. The federal government and state governments require that all ambulatory care providers maintain licensure and comply with laws. However, as ambulatory care providers continue to diversify, it is important to ensure adequate controls and standards. Controls and standards are provided through the voluntary process of accreditation. The Joint Commission provides accreditation services for most types of ambulatory care providers. However, in the past decade at least ten additional organizations have begun to provide accreditation. Some provide accreditation for more than one type of ambulatory care service. Accreditation serves many purposes, one of which is to help patients make decisions about where to receive care since accreditation can be viewed as a stamp of quality approval.

Federal and state governments and accrediting bodies all have requirements for health records as well as patient care. It is important that the HIM professional is familiar with specific state laws and the standards for all of the accrediting bodies for which her organization seeks to maintain good standing. Because these standards may change annually, it is essential that HIM professionals update themselves on at least an annual basis regarding all changes.

References

42 CFR 416.47. Revised as of October 1, 2004. Chapter IV—Centers for Medicare and Medicaid Services, Department of Health and Human Services. http://edocket.access.gpo.gov/cfr_2004/octqtr/42cfr416.47.htm.

Accreditation Association for Ambulatory Health Care (AAAHC). 2008. *2008 Accreditation Handbook for Ambulatory Health Care*. Skokie, IL: Accreditation Association for Ambulatory Health Care.

Accreditation Commission for Healthcare (ACHC). 2010. Accreditation Process. http://www.achc.org/accreditation_process.php.

American Association for Accreditation of Ambulatory Surgery Facilities (AAAASF). 2010a. About AAAASF: Mission. http://www.aaaasf.org/mission.php.

American Association for Accreditation of Ambulatory Surgery Facilities (AAAASF). 2010b. *Medicare Standards and Checklists for Accreditation of Ambulatory Care Facilities*. Gurnee, IL: AAAASF.

American College of Radiology (ACR). 2010. Breast Magnetic Resonance Imaging (MRI) Accreditation Program Requirements. http://www.acr.org/accreditation/Breast-MRI/breast_mri_reqs.aspx.

American College of Radiology (ACR). 2007. *ACR Bulletin*. http://www.acr.org/SecondaryMainMenuCategories/NewsPublications/FeaturedCategories/ACRBulletin/Archives/2007/May2007.aspx.

Benson, D. S., W. Van Osdol, and P. Townes. 1988. Quality Ambulatory Care: The Role of the Diagnostic and Medication Summary Lists. *Quality Review Bulletin* 14(6):192–97.

CARF. 2005. *Managing Your Risk with CARF Standards*. http://www.carf.org/WorkArea/DownloadAsset.aspx?id=22501.

Cofer, J., ed. 1994. *Health Information Management*, 10th ed., revised. Berwyn, IL: Physician's Record Company.

College of American Pathologists (CAP). 2010. About the CAP Accreditation Program. http://www.cap.org/apps/cap.portal?_nfpb=true&cntvwrPtlt_actionOverride=%2Fportlets%2FcontentViewer%2Fshow&_windowLabel=cntvwrPtlt&cntvwrPtlt%7BactionForm.contentReference%7D=laboratory_accreditation%2Faboutlap.html&_state=maximized&_pageLabel=cntvwr.

Commission on Cancer (CoC). 2010. Accreditation. http://www.facs.org/cancer/coc/approval.html.

Community Health Accreditation Program (CHAP). 2010. About CHAP. http://www.chapinc.org/AboutCHAP.

Illinois General Assembly. 1973. Joint Commission on Administrative Rules. Administrative Code. Title 77: Public health. Chapter I: Department of Public Health. Subchapter B: Hospital and Ambulatory Care Facilities. Part 205 Ambulatory Surgical Treatment Center Licensing Requirements. Section 205.610 Clinical Records. http://www.ilga.gov/commission/jcar/admincode/077/077002050F06100R.html.

The Joint Commission. 2008a. *Accreditation Manual for Ambulatory Surgical Centers*. Oakbrook Terrace, IL: The Joint Commission.

The Joint Commission. 2008b. Sentinel Event. http://www.jointcommission.org/SentinelEvents.

National Committee for Quality Assurance (NCQA). 2007. MCO Accreditation. http://www.ncqa.org/tabid/67/Default.aspx.

Texas Medical Board. 2010. Texas Administrative Code. Title 22: Medical boards. http://www.tmb.state.tx.us/rules/rules/bdrules.php.

US Department of Health and Human Services (DHHS). 2006. Health Information Privacy. http://www.hhs.gov/ocr/privacy/hipaa/faq/preemption_of_state_law/402.html.

Chapter 10

Long-Term Care Hospitals

Ella L. James, MS, RHIT, CPHQ

Learning Objectives

- Define long-term care hospital (LTCH)

- Describe the differences between LTCHs and acute care hospitals

- List the types of patient diagnoses commonly treated in an LTCH

- Explain the federal, state, and accreditation regulations for LTCHs

- Describe the assignment of a principal diagnosis for a patient in an LTCH

- Describe the contents of health records for long-term acute care hospitals and long-term care facilities

- Explain the health record review process in an LTCH

- Describe the current evolution of LTCH patient classification

Key Terms

Advance directives

Functional independence measures (FIM)

Health record review process

Long-term care hospital (LTCH)

Medically complex patients

Principal diagnosis

Problem list

The Joint Commission

Introduction

Long-term care hospitals (LTCHs) play an important role in the continuum of care. Patients are generally admitted to an LTCH after receiving initial treatment in an acute care hospital. If the patient's condition requires a longer length of acute care than an acute care hospital allows, the patient will often be discharged to an LTCH. The average length of stay (LOS) in an LTCH must be greater than 25 days. Although the official name for such a hospital is "long-term care hospital," they may also be called "long-term acute care hospitals" (LTACs). **Table 10.1** lists the key differences between acute care (short-term) hospitals and LTCHs. Both hospital types are reimbursed under a diagnosis-related group (DRG) or prospective payment system. Because of the significant difference in length of stay, the average base DRG rate for an LTCH stay ($38,086) is much greater than the average base rate for an acute care stay ($5,308) (CMS 2007).

TABLE 10.1. Comparison of acute care hospital and LTCH characteristics

FACILITY CHARACTERISTIC	ACUTE CARE HOSPITAL	LTCH
Populations treated	Acutely ill or injured, intensive care, inpatient surgical	Medically complex, rehabilitation, psychiatric
Medicare coverage	Acute	Acute
Length of stay criterion	None (typically 4 to 6 days)	25-day minimum
DRG base rate	$5,308	$38,086
Distinguishing physician specialties	Emergency medicine, surgeons, internists	Pulmonologists, infectious disease, internists
Nursing specialty and secondary key staff	Medical nurses, physical therapy, occupational therapy, speech pathology	Medical nurses, wound care nurses respiratory therapy, physical therapy, occupational therapy, speech pathology

Source: RTI International 2007.

This chapter describes several characteristics of the LTCH. First, the types of services provided in an LTCH are explained. Second, federal, state, and accreditation regulations are listed. Third, the professional associations that support long-term care organizations and their healthcare professionals are reviewed.

The chapter also lists and describes the content of the patient record in the LTCH, including some examples. Finally, LTCH health information management (HIM) policies and procedures for health record content and review are described.

Long-Term Acute Care Hospital Settings

LTCHs are acute care hospitals that treat patients who, on average, are hospitalized more than 25 days. They are the only Medicare providers whose patient population definition is based on an LOS rather than a diagnosis or measure of care intensity, such as inpatient nursing needs. LTCHs are certified as acute care hospitals, but unlike other acute care hospitals that specialize in certain populations, such as inpatient rehabilitation facilities (IRFs) or psychiatric hospitals, LTCHs' only distinguishing certification requirement is that their average LOS is greater than 25 days. As a result, these hospitals treat a very heterogeneous group of patients. They may specialize in patients with longer-term medical, rehabilitation, or psychiatric needs, as long as the total Medicare inpatient population's LOS is, on average, longer than 25 days (CMS 2007). Services provided by an LTCH may include comprehensive rehabilitation, respiratory therapy, cancer treatment, head trauma treatment, and pain management.

Many LTCHs specialize in treating medically complex patients who need acute inpatient medical care for a longer period than the short-term community hospital has the capacity to provide. They also specialize in treating patients on ventilators (although acute care hospitals also treat these patients in their intensive care units [ICUs] for limited periods). LTCHs, like some rehabilitation hospitals, specialize in weaning acute patients from ventilators. Unlike ICUs or inpatient rehabilitation facilities, LTCHs treat longer-term patients on a ventilator who are too frail or physically compromised to be admitted to an inpatient rehabilitation facility or whose ongoing

FIGURE 10.1. Top 10 conditions treated and care provided in the LTCH setting

Respiratory diagnosis with ventilator support
Rehabilitation
Degenerative nervous system disorders
Skin ulcers
Aftercare for musculoskeletal system and connective tissue disorders
Pulmonary edema and respiratory failure
Chronic obstructive pulmonary disease
Pneumonia
Respiratory infection
Septicemia

Source: Illinois Health Facilities Planning Board 2007.

care requirements would limit the number of ICU beds available for trauma patients in an acute care hospital (CMS 2007).

Most patients in an LTCH are considered medically complex. **Medically complex patients** require specialized care, including intensive therapies and nursing care (CMS 2007). Many medically complex cases include multisystem failure, neuromuscular damage, contagious infections, and complex wounds needing extended care. Congestive heart failure, uncontrolled diabetes, HIV and AIDS, renal failure, and methicillin-resistant *Staphylococcus aureus* (MRSA) are also treated in some LTCHs (CMS 2007). In general, LTCH patients tend to have several diagnoses on their Medicare claims, and approximately 50 percent have five or more diagnoses. **FIGURE 10.1** contains the top 10 diagnoses treated in LTCHs across the country.

Regulations

LTCHs must abide by Centers for Medicare and Medicaid Services (CMS) regulations in order to treat Medicare and Medicaid recipients. In addition, all LTCHs must operate in accordance with the laws in effect in the states where they are located. Finally, like acute care hospitals, many LTCHs seek accreditation by The Joint Commission.

Federal Regulations

LTCHs must meet state requirements for acute care hospitals and must have a provider agreement with Medicare in order to receive Medicare payments. Fiscal intermediaries verify that the LTCH meets the required average LOS of greater than 25 days (42 CFR Parts 412, 413, and 476). The federal regulations also set forth specific guidelines for designating principal diagnoses for LTCH patients. The definition for principal diagnosis is "the condition established after study to be chiefly responsible for occasioning the admission of the patient to the hospital for care" (DHHS 2005). When a patient is discharged from an acute care facility and admitted to an LTCH, the appropriate principal diagnosis at the LTCH is not necessarily the same diagnosis for which the patient received care at the acute care hospital. For example, a patient who suffers a stroke (code 436, acute but ill-defined cerebrovascular disease) is admitted to an acute care hospital for diagnosis and treatment. The patient is then discharged and admitted to an LTCH for further treatment of left-sided hemiparesis and dysphasia. The appropriate principal diagnosis at the LTCH would be a code from section 438 (late effects of cerebrovascular disease), such as 438.20 (late effects of cerebrovascular disease, hemiplegia affecting unspecified side) or 438.12 (late effects of cerebrovascular disease, dysphasia). Coding guidelines state that the residual condition is sequenced first, followed by the cause of the late effect. In the case of cerebrovascular disease, the combination code describes both the residual effect of the stroke (for example, speech or language deficits or paralysis) and the cause of the residual effect (the stroke). Code 436 is used only for the first (initial) episode of care for the stroke that was treated in the acute care setting (42 CFR Parts 412, 413, and 476).

State Regulations

State regulations for LTCHs vary greatly. It is helpful for a HIM professional to be familiar with the specific LTCH guidelines in the state where the facility operates. **FIGURE 10.2** is an example of West Virginia state guidelines. In this case, the differences between the state and federal law are primarily focused on which facilities are permitted to act as LTCHs. In West Virginia, LTCHs may only operate within an acute care facility. This type of facility is also known as a **"hospital within a hospital" (HWH)**. In most HWHs, the patient is directly transferred from an acute care bed to an LTCH bed. Although the patient remains technically within the same facility, her stays and health records must be identified clearly as either acute or LTCH. Components of the LTCH that are not specifically addressed in LTCH state guidelines generally defer to that state's acute care guidelines.

Accreditation Regulations

LTCHs are accredited by **The Joint Commission**. They do not have a specific accreditation program and are accredited in the same manner as acute care hospitals. By Joint

FIGURE 10.2. West Virginia State guidelines for LTCAHs

West Virginia Regulations for Long-Term Care Hospitals
An acute care hospital that cares for patients who have been in an intensive care or short term acute care setting that requires an extended length of stay (greater than twenty five days). LTACHs are referred to as a "hospital within a hospital." The host hospital must delicense any acute care beds used in the development of the LTACH. If the LTACH would cease to exist, would terminate its services, or would not offer its services for a period of twelve months any beds delicensed by a host hospital to establish the LTACH would revert back to the host hospital.
Development of a LTACH shall be limited to existing space within an existing general acute care facility. Space within the existing acute care facility shall be specifically designated for the LTACH and shall be designed to accommodate the treatment requirements of the LTACH patients. The applicant shall delineate the service area for the LTACH by documenting the expected areas from which it is expected to draw patients. The applicant may submit documentation on the expected service area based upon national data or statistics, or upon projections generally relied on by professionals engaged in health planning or the development of health services. The applicant shall document expected utilization for the service to be provided. The applicant shall consider the number of discharges from acute care facilities within the proposed service area that have an average length of stay greater than twenty five (25) days in making its utilization projections. After establishing expected utilization or demand, the applicant shall document the number of existing LTACH providers within the service area and the extent to which the demand is being met by existing LTACH providers.

Source: West Virginia Department of Health and Human Services Board of Review 2008.

Commission standards, LTCHs are not required to have an emergency department, an ICU, a radiology department, a pharmacy, or a laboratory. They are evaluated on their performance in the following categories:

- Ethics, rights, and responsibilities

- Provision of care

- Medication management

- Surveillance, prevention, and control of infection

- Leadership

- Management of environment of care

- Management of human resources

- Management of information

- Medical staff

Note on Future LTCH Regulations

Because of the increase in the number of LTCHs from 1995 to 2005, Medicare placed a moratorium on new LTCHs from 2007 to 2010. During that time, CMS conducted research to determine the need for LTCHs and the best way to define the LTCH patient population for quality of care and cost-effectiveness. Specific action has not yet been taken. Following are some of the recommendations made to CMS by their contractor, Research Trial Institute (RTI), regarding future regulations for LTCHs (CMS 2007):

- Restrict LTCH admissions to patients who meet certain medical conditions:

  o Their primary diagnosis must be medical, not physical functioning or psychiatric.

  o They must be medically complex as broadly defined to include a wide range of conditions, all with severe medical complications, comorbidities, or system failures, that together represent a complicated, severely ill patient.

- Develop a list of criteria to measure medical severity for hospital admissions.

- Standardize conditions of participation and set staffing requirements to ensure appropriate staff for treating medically complex patients.

- Require LTCHs to collect and submit functional impairment measures and physiologic measures on all patients receiving physical, occupational, or speech and language pathology services.

- Establish a technical advisory group to

  o Recommend a small set of criteria for defining medically complex patients appropriate for LTCH admissions.

  o Recommend measurement levels for each item that identifies medically complex patients.

- Establish a data collection mechanism to collect the data noted in the previous items

- Require LTCH patients to be discharged if not having diagnostic procedures or improving with treatment.

LTCH Health Record Content

The organization and management of the LTCH health records would be consistent with those used in a short-term acute care facility. The policies that govern the uniformity and content of the health record must be developed and maintained as they are in the short-term acute care setting. Refer to chapter 6 for details about the format of health records.

A typical LTCH health record may contain the information and forms listed in **FIGURE 10.3**. In an electronic environment, these elements will be required data fields rather than forms. Each facility determines how each data point on each form will be captured and stored to create the final electronic health record (EHR).

Many of these forms were described earlier in the book in relation to acute care settings, and their function and purpose are the same in long-term acute-care hospitals or long-term care facilities. It is extremely important to ensure that all documentation is signed, dated, and timed.

History, Physical, and Referral Information

The history and physical must be completed and placed in the health record within 24 hours of a patient's admission to the LTCH. The format of the history and physical is characteristic of a short-term acute care hospital examination. Documentation of allergies and allergic symptoms should be included in the history and physical and throughout the health record as determined by facility policy.

It is essential for physicians to understand the ICD-9-CM principal diagnosis selection guidelines and Uniform Hospital Discharge Data Set (UHDDS) definitions. Determination of the patient's principal diagnosis in the LTCH setting was addressed in the *Federal Register* in 2002 (42 CFR Parts 412, 413, and 476) and is described in this chapter.

FIGURE 10.3. Common forms in the LTCH record

History and physical	Specialty reports
Admission data	Flow sheets
Physician orders	Graphical data
Progress notes	Care plans
Problem lists	Education
Consultation records	Patient assessments
Reevaluations and assessments	Procedure records
Advance directives	Medication administration records
Laboratory reports	Discharge documentation

Principal Diagnosis

The determination of the **principal diagnosis** or the actual reason for admission to the long-term care setting is one of the most difficult documentation issues facing the long-term care environment, including the LTCH. Typically, the history and physical documentation regurgitates everything that occurred in the short-term acute care setting and tends to accentuate the acute phases of illness that have already been studied. Recent ICD-9-CM guidelines (HHS 2009) discuss the importance of determining the appropriate diagnoses in any setting. The official guidelines are updated regularly.

The admission history and physical should provide not only the history of the patient's illness but also the specific reason the patient is being admitted to the long-term care setting. The reason for admission should be clear and should reflect why the patient is coming into the LTCH. The plan of care, or impression, should discuss the specific treatments and services that will be provided for the patient's stay. It should focus on the activities of care and provide clear rationale for the admission and continued stay in the long-term care setting. As stated previously, without this documentation, the assignment of the proper diagnostic code is very difficult. In many instances, the reason for admission into the LTCH is an acute condition such as respiratory failure, complications of surgeries or devices, infections (including septicemia and pneumonia), wounds, osteomyelitis, congestive heart failure, cancer, or many other conditions or diseases. Whatever the reason for the admission to the LTCH, it should be clearly documented when the patient is admitted into the facility. Many times, the after study in the definition of the principal diagnosis has already been completed in the acute care setting, and therefore, it should be easier to determine the actual reason for the admission into the LTCH.

Admission Data

Admission data typically contain information such as nursing admission assessments, initial therapy assessments, interdisciplinary evaluation, central-line data sheets, initial pain assessment, case management assessments, nutritional screening, initial nutritional assessment, safety assessment, social services intake, general consent, and a preadmission certification. The preadmission certification helps determine if the patient is being placed in the most appropriate healthcare setting.

Physician Orders

Physician orders contain medication orders, parenteral nutrition orders, do-not-resuscitate orders, admission protocols, or orders that trigger the physician to include other orders, such as those related to diet, ventilator setting, required tests and labs, medical precautions, activities, treatment, and consults, as appropriate. These include all orders from physicians, psychiatrists, or other licensed providers.

Progress Notes

Progress notes may be written by physicians with each discipline having its own progress note section, or the progress notes may be interdisciplinary and contained in a single progress note section. If they are interdisciplinary, each discipline notes its entry as nursing, physical therapy, physician, or the like, as appropriate. See chapter 5 for sample progress notes. Progress notes capture regular and ongoing clinical data about the patient.

Problem Lists

Problem lists may be used in an LTCH to better track the extensive issues that face a chronically or critically ill patient. A **problem list** captures relevant past and current problems of each patient. It provides a mechanism to organize each of the patient's medical or physical issues. The problems are listed numerically, with the dates each problem was identified and resolved. In some LTCHs, the list may be nursing driven or physician driven. In addition to the patient-specific data, the list may also make note of the attending physician, principal diagnosis, allergies and adverse drug reactions, and symptoms of allergic/drug reactions. Not all facilities use problem lists.

Consultation Records

Consultation records include all consultations by surgeons, cardiologists, podiatrists, urologists, and other physicians, as well as dental records. These documents are similar to those used in the short-term acute care hospitals.

Reevaluations and Assessments

Reevaluations and assessments include notes from neurological, nursing, therapy, pastoral care, and social services, which support the care, treatments, and functional changes that occur over the longer LOS in the LTCH setting.

Advance Directives

Advance directives are required in the LTCH setting. An advance directive is a written document that describes the patient's healthcare preferences in the event that he is unable to communicate directly at some point in the future. The types of advance directives vary by state but typically include living wills, healthcare surrogate designation or durable power of attorney for healthcare (also called a *healthcare power of attorney*), and anatomical donation. Additional detail on advance directives can be found in chapter 5.

Laboratory Reports

Laboratory reports may become extensive in the LTCH due to a patient's LOS. These reports are sometimes divided among chemistry, hematology, urinalysis, and microbiology. Facility policy will determine how these reports are permanently filed in the patient's health record or how they are interfaced and housed in an EHR. In an electronic data management system (EDMS), if an interface cannot be developed, documents may be filed as paper or scanned into the patient's health record for easier access. An interface provides the ability for electronic systems to communicate between two or more applications using languages and codes. For example, the laboratory system used may not be a component of the EHR system and may have been purchased separately from the EHR software. In this case, an interface between the EHR and the laboratory system would be required to integrate lab data and the EHR.

Specialty Reports

Radiology reports, cardiac reports, swallow results, sleep studies, pulmonary function tests, pulse oximetry, sleep oximetry, arterial blood gas, and other specialty reports may be completed during the patient's stay in the LTCH to further diagnose health issues related to the patient's condition. Facility policy will clarify how these reports are filed or stored in the patient's health record. In the EHR environment, interfaces may be required to view the specialty reports online.

Flow Sheets

Flow sheets are used in the LTCH setting to capture valuable clinical data. These may include interdisciplinary flow sheets or discipline-specific data such as nursing flow sheets and therapy flow sheets. Other flow sheets that may be found in an LTCH health record could include those used to capture abnormal involuntary movement, antipsychotic medication, bladder training, blood glucose monitoring, hemodialysis records, critical care or code sheets, heparin injections, intake and output, monthly nursing summaries, observation sheets for one-on-one care, respiratory therapy ventilation reports, respiratory treatments, and seizure records.

Graphical Data

Graphical data typically includes blood sugar monitoring and vital signs sheets. (See figure 5.16, p. 224.) LTCH pediatric patients' records may also include growth charts. Graphical data are important because they provide a picture of data points over a grid, demonstrating increases and decreases in clinical data such as blood sugar or blood pressure, while growth chart graphs demonstrate the child's development against a norm. In an electronic environment, these data points can be displayed in list or graphical format.

Care Plans

Care plans are required documentation in an LTCH. Some LTCHs may use critical paths (or clinical pathways) for specific patients. Nursing care plans begin on admission and must be kept current throughout a patient's stay in the LTCH. Care plans are governed by the federal Conditions of Participation for Hospitals and may also be governed by state regulations.

The care plan is a snapshot of a patient's status and includes everything from social issues to disease processes. The critical paths and clinical pathways are focused on a specific disease process or pathway. For example, if the patient has pneumonia, the clinical pathway spells out the steps to take for the patient.

A care plan dictates the nursing care that will be provided to a patient. It provides the details that the nurse will apply to manage and treat problems identified by nursing assessment and not just the admitting diagnosis. There are various care plans developed for each problem for which the patient is treated. Plans are developed based on the patient's individual needs, strengths, limitations, and goals as outlined in Joint Commission standards. Care plans typically include the following:

- Patient name
- Date of initiation

- Assessed problem—usually one problem per sheet in a paper-based record or one screen in an EHR

- Subjective and objective data about the problem

- Nursing diagnoses

- Expected outcomes or goals of care and treatment and the date the expected outcomes or goals will be reached

- Interventions and the time frame for the interventions, expected date of resolution of the problem, and responsible clinical staff

- Final evaluation on the goal date to determine if the goals were met

If the goals are met, the care plan is discontinued. If the goals are not met, the care plan is reevaluated, revised appropriately, and reinstituted. As new problems arise, new care plans are created to assist the nursing staff in resolving each identified problem.

Depending on the electronic environment, care plan development may flow from assessments to help reduce duplicate documentation. Once problems have been identified, the software system may be able to open the care planning session. This process eliminates the need to reenter the problem and allows the interventions to be assigned more fluidly.

Education

Education is provided to all LTCH patients. This should include all areas of education mandated by federal and state laws and regulations and those recommended by accreditation standards. Family meetings or family conferences, where relevant to the patient's condition, may also be held in the LTCH setting.

Patient Assessments

CMS is currently considering significant changes to the LTCH system that will require significant detail about the patient's clinical condition, severity of illness, and intensity of care. RTI made the initial recommendations to CMS in 2007. Although regulations have not yet been adopted, it is likely that initial and regular patient assessments will be required in the LTCH. One form of patient assessment that may be used is the **functional independence measure (FIM)**. Although the FIM is currently used primarily in the rehabilitation setting today, there may be some LTCHs where it is appropriate to use the FIM for ongoing patient assessment.

There are 18 items measured by the FIM. For each item, the level of independence is scored on a scale of 1 to 7, with 1 being the most dependent and 7 being the most independent. Total scores range between 18 and 126. (See **FIGURE 10.4**.)

Because of the diverse nature of patients in LTCHs, the RTI recommended in its report to CMS that the current assessment items collected by LTCHs be used to create an LTCH-specific assessment. The RTI report identified 45 different assessment items commonly collected in the LTCH record. **FIGURE 10.5** lists the 45 items.

Procedure Records

Procedure records are used in the LTCH setting and must meet all Joint Commission standards for operative and invasive procedures. While many LTCHs do not have

FIGURE 10.4. Functional Independence Measures (FIMs)

FIM™ Instrument

LEVELS		
	7 Complete Independence (timely, safely) 6 Modified Independence (device)	NO HELPER
	Modified Dependence 5 Supervision (subject = 100%) 4 Minimal Assistance (subject = 75%+) 3 Moderate Assistance (subject = 50%+) **Complete Dependence** 2 Maximal Assistance (subject =25%+) 1 Total Assistance (subject = less than 25%)	HELPER

	ADMISSION	DISCHARGE	FOLLOW-UP
Self-Care			
A. Eating			
B. Grooming			
C. Bathing			
D. Dressing - Upper Body			
E. Dressing - Lower Body			
F. Toileting			
Sphincter Control			
G. Bladder Management			
H. Bowel Management			
Transfers			
I. Bed, Chair, Wheelchair			
J. Toilet			
K. Tub, Shower			
Locomotion	W Walk / C Wheelchair / B Both	W Walk / C Wheelchair / B Both	W Walk / C Wheelchair / B Both
L. Walk/Wheelchair			
M. Stairs			
Motor Subtotal Score			
Communication			
N. Comprehension	A Auditory / V Visual / B Both	A Auditory / V Visual / B Both	A Auditory / V Visual / B Both
O. Expression	A Auditory / V Visual / B Both	A Auditory / V Visual / B Both	A Auditory / V Visual / B Both
Social Cognition			
P. Social Interaction			
Q. Problem Solving			
R. Memory			
Cognitive Subtotal Score			
TOTAL FIM™ SCORE			

NOTE: Leave no blanks. Enter 1 if patient is not testable due to risk.

FIGURE 10.5. Commonly collected assessment items in LTCHs

- Conditions (medical history)
- Vital signs (includes heart rate, blood pressure, temperature, etc.; current statistics)
- Blood and plasma levels
- Arterial blood gas (S_{AO_2}, P_{CO_2}, etc.)
- Glucose levels
- IV (intravenous), including medications, antibiotics, diuretics, electrolyte replacements, and fluids
- Total or partial parenteral nutrition (TPN or PPN), enteral, or central feedings, PEG
- Chemotherapy
- GI (gastrointestinal) suctioning frequency
- Isolation
- Hemodialysis/peritoneal dialysis
- Pulse oximetry
- Progression toward goals
- Availability of laboratory services
- Psychosocial problems
- Respiratory/respiratory therapy
- Chest physiotherapy (PT)
- Tracheo-bronchial suctioning frequency/tracheostomy
- CPAP/Bi-PAP/VTM/IMV (types of ventilator support)
- Nebulized therapies
- Oxygen monitoring
- Pleural catheter management
- Tracheostomy weaning

- Pulmonary assessment
- Respiratory rate
- O_2 (oxygen) saturation
- Respiratory acidosis pH level
- F_{IO_2} titration
- Chest tubes
- Breath sounds
- Heart (cardiac)
- Left ventricular (LV) ejection fraction
- Edema
- Cardiac monitoring
- Neurological
- Neurological assessments
- Mental status/AO/cognition
- Electrocardiogram (ECG) monitoring
- Pain
- Pain management
- Analgesia/relaxant therapy
- Wounds/ulcer/stage 1-4/intensity of ulcer
- Wound dressing changes
- Wound management
- Rehabilitation
- Functional limitations/range of motion/strength/ endurance/mobility/activities of daily living

Source: RTI International 2007, 134.

operative suites, many do perform operative services such as central-line placement, chest tubes, gastrostomy tubes, tracheostomy tubes, and other services. Blood transfusions are also performed. Facility policy dictates which procedures require an informed consent. All Joint Commission standards for informed consent also apply to the LTCH setting if the facility is accredited.

Miscellaneous Data

Miscellaneous data also exist in the LTCH setting and may include some of the following data: authorizations, patient transfer records, preadmission forms, ambulance transportation forms, and interagency transfer forms (which may include specific state requirements). Many of these forms or documents may be generated by the referring facility or service agencies. In an electronic environment, many of these documents may require scanning to include them in the EHR.

Medication Administration Records

Due to the extended LOS in an LTCH setting and multiple medications that the patient is prescribed, medication administration records may be voluminous. Some LTCHs may have converted their medication records to electronic formats.

Discharge Documentation

Discharge documentation is required in the LTCH setting and includes discharge summaries, discharge instructions, discharge medication listings, discharge nursing summaries, home activity and exercise plans, skilled nursing facility placement forms, nursing home applications, and organ tissue donation, death certificate, and autopsy reports, if applicable. The LTCH discharge summary is similar to the short-term acute care hospital discharge summary requiring the same data fields. There may be state-specific criteria for the discharge summary, so it is important to include any state-specific data elements as well.

Note on EHRs in LTCHs

Similar to other providers, LTCHs are eligible for the American Recovery and Reinvestment Act of 2009 incentive payments for EHRs described in detail in chapter 6. Chapter 6 also gives examples of electronic formats for most components of the EHR. Please review the EHR sections of chapter 6 as they apply to LTCHs.

LTCH Policies and Procedures

Health information policies and procedures will encompass typical HIM practices, excluding policies on services that are not covered in the LTCH, such as birth or tumor registries. See chapter 4 for more information about registries.

Health record review activity is completed in the LTCH setting and is defined by facility policy. Open records are the focus of audits that examine clinical pertinence and health record completion. It is important to include discharge documentation monitoring in the **health record review process** to ensure that requirements and standards for discharge documentation are met as well. Health records are typically examined at the point of care by various clinical and HIM staff. Facility policy will drive the way data are gathered and disseminated. **Figure 10.6** shows a sample audit tool for open and closed records. HIM staff use such tools to examine the discharge records and ensure compliance with documentation standards for discharge summaries.

FIGURE 10.6. Sample documentation audit tool

Patient Name:				
MR#/VOL#:				
INDICATOR	YES	NO	N/A	Comment
History & Physical (H&P)				
H&P completed and on record within 24 hours of admission				
Diagnosis/impression recorded on H&P				
Reason for admission is documented				

FIGURE 10.6. (continued)

	YES	NO	N/A	Comment
Treatment plan documented in the H&P				
Family history				
Social history				
Allergies are addressed				
Review of systems				
Reflection of comprehensive physical exam				
Temperature				
Pulse				
Respiration				
Blood pressure				
Handwritten H&Ps are legible.				
Discharge Summary	YES	NO	N/A	Comment
Dictated within 14 days of patient discharge				
Final/discharge diagnoses and all other pertinent diagnoses relevant to the hospitalization				
Procedures performed				
Condition of patient at time of discharge/transfer to acute facility				
Disposition/conclusions				
Instructions to patient or family after discharge regarding discharge medications and follow-up care				
Reason for hospitalization				
Reason for hospitalization				
Significant findings				
Physician orders are dated/timed when written.				
Indication included for use of antibiotics, antipsychotics, PRN meds.				
INDICATOR	YES	NO	N/A	Comment
Orders IM				
TO/VO include time/date of receipt (nursing)				
Number of TO/VO monitored				
DATED				
TIMED				
SIGNED				
Discharge order is present.				
Physician orders are legible.				
Progress Notes	YES	NO	N/A	Comment
Notes are objective; include observations/results of therapy/ plan of action.				
Physician notes are dated/timed when written.				
If death, a final progress note is present.				
Physician progress notes are legible.				
Other	YES	NO	N/A	Comment
Allergies are present.				
Prohibited abbreviations are not used when writing orders.				

FIGURE 10.6. (continued)

INDICATOR Clinician	YES	NO	N/A	Comment
Assessments				
Nutrition screening is done within 2 working days of admission (admission or evaluations/assessment sections, progress note on COU, RCU, and PD).				
Initial pain assessment is completed.				
Initial nursing assessment within 24 hours of admission (on new admissions only)				
Physical status by nursing (monthly summary, progress notes)				
Psychological status (H&P, SW intake, psych consult, chaplain admission section as well)				
Social status (check H&P, SW intake)				
When warranted by patient need, nutritional status is assessed (nursing monthly summary, dietician progress notes, preadmission note).				
When warranted by patient need, functional status is assessed. Done for each RHB patient—chronic as needed (H&P/consults evaluations).				
Clinical progress notes are timed and dated (RN, RT, OT, PT, SLP, other).				
Need for discharge planning is assessed (case management notes/SW intake).				
Monitoring of medication effect on patient includes assessment based on collective observations, including patient's own perception of effect. (Check progress notes/MARs as necessary.)				
Clinical observations, including the results of therapy, are documented.				
Goals of treatment and treatment plans are documented.				
Care planning considers patient-specific needs, age-specific needs, and severity level of condition, impairment, or disability.				
Patient's learning needs, abilities, preferences, and readiness to learn are assessed.				
Assessment includes consideration of cultural values, religious beliefs.				
Barriers to learning are incorporated into care plans.				
Spiritual and cultural assessment is completed for the dying patient.				
INDICATOR	YES	NO	N/A	Comment
Reassessment				
Reassessment includes patient response to care.				
A significant change in the patient's condition results in reassessment.				
Have staff members integrated information from various assessments of the patient to identify and assign priorities to care needs?				
In reassessments, were care decisions based on the identified patient needs and care priorities?				
Education	YES	NO	N/A	Comment
Educational processes consider the physical, cognitive, cultural, social, and economic characteristics of the patient.				
The educational process is coordinated among appropriate staff or disciplines.				

FIGURE 10.6. (continued)

Indicator	YES	NO	N/A	Comment
Patient education is based on assessed needs, abilities, preferences, and readiness to learn, as appropriate.				
When appropriate, the patient/family is educated about safe and effective use of medications. Patient/family is preparing for self-administration of meds.				
When appropriate, the patient/family is educated about nutrition interventions, modified diets, or oral health.				
When appropriate, the patient is educated about safe and effective use of medical equipment or supplies.				
When appropriate, the patient is educated about pain and effective pain management.				
When appropriate, the patient is educated about habilitation and rehab techniques.				
When appropriate, the patient is educated about available community resources.				
When appropriate, the patient is educated regarding self-care activities.				
Education is timely (quarterly entry on patient). Family education sheet, LTC units only, excluding NB				
Patient/family education completed prior to discharge.				
When appropriate, academic education is provided to children and adolescents.				
INDICATOR	**YES**	**NO**	**N/A**	**Comment**
General Items				
Discharge summaries are completed—PT.				
Discharge summaries are completed—OT.				
Discharge summaries are completed—Other.				
Existence of advance directives NOT APPLICABLE ON PATIENTS 17 OR YOUNGER				
All diagnostic and therapeutic procedures and test results such as pathology and clinical laboratory exams are in the record.				
Face sheet is present in the record.				
All entries are signed.				
All entries are dated.				
General consent is signed and in the record.				
Pediatric Care: As appropriate, the assessment of infants, children, and adolescents includes:	**YES**	**NO**	**N/A**	**Comment**
A length/height (on nutritional evaluation—yearly) q 3 months, 0–2 yrs old, and q 6 months > 2 years old.				
Head circumference is documented on admission and then every year for patients 0–2 years old. It is done more often if deemed medically necessary. (Check growth charts, admission history database, and H&Ps.)				
Emotional, cognitive, communication, educational, social, and daily activity needs				
Developmental age				
Weight				
Immunization status				
Consideration of the patient's education needs and daily activity				
Family/guardian expectations for and involvement in the assessment, initial treatment, and continuing care of the patient are documented.				

Summary

LTCHs play an important role in the continuum of care. They provide care to patients with acute conditions that require longer LOSs than the capabilities of the acute hospital setting allow. Most patients in an LTCH are considered medically complex. Federal regulations require that LTCHs have an average LOS of at least 25 days. In addition, the Code of Federal Regulations describes how principal diagnoses should be assigned in the LTCH setting—based on the reason for admission to the LTCH, not the acute care hospital. State regulations require that same LOS, but other details may vary by state. Most LTCHs that are accredited by an outside organization choose to be accredited by The Joint Commission.

There was a moratorium on the number of LTCHs from 2007 through 2010. During that time, CMS was researching the future for LTCHs. Some of that research supports new criteria for patient admissions to LTCHs as well as the creation of patient assessments specific to the LTCH setting.

References

42 CFR Parts 412, 413, and 476. 2002. Medicare Program; Prospective Payment System for Long-Term Care Hospitals: Implementation and FY 2003 Rates; Final Rule. http://www.cms.gov/LongTermCareHospitalPPS/downloads/pp55954-56002.pdf.

Centers for Medicare and Medicaid Services (CMS). 2007. Long-Term Care Hospital (LTCH) Payment System Monitoring and Evaluation Phase II Report. https://www.cms.gov/LongTermCareHospitalPPS/Downloads/RTI_LTCHPPS_Final_Rpt.pdf.

Illinois Health Facilities Planning Board. 2007. Long-Term (Acute) Care Hospitals. http://www.idph.state.il.us/about/hfpb/pdf/LTCH%20Presentation%20%2001-08-07.pdf.

RTI International. 2007. *Long-Term Acute Care Hospital (LTCH) Payment System Monitoring and Evaluation, Phase II Report: Final.* https://www.cms.gov/LongTermCareHospitalPPS/Downloads/RTI_LTCHPPS_Final_Rpt.pdf.

US Department of Health and Human Services (HHS). 2009. ICD-9-CM Official Guidelines for Coding and Reporting. http://www.eicd.com/Guidelines/Default.htm.

US Department of Health and Human Services (HHS). 2005. The ICD-9-CM Official Guidelines for Coding and Reporting. http://www.eicd.com/Guidelines/Default.htm.

West Virginia Department of Health and Human Services Board of Review. 2008. Decision of State Hearing Officer. http://www.wvdhhr.org/oig/bor/decision%20categories/LTC%20hearings/2008%20LTC/LTC-1374-0708.pdf.

Chapter 11

Facility-Based Long-Term Care

Ella L. James, MS, RHIT, CPHQ

Learning Objectives

- Describe the different types of facility-based long-term care

- Define skilled nursing facility (SNF)

- Define nursing facility (NF)

- List the types of services provided at SNFs

- Describe the Medicare Conditions of Participation for SNFs and NFs

- Explain federal, state, and accrediting body regulations for SNFs and NFs

- Describe documentation requirements for orders for restraints

- Define the resident assessment instrument (RAI) and data collection process

- Explain documentation requirements for the RAI

- List Medicare quality indicators for SNFs

- Explain the method for obtaining and how to use Medicare's SNF Compare website

- Explain the relationship between health record documentation and Medicare quality indicators for SNFs

- Describe risk management concerns in the SNF

Key Terms

Activities of daily living

Adult foster care

Advance directives

Assisted living

Board and care homes

Commission on Accreditation of Rehabilitation Facilities (CARF)

Continuing care retirement communities

The Joint Commission

Medical necessity

Medicare Quality Indicator

Minimum Data Set (MDS 3.0)

Nursing facility (NF)

Problem list

Resident Assessment Instrument (RAI)

Resident Assessment Protocol (RAP)

Skilled-nursing facility (SNF)

State Operations Manual

Introduction

Long-term care encompasses a variety of services and supports to meet health or personal care needs over an extended period. Most long-term care is non-skilled personal care assistance, such as help performing everyday **activities of daily living (ADLs)**, which include (NCLTC 2010a):

- Bathing

- Dressing

- Using the toilet

- Transferring (to or from bed or chair)

- Caring for incontinence

- Eating

The overall goal of any long-term care services is to help patients maximize their independence and functioning.

At least 70 percent of people older than age 65 will require some long-term care services at some point in their lives. And Medicare and private health insurance programs do not pay for most long-term care services. In 2010, about 9 million Americans over the age of 65 will need long-term care services. By 2020, that number will increase to 12 million. While most people who need long-term care are age 65 or older, a person can need long-term care services at any age. Half of the people currently receiving long-term care are younger than 65 years old (NCLTC 2010b).

Many types of facility-based programs provide a range of long-term care services. Some facilities provide only housing and related housekeeping, but many also include help managing medications, assistance with personal care, supervision and special programs for individuals with Alzheimer's disease, or 24-hour nursing care. The services available in each facility are typically regulated by the state in which the facility operates. Facility-based service providers include those discussed in the sections that follow.

Adult Foster Care

Adult foster care can be provided for individuals or small groups of adults who need help functioning or who cannot live safely on their own (NCLTC 2010c). The foster family provides room and board, 24-hour availability, help managing medications, and assistance with ADLs. Licensure requirements and the terminology used for this type of facility vary greatly from state to state.

Board and Care Homes

Board and care homes, also called residential care facilities or group homes, are smaller private facilities, usually with 20 or fewer residents (NCLTC 2010c). Most board and care homes accept six or fewer residents. Rooms may be private or shared. Residents receive meals and personal care and have staff available 24 hours a day. Nursing and medical attention are usually not provided on the premises. State licensure and the terminology used for this type of facility vary greatly.

Assisted Living

Assisted living is designed for people who want to live in a community setting and who need or expect to need help functioning, but who do not need as much care as they would receive at a nursing home (NCLTC 2010c). Some assisted-living facilities are quite small, with as few as 25 residents, while some can accommodate 120 or more people. Residents often live in their own apartments or rooms but enjoy the support services that a community setting makes possible, such as (NCLTC 2010c)

- Up to three meals a day

- Assistance with personal care

- Help with medications, housekeeping, and laundry

- 24-hour security and onsite staff for emergencies

- Social programs

The cost of assisted living varies widely, depending in part on the services the resident needs and the amenities provided by the facility. Assisted living is regulated in all states, however, the requirements vary.

Continuing Care Retirement Communities

Continuing care retirement communities (CCRCs) are also called life care communities (NCLTC 2010c). They offer several levels of care in a single location. For example, many offer independent housing for people who need little or no care but also have assisted-living housing and a **nursing facility**, all on one campus, for those who need greater levels of care or supervision.

Nursing Homes

Nursing homes, also called **skilled nursing facilities (SNFs)**, nursing facilities (NFs), or convalescent care facilities, provide a wide range of services, including nursing care, 24-hour supervision, assistance with ADLs, and rehabilitation services such as physical, occupational, and speech therapy (NCLTC 2010c). Some people need nursing home services for a short period for recovery or rehabilitation after a serious illness or operation, while others need longer stays because of chronic physical, health, or cognitive conditions that require constant care or supervision. The average stay in a nursing home is about two and one-half years (Day 2011).

Skilled care is healthcare given when a patient needs skilled nursing or rehabilitation staff to treat, manage, observe, and evaluate her care. Examples of skilled care include intravenous injections and physical therapy. Skilled care is given in an SNF. Medicare covers certain skilled care services that are needed daily on a short-term basis (up to 100 days). Skilled care requires the involvement of skilled nursing or rehabilitative staff to be given safely and effectively. Skilled nursing and rehabilitation staff include (CMS 2010b):

- Registered nurses

- Licensed practical and vocational nurses

- Physical and occupational therapists

TABLE 11.1. Coverage limits of long-term care offered by health insurance

LONG-TERM CARE SERVICE	MEDICARE	PRIVATE INSURANCE (also known as Medigap)	MEDICAID	PATIENT COSTS
Nursing home care	Pays in full for days 0–20 if the patient is in an SNF following a recent hospital stay. After day 100 Medicare does not pay.	May cover the $137.50/day co-payment if the nursing home stay meets all other Medicare requirements.	May pay for care in a Medicaid-certified nursing home if the patient meets functional and financial eligibility criteria.	Patient pays only if the patient needs only personal or supervisory care in a nursing home
Assisted living facility (and similar facility option)	Does not pay	Does not pay	In some states, may pay care-related costs, but not room and board	Patient pays except as noted under Medicaid if eligible
Continuing care retirement community	Does not pay	Does not pay	Does not pay	Patient pays

Source: Adapted from NCLTC n.d.

- Speech-language pathologists

- Audiologists

This facility-based long-term care is regulated by the state where the facility operates. Any health records maintained by the facility are governed, at a minimum, by the state's department of health regulations. In some cases, facilities may seek accreditation by an external organization, which will also require that they meet those accreditation guidelines to maintain accreditation.

The only long-term care regulated and reimbursed by the Centers for Medicare and Medicaid Services (CMS) is skilled care provided in nursing homes. Of the $206 billion spent on long-term care in the United States in 2005, 49 percent was paid by Medicaid programs and 20 percent was paid by Medicare (NCLTC 2010a). Because the skilled care provided in nursing homes is the most highly regulated and the most complex, the remainder of this chapter will focus on the details of defining, regulating, and maintaining health record documentation for facilities that provide skilled nursing care.

The differences in insurance coverage for different levels of long-term care are illustrated in **TABLE 11.1**.

Skilled Nursing Care

Care provided in SNFs is regulated by the following:

- Social Security Act (Section 1819 for Medicare and Section 1919 for Medicaid)

- Medicare Conditions of Participation

- **State Operations Manual**—Guidance to Surveyors for long-term care facilities

- Quality improvement organizations

The Social Security Act (SSA) was the original legislation that addressed skilled nursing care and continues to guide all skilled nursing care reimbursed by CMS. The law is quite complex and covers about 50 pages in the SSA. The other regulating guidance noted earlier exists primarily to explain and attempt to simplify the details of the SSA.

One of the first complex issues in the SSA is the fact that skilled nursing care is addressed in two different sections—one for Medicare regulation (section 1819) and one for Medicaid regulation (section 1919). In section 1819, the SSA uses the term *skilled nursing facility* to define care provided for Medicare regulation and reimbursement purposes. In section 1919, the SSA uses the term *nursing facility* to define care provided for Medicaid regulation and reimbursement purposes. The definitions for each follow as they appear in the statute:

Skilled nursing facility (SNF) is defined as an institution (or a distinct part of an institution) which is primarily engaged in providing skilled nursing care and related services for residents who require medical or nursing care, or rehabilitation services for the rehabilitation of injured, disabled, or sick persons, and is not primarily for the care and treatment of mental diseases; has in effect a transfer agreement (meeting the requirements of §1861(1)) with one or more hospitals having agreements in effect under §1866; and meets the requirements for a SNF described in subsections (b), (c), and (d) of this section. (SSA 1992)

Nursing facility (NF) is defined as an institution (or a distinct part of an institution) which is primarily engaged in providing skilled nursing care and related services for residents who require medical or nursing care, rehabilitation services for the rehabilitation of injured, disabled, or sick persons, or on a regular basis, health-related care and services to individuals who because of their mental or physical condition require care and services (above the level of room and board) which can be made available to them only through institutional facilities, and is not primarily for the care and treatment of mental diseases; has in effect a transfer agreement (meeting the requirements of §1861(1)) with one or more hospitals having agreements in effect under §1866; and meets the requirements for an NF described in subsections (b), (c), and (d) of this section. (SSA 1992)

If a provider does not meet one of these definitions, it cannot be certified for participation in the Medicare and/or Medicaid programs (SSA 1992).

The provisions of this part of the SSA contain the requirements an institution must meet to qualify to participate as an SNF in the Medicare program and as an NF in the Medicaid program. They serve as the basis for survey activities to determine whether a facility meets the requirements for participation in Medicare and Medicaid (Medicare 2001).

SNF Health Record Content

The functions of the SNF health records are the same as those in acute care hospital settings. They function as the documentation and communication tools to facilitate the patient care delivery and legal recording of care and treatment provided to the individuals served. Unlike the acute care patient, however, the typical SNF patient has a one- to five-year length of stay. As a result, key information gathered on admission is updated on an ongoing basis. In an SNF, these data make up the resident assessment. The resident assessment describes the resident's capability to perform daily life functions and significant impairments in functional capacity. It also identifies medical problems (SSA 1992; CMS 2011b). Details of the resident assessment are addressed in the next section.

Admission paperwork includes a number of documents that need to be completed before a resident can be admitted. Requirements depend on the regulations of the state in which the facility operates. In addition to the documentation of preadmission and admission assessments, some or all of the forms, records, consents, or data fields in the electronic health record (EHR) may be created and maintained in the resident's health record. As in the acute care setting, the patient's demographic data are collected, updated, and maintained.

A completed admission application is usually kept in the admitting office. If it is electronic, it may only be accessible to those who need access. Admission applications may be scanned into the EHR because they require the resident's or surrogate's signatures for the following:

- Consent to treat

- Consent to photograph (per facility policy)

- Physician certification for Medicare

- Interagency transfer form (from the referring facility; this may be a state requirement)

- Acknowledgments

- Mental illness and mental retardation form (state specific)

- Face sheet for the health record

- Acknowledgment of the notice of privacy practices

- Resident bill of rights (depending on facility policy)

- Admission agreement (depending on facility policy)

Several different types of consent and authorization forms are used in long-term care organizations. Consents provide a means for residents to convey to healthcare providers their implied or expressed permission to administer care or treatment or other medical procedures. Authorizations, however, document the resident's formal, written permission to use or disclose his protected health information for purposes other than treatment, payment, or healthcare operations. In the electronic environment, these types of documents may have to be scanned into the resident's health record. **Advance directives** are also included in the collection of initial information for the patient's health record. An advance directive (also called healthcare directive, advance health care directive, living will, or health care directive) is a legal document used to specify whether the patient would like to be kept on artificial life support if she becomes permanently unconscious or is otherwise dying and unable to speak for herself.

Resident Assessments

As a condition of participation in both Medicare and Medicaid programs, SNFs and NFs must perform a resident assessment. The law states that an SNF (section 1819) or NF (section 1919) "must conduct a comprehensive, accurate, standardized, reproducible assessment of each resident's functional capacity, that:

- Describes the resident's capability to perform daily life functions and significant impairments in functional capacity;

- Is based on a uniform minimum data set [specified under subsection (f)]

- Uses an instrument which is specified under subsection (f)

- Includes the identification of medical problems" (SSA 1992)

Each assessment must be conducted or coordinated by a registered professional nurse, with the participation of other appropriate health professionals, who signs and certifies that the initial assessment is complete. Each individual who completes a portion of the assessment must sign and certify as to the accuracy of that portion of the assessment. The assessment must be completed no later than 14 days after the date of admission.

The assessment process is an ongoing evaluation of the resident's needs, functional abilities, and requirements, and it is used to identify and provide appropriate interventions and services. The entire assessment process is fundamental to the care-planning requirements of federal, state, and accrediting bodies.

The **Resident Assessment Instrument (RAI)** is used to collect the necessary information from and about the facility resident. The RAI consists of three basic components: The **Minimum Data Set (MDS)** Version 3.0, the Care Area Assessment (CAA) process, and the RAI utilization guidelines. The utilization of the three components of the RAI yields information about a resident's functional status, strengths, weaknesses, and preferences, and offers guidance on further assessment once problems have been identified. Each component flows naturally into the next as follows:

- **MDS.** A core set of screening, clinical, and functional status elements, including common definitions and coding categories, which forms the foundation of a comprehensive assessment for all residents of nursing homes certified to participate in Medicare or Medicaid. The items in the MDS standardize communication about resident problems and conditions within nursing homes, between nursing homes, and between nursing homes and outside agencies.

- **CAA Process.** This process is designed to help the assessor systematically interpret the information recorded on the MDS. Once a care area has been triggered, nursing home providers use current, evidence-based clinical resources to assess the potential problem and determine whether or not to make a care plan for it. The CAA process helps the clinician focus on key issues identified during the assessment process so that decisions as to whether and how to intervene can be explored with the resident. See **TABLE 11.2** for a description of comprehensive resident assessments. Specific components of the CAA process include:

  o **Care Area Triggers (CATs)** are specific resident responses for one or a combination of MDS elements. The triggers identify residents who have developed or are at risk for developing specific functional problems and require further assessment.

  o **CAA Resources** are a list of resources that may be helpful in assessing a triggered care area.

TABLE 11.2. Comprehensive resident assessments

(i) Identification and demographic information	"Identification and demographic information" refers to information that uniquely identifies each resident and the facility in which the resident resides, date of entry into the facility, and residential history.
(ii) Customary routine	"Customary routine" refers to information regarding the resident's usual community lifestyle and daily routine.
(iii) Cognitive patterns	"Cognitive patterns" is defined as the resident's ability to problem solve, decide, remember, and be aware of and respond to safety hazards.
(iv) Communication	"Communication" refers to the resident's ability to hear, understand others, make him- or herself understood (with assistive devices if they are used).
(v) Vision	"Vision" refers to the resident's visual acuity, limitations and difficulties, and appliances used to enhance vision.
(vi) Mood and behavior patterns	"Mood and behavior patterns" refers to the resident's patterns of mood and behavioral symptoms
(vii) Psychosocial well-being	"Psychosocial well-being" refers to the resident's positive or negative feelings about him- or herself or his or her social relationships.
(viii) Physical functioning and structural problems	"Physical functioning and structural problems" refers to the resident's physical functional status, ability to perform ADLs, and need for staff assistance and assistive devices or equipment to maintain or improve functional abilities.
(ix) Continence	"Continence" refers to the resident's patterns of bladder and bowel continence (control), pattern of elimination, and appliances used.
(x) Disease diagnosis and health conditions	"Disease diagnoses and health conditions"
(xi) Dental and nutritional status	"Dental condition status" refers to the condition of the teeth, gums, and other structures of the oral cavity that may affect a resident's nutritional status, communication abilities, or quality of life. The assessment should include the need for, and use of, dentures or other dental appliances. "Nutritional status" refers to weight, height, hematologic and biochemical assessments, clinical observations of nutrition, nutritional intake, resident's eating habits and preferences, dietary restrictions, supplements, and use of appliances.
(xii) Skin conditions	"Skin conditions" refers to the resident's development, or risk of development, of a pressure sore.
(xiii) Activity pursuit	"Activity pursuit" refers to the resident's ability and desire to take part in activities that maintain or improve, physical, mental, and psychosocial well-being. Activity pursuits refer to any activity outside the ADLs that a person pursues to obtain a sense of well-being. Also, it includes activities that provide benefits in self-esteem, pleasure, comfort, health education, creativity, success, and financial or emotional independence. The assessment should consider the resident's normal everyday routines and lifetime preferences.
(xiv) Medications	"Medications" refers to all prescription and over-the-counter medications taken by the resident, including dosage, frequency of administration, and recognition of significant side effects that would be most likely to occur in the resident. This information must be in the resident's clinical record.

TABLE 11.2. (continued)

(xv) Special treatments and procedures	"Special treatments and procedures" refers to treatments and procedures that are not part of basic services provided. For example, treatment for pressure sores, nasogastric feedings, specialized rehabilitation services, respiratory care, or devices and restraints.
(xvi) Discharge potential	"Discharge potential" refers to the facility's expectation of discharging the resident from the facility within the next three months.
(xvii) Documentation of summary information regarding the additional assessment performed on the care areas triggered by the completion of the MDS.	"Documentation of summary information (xvii) regarding the additional assessment performed" through the CAAs refers to documentation concerning which CAAs have been triggered, documentation of assessment information in support of clinical decision making relevant to the CAAs, documentation regarding where, in the clinical record, information related to the CAAs can be found, and for each triggered CAA, whether the identified problem was included in the care plan.
(xviii) Documentation of participation in assessment	"Documentation of participation in the assessment" refers to documentation of who participated in the assessment process. The assessment process must include direct observation and communication with the resident, as well as communication with licensed and nonlicensed direct care staff members on all shifts.

Source: CMS 2011b, 121–123.

- o **CAA Summary (Section V of the MDS 3.0)** provides a location for documentation of the care areas that have been triggered from the MDS and the decisions made during the CAA process regarding whether or not to proceed to care planning (CMS 2010a).

   CAAs are not required for Medicare assessments. They are required only for comprehensive clinical assessments (that is, admission assessments, annual assessments, significant change in status assessments, or significant correction of a prior full assessments). "However, when a Medicare assessment is combined with a comprehensive clinical assessment, the CAAs must be completed in order to meet the requirements of the comprehensive clinical assessment. A CAA should provide nursing home staff with comprehensive information for evaluating factors that may cause, contribute to, or exacerbate the triggered condition" (CMS 2010a).

- • **Utilization Guidelines.** The Utilization Guidelines provide instructions for when and how to use the RAI. These include instructions for completing the RAI and structured frameworks for synthesizing MDS and other clinical information. (CMS 2010a).

Resident Assessment Protocols

Resident Assessment Protocols (RAPs) "are problem-oriented frameworks for additional assessment based on problem identification items (triggered conditions). They form a critical link to decisions about care planning. The RAPs guidelines provide guidance on how to synthesize assessment information within a comprehensive assessment. The triggers target conditions for additional assessment and review, as warranted by MDS item responses. The RAPs guidelines help facility staff evaluate 'triggered' conditions" (CMS 2010a).

The RAPs include the principal components of a long-term care resident's care plan. They are used to further define the resident's care-planning needs and treatment. Moreover, they are used in conjunction with the MDS to ensure that the resident's assessment is comprehensive and the care-planning process is complete. Currently, long-term care facilities are required to use the RAI version 2.0. CMS recently released MDS 3.0 (CMS 2011a).

During the RAI process, several assessments should be considered to support the MDS documentation and may include the following:

- Physician history and physical exam
- Nursing assessment
- Wound and skin assessment
- Fall assessment
- Bowel and bladder assessment
- Pain assessment
- Basic mental/cognitive examination
- Restraint assessment (only if applicable)
- MDS assessment
- Nutritional assessment
- Therapy assessments, as required
- Therapeutic recreation assessment
- Pastoral care assessment

The MDS is a primary document in the resident's health record. The RAI is used to evaluate new residents of long-term care facilities within 14 days of admission, but the interdisciplinary team must complete further assessments and reassessments to enhance the MDS data-gathering process. Evaluations are conducted every quarter, every year, and whenever there is a significant change in the resident's status.

The completion schedule for residents who are eligible for Medicare benefits is slightly different from the schedule for other residents. Note that the "assessment type" is the time frame for which an assessment is completed, while the "assessment window" is how long a facility has to complete the assessment. See also "MDS 3.0 for Nursing Homes and Swing Bed Providers" for more information (CMS 2011a).

Physician Documentation

In addition to the RAI, physicians must comply with specific documentation requirements in the SNF. These requirements are outlined in the Social Security Administration and the Medicare Conditions of Participation, with the exception of history and physical documentation requirements, which are outlined by The Joint Commission.

Each resident must remain under the care of a physician (CMS 2010a). The facility also must demonstrate that a physician oversees the medical care of each resident at all times. This is done through physician documentation. The documentation verifies that the medical oversight or supervision of care for long-term care residents has occurred. The interdisciplinary team and care-planning process must involve the physician. In the long-term care environment, the physician is not required to visit the resident every day but, rather, as the resident's needs dictate. However, the physician must be informed of the resident's status changes and identified medical problems to ensure that proper care is provided in a timely manner (James 2007).

The physician documentation requirements are addressed in the sections that follow.

Admission Order

A physician must personally approve in writing a recommendation that an individual be admitted to a facility. Each resident must remain under the care of a physician.

Physician Visit Documentation

The physician must

- Review the resident's total program of care, including medications and treatments, at each visit required

- Write, sign, and date progress notes at each visit

- Sign and date all orders with the exception of influenza and pneumococcal polysaccharide vaccines, which may be administered per physician-approved facility policy after an assessment for contraindications.

Physician Visit Frequency

The physician must comply with the following patient visitation schedule:

- The residents must be seen by a physician at least once every 30 days for the first 90 days after admission, and at least once every 60 days thereafter.

- A physician visit is considered timely if it occurs no later than 10 days after the date the visit was required.

History and Physical

The physician history and physical must be completed as specified by state regulations. In addition, if a facility chooses to be accredited by The Joint Commission, it must adhere to those regulations. The Joint Commission requires that the history and physical or medical assessment be completed within 24 hours before admission or within 72 hours after admission (Joint Commission 2007). A history and physical that is received from the attending physician or licensed independent practitioner and completed within 30 days prior to admission may be used as long as it summarizes the patient's condition and care prior to admission and describes the resident's current physical/psychosocial status (Joint Commission 2007).

While there are no federal time-frame requirements for completing the admission nursing assessments, states may have their own regulations and accreditation bodies. In 2007, The Joint Commission stipulated that "the organization initiates nursing assessments within 24 hours of admission…At minimum, the organization completes assessments within five calendar days after admission for all disciplines pertinent to the reason for admission or as required by law and regulation" (Joint Commission 2007).

Initial nursing assessments must be completed as established by law or facility policy, but no later than 14 days after admission. In addition, several Joint Commission requirements address the assessment of each resident. The organization must have a process for assessing and reassessing residents, and reassessments must be conducted at regular intervals. These assessments must be overseen by a registered nurse. Initial assessments also must specifically address the status, needs, and potential of each resident and include information on his or her medical, physical, functional, psychosocial, and nutritional status (see **FIGURE 11.1**).

FIGURE 11.1. Relevant past medical history and medical status

- Diagnoses
- Medications
- Allergies
- Treatments
- Results of diagnostic or laboratory studies
- Prognosis
- Limitations
- Precautions
- Neuropsychiatric status: Mental, affective, cognitive, sleeping patterns or memory, recall ability, decision-making ability, and behavior
- Communication status: Hearing, speech, language, voice, and modes of expression
- Rehabilitation status: Previous and current functional status, ADLs, mobility, balance, strength, bowel and bladder function, sensory capacity and impairments, vision, ability to swallow, orientation, and rehabilitation potential
- Psychosocial status: Level of functioning, cultural and ethnic factors, current emotional status, social skills, family circumstances, family relationships, current living situation, relevant past history, past roles, and response to current status
- Spiritual status: Spiritual orientation, including the dying individual's self-esteem
- Physical status: Musculoskeletal, cardiorespiratory, gastrointestinal, integumentary, and foot care
- Level of activity: Use of free time; personal preferences; preadmission hobbies, interests, and lifestyle; past and current activities; and ability to participate
- Nutritional and hydration status: Potential nutritional risk and deficiencies; cultural, religious, or ethnic food preferences; special dietary requirements; and nutrient-intake routines
- Dental status and oral health: Condition of the oral cavity, teeth, and tooth-supporting structures; natural teeth or dentures; functioning with or without natural teeth or dentures
- Level of pain: Origin, location, severity, alleviating and exacerbating factors, and current treatment and response to treatment
- Response to stress caused by present situation, illness, and treatment
- Educational needs: Needs, preferences, abilities, and readiness to learn to include family members

Source: James 2007.

Discharge Summary

When the facility anticipates discharge a resident must have a discharge summary that includes

- A recapitulation of the resident's stay

- A final summary of the resident's status at the time of the discharge that is available for release to authorized persons and agencies, with the consent of the resident or legal representative

Progress Notes

An admission progress note is completed when the resident is admitted to the long-term care facility. An "admission note should be entered into the resident's health record that includes the date and time of admission, how the resident arrived at the facility (for example, by ambulance), the reason for the admission, and the resident's current condition and health status. State regulations include specific requirements for admission documentation, time frame for completion, and other specified requirements" (James 2007). Often these notes are very short and succinct, but they should reflect and support the reason for admission to the long-term care setting.

Additional progress notes are entered as determined by federal, state, and accrediting body regulations and standards. Each time the resident is seen by a physician, a progress note should be entered.

Physician Orders

The physician's order must include the frequency, duration, and scope of treatment and be dated and signed. These orders are written when changes, additions, or deletions are required in care and treatment of the resident. They include but are not limited to medications (pharmacy orders), treatments such as dressing changes, services such as therapies, ancillary tests such as laboratory blood draws and cultures or radiology studies, and diet orders (James 2007).

Physician Consultations

Consultations may be required when the resident's health status dictates that a specialist examine identified problems encountered in her care and treatment. Such specialists may include podiatrists, cardiologists, pulmonologists, or surgeons. Consultations are usually kept for easy access in a separate section in the resident's health record. In an electronic environment, consultants who make visits to the resident in the facility require access to the EHR to complete the consult documentation. If the resident is sent outside the facility for the consultation, the consult may need to be scanned into the health record so that staff has easy access to the information. Consultations in a long-term care facility contain the same data elements as those in the short-term acute care and long-term acute care hospital.

Other Documentation

Other documentation—electronic, hybrid, or paper—includes monthly summaries, education records, ADLs, therapy, flow sheets, laboratory and special reports, medication administration records, discharge documentation, accident and incident reports, and organization/management.

Monthly Summary

A monthly summary may be completed in the long-term care setting to help summarize the care given to the resident over time. There are no federal requirements for a summary note; however, state laws may be more specific. The monthly summary is a mechanism to capture concise monthly updates reflecting gains and declines in the resident's condition and health status. The monthly summary should correlate with the resident's care-planning process and further support the MDS assessments.

Education Records

Education of the resident should be documented as provided and completed by the time of discharge. The documentation should be an interdisciplinary team effort. Based on Joint Commission documentation requirements, the resident is assessed for needs, abilities, preferences, and readiness to learn, as appropriate, and the education plan considers the physical, cognitive, cultural, social, and economic characteristics of the resident. The education documentation should include the following (James 2007):

- Available community resources
- Habilitation and rehabilitation techniques
- Nutrition interventions, modified diets, or oral health, when applicable
- Pain and effective pain management
- Safe and effective use of medical equipment or supplies
- Safe and effective use of medications
- Self-administration of medications
- Self-care activities

Activities of Daily Living

ADLs should be documented. Although there is no federal requirement for this documentation, ADLs are part of the MDS, and many long-term care facilities capture this information as supporting documentation. The resident's ADLs indicate his functional status. The documentation of ADLs supports the MDS assessments. Functional ability can be divided into the following categories:

- Bed mobility
- Transfer
- Walking
- Locomotion
- Dressing
- Eating
- Toilet use
- Personal hygiene
- Bathing

Therapy

Rehabilitative therapy is made up of those services provided by the licensed therapist staff. These individuals are allied health professionals in physical therapy, occupational therapy, speech-language therapy, and respiratory therapy. Rehabilitative therapy should not be confused with nursing restorative care. The federal government sets stringent standards for nursing homes "to attain or maintain the resident's highest practicable physical, mental, and psychosocial well-being" (CMS 2011). Rehabilitative therapy provides another mechanism to ensure that residents achieve the best quality outcomes of care. Rehabilitative therapy services documentation includes the assessments, daily flow-sheet charting, diagnostic evaluation, education, management, and treatments.

Flow Sheets

Flow sheets are used in various ways in the long-term care setting and are used by all clinical staff to capture the health and functional status and responses to treatment, and "the common purpose of all of these flow sheets is to document that required services were delivered to the facility's residents and to provide a means of communication among healthcare workers" (James 2007). In the long-term care setting, flow sheets are usually discipline specific rather than interdisciplinary.

Laboratory and Special Reports

Laboratory reports contain information gathered from many kinds of laboratory and diagnostic test results. These reports help establish the correct diagnosis and treatment plan for each resident and assess changes in residents' health conditions and status.

Special reports include the results of imaging and pathology testing, among other procedures. Imaging may include a full range of radiological service diagnostic test results, including the more common X-ray, electrocardiogram, Holter monitor, magnetic resonance imaging, computed tomography scan, and respiratory therapy reports (such as pulmonary function testing and pulse oximetry results). X-ray reports are the most common test result found in the resident's health record (James 2007).

Medication Administration Records

Medication administration records (MARs) are used to capture the delivery of each drug to the resident. The MAR identifies medications a resident is scheduled to take, how often they should be administered, and at what dose (James 2007).

Discharge Documentation

Federal regulations require that the reason or need for the transfer or discharge be documented in the resident's health record. In addition, each resident must be notified in writing of the reasons for the transfer or discharge and the facility bed-hold policy. Discharge documentation refers to those records that must be completed at the time the resident is transferred to another facility or discharged from the facility. These documents include the following:

- Medication education and drug discharge documentation

- Clinical discharge summaries for all disciplines treating the resident

- Comprehensive assessment (MDS)

- Discharge plan of care

- Discharge instructions to the resident or resident's family as appropriate

- Transfer forms or interagency transfer forms

- Physician discharge summary

SNF Accreditation Standards and Regulations

A major change for long-term care occurred in 1987, when President Ronald Reagan approved a revision to Medicare and Medicaid that requires long-term care providers to provide services so each resident can "attain and maintain [the] highest practicable physical, mental, and psychosocial well-being" (National Long-Term Care Ombudsman Resource Center 2001).

Long-term care facilities are subject to several intricate operating requirements. These include both voluntary and mandatory requirements, which can include the following:

- Federal statutes and regulations

- State licensure

- State health record regulations

- State public health codes

- State regulations for Medicaid qualifications

- County and municipal building safety codes

- Federal health information privacy and security standards

- Joint Commission standards (voluntary)

It is imperative that long-term care facilities consult all of these areas to ensure compliance with all regulations and standards.

Medical Necessity and Medicare Documentation

The federal government requires accurate, timely, and complete health record documentation of the skilled nursing and therapeutic services provided to Medicare beneficiaries. The resident's health record must substantiate the clinical indications and **medical necessity** for Medicare Part A coverage as well as the skilled services required and the resident's continued need for coverage. Documentation that supports that skilled services are medically reasonable and necessary is required for all charges submitted on the UB-04 (CMS 2002).

Medicare's Conditions of Participation require that a physician's orders describing the resident's immediate care requirements be provided to the facility at the time of admission. A physician's certification of the resident's need for long-term care services is also required at any time the resident is eligible for Medicare benefits. In addition, Medicare regulations stipulate that a health record must be established for every resident at the time of admission.

Each Medicare resident must have a Medicare Part A certification and recertification executed and signed by the physician who knows the resident's care and treatment requirements. Certification/recertification includes the reasons for Medicare coverage and the skilled services that will be provided. Certification is mandated upon admission; recertifications are mandated for as long as the resident continues to receive Medicare Part A benefits. The recertification is also required when a resident returns to a long-term care facility after a temporary acute care hospital stay, as long as the resident still qualifies for Medicare coverage.

Physician Certification

Staff and attending physicians must periodically certify the need for long-term care services within an SNF. **Physician certification** is required on admission or as soon as possible thereafter. The first recertification is required no later than the 14th day of the patient's stay, and additional recertifications are required every 30 days (CMS 2011).

Standards Governing Assessments

Documentation of the assessments conducted in the long-term care setting is driven by federal and state regulations and accreditation standards. **Medicare prospective payment system** requirements also affect clinical documentation efforts. Depending on state requirements, the admission process may start when potential residents are placed on the facility's waiting list. The waiting list may be a state-specific requirement. All states, however, require that residents of long-term care facilities remain under the care of a physician throughout their stay. This is demonstrated through the documentation process of the long-term care health record.

The Joint Commission states that the long-term care facility should admit and treat only those residents whose "identified care, treatment, and services needs it can meet" (Joint Commission 2007). Additionally, information about each potential patient is used "to match an individual's need with the appropriate setting, care level, and intervention" (Joint Commission 2007).

The **Commission on Accreditation of Rehabilitation Facilities (CARF)** accreditation recognizes facilities not only for rehabilitation but also for retirement living, disability, addiction, and substance abuse (CARF 2011). Consumer satisfaction is at the forefront of CARF accreditation. CARF standards focus on the goals and activities of the resident and the outcomes of care. Thus, CARF standards look at the needs of the resident, proper placement, and the outcomes of care.

Medicare Quality Indicators for SNFs

One of the results of the data that are collected by SNFs for the MDS through the RAI described earlier is the ability to compare the quality of care provided by two or more SNFs. CMS has made this information readily available to healthcare consumers on the Medicare Nursing Home Compare website. The website guides the user through a simple process of first identifying which nursing homes she wants to compare. The user is given a choice of using zip code, city, state, or nursing home name. The site returns all SNFs that met the search criteria, and the user identifies which SNFs she would like to compare. The detailed report contains a list of all of the criteria used to determine how an SNF is rated. **TABLE 11.3** lists the Medicare Quality Indicators used to rate the quality of each SNF.

TABLE 11.3. Medicare Quality Indicators

- Long stay residents given influenza vaccination during the flu season
- Long stay residents who were assessed and given pneumococcal vaccination
- Residents whose need for help with daily activities has increased (since admission)
- Residents who have moderate to severe pain
- High-risk long stay residents who have pressure sores
- Low-risk long stay residents who have pressure sores
- Residents who were physically restrained
- Residents who become depressed or anxious
- Residents who lose control of their bowels or bladder
- Residents who have/had a catheter inserted and left in their bladder
- Residents who spend most of their time in bed or in a chair
- Residents whose ability to move about in and around their room got worse
- Residents who had a urinary tract infection
- Residents who lose too much weight
- Short stay residents given influenza vaccination during the flu season
- Short stay residents who were assessed and given pneumococcal vaccination
- Short stay residents who have delirium
- Short stay residents who had moderate to severe pain
- Short stay residents who have pressure sores

Source: Medicare n.d.

In addition to a detailed report, the user is also provided with a summary report that rates each SNF using the following star ratings (Medicare n.d.):

- One star: much below average

- Two stars: below average

- Three stars: average

- Four stars: above average

- Five stars: much above average

Risk Management and Liability

Identical liability issues exist in the long-term acute care and long-term care settings as in short-term acute care. Long-term care facilities also look at risk management concerns, incident reporting, and medical staff credentialing and privileging and rely on the health record documentation to support these areas. While long-term care may have more issues with longer stays and accidents or injuries within the facility, the liability factors discussed under short-term acute care also apply in these care settings.

Accidents or incidents may occasionally occur in the long-term care setting. When they do, they must be reported in an accident or incident report. The facts of the event must also be documented in the resident's health record. The actual accident or incident report does not get filed into the resident's health record. Facility policy must outline how the facts of the occurrence should be documented: "documentation does not indicate that an incident report has been filed, nor does it refer to the report in the documentation. However, the resident's health record must reflect the facts of the injury and how it was received" (James 2007).

The same standards for documentation and management of the acute care setting apply in the long-term care setting. The resident's health record is the principal communication instrument for planning, coordinating, and managing the resident's care. It is the legal business record of the facility. Moreover, it is the facility's defense against malpractice claims.

Summary

Long-term care encompasses a variety of services and supports to meet health or personal care needs over an extended period of time. The overall goal of any long-term care services is to help patients maximize their independence and functioning. Numerous types of facility-based programs provide long-term care services that range from room and board with medication administration to skilled nursing care. Skilled nursing care is the only type of care that is regulated and reimbursed by CMS. Skilled care is healthcare given when a patient needs skilled nursing or rehabilitation staff to treat, manage, observe, and evaluate his care. Examples of skilled care include intravenous injections and physical therapy. Because the average length of stay in an SNF ranges from one to five years, the type of information collected and maintained on SNF residents is more comprehensive than that collected on patients in the acute care setting. The SNF staff must complete a resident assessment by collecting data items consistent with the MDS necessary for SNF CMS requirements. Both care and documentation and data requirements are regulated by the federal government and state governments. For facilities that choose to be accredited by The Joint Commission, additional documentation requirements apply. One use for the data that are collected on SNF residents is to populate the Medicare Nursing Home Compare website. The site allows healthcare consumers to compare SNFs and view detailed data on the SNFs' Medicare Quality Indicators. This process is designed to create incentives for SNFs to continuously improve the quality of care and the quality of data and documentation they collect and record for each resident.

References

Centers for Medicare and Medicaid Services (CMS). 2011a. MDS 3.0 for Nursing Homes and Swing Bed Providers. https://www.cms.gov/nursinghomequalityinits/25_nhqimds30.asp.

Centers for Medicare and Medicaid Services (CMS). 2011b. *State Operations Manual: Appendix PP—Guidance to Surveyors for Long Term Care Facilities.* https://cms.gov/manuals/Downloads/som107ap_pp_guidelines_ltcf.pdf.

Centers for Medicare and Medicaid Services (CMS). 2010a. *CMS' RAI Version 3.0 Manual: Medicare SNF PPS.* https://www.cms.gov/SNFPPS/.

Centers for Medicare and Medicaid Services (CMS). 2010b. *Medicare Coverage of SNF Care.* http://www.medicare.gov/publications/pubs/pdf/10153.pdf.

Centers for Medicare and Medicaid Services (CMS). 2002. Long-Term Care Hospital PPS Training Guide. http://www.cms.hhs.gov/LongTermCareHospitalPPS/03_ltch_train.asp.

Commission on Accreditation of Rehabilitation Facilities (CARF). 2011. Providers Earn Recognition for Accredited Services. http://www.carf.org/Providers/.

Day, T. 2011. National Care Planning Council (NCPC): About Nursing Homes. http://www.longtermcarelink.net/eldercare/nursing_home.htm.

James, E. 2007. *Documentation and Reimbursement for Long-term Care*, 2nd ed. Chicago: AHIMA.

The Joint Commission. 2007. *Comprehensive Accreditation Manual for Long-Term Care*. Oakbrook Terrace, IL: Joint Commission.

Medicare. n.d. Nursing Home Compare. http://www.medicare.gov/NHCompare/Include/DataSection/Questions/ProximitySearch.asp.

Medicare. 2001. Medicare Conditions of Participation for Skilled Nursing Facilities. http://frwebgate.access.gpo.gov/cgi-bin/get-cfr.cgi?TITLE=42&PART=483&SECTION=1&YEAR=2001&TYPE=TEXT.

National Clearinghouse for Long Term Care (NCLTC). 2010a. Definitions & Need for LTC. http://www.longtermcare.gov/LTC/Main_Site/Understanding/Definition/Index.aspx.

National Clearinghouse for Long Term Care (NCLTC). 2010b. Who Needs LTC? http://www.longtermcare.gov/LTC/Main_Site/Understanding/Definition/Who.aspx.

National Clearinghouse for Long Term Care (NCLTC). 2010c. Facility Based Services. http://www.longtermcare.gov/LTC/Main_Site/Understanding/Services/Facility_Based_Services.aspx.

National Clearinghouse for Long Term Care (NCLTC). n.d. Who Pays for LTC Services? http://longtermcare.gov/LTC/Main_Site/Paying/Costs/Who_Pays.aspx.

National Long-Term Care Ombudsman Resource Center. 2001. Federal Nursing Home Reform Act from the Omnibus Budget Reconciliation Act of 1987. http://www.ltcombudsman.org/about.

US Social Security Administration (SSA). 1992. Payment to hospitals for inpatient hospital services Sec. 1886. [42 U.S.C. 1395ww] (d)(II)(B)(iv). *United States Code*. http://www.ssa.gov/OP_Home/ssact/title18/1886.htm.

Chapter 12

Home Care and Hospice Documentation, Accreditation, Liability, and Standards

Margaret J. White, MS, NHA, RHIA, CPHQ

Learning Objectives

- Identify the key components of the home care and hospice health record database

- Develop an understanding of Medicare home care and hospice benefits

- Introduce the Medicare home care survey process

- Discuss the documentation challenges for the prospective payment system and Outcome and Assessment Information Set (OASIS)

- Provide the quantitative record review guidelines

- Introduce the home care and hospice legal issues

- Define outcomes management and quality requirements of home care and hospice

- Reinforce the importance of confidentiality of performance improvement activities and OASIS

Key Words

Advance directive

Analysis

Application

Civilian Health and Medical Program of the Uniformed Services (CHAMPUS)

Collection

Community Health Accreditation Program (CHAP)

Comprehensive assessment

Do-not-resuscitate (DNR) order

Durable power of attorney

Home Assessment Validation and Entry (HAVEN)

Home care

Home health

Home health agency (HHA)

Home health resource group (HHRG)

Living will

Masking

Medicare certified

National Association for Home Care & Hospice (NAHC)

OASIS

Omnibus Budget Reconciliation Act of 1987 (OBRA)

Outcome and Assessment Information Set (OASIS)

Outcomes

ORYX

Patient outcome measures

Patient Self-Determination Act

Patient's rights

Performance improvement (PI)

Performance measurement

Plans of care

Prospective payment system (PPS)

Regional Home Health Intermediary (RHHI)

Request for anticipated payment (RAP)

RHHI Outcomes and Assessment Information Set Verification (ROVER) protocol

Risk-adjusted outcome

Tax Equity and Fiscal Responsibility Act of 1982 (TEFRA)

Warehousing

Introduction

Home care in the United States is a diverse and dynamic service industry. Within this industry, home health agencies, home care, personal-care providers, and hospices have come to be known collectively as home care organizations. More than 20,000 providers deliver home care services to some 8 million individuals who require services because of acute illness, long-term health conditions, permanent disability, or terminal illness. The term *home care* is interchangeable with **home health**. Annual expenditures for home health were estimated to be $2 trillion in 2010. The growth of the agencies themselves has also been dramatic. The first home care agencies were established in the 1880s. By 1963, the number of agencies was nearly 1,100. Today that number is approximately 11,000 (NAHC 2010).

According to 2010 **National Association for Home Care and Hospice (NAHC)** data, **Medicare-certified** home health agencies grew more than threefold between 1967 and 1985, from 1,753 to 5,983. However, in the 1980s, the number of Medicare-certified home care agencies leveled off to approximately 5,900 as a result of increasing Medicare paperwork and unreliable payment policies. Both of these problems led to a 1987 lawsuit brought against the Centers for Medicare and Medicaid Services (CMS) by a coalition of US congressional members, consumer groups, and the NAHC. After the successful conclusion of the lawsuit, Medicare's annual home care benefit increased significantly, and the number of agencies rose to more than 10,000. Yet, once again, the number of Medicare-certified agencies has declined to 7,265 since 2003. NAHC believes the 31.5 percent decline in agencies between 1997 and 2001 is the direct result of changes in Medicare home health reimbursement enacted as part of the Balanced Budget Act of 1997 (BBA) (NAHC 2001).

Medicare added hospice benefits in October 1983, 10 years after the first hospice was established in the United States. The number of Medicare-certified hospices has grown from 31 in January 1984 to 3,407 as of December 2009. Home care and hospice growth occurred in a competitive, managed-care environment. This environment challenges providers to develop information management systems that encourage documentation of standardized, high-quality, and accessible data and information to support patient and family care, quality improvement efforts, strategic planning, and other essential activities (NAHC 2010).

Background

Various factors have driven the need for improved health information management (HIM) in home care and hospice organizations.

Compliance with Federal Regulations

The CMS, through its Home Health Initiative, developed a quality-monitoring system that makes highly specific data collection and information management demands on home care providers. The BBA and the **Omnibus Budget Reconciliation Act of 1987 (OBRA)** mandated the implementation of a new prospective payment system for skilled nursing facilities, home healthcare agencies, outpatient rehabilitation services, and other outpatient services provided to Medicare beneficiaries. The **prospective payment system (PPS)**, which became effective on October 1, 2000, changed Medicare and Medicaid home care reimbursement from a cost-based system to a fixed-fee system based on a patient-need classification system. The BBA bundled all services covered and paid for on a reasonable cost basis under the Medicare home health benefit, including medical supplies, into the prospective payment.

Standard Core Assessment Tool

One of several challenges in revising the home health Conditions of Participation (COP) was the development of a standard core assessment tool. The management tool is designed to be used by providers and, eventually, by government agencies and healthcare consumers to compare patient indicators and outcomes across providers. CMS made outcome-based quality management reports available to providers in early 2000.

Conditions of Participation and The Joint Commission Standards

CMS revised its COP and the The Joint Commission revised its standards to focus on outcomes of care and to eliminate unnecessary procedural requirements. The challenge for these revisions was to standardize assessments and develop data collection methods that providers could use as management tools. In addition, the revisions were meant to enable government agencies, accreditation and licensure organizations, surveyors, and healthcare consumers to compare indicators and outcomes across home health organizations.

Standardized Definitions for Data Elements

In 1993, NAHC's board of directors charged the information resources and quality assurance committee with the task of developing standardized definitions for home care and hospice data elements through a consensus conference process. The board recognized that a uniform minimum data set was a necessary first step toward achieving standardized, comparable home care and hospice data. The conference was held in December 1993. In 1997, the information resources and quality assurance committee added the **Outcome and Assessment Information Set (OASIS)** to the uniform minimum data sets. OASIS is a group of data elements that represent core items in a comprehensive assessment for an adult home care patient. The data elements form the basis of measurements used for outcome-based quality improvement.

Uniform Minimum Data Sets

A uniform minimum data set (UDS) is a minimum set of informational items that have uniform definitions and predefined categories. UDSs are designed to meet the essential information needs of multiple users in the healthcare system. The framework adopted to guide development of the data set for home care and hospice services was based on the US Department of Health and Human Services' concept of a UDS. While the UDS will not necessarily meet the total data needs of any one organization, neither does it limit additional data collection. It addresses data documentation and collection at the organizational level and at the individual patient level. This data set is being used for data collection efforts conducted by the NAHC. Other entities involved in home care and hospice are encouraged to use these definitions when constructing surveys and questionnaires (NAHC 2010).

Compliance with Accreditation Standards

Organizations that choose to be accredited by The Joint Commission must meet its management of information (IM) standards (Joint Commission 2011b). Home care and hospice organizations may also decide to participate in the **Community Health Accreditation Program (CHAP)**, whose core standards are related to information management, clinical records, and management information systems.

Framework for Providers

Through the management of information standards in The Joint Commission's 2011 *Comprehensive Accreditation Manual for Home Care (CAMHC)*, a series of required processes provide a framework for home care and hospice providers to more effectively and productively manage their information. The 2011 standards are functionally based, and IM is viewed as a function integral to the provision of care and services. The Joint Commission IM standards describe the effective and continuous improvement of information management in healthcare organizations. The organization's leaders are responsible for achieving, maintaining, and improving an organization-wide approach to information management and ensuring that the staff is educated and trained in managing and using information.

The Managed-Care Environment

To vie for managed-care contracts and to survive in the current competitive healthcare environment, home care and hospice providers need data and information to document the quality, outcomes, and costs of services provided. Providers who can demonstrate that their services and outcomes are superior (through comparisons with norms or comparative data) have a competitive edge.

Increasingly Complex Organizations

As healthcare organizations become more diverse, the need for available organization- and patient-level process and outcome data and information grows. Reliable, standardized systems for data documentation are essential, as are efficient methods for sharing data and information among providers within an organization.

Government Influences

State and federal governments need home care and hospice information to examine such issues as access to healthcare services and the quality, outcome, utilization, and costs of services provided. Having such information is especially vital when reformed systems are introduced.

This trend is illustrated by two initiatives to capture outcome data: The Joint Commission's **ORYX** and CMS's OASIS. Both data function as benchmarks of **performance improvement (PI)** within and among organizations. However, the raw data that each data set gathers must be collected in a way that ensures data quality. Organizations must invest in quality technology and quality staff. Attaining quality comes under the practice of data quality management (DQM). DQM functions involve continuous improvement for data quality throughout an organization and include four key processes for data (AHIMA 2007, 20):

1. **Application:** The purpose for which data are collected

2. **Collection:** The processes by which data elements are accumulated

3. **Warehousing:** The processes and systems used to archive data and data journals

4. **Analysis:** The process of translating data into information used for an application

Home Health and Hospice Record Content

The information provided upon referral is essential when determining whether a patient is suitable for admission to home care or hospice. Admission criteria depend on the types of care and services the organization provides, its care philosophies, and Medicare coverage guidelines. In hospices, typical criteria include a terminal prognosis, the inappropriateness of curative treatment, a patient's desire for palliative treatment, a physician's order, and, depending on hospice philosophy, the availability of a willing and able caregiver. Four general categories govern admission criteria (Haddad 1987):

1. Medical stability (with the exclusion of hospice patients)

2. Desire for home care (or hospice)

3. The suitability of the home environment

4. Financial resources

The health record originates with intake/referral data, and these data form the basis for initial care planning. Intake personnel commonly receive referral data via telephone or facsimile. Some organizations have nurses working in hospitals to assist in discharge planning and admitting patients to home or hospice care. Such early collaborative efforts result in accurate referral data, which are vitally important for continuity of care, especially in cases where patients are receiving clinical respiratory or pharmaceutical/infusion therapy.

At times, referral information received via telephone is not complete. The ideal method for providing patient referral information is to transmit it electronically. This will become more common as home care and hospice organizations develop links with managed-care organizations or healthcare networks. Faxing is also an efficient method of sending data from healthcare facilities and is preferred over telephone transmission, because the resulting data are more accurate and complete.

The intake or clinical record documentation must specify a start-of-care date. According to the Medicare COP 484.55, the initial assessment visit must be held within either 48 hours of referral or 48 hours of the patient's return home or on the physician-specified start-of-care date. In the absence of a physician-specified start-of-care date, the initial assessment visit is conducted within 48 hours of the referral. When the physician specifies a start-of-care date, this supersedes the 48-hour time frame. The intake or clinical record documentation must specify a start-of-care date.

Recommendations for the content of referral and intake data in home care and hospice are listed in **FIGURE 12.1**.

Documentation of a patient's physical limitations (such as blindness) is also desirable so that any problems with delivery of services can be anticipated.

Within 10 days, written transfer information, including transfer discharge summaries and other pertinent portions of the clinical record, should be received from the transferring facility (CMS 2011a).

FIGURE 12.1. Home care and hospice documentation requirements

A. Documentation requirements for professional home care services

1. Admission/referral/general information should include the following:

   a. Patient-identifying data and social information

   b. Name, address, and telephone number of next of kin or significant other

   c. Emergency contact

   d. Referral source

   e. Attending physician identification

   f. Reimbursement information

2. Initial clinical information should be received from the attending physician, referral source, and/or patient or family, and documented prior to the first home visit. This includes the following:

   a. Admitting diagnosis(es), principal and other

   b. Surgical procedures related to home care admission

   c. Significant history and presenting problems, including the patient's social and emotional status, activity limitations, and limitations to healthcare access

   d. Allergies

   e. Initial medication and treatment orders, including type and frequency of services to be provided and the supplies and equipment needed, in the form of verbal orders until signed orders are received

   f. Any dietary restrictions

   g. Patient's living arrangements

   h. Availability of an able and willing caregiver

   i. Other agencies involved in care

B. Documentation requirements for hospice patient services

1. Admission/referral/general information should include the following:

   a. Patient-identifying data and social information

   b. Name, address, and telephone number of next of kin or significant other

   c. Primary-care person's name, when applicable

   d. Referral source

FIGURE 12.1. (continued)

---

    e. Physician identification

    f. Referral information

    g. Any other information that standards/regulations require

2. Initial clinical information should be received from the attending physician (directly or through approved personnel) and documented prior to admission. This includes the following:

    a. Admitting diagnosis(es), principal and other

    b. Prognosis

    c. Current medical findings, including present physical, social, and emotional status of the patient

    d. Allergies

    e. Pain status

    f. Initial medical and treatment orders, including medications

    g. Input in establishing, and concurrence with, tentative treatment plan

    h. Any dietary restrictions

    i. History and physical examination

    j. For Medicare hospice patients, physician certification of a life expectancy of one year or less

    k. Any other information that standards/regulations require

C. Nonmedical services

1. The following information should be received regarding homemaking services or durable medical equipment with no professional services provided.

    a. Client-identifying information, including client's name, address, and telephone number

    b. Demographic and social information, including sex, birth date, race, ethnicity, marital status, and usual living arrangement

    c. Emergency contact

Face-to-Face Requirement

In January 2011, the requirement was added that "a physician who certifies a patient as eligible for Medicare home health services must see the patient. The law also allows the requirement to be satisfied if a non-physician practitioner (NPP) sees the patient, when the NPP is working for or in collaboration with the physician. As part of the certification form itself, or as an addendum to it, the physician must document that the physician or NPP saw the patient, and document how the patient's clinical condition supports a homebound status and need for skilled services. The face-to-face encounter must occur within the 90 days prior to the start of home healthcare, or within the 30 days after the start of care" (CMS 2011a). Additional guidance has been made available via a 2010 special edition article on the Medicare Learning Network website.

OIG Work Plan

The Office of Inspector General (OIG) started monitoring all Medicare beneficiary access to **home health agencies (HHAs)** in 1999. In 1999, the OIG concluded that there appeared to be no widespread problem with placing Medicare hospital patients with HHAs.

The 2007 OIG work plan continued to monitor home health outliers, enhanced payments for home health therapy, cyclical noncompliance, accuracy of data on the Home Health Compare website, and accuracy of coding claims for Medicare Home Health Resource groups and home health rehabilitation therapy services. Many HHAs use select OASIS questions to screen potential referrals. With the OIG work plan, documenting referrals that are not admitted is even more important.

The OIG work plan is now focusing on the Outcome and Assessment Information Set (OIG 2010, 11).

> Oversight of Home Health Agency Outcome and Assessment Information Set Data: We will review CMS's oversight of Outcome and Assessment Information Set (OASIS) data submitted by Medicare-certified HHAs. Federal regulations at 42 CFR § 484.55 require HHAs to conduct accurate comprehensive patient assessments that include OASIS data items and submit the data to CMS. OASIS data reflect HHAs' performance in helping patients to regain or maintain their ability to function and perform activities of daily living. OASIS data also include measures of physical status and use of services, such as hospitalization or emergent care. CMS has used OASIS data for its HHA PPS since 2000; began posting OASIS-based quality performance information on its Home Health Compare website in the fall of 2003; and conducted a home health pay-for-performance demonstration based on OASIS data during 2008 and 2009. We will review CMS's process for ensuring that HHAs submit accurate and complete OASIS data.

Home Care and Hospice Assessment Information

Although the initial assessment may begin in the hospital or long-term care facility from which the patient is referred, it more commonly begins on the first home care visit or admission to hospice. The type, content, and comprehensiveness of the assessment should correspond to the types of care and services to be provided. The suitability of a home environment must be included in the assessment, as well as any safety measures that are needed, especially relating to the placement of durable medical equipment (DME) and the provision of infusion therapy. The ability of the patient and her family to use the equipment provided also needs to be assessed. In addition, the assessment should include the availability of an able and willing caregiver, living arrangements, and family composition. This information, together with an assessment of activity and functional limitations (including mental health and emotional status), helps determine the extent of required support. Nonhospice home care also uses this information to plan for discharge.

Home Care and OASIS

Before comprehensive assessment and OASIS data collection can occur, the HHA must inform Medicare and Medicaid patients about OASIS and explain their rights with respect to the collection and reporting of the data. (Note: OASIS data collection is not required for non-Medicare or non-Medicaid patients.) These rights include the following:

- The right to be informed that OASIS information will be collected and for what purpose

- The right to have the information kept confidential and secure

- The right to be informed that OASIS information will not be disclosed except for legitimate purposes allowed by the Privacy Act

- The right to refuse to answer a specific question

- The right to see, review, and request changes on their assessment

A standard notice to patients that explains these rights in plain language was published in the *Federal Register* on June 18, 1999, and is available in English and Spanish on the OASIS website. HHAs must present and explain this required notice to beneficiaries before their initial OASIS assessment (CMS 2011e).

When professional home care services are provided, the assessment becomes more comprehensive, documenting the presence and absence of problems. In years past, the OIG work plan included a determination on how assessment information helps establish the case-mix adjustment used in determining the level of Medicare payment to an HHA for a particular patient.

Medicare COP 484.55 requires that each patient receive, and an HHA provide, a patient-specific, **comprehensive assessment** that accurately reflects the patient's current health status and includes information that may be used to demonstrate the patient's progress toward desired outcomes. The comprehensive assessment must identify the patient's continuing need for home care and meet the patient's medical, nursing, rehabilitative, social, and discharge planning needs. For Medicare beneficiaries, the HHA must verify the patient's eligibility for the home health benefit, including homebound status, both at the time of the initial assessment visit and at the time of the comprehensive assessment. The comprehensive assessment must also incorporate the current version of OASIS items, using the language and groupings as specified by the secretary. The comprehensive assessment includes the collection of OASIS data items by a qualified clinician, such as a registered nurse, physical therapist, occupational therapist, or speech–language pathologist.

Additional requirements apply to Medicare patients. Agencies are expected to conduct an assessment that accurately reflects the patient's current health status and includes information to establish and monitor a plan of care. The plan of care must be reviewed and updated at least every 60 days or as often as the severity of the patient's condition requires. The requirement to conduct a drug regimen review applies to all patients serviced by the HHA.

Federal regulations require a comprehensive assessment, with OASIS data items integrated, for all patients who receive skilled services except for those who are younger than age 18, receiving maternity services, receiving only housekeeping or chore services, or receiving only personal care services. This includes Medicare, Medicaid, managed care, and private pay patients accepted by the HHA. It also includes Medicaid patients receiving services under a waiver program. Although comprehensive assessments are required for all patients, the OASIS is required only for Medicare and Medicaid patients.

Subsequent updates on the comprehensive assessments must be conducted at certain intervals after admission. These updates must include specific data items in the current OASIS data set. OASIS data items are not meant to be the only items included in an agency's assessment process. They are standardized health assessment items that must be incorporated into an agency's own comprehensive assessment tool. For therapy-only cases, the comprehensive assessment should incorporate OASIS data items with other assessment data that the HHA currently collects for therapy patients, as opposed to simply adding them at the beginning or end (CMS 2011e).

Hospice and Assessment

Hospice care requires a patient and family assessment. This involves a psychosocial assessment of patient and family needs, including adaptive and coping abilities. A spiritual assessment is also performed. This may be included on a psychosocial assessment form or on a separate assessment form. The assessment of bereavement support needs begins on hospice admission.

When a hospice patient is experiencing pain, a pain assessment is performed to document the effectiveness of pain medication. The Joint Commission (1995) considers pain the fifth vital sign (after blood pressure, temperature, pulse, and respiration rate), and it should be assessed whether the patient has a history of pain or not. As discussed earlier, the content of assessment forms for particular categories of patients may conform to information items indicated by a critical path, with opportunity for individualization. A large number of home care and hospice organizations record pain assessment information electronically, via handheld devices or portable computers.

FIGURE 12.2 lists the recommendations for the content of initial assessment information for home care and hospice patients.

FIGURE 12.2. Content of initial assessment information for professional home care and hospice patient services

---

A. Content of initial assessment information for professional home care services

  1. The health record documents, including the following initial nursing assessment information:

    a. Diagnoses and problems

    b. Past medical history and present illness

    c. Review of systems

    d. Present medications and treatment

    e. Activities of daily living and functional limitations

    f. Patient-care requirements, including equipment and supplies needed

    g. Dietary and nutritional information

    h. Suitability of the patient's residence and safety measures required to protect the client from injury

    i. Composition of household and relevant information regarding the family and caregiver

  2. When skilled nursing is required, the home care nursing staff obtains the initial nursing assessment on the first day of admission; when skilled nursing care is ordered later during admission, the assessment is obtained at the first skilled-care visit. Be aware that some states require a nursing assessment even when skilled nursing care is not provided. The record should also include documentation of the initial clinical evaluations of other disciplines or services that may have been involved in care of the patient (for example, physical therapy, occupational therapy, and pharmacy). The start of care begins at the first billable visit according to PPS regulations.

  3. Relevant X-ray, pathology, laboratory, or other test findings are documented.

B. Content of initial assessment information for hospice patient services

  1. The hospice record, including the following relevant information:

    a. Diagnoses

    b. Past medical history

    c. Review of systems

FIGURE 12.2. (continued)

    d. Present treatment

    e. Activities of daily living

    f. Functional limitations

    g. Patient-care requirements

    h. Dietary or nutritional information

    i. Pain assessment

    j. Psychosocial assessment

    k. Spiritual assessment

    l. Safety measures required to protect the patient from injury

    m. Equipment needed in the home

    n. Suitability of the patient and family residence

    o. Relevant information regarding the primary caregiver

2. The appropriate hospice clinical staff obtains the initial assessment on the first day of admission or on the first home visit. The record should also include documentation of the initial clinical evaluations of other disciplines involved in the care of the patient (for example, physical therapy, occupational therapy, and pharmacy).

3. Relevant X-ray, pathology, laboratory, or other test findings are documented.

4. A problem list, based on the initial assessment, is documented.

C. Nonmedical services

1. When nonmedical services, such as homemaker/chore services or DME are administered with no professional service provision, assessment information is much more limited than in the preceding cases. Referencing Joint Commission (2007) requirements is recommended in these instances.

Home Health Plans of Care

In this section, the term *plans of care* refers to the Medicare-required home health plans of care documented on CMS form 485. Although the form is no longer required and references to it have been removed from the CMS website, the information contained in the form is required as noted in the *Federal Register*, § 409.32. Agencies may choose to use form 485 to meet the required documentation and as guidance in electronic format. (See **FIGURE 12.3**.) Plans of care may also be referred to as *physician's orders*. A description of care plans follows.

Based on the problems and needs identified during assessment and documented on the problem list, care plans are comprehensive and include documentation of care or services to be provided by all disciplines, independent contractors, organizations, and volunteers. The Joint Commission (2011a) requires that an organization design the process, including required documentation, for care planning, review, and, when necessary, revision. Care plans include goals and objectives and indicate the person/discipline responsible for implementing the plan(s), frequency of services to be provided, and medications prescribed. Hospice care plans are interdisciplinary. Record documentation reflects the participation of patients, physicians, and pharmacists in care planning (Joint Commission 2011b).

FIGURE 12.3. Example of a home health certification and plan of care

Department of Health and Human Services Centers for Medicare & Medicaid Services	Form Approved OMB No. 0938-0357

HOME HEALTH CERTIFICATION AND PLAN OF CARE

1. Patient's HI Claim No.	2. Start Of Care Date	3. Certification Period From: To:	4. Medical Record No.	5. Provider No.

6. Patient's Name and Address	7. Provider's Name, Address and Telephone Number

8. Date of Birth	9. Sex ☐ M ☐ F	10. Medications: Dose/Frequency/Route (N)ew (C)hanged

11. ICD-9-CM	Principal Diagnosis	Date
12. ICD-9-CM	Surgical Procedure	Date
13. ICD-9-CM	Other Pertinent Diagnoses	Date

14. DME and Supplies	15. Safety Measures:
16. Nutritional Req.	17. Allergies:

18.A. Functional Limitations

1	☐ Amputation	5	☐ Paralysis	9	☐ Legally Blind
2	☐ Bowel/Bladder (Incontinence)	6	☐ Endurance	A	☐ Dyspnea With Minimal Exertion
3	☐ Contracture	7	☐ Ambulation	B	☐ Other (Specify)
4	☐ Hearing	8	☐ Speech		

18.B. Activities Permitted

1	☐ Complete Bedrest	6	☐ Partial Weight Bearing	A	☐ Wheelchair
2	☐ Bedrest BRP	7	☐ Independent At Home	B	☐ Walker
3	☐ Up As Tolerated	8	☐ Crutches	C	☐ No Restrictions
4	☐ Transfer Bed/Chair	9	☐ Cane	D	☐ Other (Specify)
5	☐ Exercises Prescribed				

19. Mental Status:

1	☐ Oriented	3	☐ Forgetful	5	☐ Disoriented	7	☐ Agitated
2	☐ Comatose	4	☐ Depressed	6	☐ Lethargic	8	☐ Other

20. Prognosis:

1	☐ Poor	2	☐ Guarded	3	☐ Fair	4	☐ Good	5	☐ Excellent

21. Orders for Discipline and Treatments (Specify Amount/Frequency/Duration)

22. Goals/Rehabilitation Potential/Discharge Plans

23. Nurse's Signature and Date of Verbal SOC Where Applicable:	25. Date HHA Received Signed POT
24. Physician's Name and Address	26. I certify/recertify that this patient is confined to his/her home and needs intermittent skilled nursing care, physical therapy and/or speech therapy or continues to need occupational therapy. The patient is under my care, and I have authorized the services on this plan of care and will periodically review the plan.
27. Attending Physician's Signature and Date Signed	28. Anyone who misrepresents, falsifies, or conceals essential information required for payment of Federal funds may be subject to fine, imprisonment, or civil penalty under applicable Federal laws.

Form CMS-485 (C-3) (02-94) (Formerly HCFA-485) (Print Aligned)

Source: CMS 1994.

For reimbursement purposes, the physician uses CMS form 485 to certify the patient's need for home health service. Most HHAs have computer-based applications to assist them in completing the form and tracking the need for recertification, which is required every 60 days. Hospice certifications are required after the first 90 days, after the second 90 days, and every 60 days thereafter.

When a Medicare-certified hospice contracts with an inpatient facility, the inpatient care must be based on the hospice's interdisciplinary care plan. The hospice maintains control of the care, and this must be clearly stated in the health record. Policies, procedures, and contracts define the relevant information to be shared among providers so that gaps in care are prevented, and the hospice record documents all services provided. Procedures should provide for written and oral communication among hospice team members and inpatient care providers throughout the inpatient care episode.

Standardized care plans and protocols are available for provision of specific services and for medical and nursing diagnoses. Any standardized care plans that are used must be individualized for each patient and caregiver. When clinical pathways are used, standardized or structured care plans may also be used for documentation.

Regardless of an organization's Medicare certification status, a care plan conforms to the physician's plan-of-care orders. The plan is based on the nursing initial assessment and the initial assessments of other disciplines involved in the care of the patient. An interdisciplinary care plan is recommended, but separate discipline care plans may be documented when they are filed together in the health record.

Figure 12.4 lists the content of interdisciplinary care plans for professional home care and for hospice patients.

Physician's Orders

The health record includes legible, complete, signed, and dated physician's diagnoses and therapeutic orders. The person authorized to accept the orders must record, date, and sign all verbal or telephone orders, and the attending physician must countersign and date the orders within the time period specified by organization policy and required by state regulations. The use of electronic signatures is addressed later in the chapter. When pharmaceutical care is provided, the pharmacist reviews paper and electronically generated prescriptions and verbal orders before dispensing medication.

CMS views the initial percentage payment as a **request for anticipated payment (RAP)** rather than a Medicare claim for home health PPS purposes. The payment does not require a physician-signed plan of care before submission. To request anticipated payment for the initial percentage based on a physician's verbal orders, a copy of the plan of care with all the orders—in writing with the date of receipt by the registered nurse or qualified therapist responsible for furnishing or supervising the ordered services—must be completed and immediately sent to the physician for signature. The RAP may be submitted when the HHA has a signed referral prescribing the physician's detailed orders for services and the patient's condition. Signed orders must be obtained as soon as possible and before the claim for services is submitted for the final percentage payment of each episode. The claim for the final percentage payment requires a signed plan of care prior to billing.

The RAP will be canceled and recovered unless the claim for the episode is submitted within 60 days of the end of the episode or the issuance of the anticipated payment. This split-percentage payment approach helps alleviate cash flow concerns but increases the need for timely signed orders.

Hospice Clinical and Progress Notes

For this discussion, the term *clinical note* refers to a note documenting care services provided, and *progress note* refers to a summary note. A progress note may be documented on any transfer between hospice care levels, on discharge, or when physicians or others need a summary of recent services provided.

FIGURE 12.4. Content of interdisciplinary care plans for professional home care services and for hospice patient services

A. Content of interdisciplinary care plan for professional home care services

  1. The care plan documents the following information:

    a. Identified patient problems

    b. Expected outcomes, long- and short-term goals

    c. Plans and interventions, including medications prescribed and required medical equipment to be provided to meet the identified goals

    d. Discipline responsible for carrying out plans and achieving goals

    e. Dates when expected outcomes are met

    f. Signature of the nurse or care coordinator for the patient

  2. Verbal orders should be appropriately documented and signed by the attending physician within the required time and prior to billing; care plan should be updated when an additional discipline enters the care of the patient or when change occurs in care management.

  3. The care plan should undergo interdisciplinary review, even when separate discipline care plans may be documented. The service providers and, whenever possible, the attending physician, should perform this review. When care services are provided through contractual agreement, persons who provide these services should also participate in care plan review.

  4. Care plan reviews should be individualized to each patient and occur at least every 60 days. Reviews should be documented in case conference minutes or elsewhere in the health record. Care plan changes should also be documented.

  5. The record should clearly reflect coordination of care planning between all disciplines, paraprofessionals, organizations, and other care providers, as well as between the organization, the attending physician, and the patient.

B. Content of interdisciplinary care plan for hospice patient services

  1. It is recommended that, within one week of admission, an interdisciplinary care plan be developed for the patient and the patient's family. This plan should conform to physician's orders and be based on clinical information in the initial database and problem list. The care plan documents the following information:

    a. Identified patient and family problems and needs

    b. Identified goals that are realistic, achievable, and measurable

    c. Care and services to be provided to meet identified goals, including medications prescribed and required medical equipment

    d. The signature of the attending physician and team coordinator for the patient and family

  2. Verbal orders should be appropriately documented and signed by the attending physician; care plan should be updated when an additional discipline enters the care of the patient and family or when change occurs in care management.

  3. The planned frequency of interdisciplinary care plan review should be documented. Although each care plan is individualized to the patient, reviews should occur no less than every two weeks after admission. Care plan changes should be documented, and when appropriate, there must be documentation of new orders signed by the attending physician.

  4. Record documentation should include the findings and conclusions of team case conferences.

  5. Continuing discussions among the attending physician and members of the interdisciplinary team should be documented.

C. Nonmedical services

  1. When nonmedical services are provided, the health record should contain documentation of the services performed. Refer to Joint Commission (2007) standards for additional guidance.

Clinical Notes and Visit Documentation

Clinical and visit notes are designed to give a clear, comprehensive picture of the patient's clinical status, the care being provided, and the patient's response to that care. Policies, procedures, and forms, whether paper-based or electronic, can ensure that documentation is efficiently entered into the record and that such important aspects of care as supervision of care and education of the patient and family are documented. Documentation incorporates conversations with physicians, pharmacists, relatives, and others who have an impact on patient care.

When nonmedical services are being provided and there is no professional service provision, a checklist may be used to document the services provided.

When professional services are provided, visits by licensed certified staff are documented in a signed and dated clinical progress note or flow-sheet entry, which includes the following information:

- A description of the patient's physical and psychosocial signs and symptoms or changes in signs and symptoms

- Any treatment, service, or medication rendered and the patient's reaction

- Any changes in the patient's condition or the patient's and family's psychosocial status

- Any patient and family instruction given, as well as patient and family demonstration or verbalization of knowledge of instructions given

- Plans for future visits

When flow sheets are used to document interventions or progress toward care goals, clinical notes are then used to record supplemental information such as assessment of findings, interventions and plans, telephone conversations, and nursing supervisory visits every 14 days. When flow sheet documentation uses a coding system, a legend should appear on the form.

The comprehensive assessment must include a review of all medications the patient is currently using to identify any potential adverse effects and drug and food reactions, including ineffective drug therapy, significant side effects, significant drug and food interactions, duplicate drug therapy, and noncompliance with drug therapy. This requirement applies to all patients being serviced by the HHA, regardless of whether OASIS-specific requirements apply.

When authorized home care or hospice staff administers medications, the action is documented in the health record along with any beneficial effects or presumed adverse drug reactions. When pharmaceutical and infusion therapy services are provided, patients are continually monitored for medication effectiveness and actual or potential medication-related problems. This is a collaborative process involving the pharmacist, and documentation will show evidence of this collaboration. The health record provides evidence that conclusions and findings of medication monitoring are communicated to all healthcare professionals involved in the patient's care (Joint Commission 2011a). When pharmaceutical services are provided, pharmacy records are filed with health records (Joint Commission 2011a). The American Society of Health-System Pharmacists (2003) has developed educational materials on the health record and the pharmacist's record documentation.

Home Health Aide Documentation

Agencies must provide enough home health aide services to meet the patient's needs. Home health aides who are employees of the home care or hospice facility and aides used by the agency hospice under an arrangement or contract must meet the personnel qualifications specified by the COP. Home health aides are selected on the basis of such factors as a sympathetic attitude toward the care of the sick; ability to read, write, and carry out directions; maturity; and ability to deal effectively with the demands of the job. They are closely supervised to ensure their competence in providing care. A registered nurse provides written patient-care instructions and monitors the services provided by the home health aide. This nurse also visits the patient's residence at least once every two weeks to assess aide services and relationships and determine whether goals are being met. The visit need not be made while the aide is furnishing services. Home health aide services should be adequately documented in the health record, including nursing orders for the aide and an assignment sheet, a flow sheet, and narrative notations documenting services rendered. The nurse or therapist should also include documentation of coordination of care with the aide and continuing supervision of the aide's services. It is recommended that home health aides record the services they provide in a checklist format. Aides should document short narrative notes only when reporting unusual occurrences (for example, changes in the condition of the patient or phone calls) or when state regulations require it.

Dietary and Nutritional Information

Health record documentation should reflect, as appropriate, the patient's nutrient intake, dietary instructions to the patient and family, and demonstration or verbalization from the patient and family of dietary instructions given. A diet history and nutritional evaluation by a dietitian should be completed when appropriate as defined in organization policy.

Progress Notes and the Discharge Transfer Record

Upon a patient's discharge or death, a summary is documented. This report includes the following information:

- Admission and discharge dates and type of discharge

- Care and support provided by each discipline

- Status of goal attained upon discharge or death

- When discharged alive, the status of the patient and the reason for discharge

- Discharge diagnoses or problems

- Any unmet needs and referrals for continuing care

- For hospice settings, time (if known) and place of death, as well as plans for bereavement follow-up

Home care or hospice organizations may include additional outcome-monitoring information on their discharge summaries. OASIS data are collected and completed by the qualified clinician when a patient transfers to an inpatient facility with or without discharge, in the case of a discharge to community, or when the patient dies at home. Agencies may take up to seven calendar days after the date of completion of the comprehensive assessment to enter (encode) the OASIS data into their computers using **Home Assessment Validation and Entry (HAVEN)** software or a similar application. The day the clinician completes the assessment is day zero for the purpose of calculating the seven-day window. Encoding of all OASIS data items must be complete, or locked, to accurately compute the information (Health Insurance Prospective Payment System [HIPPS] code set) necessary for billing Medicare patients under the PPS.

When hospice patients are transferred between home and inpatient care, a transfer note is created. The documentation summarizes the patient's status, the care and support being provided, and the reason for transfer.

For Medicare-certified HHAs, a discharge summary that includes a patient's medical and health status at discharge must be made available to the patient's attending physician, and physicians must be informed of this availability. The discharge summary may be incorporated into the routine summary reports already furnished by the physician (CMS 2011a).

Notations should be appropriately labeled and should provide an overall, comprehensive view of the patient's total progress and current summary report, including social, emotional, and behavioral adjustments relative to the diagnosis, treatment, rehabilitation potential, and anticipated outcomes. Medicare regulations do not dictate the frequency with which progress notes must be written.

Facsimile Signatures

The plan of care or verbal order may be transmitted by facsimile machine. The HHA is not required to have the original signature on file. However, it is responsible for obtaining original signatures if an issue surfaces that would require verification of an original signature. When the fax date is used to indicate when the document was received from the physician, the faxed copy must clearly indicate that the faxed date is the date the document was faxed from the physician to the agency.

Electronic Signatures

HHAs that maintain electronic beneficiary records rather than hard copies may use electronic signatures. However, all such entries must be appropriately authenticated and dated. Authentication must include signatures, written initials, or computer secure entry by a unique identifier of a primary author who has reviewed and approved the entry. The HHA must have safeguards to prevent unauthorized access to the records and a process for reconstruction of the records in the event of a system breakdown. Providers using alternative signature methods should check federal, state, and local law requirements to ensure compliance and should recognize the potential for misuse or abuse with alternative methods (CMS 2011c).

The Medicare Hospice Benefit

It is essential that health information managers working in hospice know what makes a patient eligible for the Medicare hospice benefit and how to document provision of care. Most hospice reimbursement hinges on meeting those requirements. Medicare coverage for hospice care began with enactment of section 122 of Public Law 97–248, the **Tax Equity and Fiscal Responsibility Act of 1982 (TEFRA)**. The Code of Federal Regulations (Medicare COP 484.55) defines the Medicare hospice benefit and documentation requirements. Interpretive guidelines provide additional guidance on required documentation. Throughout this section, definitions and requirements have been abstracted from these sources. Patients must elect hospice care from a Medicare-certified hospice to be eligible for Medicare reimbursement. When patients elect hospice care, they waive their rights to Medicare reimbursement for treatment of their principal (terminal) diagnosis and related conditions outside of care provided by the designated hospice, by another hospice provided under arrangements made by the designated hospice, or by the individual's attending physician when that physician is not an employee of the designated hospice or receiving compensation from the hospice for those services. An individual can revoke the Medicare hospice benefit and then reelect the benefit after revocation. An individual can also elect to change the designated hospice program. Election, revocation, and reelection of the Medicare hospice benefit—as well as change of the designated hospice—must be documented in the health record, and that documentation should clearly show that the patient or the patient's legal representative was well informed. Patients can elect the hospice benefit at any time. The periods consist of the following:

1. The initial 90-day period

2. The subsequent 90-day period

3. The subsequent extension of an unlimited number of 60-day periods when the patient is certified terminally ill with a six-month prognosis if the disease runs its normal course

To be eligible for the hospice benefit, a patient must have a physician-certified terminal illness. A written certification must be obtained for each of the three periods in the preceding list, and the certification must indicate a life expectancy of six months or less if the terminal illness runs its normal course. The health record should contain evidence of this certification.

Medicare hospice fiscal intermediaries focus on medical reviews of hospice claims. One area these intermediaries question concerns the validity of the terminal certification of some patients. Some cases of long lengths of stay for patients with chronic diagnoses have led to this questioning.

To prevent denials, coding personnel are advised to use the most specific diagnosis codes and to ensure that the terminal diagnosis is always listed as the principal diagnosis. All complications of chronic conditions should be documented and coded as appropriate. In addition, health record documentation on admission and throughout a hospice episode must support a patient's terminal status. When a claim is selected for medical review, it is recommended that copies of all health record documentation, including the admission assessment, be submitted to a fiscal intermediary for review (HAA 2005).

The Hospice Association of America (HAA), in conjunction with CMS and the National Hospice Organization, has developed guidelines on screening hospice patients who have illnesses other than cancer for admissions and recertifications. Guidelines address how to determine a patient's prognosis, what to look for, and what to document (HAA 2005).

Provision of Care Under the Medicare Hospice Benefit and Documentation

Medicare has defined four general hospice care levels and assigned different reimbursement rates to each:

1. Routine home care

2. Continuous home care

3. Inpatient respite care

4. General inpatient care

A hospice must maintain management control of a patient's care, regardless of the treatment setting, and the health record must contain evidence of this control. According to Medicare regulations, hospices that cannot provide inpatient care directly must contract with an inpatient care provider.

Hospice regulations require an interdisciplinary group to plan and provide or supervise the care and services provided to patients and families. This group includes at least the following hospice employees:

- A doctor of medicine

- A doctor of osteopathy

- A registered nurse

- A social worker

- A pastoral counselor or another type of counselor

The care plan becomes the basis for team decision making and can be considered the map for team interventions.

Medicare requires that volunteers be used in administrative or direct patient care roles. In many hospices, volunteers provide services and support to the patient, family, or significant other. Volunteers are considered members of the interdisciplinary team.

Following is a summary of the advice included in this chapter regarding documentation and the Medicare hospice benefit:

- The health record must contain evidence that the interdisciplinary team plans and manages a patient's care across all settings of care.

- The health record must contain evidence that hospice interdisciplinary care continues when a patient is admitted for inpatient hospice care.

- Health record documentation must justify the level of hospice care the patient is receiving. When the status of a patient changes such that he requires continuous home care or inpatient care, clinical notes must document this change, and the care plan must be revised to indicate any new problems or changes in plans.

Volunteer Documentation

Volunteers are defined in 42 CFR 418.3 as hospice employees who facilitate compliance with the hospice core services requirement. The hospice uses volunteers, in defined roles, under the supervision of a designated hospice employee. The hospice must provide appropriate volunteer training consistent with the specific tasks that volunteers perform. The interdisciplinary group assesses the patient's and caregiver's need for a volunteer. Volunteers must be used in administrative or direct patient care roles. Agencies must document the roles assigned to that hospice's volunteers. Hospices use volunteers to supplement the care provided by the paid staff who work directly with patients and their family members, both in the patients' homes and in the inpatient setting. Hospices must document the cost savings of volunteers, which must include the identification of necessary positions occupied by volunteers, work time spent by volunteers, and estimates of the dollar costs that the hospice would have incurred if paid employees occupied the positions. Hospices must document a continual level of volunteer activity and expansion of care and services achieved through the use of volunteers, including the types of services and the time worked (CMS 2011c).

In hospice settings, volunteers write notes after each visit and include them in the hospice record using separate volunteer documentation forms. The volunteer coordinator or nurse team coordinator reviews the volunteer's notes and initials them before they are filed. Volunteer's notes include the following information:

- New issues, special concerns, or significant changes observed in the patient or family since last contact

- The volunteer's response and interventions to changes or concerns at this contact

- The volunteer's plan for next contact

- The request for special consultation or contact from other staff when needed

Bereavement Documentation

Bereavement counseling services are often provided to the family and caregivers after a patient's death. Counseling is provided on the basis of an assessment of the family's and caregiver's needs, the presence of any risk factors associated with the patient's death, and the ability of the family and caregivers to cope with grief. The supervisor of bereavement services may be the interdisciplinary group social worker or an other professional with documented evidence of training and experience in dealing with grief. Documentation for bereavement counseling does not necessarily have to be contained in the clinical record, but it must be maintained by the hospice in an organized, easily retrievable manner for a specified period.

The hospice record includes initial and follow-up bereavement assessments of the family and significant other that documents their physical and emotional status. It is recommended that the initial bereavement assessment be completed at the team meeting following the patient's death. The bereavement follow-up assessment is completed within four weeks of the patient's death. Subsequent bereavement assessments are completed as deemed necessary by the hospice bereavement staff and as stated in hospice policy. Notes are written after each bereavement visit. These notes document the general emotional and physical status of the family and significant other at that visit, any counseling that was performed or follow-up action taken, and any changes in plans. On discharge from bereavement follow-up, a summary is written. This summary includes appropriate information regarding services provided to the family and significant other as well as the status of the family and significant other during the last bereavement contact.

Justification of Hospice Skilled Care Levels

Employees in Medicare-certified hospices must be conscientious when documenting a patient's need for inpatient and continuous home care and the actual provision of services. To be considered continuous by Medicare, home care must be provided for at least 12 hours in one 24-hour period (for example, 12:00 a.m. to 11:59 p.m.), and care must be predominantly skilled nursing care. Continuous care is initiated during periods of crisis (such as severe pain, hemorrhaging, and imminent death) or when active palliation or management of acute medical symptoms is needed. Record documentation must describe the crisis and include the date and time it occurred. In conjunction with this, the patient's care plan is revised to reflect the changes in the problems and care provision. During continuous care, an extensive nursing note is written at least hourly, and it is signed with the date and time, as are all record notations during this period. When inpatient care is required, a medical crisis such as "symptoms out of control" is documented. On admission and continuously throughout the inpatient care period, documentation reflects the patient's need for acute care. As with continuous care, the interdisciplinary care plan is modified to reflect new or exacerbated problems and any changes in care provision. The hospice furnishes a copy of the patient's plan of care to the inpatient provider and specifies the inpatient services to be provided.

Short-term inpatient care may be provided in a Medicare hospice inpatient unit. The Medicare conditions for each of these service providers apply to all patients, regardless of payment source, unless a specific exception is provided in the regulations. Services provided in an inpatient setting must conform to the hospice patient's written plan of care and must be reasonable and necessary for the palliation of symptoms or the management of the terminal illness. General inpatient care may be required to adjust and monitor the patient's pain control or manage acute or chronic symptoms that cannot be managed in another setting. Inpatient admission may also be furnished to provide respite for the patient's family or other persons caring for the individual at home. Respite care is the only type of inpatient care that may be furnished in a nursing facility. The hospice is accountable for all hospice services provided under arrangement at nursing facilities. The hospice furnishes the inpatient provider with a copy of the patient's plan of care and specifies the inpatient services to be furnished. The hospice health record includes a record of all inpatient services and events and a copy of the discharge summary (CMS 2011a).

The Medicare Home Care Benefit

Successful health information managers working in home health often refer to chapter 7 of the Medicare *Benefit Policy Manual*, "Home Health Services" (CMS 2011c). The policy manual is key to understanding how the Medicare home care benefit drives documentation requirements for patient care, home health certification, CMS form 485, Medicare home care surveys, and the PPS. The following sections describe some of those requirements.

Home Health Prospective Payment System

Medicare reimburses all HHAs under a PPS. PPSs are designed to promote efficiency and help prevent waste and abuse within the home health payment system.

Between 1990 and 1997, home healthcare expenditures grew from 2.9 percent to nearly 9 percent of all Medicare payments. The earlier cost-based system was creating growth in home health spending, due in large part to the lack of incentives to efficiently provide care. Previously, HHAs had been paid based on the costs of providing care, which was only subject to a per-visit limit. The more visits HHAs provided, and the greater the cost increases, the greater the payments to those HHAs. The old system encouraged abuse, as evidenced by the increase in per-beneficiary visits, which more than doubled

FIGURE 12.5. Home healthcare services PPS

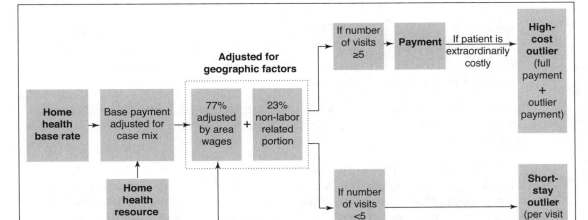

*The home healthcare services PPS uses a version of the hospital wage index called the "pre-floor, pre-classification hospital wage index."

Source: Medpac 2010, 3.

from 36 in 1990 to 80 in 1997. The General Accounting Office (GAO) reported in 2002 that Medicare payments to HHAs were considerably higher than payments for full home healthcare episodes (on average, about 35 percent higher for the first six months of 2001) (GAO 2002). In 2005, according to CMS Health Care Information System (HCIS) data, the average number of beneficiary visits was 31, with an average payment per patient of $4,050. The most recent data available, the 2009 HCIS data, indicates little change. The average number of beneficiary visits was 34, with an average payment of $4,930.

The interim payment system, which was mandated by the Balanced Budget Act of 1997 and replaced three years later with the PPS, was based on the lowest of reasonable costs, an aggregate cost limit per visit, or an aggregate cost limit per beneficiary. Such limits removed incentives to increase payment by providing unnecessary visits.

Under the PPS, HHAs are now paid a predetermined base payment that may vary per each 60-day episode of care depending on the patient's severity of illness and home health needs. As identified through completion of the OASIS documentation, the services that are reimbursed include home health aide visits, skilled nursing visits, supplies, medical social services, and therapy. CMS is currently refining the PPS for home health due to the rising costs within the program. **FIGURE 12.5** illustrates the PPS payment determination factors. The reader is encouraged to keep an eye toward these changes. Key points of the PPS include the following:

- Medicare pays for home healthcare with both Part A and Part B funds; in 2007, total payments were $16.9 billion.

- Medicare will reimburse HHAs for each 60-day episode of care as long as the patient remains eligible and the services are medically necessary.

- Beneficiaries who have greater home healthcare needs will warrant higher payment rates to their HHAs.

- Payment is determined by the intensity of care provided. Data documented from patient assessments (which is already a requirement for all Medicare-participating HHAs) will be used to support payment rates. Payment rates are also adjusted by area wage differences.

- In cases where the patient's care results in unusually high home healthcare costs, outlier payments will be made for a portion of the amount of costs beyond the set threshold.

- To streamline the approval process and ensure adequate payment when an HHA accepts a new Medicare patient, the CMS will pay up front 60 percent of the initial episode reimbursement. The HHA will receive the remaining 40 percent of payment at the end of that initial episode of care. Episodes of care that follow will be paid based on equally divided payments between the beginning and end of those care episodes.

- Patients who have a significant change in their condition during an episode of care will have an adjustment made to their payment rate.

- HHAs will get a partial episode payment according to PPS regulations when a patient chooses to transfer or discharge from and return to the same agency, warranting a new clock for payment. This is considered a beneficiary-elected transfer. When a new 60-day episode begins, the original 60-day payment is proportionally adjusted to reflect the time the beneficiary remained under the agency's care before the intervening event.)

- HHAs and suppliers will be paid separately for DME if it is medically necessary.

The Medicare Home Care Benefit and Documentation of Eligibility

Medicare certification of Part A home care providers includes the HHA. Because Medicare Part B providers (such as DME and pharmacy) are considered vendors, they are not certified. The *Home Health Agency Manual* defines the Medicare home care benefit and documentation in relation to such. Interpretive guidelines provide additional directions concerning required documentation. Throughout this section, definitions and requirements have been abstracted from these sources (all other sources are referenced).

To be eligible for Medicare-reimbursed home healthcare, a Medicare beneficiary must meet the following conditions:

- The beneficiary is confined to home.

- The beneficiary is under the care of a physician, who establishes and approves the plan of care for the individual.

- The beneficiary needs intermittent, skilled nursing care, physical therapy, speech therapy services, or continuing occupational therapy.

Home Confinement (Homebound Status)

Patients should be essentially homebound. This does not mean that the patient must be bedridden, but leaving home must present considerable difficulty and be infrequent and of short duration unless for medical reasons. The reason(s) for homebound status and the fact that the patient is homebound must be recorded on CMS form 485 or facsimile, on the comprehensive assessment, and periodically in the clinical notes. Documentation regarding homebound status should be descriptive. Why is a patient homebound? What happens when a patient walks too far? When the patient visits the doctor, what type of assistance is provided? Nursing and therapy documentation should be congruent, not conflicting. OASIS items MO350–MO380 and Life System Profile items MO640–MO820 should also support the patient's homebound status. According to CMS regulations, the patient's inability to drive does not necessarily render the patient homebound (CMS 2011c).

Home Health Under the Care of a Physician

The beneficiary's physician is responsible for signing the home health certification CMS form 485 at the initiation of any plan of care. On completion of every 60-day episode during which the patient received continuous home healthcare from the same HHA, the beneficiary's physician is responsible for home health recertification. The home health PPS should not have changed the plan of care. It remains the responsibility of the beneficiary's physician to develop a plan of care based on her intimate knowledge of the medical condition of the home health patient. The plan of care developed in consultation with the agency staff covers all pertinent diagnoses, mental status, types of services and equipment required, frequency of visits, prognosis, rehabilitation potential, functional limitations, activities permitted, nutritional requirements, medications and treatments, safety measures to protect against injury, instructions for timely discharge or referral, and any other appropriate items.

The patient's physician approves the patient's plan of care and certifies the need for home health services by signing a home health certification and plan of care, CMS form 485 (figure 12.3). CMS now allows for physician review, care plan oversight, and certification update reimbursement. On completion of each 60-day episode, if the patient continues to receive continuous home healthcare from the same HHA, the beneficiary's physician is responsible for recertifying the plan of care.

Skilled Services Requirement for Benefit Eligibility

A home care patient must require skilled services. The three required skilled services include intermittent skilled nursing care, physical therapy, and speech therapy. Patients receiving one of these three services are also eligible to receive medical social services and occupational therapy; the occupational therapy may be continued if required after other skilled services have been discontinued.

A fiscal intermediary's decisions must be based on the individual patient's health status and medical need as reflected in her plan of care and health record. Although intermediaries have edit screens to detect questionable claims, the information from these screens cannot be the only reason for denying coverage, and documentation must also be reviewed.

According to CMS, reimbursable skilled nursing care consists of services that are reasonable and necessary to the treatment of illness or services that must be performed by or under the direct supervision of a licensed nurse to ensure the safety of the patient and achieve the desired result. General categories of reimbursable skilled services include the following:

- Observation and assessment when significant changes in the patient's condition could occur that would require the skills or evaluation of a skilled nurse and that may result in changes in the client's plan of treatment or in possible institutionalization

- Teaching and training activities that require nursing skills or knowledge

- Performance of skilled procedures such as the insertion and sterile irrigation of catheter, intravenous and intramuscular injections, and wound care

- Management and evaluation of the care plan

Chapter 7 of the Medicare *Benefit Policy Manual* includes additional discussion regarding coverage for skilled care services and other reimbursable services (CMS 2011c). Documentation throughout the record must continually confirm the need for and provision of skilled services.

When a patient begins receiving one of these skilled services, he qualifies for other reimbursable services. These other services include medical social services provided to patients under direction of a physician, part-time or intermittent home health aide services, medical supplies (other than drugs or biologicals), and DME available from the agency. Recent changes to Medicare home care regulations allow medical social services of a brief duration to be provided to families of patients.

Intermittent or Part-Time Home Care Benefits

For coverage of home care benefits, skilled nursing and aide services must be provided on an intermittent or part-time basis. The Medicare *Benefit Policy Manual* (CMS 2011c) defines the terms *intermittent* and *part-time* in detail.

Home Health Certification and Plan of Care

Home Health Certification and Plan of Care, CMS form 485, is designed to meet regulatory requirements for the physician's plan of care, although, as previously stated, it is not a mandated form. It documents a physician's certification and recertification that a patient needs home health services and meets the Medicare requirements for receipt of home health services. Chapter 7 of the Medicare *Benefit Policy Manual* offers detailed instructions on how to provide this information (CMS 2011c). The agency must document this before the final claim for each episode can be submitted to the Medicare fiscal intermediary. The patient's physician must review, update, and recertify the plan of care at least every 60 days.

Medicare Home Care Surveys

Medicare home care surveyors use medical, nursing, and rehabilitative care indicators to determine the quality of a patient's care and the scope of the HHA services provided to the client. These surveyors use the CMS Home Health Functional Assessment to document data from home care record reviews and patient visits. During a standard

FIGURE 12.6. Information documented by Medicare surveyors from home care record reviews and patient visits

Partial or extended Medicare surveys can focus on the following standards:

- COP 484.10 Patient's rights

- COP 484.11 Release of patient-identifiable OASIS information

- COP 484.12 Compliance with federal, state, and local laws; disclosure and ownership information; and accepted professional standards and principles

- COP 484.14 Organization, services, and administration

- COP 484.14(g) Coordination of services

- COP 484.16 Group of professional personnel

- COP 484.18 Acceptance of patients, plans of care, and medical supervision

- COP 484.30 Skilled nursing services

- COP 484.32 Therapy services

- COP 484.34 Medical social services

- COP 484.36 Home health aide services

- COP 484.38 Qualification to furnish outpatient physical therapy or speech therapy

- COP 484.48 Clinical records

- COP 484.55 Comprehensive assessment of patients

Medicare survey, an agency's admission volume determines the number of records to be reviewed, and surveyors review a stratified sample of clinical records.

Based on record review, employee interviews, and home visits to patients, Medicare surveyors make their conclusions about the areas listed in **FIGURE 12.6**.

Medicare guideline COP 484.20(a) instructs surveyors on presurvey and on-site survey activity related to OASIS data collection. Before the survey, surveyors check with the state OASIS education or automation coordinator and review OASIS data management reports to determine whether encoding is completed within seven days after completing the OASIS data set. Surveyors check to see if the HHA is transmitting its own data or has an arrangement with an outside entity acting on its behalf to submit OASIS data to the state agency electronically. If the latter is the case, surveyors confirm the existence of a written contract that describes the HHA's arrangement with the outside entity. Surveyors determine the process for encoding and locking OASIS data being readied for transmission to the state. When questions are raised through interview or record review, surveyors review the HHA's policies regarding encoding time frames. New HHAs seeking initial certification must apply for appropriate state and federal HHA identification and passwords and be able to demonstrate compliance with collecting, completing, encoding, and reporting OASIS data for all applicable patients in an electronic format that meets CMS specifications prior to the initial survey (CMS 2011e).

Home Care Medicare Reimbursement Documentation Guidelines

Whether federally or privately funded, insurance programs employ specific guidelines to determine patient eligibility for home care benefits. When a home care organization accepts a client for care, it also assumes the responsibility for documenting that the client meets the eligibility guidelines at the time of admission and throughout the period during which the client receives care. Failure to do so can lead to additional costs for the agency should claims be denied.

Medicare is the largest single payer for home care services. Other public funding sources for home care include Medicaid, the Older Americans Act, Title XX social services block grants, the Veterans' Administration, and the **Civilian Health and Medical Program of the Uniformed Services (CHAMPUS)**. Private insurance accounts for only a small portion of home care payments. Slightly more than one-fifth of home care services is financed through out-of-pocket payments. Clearly, it serves the best interests of home care organizations to be familiar with the requirements of the various third-party payers and design documentation systems that not only facilitate the provision of high-quality care but also ensure documentation of specific information required for reimbursement.

Initial Agency Contact Documentation

Documentation of the initial agency contact must establish that the client is eligible for services that are reimbursed by the third-party payer and that the professional caregiver has rendered a medically necessary service during the contact. Many third-party payers will only reimburse for conditions of an acute nature. The assessment must give a clear picture of the patient's status before the onset of the acute illness, report the date of onset of the acute illness, and describe the patient's limitations that resulted from the illness. All of these factors are necessary to support the provision of home care services.

Physician Plan of Care

Third-party payers require that professional services be provided under a plan of care that a physician has established. The plan of care, which documents physician's orders, should reflect an accurate diagnosis and list treatments and services to be provided. In addition, the plan of care should indicate the frequency and duration expected for each treatment modality. Subsequent documentation should note that services have been provided within the bounds of the plan of care and any subsequent physician's orders. The third-party payer has no obligation to reimburse for services that have not been specifically ordered or were provided more frequently or for a longer duration than ordered. It is important to note that the services provided must be appropriate to the patient's diagnosis. For example, when physical therapy services are ordered, the patient's diagnosis must reflect that the client has a problem that requires the services of a physical therapist.

Homebound status must be established during the initial visit. The Medicare *Home Health Agency Manual* states that, by definition, homebound status is retained when the patient can leave home only with some difficulty for medical appointments or for occasional other purposes. Continuing documentation substantiates this homebound status.

First Visit Criteria

It is also important for the professional caregiver to document any care given during the initial visit to the client. Most third-party payers will not reimburse a visit made for assessment purposes alone. If the nurse assesses a healing wound during an initial assessment and then changes the dressing, the assessment and change of dressing must be documented. Documentation language is important. The third-party payer wants to see that the client is receiving the care that the skilled professional is trained to give; so record documentation must demonstrate that the care has been provided. Need-based charting is a must. Each entry must stand alone in its ability to demonstrate that a problem or need existed, that it was within the realm of reimbursable services, that intervention was taken by a skilled professional, and that the effects of the intervention were assessed. Instead of simply saying that a leg wound was dressed, nurses must describe the wound, the amount and type of drainage, any odor, and the diameter and depth. Documentation must specifically indicate what kind of wound dressing was used, the client's response to the procedure, the client's understanding of his or her role in the care of the wound, and the plan for future visits. Many states have local coverage determinations specific to wound care that further list documentation requirements.

Because of the need for detailed, specific documentation, it has become increasingly important that the format of the record expedite this documentation. However, some third-party reviewers have not been receptive to forms that use a checklist format. The professional caregiver must be acutely aware of how entries in the record are documented. Simple remarks such as "walks with walker" may signify to the reviewer that the patient is no longer homebound when the caregiver may have meant that the patient requires the use of a walker to ambulate from the bed to the living room or that the patient continues to be unable to ambulate without the assistance of a walker. Specific statements about the extent to which the client is able to ambulate are also important in documenting homebound status: for example, the caregiver could state that the patient is unable to ambulate more than 10 feet without stopping to rest.

Premature Judgments and Ambiguity

Care should be taken to avoid making premature judgments about the client's condition. For example, if the nurse on the second visit finds that the client's blood pressure is within normal limits, a statement such as "blood pressure stable on medication" could indicate to the reviewer that the client no longer requires nurse visits. The nurse would be better advised to record that the client's blood pressure is responding to diet and medication intervention and then go on to describe what continuing needs for nursing care are present. On the next visit, documentation could reflect that the client is continuing to respond to diet and medication intervention. As a general rule, it will be easier to convince a reviewer to acknowledge that a problem continues when the caregiver focuses on what else needs to occur before the client is ready for discharge, rather than on progress made to date.

Ambiguity can also cause denial of a benefits claim when the reviewer does not have enough information to substantiate that skilled care was given. For instance, if a nurse was seeing a patient newly diagnosed with diabetes and wanted to indicate that diet was assessed and instructions were given on specific food exchanges during the visit, documentation should specifically reflect these details rather than simply stating that the diet was reviewed and food exchanges discussed. Most third-party payers will not reimburse for reviews and discussions; however, they will pay for assessments and instructions.

At the time of discharge, the record should include the skilled services that were rendered on the final day of care. If the client no longer needed assistance to ambulate, a question could arise as to whether the client continued to be homebound and in need of home healthcare. It could be argued that such details are trivial and foolish. However, claims have been denied because documentation lacked details.

The burden of proof lies with the home care organization. Although an organization has the right to appeal a claim denial, such appeals are costly in terms of delays in receiving reimbursement and the staff time required to complete the paperwork. Potential denials are best avoided by following the rules and providing details up front. Denials should be categorized and reported by reason so that corrective action may be taken. Medicare regional home health intermediaries can provide quarterly cumulative denial data. Audit and billing activities should be set up accordingly.

Timeliness of Documentation

Documentation must be timely, or payment may be jeopardized. An organization can better accomplish this task by being aware of paperwork submission deadlines for services payment and sharing this information with the staff who submits claims for reimbursement.

Documentation Challenges for PPS and OASIS

Many home health providers are overwhelmed by the burden of documentation for the PPS and OASIS. For patients to whom OASIS applies, Medicare COP 484.55 requires that the comprehensive assessment must be completed in a timely manner, consistent with the patient's immediate needs, but no later than five calendar days after the start of care. Item M0090 on the OASIS data set reflects the final date the qualified clinician completed the actual patient assessment. This is usually the date of the last home visit made to complete the comprehensive assessment, but it may reflect a date subsequent to the on-site visit when the qualified clinician needs to follow up with the patient's family or physician to complete a data item. The agency has 30 additional days from the date that the patient assessment is completed to encode, enter, edit, check, lock, and export the data for future submission to the state survey agency.

Every month, agencies must electronically report all OASIS data collected on all applicable patients in a format that meets CMS electronic data and editing specifications. OASIS data on non-Medicare and non-Medicaid patients receiving skilled services must be reported once the masking requirement is effective. Agency software must mask non-Medicare and non-Medicaid OASIS data so that the patient-identifiable information remains anonymous, except to the reporting HHA. If an HHA is using software developed by a private vendor, that software must appropriately mask non-Medicare and non-Medicaid records for all assessments in a manner similar to the functionality provided by the HAVEN software.

Medicare COP 484.20 requires OASIS data collection by a qualified clinician as part of the comprehensive assessment at start of care, resumption of care, follow-up, transfer to inpatient facility with or without discharge, significant change in clinical condition, discharge to community, and death at home. Encoding of OASIS data items must be complete and locked to accurately compute the information (HIPPS code) necessary for billing Medicare patients under the PPS (CMS 2010a).

As the experiences of home care and hospice providers make evident, the paperwork burden is not abating, although the OASIS is not required for hospice patients. Home care and hospice organizations are addressing the paperwork burden by implementing more efficient documentation systems. However, the process for reducing the time needed for documentation is complex and time consuming. Computerizing the record alone is no panacea for reducing the documentation burden. Gains in productivity can arise from computerization, or even a new manual system, when organizations plan carefully through an assessment of needed data, revised processes, staff education, and monitoring of the effectiveness of the new system. Regardless of whether an organization's health record is in a paper-based or electronic format, efficiency can be gained through well-designed forms and data-entry screens that are logically sequenced and discourage redundant data entry.

Communication and Timeliness of Documentation

To offer well-coordinated care, an individual care provider needs ready access to information on the care and services that all disciplines and organizations provide to patients. In addition, providers need information on patients' response to care and any changes in care plans and goals.

The possibility of inadequate transmission of treatment-related information among home care staff and between home care programs and other organizations providing patient care is a negligence risk. This risk is equally high for hospice programs, perhaps more so when hospices contract for inpatient or skilled nursing facility services. Maintaining timely communication can be challenging, because physicians, the actual care setting, and many individual care providers are physically distant from the home care or hospice organization. The health record is one vehicle for communication. Other vehicles include computer terminals, portable computers (laptops and tablets), handheld devices, telemedicine devices, telephones, and facsimile machines. The health record also contains evidence of continuing communication. A good standard of practice obligates the home care and hospice program to provide information to patients and their families.

Timely health record documentation affects communication and the coordination of care. An organization's policies address the time requirements for incorporating OASIS, encounter information, and signed orders into the health record. Healthcare practitioners should record their findings at the point of care or within 24 hours of an encounter to adequately support patient care. State laws frequently define timeliness, especially in relation to signatures on physician's orders. Failure to obtain signed orders in accordance with policies and state laws puts an organization at a liability risk and raises red flags for payers and surveyors. Additionally, Medicare and some third-party payers cannot be billed unless signed orders are present.

Home care and hospice organizations must go to great lengths to promptly incorporate documentation and signed orders into paper-based health records, and it may be difficult to meet state requirements for timely documentation. Computer-based record systems can make it possible for care providers to document at the point of care on handheld devices or portable computers brought to the patient's home and to transmit current patient information to the organization's centralized computer through wireless technology or modems in the individual caregiver's home. Such computer systems are becoming increasingly common in the home care and hospice settings. Computer networks to physician offices are also useful, so that information can be efficiently shared and orders can be signed electronically. This application is currently far less common, except when all healthcare providers are part of a larger health system.

Consistent and Complete Documentation

A litmus test for an accurate and up-to-date health record is whether an alternative care provider can review the record on any given day and obtain a clear, consistent picture of the patient's status, her care plans and goals, and the care and services recently provided. Although passing this litmus test takes some effort, the alternative could be incomplete and inconsistent documentation that might lead to serious problems involving care, legal, reimbursement, licensure, and accreditation issues. Timely documentation and reference-based, up-to-date documentation policies, procedures, and practices promote completeness and consistency in documentation. In addition, ongoing record reviews that monitor record completeness and consistency can target problem areas needing improvement.

Because home care and hospice programs have come under increased scrutiny during investigations for Medicare fraud, incomplete or inconsistent documentation poses particular legal concerns (Harrison and Cole 2005). Section 1128B of the US Social Security Act prohibits obtaining money from the federal government to which one is not entitled by submitting inaccurate information, overutilizing services, or falsifying the information provided. Billing for services not provided may be alleged under this prohibition when documentation does not agree with claims that have been submitted. For example, documentation may not be present for services provided, or documentation of a patient's status may not be consistent. Complete, consistent documentation that includes dates of service provided and signatures of providers goes a long way toward avoiding (and when necessary, defending against) fraudulent claim allegations. Complete records also protect an organization from unsubstantiated lawsuits and judgments.

Development of Documentation Policies and Procedures

When documentation policies and procedures are specific and clear, health records reflect care and service provision in keeping with community standards. Policies and procedures guide the practice and documentation of a home care or hospice organization. When based on community standards and reimbursement regulations, they also define what disciplines can and cannot do and give directions for performing and documenting a particular responsibility. For example, a policy and procedure would delineate who notifies a physician of a change in a patient's condition, when this notification is necessary, and how it should be conveyed and documented.

A discipline's professional practice standards reflect community standards and define the discipline's scope and practice. Professional practice standards are developed and published by such professional organizations as the American Nurses Association (ANA), National Association of Social Workers, American Occupational Therapy Association, American Physical Therapy Association, and American Speech and Hearing Association. The ANA has standards for home health nursing practice. States have practice acts or statutes that define professional practice for advanced practice nurses and other disciplines. CHAP and Joint Commission (2011a) standards and federal and state regulations also reflect community standards. These standards and regulations may be referenced in a court of law even when an organization has chosen not to be accredited or Medicare certified. The Joint Commission standards (2011a) require numerous documentation policies and procedures.

Up-to-date, standard operating procedures that are monitored for compliance help to ensure high-quality, consistent care and legally protect the individual provider and the organization. Policies and procedures that are consistently reviewed and updated to reflect changes in community standards, laws, organizational structure, and technology are an organization's key to risk management (Harrison and Cole 2005).

Quantitative Record Review Guidelines

Quantitative record review should be conducted at regular intervals. Routine quantitative review of all hospice and home care records ensures that the required documentation is present, accurate, consistent, and timely.

The quantitative record review described in this section differs from the qualitative home care clinical record review that Medicare requires. Clinical record review may focus on completeness, but it also examines quality and utilization of services. Requirements call for it to be completed only quarterly, on a sample of health records.

Trained staff or HIM professionals, known as registered health information technicians (RHITs) and registered health information administrators (RHIAs), often perform quantitative record review. Health records should be reviewed on admission, at discharge, and every 30 to 60 days. Monitoring processes should ensure timely documentation of the services provided and the timely signature of physician's plans of care and orders. Policies and procedures should address the process of record review and administrative mechanisms for ensuring staff compliance in completing records.

The fact that the Medicare PPS is reimbursed on the basis of the home health resource group is not a reason to skip the review of Medicare documentation. The OIG's compliance program guidance stresses that accurate documentation of care is reflected in charges. Annual updating and calculation of norms for the PPS are driven by actual charges. As with compliance, tracking actual charges makes good business sense; it helps the organization measure its efficiency in resource utilization. For compliance purposes, all documentation used to generate a bill for patient care should be reviewed. This type of review is different from a review for coding purposes. Documentation monitoring, performed concurrently, ensures that the documentation reflects the full extent of the care provided. At a minimum, the following types of documentation should be monitored concurrently:

- Documentation generating charges (especially higher dollar amounts, as with infusion care)

- Documentation for any physician charges

- Documentation for ancillary service billing

The HIM department should manage documentation monitoring. However, involving expert clinical staff when necessary validates the process and involves more of the organization's staff in compliance. Clinical staff expertise may be needed for some parts of the review or for the clinical record review process (Krouth 2000).

Part of The Joint Commission's assessment of an ongoing record review process will be determining whether problems were identified and corrected (2011a). Copies of minutes are good pieces of evidence that action was taken. In addition, agencies should review about 5 percent of their discharges. For example, if an agency discharges 1,000 patients each quarter, the ongoing record review should include 50 records each quarter, or about 17 records per month (HCPro 2000).

FIGURE 12.7. Information reviewed after hospice admission

• Dates and signatures on all documents	• Advance directives
• Patient's name on all documents	• Do-not-resuscitate (DNR) and other applicable "do not" orders
• Correct filing of all documents	
• Referral information	• Required assessments
• Patient and family identification data	• Current physical examination
• Properly completed consent forms	• Interdisciplinary care plan
• Patient's rights documentation	• Copies of documents from the transferring facility
	• Other documents as required by an individual hospice

Hospice Inpatient Record Review

All hospice inpatient records should be reviewed shortly after admission to and on discharge from inpatient care. The records of patients who are inpatients for extended periods should also be reviewed every 30 to 60 days. Shortly after the admission of the patient, the health record is reviewed for the information listed in **FIGURE 12.7**. On discharge of the patient and on an ongoing basis, the health record should be reviewed for the information listed in **FIGURE 12.8**.

Home Care Record Review

Clinical record review is a concurrent process at home health organizations. Records are reviewed for completeness, timeliness, and accuracy at admission, as visits are made, and at discharge. In addition, home health organizations must have a tracking process to ensure the prompt return of physicians' plans of care and orders.

Admission Review

Shortly after a patient's admission to home care or hospice, the health record should be reviewed for the information listed in **FIGURE 12.9**.

Discharge and Ongoing Review

On discharge and on an ongoing basis (every 30 to 60 days), the home care health record should be reviewed for the information listed in **FIGURE 12.10**.

Visit Documentation Review

To ensure that records are complete, many home care and hospice providers monitor visit documentation. The HIM professional or trained staff can accomplish visit reviews

FIGURE 12.8. Information reviewed upon hospital discharge

• Date and signature on all documents	• Team case conference documentation
• Patient's name on all documents	• Clinical/progress notes
• Correct filing of all documents	• A discharge summary to include discharge diagnosis and the applicable bereavement assessments
• Updated care plans	

FIGURE 12.9. Information reviewed upon home care admission

- Dates and signatures on all documents
- Patient's name on all documents
- Correct filing of all documents
- Referral information
- Patient identification data
- Properly completed consent forms and service agreements
- Documentation of provision of patient's rights and advance directive information
- Copies of advance directives, when applicable
- Required comprehensive initial assessments
- Signed physician plan of care and physician orders
- Care plan for each discipline providing service and/or for each type of service being provided (interdisciplinary for hospice)
- Copies of documents from transferring agencies
- Other documents as required by the individual organization

by documenting visits against itineraries or schedules. To ease the process, individual providers can attach or consolidate clinical notes to their itineraries and provide this documentation to review personnel for verification before filing. Alternatively, review personnel can be presented with itineraries and schedules to check against handwritten or typed notes before filing. When the notes are computer based, the review personnel can compare itineraries and schedules against the computer-based documentation. A computer-based system also makes it possible to routinely check schedules against clinical progress note documentation. Visit documentation review should be included in routine processes, so that the review does not delay the filing of clinical progress notes.

Physician's Documentation Review

Home care organizations can rely on the mail or the fax machine to obtain required physician signatures on plans of care and orders. A system should be put in place to monitor the timeliness of signatures and to follow up when signatures are late. When problems persist, even with a monitoring system, the entire process should be reviewed to determine how to better achieve timeliness. Although the organization has little control over the behavior of physicians, it can reduce its own time lags. A monitoring system should address the points detailed in **FIGURE 12.11**.

FIGURE 12.10 Information reviewed upon home care discharge and ongoing review

- Date and signature on all documents
- Patient's name on all documents
- Correct filing of all documents
- Team case conference documentation (interdisciplinary for hospice and interdisciplinary preferred for other providers)
- Updated and signed plans of care and orders by the attending physician
- Updated care plans for all disciplines providing service and for each type of service being provided (interdisciplinary for hospice)
- Clinical progress notes, home health aide notations, or volunteer documentation for each visit made
- Home health aide supervisory visits by a nurse or therapist
- Evidence of review of volunteer notes
- Discharge summary documenting care and support provided by each discipline, whether goals were met, discharge type, discharge medical and health status and reason for discharge when patient is discharged alive, unmet needs and plans for follow-up care, discharge diagnoses and problems, admission and discharge dates; and, for hospice, applicable bereavement assessments

FIGURE 12.11. Physician's documentation review monitoring guidelines

- Physician's offices should be notified about any items not returned within a specific time period.

- Staff must confirm that the orders were sent to the correct physician at the correct office before resending orders for signature.

- Establishing trends in delinquent orders by physician groups will allow the organization to determine whether some referral relationships continually put the agency at financial or compliance risk.

- Agency managers should know how many claims are on hold due to unsigned orders.

- The following methods can be used to monitor return of plans and orders from physicians.

  o Copies of mailed or faxed documents should be kept in a tickler file by order date. Upon return of the signed order, the tickler file copy can be pulled and appropriately destroyed. A specified time frame should be established to review and resend orders.

  o A manual or computer-based log of unsigned documents should be maintained, in which attempts to retrieve signed orders are logged. A review of report details will help identify delinquent signatures.

  o Home health order-generating software that includes documentation tracking modules can be employed. Some software systems even allow document tracking through bar codes and bar code readers.

Home Care and Hospice Legal Issues

In home care and hospice, patient's rights, advance directives, do-not-resuscitate orders, and issues related to the withholding of life-sustaining treatment are pertinent legal issues. To avoid pitfalls, organizations should review written policies, procedures, and organization-specific documentation requirements carefully for redundancy.

Patient's Rights

Home health organizations have a responsibility to inform patients of their rights with respect to care provided. Patients whose data will be collected and used by the federal government must receive a notice of their privacy rights. The health record provides evidence that patients are fully informed consumers, actively involved in their care. The protection and promotion of patient and family rights and responsibilities in home care and hospice programs is addressed by CHAP and The Joint Commission (2011a) standards, as well as by Medicare home care and hospice COP.

OBRA requires organizations receiving Medicare and Medicaid funds to document that home care and hospice patients are informed of their rights and that they agree to their care plans. To this end, patients are provided with a bill of rights. This form can be used as is or modified to reflect state licensure requirements, any new accreditation standards, or references to hospice instead of home care.

Medicare COP 484.10 confirms a **patient's right** to be informed about and participate in planning care and treatment, and the right to be informed, in advance, about the care to be furnished, any financial liability, and any changes in the care plan. The patient is also to be informed of any financial liability for care rendered and any changes to that liability. The HHA must advise the patient in advance of the disciplines that will furnish care and the proposed frequency of visits. The HHA must advise the patient in advance of any change in the plan of care before the change is made. The patient has the right to participate in the planning of care. The HHA must advise the patient in advance of the right to participate in planning the care or treatment and planning changes in the care or treatment (CMS 2011a).

The OASIS database is subject to the requirements of the federal Privacy Act of 1974 (5 USC § 552a). The privacy act allows the disclosure of information from a system of records without an individual's consent if the information is to be used for a purpose that is compatible with the purposes for which the information was collected. However, under patient's rights regulations, the HHA must provide the patient with a written notice of the collection of OASIS information in advance of furnishing care to the patient.

Determining care includes the right of a patient to refuse treatment, which the US Supreme Court supported in *Cruzan v. Director of the Missouri Department of Health* (1990). In the Cruzan decision, the court affirmed both the right of a patient to refuse medical treatment and the status of artificial tube feeding as medical treatment. The decision affirmed a patient's right to refuse both life-sustaining treatment and life-saving treatment (Brent 2005).

Patient Self-Determination Act of 1990

In 1990, OBRA's **Patient Self-Determination Act** was enacted. It requires home care and hospice organizations receiving Medicare and Medicaid funds to inform patients of their rights under state law to make advance decisions concerning medical care by activating advance directives. **Advance directives** are instruments patients can use to clarify treatment choices in the event that they lose the ability to do so. State laws recognize different types of advance directives. Two common types are living wills and durable powers of attorney. A home care and hospice organization's written policies and procedures on advance directives should reflect required documentation, including the following (Brent 2005):

- A discussion with the patient regarding the presence of advance directives

- Provision of written information to the patient on state laws and the organization's advance directive policies

- Medical orders to carry out the patient's wishes

- The physical presence in the record of the advance directive itself

When an existing advance directive is not filed in the health record, documentation explains the reason why, such as patient refusal.

Do-Not-Resuscitate Orders

A **do-not-resuscitate (DNR)** order is a physician's order documenting a patient's (or a substitute decision maker's) desire for no resuscitation attempts. (See **FIGURE 12.12**.) Although a DNR order results from a desire expressed in an advance directive, it does not replace the need for that directive. In hospice care cases, routine-care-only orders (or consent for care that indicates routine care only) are not substitutes for a specific DNR order. Prior to writing a DNR order, a discussion should take place between the attending physician and other team members, the patient, and the next of kin or significant other. The health record contains documentation of the content and outcome of this discussion, and the record must also be clearly flagged to indicate the presence of a DNR order. This is especially important in the hospice inpatient setting. If the DNR form is missing, there is a risk of resuscitating a person in error.

In relation to other life-sustaining measures, "do not" orders are necessary in home care and hospice. "Do not" orders include such orders as "do not hospitalize" and "do not treat." These orders should also be documented and flagged, as appropriate. When

FIGURE 12.12. Sample do-not-resuscitate (DNR) order

DO-NOT-RESUSCITATE • DNR • DO-NOT-RESUSCITATE • DNR • DO-NOT-RESUSCITATE • DNR

(Page 1 of 2)

Illinois Department of Public Health
UNIFORM DO-NOT-RESUSCITATE (DNR) ADVANCE DIRECTIVE

Patient Directive

I, _____, born on _____, hereby direct the following in the event of:
   (print full name)   (birth date)

1. **FULL CARDIOPULMONARY ARREST (When both breathing and heartbeat stop):**

   ☒ **Do Not Attempt Cardiopulmonary Resuscitation (CPR)**
   (Measures to promote patient comfort and dignity will be provided.)

2. **PRE-ARREST EMERGENCY (When breathing is labored or stopped, and heart is still beating):**

   SELECT ONE

   ❑ **Do Attempt Cardiopulmonary Resuscitation (CPR) -OR-**

   ❑ **Do Not Attempt Cardiopulmonary Resuscitation (CPR)**
   (Measures to promote patient comfort and dignity will be provided.)

   Other Instructions _____

   _____

Patient Directive Authorization and Consent to DNR Order (Required to be a valid DNR Order)
    I understand and authorize the above Patient Directive, and consent to a physician DNR Order implementing this Patient Directive.

_____   _____   _____
Printed name of individual   Signature of individual   Date

-OR-

_____   _____   _____
Printed name of (circle appropriate title):   Signature of legal representative   Date
legal guardian
OR agent under health care power of attorney
OR healthcare surrogate decision maker

Witness to Consent (Required to have a witness to be a valid DNR Order)
    I am 18 years of age or older and acknowledge the above person has had an opportunity to read this form and have witnessed the giving of consent by the above person or the above person has acknowledged his/her signature or mark on this form in my presence.

_____   _____   _____
Printed name of witness   Signature of witness   Date

Physician Signature (Required to be a valid DNR Order)
    I hereby execute this DNR Order on _____.
                        Today's date

_____   _____   _____
Signature of attending physician   Printed Name of attending physician   Physician's telephone number

◆ *Send this form or a copy of both sides with the individual upon transfer or discharge.* ◆

DNR • DO-NOT-RESUSCITATE • DNR • DO-NOT-RESUSCITATE • DNR • DO-NOT-RESUSCITATE

FIGURE 12.12. (continued)

(Page 2 of 2)

Illinois Department of Public Health
UNIFORM DO-NOT-RESUSCITATE (DNR) ADVANCE DIRECTIVE

Patient's name _____

Summarize medical condition:

When This Form Should Be Reviewed

This DNR order, in effect until revoked, should be reviewed periodically, particularly if –

- The patient/resident is transferred from one care setting or care level to another, or
- There is a substantial change in patient/resident health status, or
- The patient/resident treatment preferences change.

How to Complete the Form Review

1. Review the other side of this form.
2. Complete the following section.
   If this form is to be voided, write "VOID" in large letters on the other side of the form.
   After voiding the form, a new form may be completed.

Date	Reviewer	Location of review	Outcome of Review
			❏ No change
			❏ FORM VOIDED; new form completed
			❏ FORM VOIDED; **no** new form completed

Date	Reviewer	Location of review	Outcome of Review
			❏ No change
			❏ FORM VOIDED; new form completed
			❏ FORM VOIDED; **no** new form completed

Date	Reviewer	Location of review	Outcome of Review
			❏ No change
			❏ FORM VOIDED; new form completed
			❏ FORM VOIDED; **no** new form completed

Advance Directives

I also have the following advance directives: **Contact person** (name and phone number)

❏ Health Care Power of Attorney   _____

❏ Living Will   _____

❏ Mental Health Treatment
   Preference Declaration   _____

◆ *Send this form or a copy of both sides with the individual upon transfer or discharge.* ◆

IOCI 0741-10

Source: Illinois Department of Public Health 2010.

hospices document routine-care-only orders to cover "do not" orders, policy must clearly reflect the meaning of the routine-care-only orders, and their meaning should be conveyed to the patient and/or family.

Hospices and other healthcare providers need to develop mission statements reflecting their care philosophies. These mission statements must be shared with patients and their families or significant others. The sharing of an organization's care philosophies should be documented, especially in relation to DNR orders, other "do not" orders, and philosophies regarding other life-sustaining measures. The Joint Commission standards and Medicare home care and hospice regulations require that patients and their families be informed of healthcare providers' care philosophies.

Written policies and procedures on DNR orders, other "do not" orders, and the withholding or withdrawing of other life-sustaining treatment should specify the documentation required and reflect an organization's care philosophies, review of legal requirements, and input from legal counsel. State laws vary significantly regarding DNR orders and the withholding or discontinuance of other life-sustaining treatment. Organizations should be cognizant of their state laws and the legal climate surrounding them.

Home Health Initiative and Home Care Outcome Monitoring

In 1994, CMS began the Medicare home health initiative to identify opportunities for improvement in the Medicare Home Health Benefit. Among the primary recommendations, CMS was advised to develop home health COP that include a core standard assessment data set and patient-centered, outcome-oriented performance expectations that stimulate continuous quality improvement. OASIS has become part of the information system that was designed to collect and report beneficiary-specific outcomes and provider performance across a multitude of delivery sites (CMS 2011d).

On the basis of comments received, minor modifications were made to the Outcome and Assessment Information Set (OASIS-A2). CMS published the Outcome and Assessment Information Set (OASIS-B1) in June 1998. OASIS is a group of data elements that represent core items of a comprehensive assessment for an adult home care patient. In addition, OASIS forms the basis for measuring patient outcomes for purposes of outcome-based quality improvement (OBQI). OASIS serves as a key component in fostering and monitoring improved home healthcare outcomes in the partnership between Medicare and the home care industry. It is also an integral part of the revised COP for Medicare-certified HHAs. Outcome measures are the crux of OBQI, which is a systematic approach HHAs can implement and follow to continuously improve the quality of care they provide. OASIS data improve each state's ability to identify areas of potential quality concerns. See the CMS OASIS data sets website for further information.

Most data items in the OASIS were derived in the context of a national research program to develop a system of outcome measures for home care. Outcome-based quality improvement and OASIS evolved over a 10-year developmental period. The core items were refined through several iterations of clinical and empirical research. A group of home care experts added other items to augment the outcome data set. The goal was not to produce a comprehensive assessment instrument, but to provide a set of items for measuring patient outcomes and for assessment, which HHAs could augment as needed. OASIS items are used in outcome monitoring, clinical assessment, care planning, and other internal agency-level applications.

OASIS encompasses sociodemographic, environmental, support system, health status, and functional status attributes of adult (nonmaternity) patients. In addition, selected attributes of health service utilization, such as therapy utilization, are included. These different attributes should be part of a comprehensive patient assessment.

More recently, CMS has begun using the OASIS to determine patient outcomes. The OBQI approach (CMS 2010a)

> entails collecting patient data using the OASIS at regular intervals (at start of care and every 60 days until and including time of discharge). OASIS data are computerized, edited, and transmitted to a central source (the central source for Medicare is the State agency specified by CMS). An Outcome Report that compensates for differences between the agency and the comparison or benchmark group is then produced, completing the outcome analysis component of OBQI. Upon completion of the evaluation, a plan of action is documented that specifies which care processes will be changed, how they will be changed, who will be responsible for monitoring the implementation of the change, and how the change process will be evaluated.

More information is available at the CMS Home Health Quality Initiative page of the CMS website.

Currently, there are 41 Home Health Quality Initiative measures (CMS 2010a), which are risk-adjusted quality measures.

Patient Outcome Measures

Patient outcome measures are calculated on a completed episode of care that begins with admission to an HHA (or a resumption of care following an inpatient facility stay) and ends with discharge or transfer to an inpatient facility. This is different from a home health prospective payment episode of 60 days. A patient **outcome** is defined as a change (or lack of change) in a patient's condition during an episode of care.

Risk-adjusted outcome rates are adjusted to compensate for differences in the patient population served by different HHAs, including differences between states. See **FIGURE 12.13**.

FIGURE 12.13. Home health quality measures (OBQI outcomes)

UTILIZATION OUTCOMES	END-RESULT OUTCOMES
• Discharged to community	• Improvement in grooming
• Acute care hospitalization (lower values preferred)	• Stabilization in grooming
• Any emergent care (lower values preferred)	• Improvement in upper-body dressing
	• Improvement in lower-body dressing
	• Improvement in bathing
	• Stabilization in bathing
	• Improvement in toileting
	• Improvement in transferring
	• Stabilization in transferring
	• Improvement in ambulation/locomotion

FIGURE 12.13. (continued)

	• Improvement in eating
	• Improvement in light meal preparation
	• Stabilization in light meal preparation
	• Improvement in laundry
	• Stabilization in laundry
	• Improvement in housekeeping
	• Stabilization in housekeeping
	• Improvement in shopping
	• Stabilization in shopping
	• Improvement in phone use
	• Stabilization in phone use
	• Improvement in management of oral medications
	• Stabilization in management of oral medications
	• Improvement in dyspnea
	• Improvement in urinary tract infection
	• Improvement in urinary incontinence
	• Improvement in bowel incontinence
	• Improvement in pain interfering with activity
	• Improvement in number of surgical wounds
	• Improvement in status of surgical wounds
	• Improvement in speech and language
	• Stabilization in speech and language

Source: CMS 2010.

Quality Requirements

Home care and hospice programs that seek accreditation through the CHAP or The Joint Commission (2011a) or elect to seek Medicare (CMS 2011e) certification must meet the PI requirements of these groups. Organizations in states with licensing regulations that require quality management must also meet state requirements.

CHAP Performance Improvement Standards

CHAP standards emphasize the need for healthcare organizations to establish an organizational structure that supports a consumer-oriented philosophy and consistently provides high-quality services and products. CHAP standards also stress the need for adequate resources and a strong potential for long-term viability. The organization's focus on quality must be reflected in its strategic plans, staff orientation and development programs, and quality commitment (CHAP 2011).

CHAP standards require planned efforts to ensure continuous quality improvement. In addition, the organization must develop quality improvement measures and monitoring processes for the following factors (CHAP 2011):

- Client outcome data

- Client satisfaction assessment

- Clinical record reviews

- Peer reviews

- Program evaluations

The standards address the required content of the quality improvement plan and specifics regarding expectations for monitoring. The standards also require that organizations document evidence illustrating how the organization used quality improvement results in service planning and problem resolution. Evidence should also show that the organization's quality improvement efforts resulted in actual improvements (CHAP 2011).

The Joint Commission Performance Improvement Standards

The Joint Commission standards, when followed, lead to positive outcomes. Performance expectations for each function are addressed in the *Comprehensive Accreditation Manual for Home Care* (Joint Commission 2011a). The standards for improving organizational performance provide a framework for improving the functions addressed in the manual. This framework emphasizes quality and focuses on the common causes of problems and processes. Although The Joint Commission's standards do not require continuous quality improvement per se, they do require a process in which planning, design, measurement, assessment, and improvement focus on and lead to PI. A brief discussion of the requirements for each of these components follows. The standards themselves should be referenced for specifics.

Planning Standards

Standards require evidence of a planned, systematic, and organization-wide approach to PI (Joint Commission 2011a). Planning must address the processes for conducting PI. Collaboration among disciplines and services should be evident in PI efforts, and contracted services should be included in planned PI activities (Joint Commission 2011a).

Design Standards

Design standards address the concept of building in quality at the front end of the process, and thus they focus on new processes. Standards require that the design of new processes take into consideration the following factors:

- The organization's mission, vision, and plans

- Needs and expectations of patients, staff, and others

- Up-to-date sources of information related to designing processes, such as practice guidelines or parameters

- Performance of the processes and their outcomes in other organizations, such as information from reference databases

Measurement of Performance

Performance measurement is at the heart of all PI activities. Through evaluation of measurement data, home care and hospice organizations address the need for improved processes. The Joint Commission (2007) requires certain measurements to be systematically conducted for the following factors:

- Processes and outcomes

- Performance of processes pertaining to the functions addressed in the accreditation manual

- Quality control activities in at least the following areas, where applicable:

  o Clinical laboratory services

  o Equipment provided to patients

  o Equipment used in providing care

  o Pharmacy equipment and preparations

Data collection can focus on high-priority improvement issues and measurement of the stability of a particular process or the predictability of a particular outcome (also known as a *continuous measurement*). Performance measurement of the functions addressed in the accreditation manual must be continual and focus on processes that meet the following characteristics (Joint Commission 2011a):

- Affects a large percentage of patients

- Places patients at serious risk when not performed well, or when performed when not indicated, or when not performed when indicated

- Has/have been or are likely to be problem prone

Assessment of Measurement Data

The Joint Commission requires organizations to have a systematic process in place for assessment of measurement data. This assessment should incorporate statistical quality-control techniques and internal and external comparisons of organization process and outcome data over time. External comparisons include sources such as practice guidelines, data from other organizations, and reference databases. Home care and hospice organizations are advised to obtain Joint Commission input on the expected level of compliance regarding required comparisons.

The Joint Commission standards require intensive assessment of any undesired variation in performance. This variation may be represented by an important single event (The Joint Commission uses the term *sentinel event*), such as a blood transfusion reaction, or by a significant variation from either the standards or comparative performance of other organizations. The Joint Commission requires intensive assessment when any of the following sentinel events occur: confirmed transfusion reactions, significant adverse drug reactions, or significant errors related to medication use. In addition, organizations may choose to perform intensive review to further improve performance. When systematic data assessment reveals that an individual's

FIGURE 12.14. Standards-based performance areas for home care organizations

- Emergency management
- Environment of care
- Equipment management
- Human resources
- Infection prevention and control
- Information management
- Leadership
- Life safety

- Medication management
- National patient safety goals
- Performance improvement
- Provision of care, treatment, and services
- Record of care, treatment, and services
- Rights and responsibilities of the individual
- Waived testing

Source: The Joint Commission 2011b.

performance presents an opportunity for improvement, the person responsible for patient services ensures that steps for assessing and improving competence are followed (Joint Commission 2011a).

Performance Improvement Process

The last component of The Joint Commission's standards for improving organizational performance concerns the PI process itself. Standards require the PI process to be systematic and standardized throughout the organization. Because every opportunity for improvement cannot be addressed, the standards require organizations to establish criteria for prioritizing. They specify considerations that the criteria should address, operational issues that must be considered when designing or improving an activity, and the planning, measurement, and assessment that must occur before an improved process is fully implemented (Joint Commission 2007). The 2011 standards-based performance areas for home care organizations are shown in **FIGURE 12.14**.

Medicare Conditions of Participation for Home Care

OBRA had a major impact on the delivery of home healthcare services. The revised COP focused on the health and safety of patients and emphasized patient's rights and the competency of home health aides. Initially published in the *Federal Register* in 1989, the COP were revised in 1990, 1991, and 1995. In 1999, CMS added a new condition on comprehensive assessment and the OASIS. In 2000, CMS revised some conditions as part of the final rule for the PPS. The interpretive guidelines define the conditions and provide surveyors with direction for the survey process. The guidelines were originally published in the State Operations Manual in 1991 and revised in 1993, 1997, 2000, 2007, and 2010. The reader should refer to the most current version.

The Home Health Initiative

The revised COP for Home Health Agencies include requirements for an internal quality improvement system based on OASIS data. These outcome measures are both global and focused on specific patient groups. Monitoring clinical progress and financial exposure by episode under the PPS requires effective, time-efficient reviews week after week.

OASIS is intended to support home care assessment and outcome monitoring. It gave **Regional Home Health Intermediary (RHHI)** auditors a new audit tool. The **RHHI Outcomes and Assessment Information Set Verification (ROVER) protocol** is an automated accuracy software application used to assist in the medical review of home health claims submitted by HHAs that are paid under the HHA PPS. According to the CMS *Medicare Claims Processing Manual,* updated 2010, ROVER uses health records to verify that the information on an HHA-completed OASIS reflects the patient's condition and the services actually delivered during a particular episode. The program guides medical review staff through a review of information in the clinical record. The reviewer can document whether the case-mix OASIS items have been validated by the information contained in the record. The end results are twofold: a recommended **home health resource group (HHRG)** classification based on the input data and a reporting database containing information from the reviews. There are 153 HHRGs, determined by clinical, functional, and service utilization factors (**FIGURE 12.15**). Therefore, the information gained by the use of ROVER applies not only to data verification but also to intermediary data analysis and provider education (CMS 2010b). The reader is encouraged to read the CMS *Medicare Claims Processing Manual.*

Case-Mix and Adverse Event Reports for Outcome-based Quality Management

CMS recommends a two-stage outcome-based quality improvement process. The first stage includes conducting outcome analysis; collecting needed OASIS data; processing, editing, and transmitting data; and reviewing risk-adjusted outcome reports. The second stage involves targeting outcomes for enhancement, evaluating the care for targeted outcomes, and developing a plan of action to change care. CMS prescribes the quality management process shown in **FIGURE 12.16**.

Agencies should prioritize the adverse events and outcomes by the highest incidence and then investigate those most clinically relevant to the organization. After reviewing comparison charts and listing the clinical actions expected to prevent adverse events, HHAs can design chart audit tools. They can use record review findings to refine subsequent investigations and identify appropriate and problematic care.

CMS warns HHAs against assuming that change will happen. Instead, they should develop improvement plans to proactively change care. As part of the plan, the HHA states the care delivery expectations, implements the improvement activities, and monitors the care provided. CMS also encourages HHAs to incorporate monitoring plans into other record activities and determine what positions should receive monitoring results. Only then can HHAs expect incremental changes.

State Survey Agencies

State survey agencies will periodically review case-mix and adverse event reports. Reports may also be used during the survey process under the COP 484.52 agency and program evaluation, policy and administrative review, and clinical record review.

The COP for Medicare-certified HHAs require an annual evaluation of the agency's overall program and a quarterly clinical record review. Patient care services are one component of the agency's total program that must be included in this evaluation. The use of the case-mix and adverse-event outcome reports to review and improve patient care delivery is congruent with these program evaluation components. State survey agencies are

FIGURE 12.15. HHRG determination

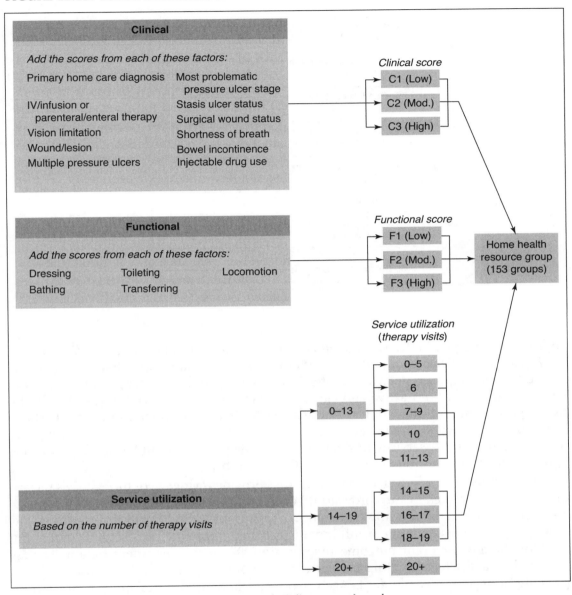

Note: OASIS (Outcome and Assessment Information Set), IV (intravenous), mod.

Source: Medpac 2010, 2.

also expected to incorporate the adverse-event outcome reports into the off-site presurvey preparation and the on-site survey.

Written Policies

Home health regulations state that agencies must have written policies requiring an annual evaluation of their overall program. The evaluation assesses the program's appropriateness, adequacy, effectiveness, and efficiency. Results of the evaluation are reported to and acted on by those responsible for the operation of the agency and are maintained separately as administrative records. As part of the evaluation process, the agency's policies and administrative practices are reviewed to determine the extent to which they promote

FIGURE 12.16. Quality management process

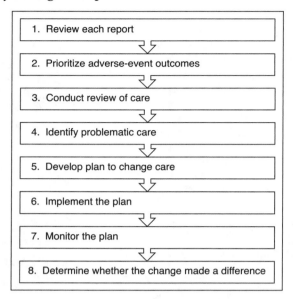

1. Review each report
2. Prioritize adverse-event outcomes
3. Conduct review of care
4. Identify problematic care
5. Develop plan to change care
6. Implement the plan
7. Monitor the plan
8. Determine whether the change made a difference

appropriate, adequate, effective, and efficient patient care. Mechanisms are established in writing for the collection of pertinent data to assist in evaluation (COP 484.52a). On a quarterly basis, appropriate health professionals who represent the scope of the program review a sample of both active and closed clinical records to determine whether established policies are followed in furnishing services directly or under arrangement. There is a continuing review of clinical records for each 60-day period over which a patient receives home health services to determine the adequacy of the plan of care and the appropriateness of continuation of care (COP 484.52b).

The investigation of adverse-event outcomes provides evidence of the agency's review of potential problems in care provision. When problems in care provision are discovered, the development and implementation of the improvement plan demonstrates the agency's goals of overcoming or minimizing existing problems. The use of a chart audit tool for the adverse-event outcome investigation shows that pertinent data are being collected to assist in evaluating patient care. The adverse-event outcome investigation partially addresses this standard. Agency policies and procedures must address how reports are incorporated into the program evaluation.

Quarterly Record Review

Quarterly record review is required to determine whether established HHA policies are being followed in the provision of care. Two aspects of the adverse-event outcome report investigation address this standard. The chart audit tool used to investigate adverse outcomes and the monitoring of clinician compliance with new or revised care practices are expected to incorporate any relevant HHA policies for care provision. When the investigation process is phased, the adverse events can be investigated and monitored on a quarterly basis, and the associated record review is incorporated into the HHA's current quality monitoring requirements. Investigation of adverse outcomes thus becomes part of the overall quality monitoring program. Although these reports represent many HHAs' first exposure to the use of outcomes for quality improvement activities, the utility of the reports for the HHA's overall quality monitoring program is clear. The benefit to patients is also evident as agencies focus on continuous quality of care improvement.

Adverse-Event Outcome Reports

Both state survey agencies and HHAs have access to the adverse-event outcome reports. State survey agencies review available reports as part of their presurvey preparation. The reports help surveyors identify focus areas for the on-site survey. Surveyors expect HHAs to use the information in the reports to improve patient outcomes. They assess the HHA's use of the reports for quality monitoring, including how the HHA addresses any systemic issues, to reduce the incidence of similar adverse events in the future. For example, surveyors may review the specific patient situations included in the adverse-event outcome reports to determine whether any of these events might have been prevented. The surveyor's review may also be used to determine whether any of the adverse event outcomes resulted from the HHA's noncompliance with the COP. HHAs are strongly encouraged to apply the information presented in their reports to their ongoing quality-monitoring program.

Medicare Conditions of Participation for Hospices

Medicare COP reads as follows (CFR 2011):

> The hospice must develop, implement, and maintain an effective, ongoing, hospice-wide data-driven quality assessment and performance improvement program. The hospice's governing body must ensure that the program: Reflects the complexity of its organization and services; involves all hospice services (including those services furnished under contract or arrangement); focuses on indicators related to improved palliative outcomes; and takes actions to demonstrate improvement in hospice performance. The hospice must maintain documentary evidence of its quality assessment and performance improvement program and be able to demonstrate its operation to CMS.

a. Standard: Program scope.

1. The program must at least be capable of showing measurable improvement in indicators related to improved palliative outcomes and hospice services.

2. The hospice must measure, analyze, and track quality indicators, including adverse patient events, and other aspects of performance that enable the hospice to assess processes of care, hospice services, and operations.

b. Standard: Program data.

1. The program must use quality indicator data, including patient care and other relevant data, in the design of its program.

2. The hospice must use the data collected to do the following:

i. Monitor the effectiveness and safety of services and quality of care.

ii. Identify opportunities and priorities for improvement.

3. The frequency and detail of the data collection must be approved by the hospice's governing body.

c. Standard: Program activities.

1. The hospice's performance improvement activities must:

   i. Focus on high-risk, high-volume, or problem-prone areas.

   ii. Consider incidence, prevalence, and severity of problems in those areas.

   iii. Affect palliative outcomes, patient safety, and quality of care.

2. Performance improvement activities must track adverse patient events, analyze their causes, and implement preventive actions and mechanisms that include feedback and learning throughout the hospice.

3. The hospice must take actions aimed at performance improvement and, after implementing those actions, the hospice must measure its success and track performance to ensure that improvements are sustained.

d. Standard: Performance improvement projects. Beginning February 2, 2009 hospices must develop, implement, and evaluate performance improvement projects.

1. The number and scope of distinct performance improvement projects conducted annually, based on the needs of the hospice's population and internal organizational needs, must reflect the scope, complexity, and past performance of the hospice's services and operations.

2. The hospice must document what performance improvement projects are being conducted, the reasons for conducting these projects, and the measurable progress achieved on these projects.

e. Standard: Executive responsibilities. The hospice's governing body is responsible for ensuring the following:

1. That an ongoing program for quality improvement and patient safety is defined, implemented, and maintained, and is evaluated annually.

2. That the hospice-wide quality assessment and performance improvement efforts address priorities for improved quality of care and patient safety, and that all improvement actions are evaluated for effectiveness.

3. That one or more individual(s) who are responsible for operating the quality assessment and performance improvement program are designated.

Surveyors examine structures and processes that contribute to the quality of hospice services. The principal survey focus is the how the hospice's practices implement hospice requirements and the effect of the hospice's services on the patients. Home visits must be made to a sample of Medicare and Medicaid hospice patients if the surveyor determines that such visits are necessary to confirm compliance with all conditions and standards. The hospice self-assessment should include all provided services and the patients' and caregivers' responses to those services. It should also include those services that could have been provided but were omitted. Special attention should be given to the hospice's ability to deal with symptom management, pain control, stress management, continuity of care, and inpatient care. Suggestions for improving care and any problems identified in providing hospice care should receive appropriate consideration from the hospice management or governing body (CMS 2010c).

Interpretive CMS *State Operations Manual* (2010c) guidelines indicate that a hospice have a system for evaluating the care and services provided as well as services that might appropriately have been provided but were not. The governing body should support the quality assurance program, and the program should encompass critiques by the patients' families, monitoring of staff performance, and an annual program evaluation of the hospice's total operation. Annual studies should be done of at least the following areas:

- Symptom management

- Stress management

- Continuity of care

- Inpatient care

A representative of the governing body must be involved in the annual program evaluation, as should representatives from the various disciplines and representatives from home care inpatient services. Throughout the process, a reporting mechanism to the governing body is required (CMS 2010c).

The Joint Commission's Performance Measurement Data

Joint Commission surveyors assess how home care organizations have integrated and used ORYX performance measurement data in their PI activities. During the PI interview, surveyors ask organization leaders what process they used to select performance measures, how ORYX data have been integrated into internal PI activities, and what results emerged from these activities. ORYX initiatives are designed so that expectations should increase over time. The initial phase of the ORYX initiative offers accredited healthcare organizations significant flexibility by allowing them to select the performance measurement system and individual measures that best serve their strategic measurement goals. More than 15,000 performance measures from nearly 300 performance measurement systems have already been cataloged in The Joint Commission's database as part of this initiative.

The next phase of the ORYX initiative includes the identification of specific core performance measures and the opportunity for listed systems to embed some or all of these measures in their own systems. Core measures are grouped into measure sets. In time, measure sets may include clinical performance, client perception of care, health status, and administrative or financial measures. The initial core measures focus primarily on clinical performance. Core measures allow comparisons of processes and outcomes of patient care among healthcare organizations, regardless of which performance measurement system the organization is using. The Joint Commission is gradually transitioning core measure sets into ORYX requirements (Joint Commission 2010).

The ORYX Initiative

ORYX is the name of The Joint Commission's initiative, introduced in 1997, to integrate performance measures into the accreditation process. The ORYX initiative requires organizations to collect quarterly performance measurement data and submit the information to The Joint Commission. ORYX integrates outcomes and other performance measurement data into the accreditation process. The goal is to provide a continuous, data-driven accreditation process that focuses on the actual results of care (performance measurement) and is more comprehensive and valuable to all stakeholders. The Joint Commission strives toward its primary mission of improving the quality of care provided to the public through the provision of healthcare accreditation and related services that support PI in healthcare organizations. As the critical link between accreditation and the outcomes of patient care, ORYX allows The Joint Commission to review data trends and patterns and to work with organizations as they use data to improve patient care. ORYX performance measures supplement and help guide the standards-based survey process by providing more targeted bases for the regular accreditation survey, continuously monitoring actual performance, and guiding and stimulating continuous improvement in healthcare organizations.

Home health organizations with an average annual census of 120 patients or more, accredited prior to January 1, 2001, were required to select and participate in a performance measurement system. The organizations chose six clinical or perception-of-care measures and began data collection on January 1, 2001. They selected the measures most relevant to their patient populations and strategic measurement objectives. The resulting data were reported by the performance measurement system to The Joint Commission by July 31, 2001.

Selecting or participating in a performance measurement system was optional for home health organizations with an average annual census of less than 120 patients or organizations undergoing their initial survey in 2001. Organizations that opted in chose six existing performance measures that were most relevant to their patient populations and strategic measurement objectives. Sources included listed performance measurement systems, the professional literature, internally developed measures, and measures from professional associations. Measure selections were reported to The Joint Commission on a standardized reporting form.

Surveyors assessed organizations' use of selected measures in their PI activities during the on-site survey process. Organizations were expected to demonstrate, for each measure, the ability to collect data reliably, conduct credible analyses of the data, and initiate appropriate system and process improvements.

Today, this remains true. Home care agencies are encouraged to submit data to The Joint Commission "until such time that relevant core measures are identified and implemented by The Joint Commission. Participation in a listed performance measurement system will provide comparative data that may not otherwise be readily available and help facilitate ongoing compliance with performance measurement and improvement requirements" (Joint Commission 2010).

Summary

It is important for the HIM practitioner to understand the key components of the home care and hospice health record database and the regulatory environment under which home care agencies and hospices operate. Although many of the health record database components will be familiar to practitioners from other healthcare settings, some components are unique to each home care and hospice organization. CMS has identified core components that present many documentation challenges related to the Medicare home care PPS, the OASIS, and the provision of care under the Medicare hospice benefit, all of which clinicians in home care and hospice settings strive to meet while caring for their patients.

The HIM practitioner must understand the importance of continually reviewing the documentation to confirm that health records meet all applicable regulations and standards. Additionally the HIM practitioner must assist her agency in understanding the outcomes management and quality initiatives under way by CMS and other accrediting organizations. The HIM practitioner must recognize the ever-changing regulatory environment and keep abreast of the changes and challenges faced by home care and hospice agencies.

References

AHIMA. 2007. Position Statement: Quality Healthcare Data and Information. *Journal of American Health Information Management Association* 78(1):20.

American Society of Health-System Pharmacists. 2003. Medication Therapy and Patient Care: Organization and Delivery of Services–Guidelines. http://www.ashp.org/DocLibrary/BestPractices/OrgGdl-DocPMR.aspx.

Brent, N.J. 2005. Protecting the AIDS Patient's Right to Make Treatment Decisions. *Home Healthcare Nurse* 12(2):10–11.

Centers for Medicare and Medicaid Services (CMS). 2011a. Home Health PPS. http://www.cms.gov/Home-HealthPPS/Downloads/f2f_listserv.pdf.

Centers for Medicare and Medicaid Services (CMS). 2011c. Home Health Services. In *Medicare Benefit Policy Manual*, Rev. 37. https://www.cms.gov/manuals/Downloads/bp102c07.pdf.

Centers for Medicare and Medicaid Services (CMS). 2011d. Inpatient Rehabilitation Facility PPS: IRF Patient Assessment Instrument. http://www.cms.hhs.gov/InpatientRehabFacPPS/04_IRFPAI.asp.

Centers for Medicare and Medicaid Services (CMS). 2011e. OASIS User Manuals. http://www.cms.hhs.gov/HomeHealthQualityInits/14_HHQIOASISUserManual.asp#TopOfPage.

Centers for Medicare and Medicaid Services (CMS). 2010a. Home Health Agency Billing. In *Medicare Claims Processing Manual*. http://www.cms.hhs.gov/manuals/downloads/clm104c10.pdf.

Centers for Medicare and Medicaid Services (CMS). 2010b. *Outcome-Based Quality Improvement (OBQI) Manual*. https://www.cms.gov/HomeHealthQualityInits/Downloads/HHQIOBQIManual.pdf.

Centers for Medicare and Medicaid Services (CMS). 2010c. *State Operations Manual*. http://www.cms.hhs.gov/Manuals/IOM/list.asp.

Centers for Medicare and Medicaid Services (CMS). 2003. CMS Medicare Manual System, Pub. 100-8 Program Integrity, Transmittal 42. http://www.cms.hhs.gov/Transmittals/Downloads/R42PI.pdf.

Centers for Medicare and Medicaid Services (CMS). 2000. Medicare program; Prospective payment system for home health agencies; Final Rule. 42 CFR Parts 409, 410, 411, 413, 424, and 484. *Federal Register* 65(128):41127–41214. http://www.thefederalregister.com/d.p/2000-07-03-00-16432.

Centers for Medicare and Medicaid Services (CMS). 1999. Reporting outcome and assessment information set (OASIS) data; Final rule. 42 CFR Part 484. *Federal Register* 64(15):3748–63. http://www.cms.hhs.gov/OASIS/Downloads/reporting.pdf.

Code of Federal Regulations (CFR). 2011. Title 42: Public Health. Part 418—Hospice care. 418.58 Condition of participation: Quality assessment and performance improvement. http://ecfr.gpoaccess.gov/cgi/t/text/text-idx?c=ecfr&sid=009d7a8f47e1232ab64f843034cf7275&rgn=div5&view=text&node=42:3.0.1.1.5&idno=42#42:3.0.1.1.5.3.3.4.

Community Health Accreditation Program (CHAP). 2011. *Standards of Excellence for Home Care Organizations*. New York: National League for Health Care and Community Health Accreditation Program.

Cruzan v. Director, Missouri Department of Health, 497 U.S. 261 (1990).

General Accounting Office (GAO). 2002. Report to Congressional Committees: Medicare Home Health Care; Payments to Home Health Agencies Are Considerably Higher Than Costs. GAO-02-663. http://www.gao.gov/new.items/d02663.pdf.

Haddad, A.M. 1987. *High Tech Home Care: A Practical Guide*. New York: Aspen Publishers.

Harrison, B.A., and D. Cole. 2005. Managing Risk to Minimize Liability. *Caring* 13(5):26–30.

HCPro. 2000. Ongoing Record Review: One Hospital's Pathway to Success. *Medical Records Briefing* 15(11):1–3.

Hospice Association of America (HAA). 2005. Region IV Hospices Face New Claims Review Edit and New Policy Regarding Limitation of Liability. *Hospice Forum* 9(13):1–2.

Illinois Department of Public Health. 2010. Uniform Do-Not-Resuscitate (DNR) Advance Directive. http://www.idph.state.il.us/public/books/dnrform10.pdf.

The Joint Commission. 2011a. *Comprehensive Accreditation Manual for Home Care* (*CAMHC*). Oakbrook Terrace, IL: The Joint Commission.

The Joint Commission. 2011b. Facts about Home Care Accreditation. http://www.jointcommission.org/assets/1/6/Home_Care_Facts_2_17_11.pdf.

The Joint Commission. 2010. ORYX Non-Core Measure Information. http://www.jointcommission.org/oryx_non-core-measure_information.

The Joint Commission. 2007. *Comprehensive Accreditation Manual for Home Care* (*CAMHC*). Oakbrook Terrace, IL: The Joint Commission.

The Joint Commission. 1995. *Understanding the Patient's Perspective: A Tool for Improving Performance*. Oakbrook Terrace, IL: The Joint Commission.

Krouth, M. 2000. Monitoring Content and Quality of Documentation. *HIM Connection* 2(43):2–4.

Medicare Learning Network. 2010. MLN Matters: Information for Medicare Fee-for-Service Health Care Professionals. http://www.cms.gov/MLNMattersArticles/downloads/SE1038.pdf.

Medpac. 2010. Home Health Care Services Payment System: Payment Basics. http://www.medpac.gov/documents/MedPAC_Payment_Basics_10_HHA.pdf.

National Association for Home Care and Hospice (NAHC). 2010. Home Care & Hospice Facts & Stats. http://www.nahc.org/facts.

National Association for Home Care and Hospice (NAHC). 2001. Basic Statistics About Home Care. http://www.nahc.org/consumer/hcstats.html.

Office of Inspector General (OIG). 2010. Work Plan: Fiscal Year 2010. http://oig.hhs.gov/publications/docs/workplan/2010/Work_Plan_FY_2010.pdf.

Office of Inspector General (OIG). 2007. Work Plan: Fiscal Year 2007. http://www.oig.hhs.gov/ publications/docs/workplan/2007/Work%20Plan%202007.pdf.

Omnibus Budget Reconciliation Act of 1987 (OBRA). 1987. Public Law 100-203, (101 Stat. 1330), SEC. 4001 [2 USC 902 note]. United States Code. http://www.ssa.gov/OP_Home/comp2/F100-203.html.

Patient Self-Determination Act. 1990. Public Law 9621, (1395aa. 1395cc. 1395dd. and 1395hh) and sec. 602 (k) of Pub. L. 962), [42 U.S.C. 1302.1395x. 1395ww note]. United States Code.

US Department of Justice. 2004. Federal Privacy Act; Final Rule. 5 USC 552a.

Chapter 13

Behavioral Healthcare

Kathleen M. Munn, RHIA, and Diana M. Warner, MA, RHIA, CHPS, FAHIMA

Learning Objectives

- List and explain the sources of regulations and standards that apply to behavioral healthcare records

- Describe the variety of settings for behavioral healthcare services

- List and describe the documentation issues unique to behavioral healthcare settings

- Describe the content of the behavioral health record

- Define and describe psychotherapy notes and their special protection under Health Insurance Portability and Accountability Act (HIPAA) privacy regulations

- List and describe the many outside forces affecting behavioral healthcare

Key Words

Advance directive

Conservatorship

Covered entity (CE)

Day treatment

Diagnostic and Statistical Manual of Mental Disorders, fourth edition (DSM-IV)

Durable power of attorney

Early childhood intervention (ECI)

Employee assistance program (EAP)

Family Educational Rights and Privacy Act of 1974 (FERPA)

Global assessment of functioning (GAF)

Health Insurance Portability and Accountability Act of 1996 (HIPAA)

Inpatient facility

Integrated delivery system (IDS)

Living will

Managed behavioral healthcare organization (MBHO)

Managed care organization (MCO)

Mental Health America (MHA)

National Committee for Quality Assurance (NCQA)

Outcomes assessment

Outpatient facility

Partial stay

Personal health information (PHI)

Process note

Residential program

Standards and Guidelines for the
Accreditation of Managed Behavioral
Health Organizations

Substance Abuse and Mental Health
Services Administration (SAMHSA)

Introduction

An estimated one in four Americans, roughly 26 percent, will suffer from a diagnosable mental illness in any given year (NIMH 2010a). These conditions, which encompass a wide variety of cognitive, emotional, and behavioral illnesses, along with mental retardation, developmental disabilities, and substance abuse, are classified in the ***Diagnostic and Statistical Manual of Mental Disorders, fourth edition*** *(Text Revision 2000)*, or *DSM-IV-TR*. *DSM-IV* is the classification system used in the United States to diagnose and classify mental illness (APA 2000).

Behavioral health has unique documentation challenges. Clients may be at high risk for suicidal or homicidal behavior. Often they are committed to a behavioral healthcare facility involuntarily or are required to receive treatment against their wishes. Clients who complain of suicidal thoughts or display overtly suicidal behaviors, yet persist in refusing care, present healthcare providers with significant care and safety challenges. Complete and timely documentation of these situations is critical. Consequently, staff must have an organized system for documenting and addressing such behavior.

Behavioral healthcare also poses unique challenges in the area of patient rights. Even though mental illness may put clients at high risk for suicidal or homicidal behavior, they have the right to refuse psychiatric treatment. Psychiatric institutions to which clients are committed involuntarily must draw a fine line between safeguarding the client's rights and protecting the interest of society.

The Recipients of Behavioral Healthcare Services

More than 57 million Americans are currently diagnosed with a mental health disorder (Kessler et al. 2005). As shown in **FIGURE 13.1**, mental illness is prevalent in all races, ages, and social settings and affects almost every family in the United States (HHS 2001).

Today's healthcare system offers a number of mental health or behavioral healthcare services to individuals living with these conditions. The terms *mental health* and *behavioral health* are used interchangeably throughout this chapter, as both are frequently used in treatment settings around the country.

Individuals who seek these services are most commonly referred to as *clients*, although they are also referred to as *patients, consumers,* or *recipients*. These terms are used interchangeably throughout this chapter as well.

Behavioral healthcare services may be initiated through court-ordered treatment. The need for treatment in the forensic population (jails and prisons) continues to grow, and the provision of behavioral healthcare services is increasing to forensic populations as funding for these special-needs clients increases.

Organization and Operation

Behavioral healthcare facilities may be private, stand-alone entities, or they may be affiliated with an area hospital or larger healthcare organization. In addition, some behavioral organizations are part of a chain, with a main corporate office and facilities in a

FIGURE 13.1. Prevalence of serious mental illness among US adults by age, sex, and race in 2008

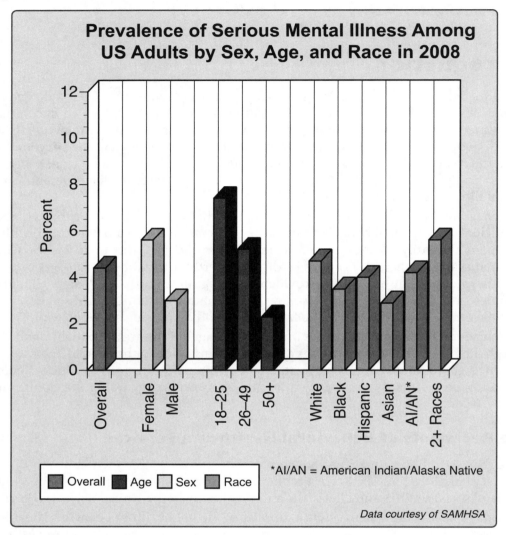

Source: NIMH (2010a).

specific region or throughout the nation. Many organizations today are owned, operated, and funded by individual states or counties.

In most states, healthcare plans such as Medicaid or plans run by individual counties provide the funding for treatment of individuals with behavioral healthcare problems. If an individual has private insurance that covers behavioral healthcare services, the state or local government may be responsible for paying the difference.

Settings

The present behavioral healthcare environment allows for an individualized approach to treatment and for provision of treatment in the least restrictive setting possible. Treatment may be provided by a psychiatrist, a psychologist, an advanced nurse practitioner, or a variety of rehabilitative or social work specialists. In many settings, a combination of these individuals provides treatment. After a diagnosis has been established, careful consideration is given to the individual's social, medical, and financial circumstances and service needs. The provider or provider team develops a treatment or service plan in response to the individual's needs. The client and the client's family, if available, are often encouraged to actively participate in development of the treatment or service plan.

Additionally, an organization's medical staff rules and regulations must address unique areas in behavioral healthcare, such as the use of seclusion and restraint, psychotropic medication, and suicide watch, which may be forced on a patient due to self-imposed danger or threat to others. Documentation for these issues is discussed later in this chapter.

Although terminology, licensure, documentation, and staffing requirements may vary from state to state, behavioral healthcare settings have three basic types: inpatient, residential, and outpatient. Special settings include community mental health entities, employee-assistance programs, and schools and universities.

Inpatient Facilities

Inpatient facilities provide patients with around-the-clock care. Of the 5.4 million people who sought mental health treatment in 1990, less than 7 percent required hospitalization. More than half of those who needed inpatient care had schizophrenia, one of the most severe forms of mental illness (MHA 2011).

Inpatient facilities may be a dedicated portion of a hospital or may stand alone. Clients whose needs fall between inpatient and outpatient services, and who would benefit from a short stay at in inpatient facility or hospital, have need of partial-stay services or partial hospitalization. **FIGURE 13.2** lists some of the elements to review

FIGURE 13.2. Elements to review for inpatient behavioral facility hospitalization

- Any evidence of self-injurious behavior?
- Any evidence of threatening behavior?
- Any evidence of disorganized behavior?
- Any evidence of disordered thinking?
- Description of mood and affect.
- Is patient compliant with treatment plan?
- Is patient eating? How much?
- Is patient sleeping adequately? How many hours?
- Is patient attending to activities of daily living appropriately?
- Is patient compliant with medication? Medication education provided?
- Use of PRNs and response
- Documentation of severity of symptoms, whether they have increased or decreased, or whether different symptoms have emerged.
- Does patient require 24-hour professional observation?
- Passes: Documentation of why passes are needed and response to pass
- Groups: Attendance and participation level
- Patient's ability and willingness to participate in discharge planning
- Is family/significant other participating in patient's treatment?
- If patient has substance misuse or abuse issues, is the patient willing to address this in treatment?

Source: Martins and Nicholson 2008, 241.

regarding medical necessity for inpatient behavioral facility hospitalization (Martins and Nicholson 2008).

Partial Stay or Day Treatment

Partial stay or **day treatment** programs provide individuals with mental health treatment that is more intense than the services provided on an outpatient basis. Most payers (including Medicare) cover this service when the physician determines it to be medically appropriate (CMS 2010a). Typically, partial hospitalization is a four-hour-a-day, Monday through Friday program in which treatment may be provided in the morning, afternoon, or even early evening. Day treatment is typically provided eight hours a day, Monday through Friday, during the work day.

Day treatment/day care/partial hospitalization services include the following:

- Social and recreation activities for individuals who require general supervision during the day

- Psychosocial programs for social interaction

- Family counseling services directed toward a family member's problem in relation to the patient's condition

- Vocational training for employment opportunities, work skills, or work settings

Residential Programs

These programs provide a homelike environment and help residents build self-esteem, develop relationships, and improve life skills. Residents benefit from daily professional treatment provided on the premises. Treatment can include individual psychotherapy, group therapy, vocational/educational counseling and support, and treatment for co-occurring addictions.

Group Residential Communities

Also called "group homes," these family-like surroundings provide tools through which residents repair self-esteem, build skills, develop relationships, and learn to manage symptoms. They create a stable, long-term living arrangement that increases quality of life and continued growth as defined for each client. Clinical treatment may be optional and occurs off-site. Length of stay varies, and the treatment period can be extensive.

Apartment-Based Communities

Residents live in apartments while participating in a program of therapeutic activities, supportive relationships, and treatment. Clinicians may visit resident apartments to gain insight that enhances treatment and recovery. This style of residence may offer a greater degree of independence than other settings (ARTAUSA 2011).

Outpatient Facilities

Outpatient facilities provide clients with access to a stable treatment provider on an outpatient basis. Such care may occur in a formal office setting or in the comfort of the patient's residence. In some circumstances, outpatient services are provided in homeless shelters in an effort to reach the estimated hundreds of thousands of homeless individuals in America who suffer from mental illness (SAMHSA 2010). Intensive outpatient services, where patients are seen a few hours a day until stabilized, are also available.

Community Behavioral Health Centers

The Mental Retardation Facilities and Community Mental Health Centers Construction Act of 1963 led to the establishment of more than 750 comprehensive community mental health centers throughout the United States. This helped people with mental illnesses, who were formerly secluded in hospitals and isolated institutions, move back into their communities. The development of new medications and treatments contributed to this shift. The populations of state inpatient hospitals have dropped from near 600,000 in 1955 to fewer than 70,000 today. Community-based organizations provide comprehensive behavioral healthcare services for mental illness and intellectual and developmental disabilities. Some provide substance addiction services as well. Community-based behavioral care is delivered by a mix of government and county-operated organizations as well as private nonprofit and for-profit organizations. Funding for services comes from Medicaid (up to 70 percent of services); county, state, and federal programs; Medicare; and private insurance (NCBBH 2011).

Employee Assistance Programs

Employers acknowledge the need for mental health services for their employees by providing access to **employee assistance programs (EAPs)**. These outpatient programs are designed to provide employees with immediate access to psychological counseling on a limited basis and may be provided on-site or through local providers. Assistance provided may include counseling psychology, social work, organizational development, chemical dependency services, and marriage and family therapy.

Schools and Universities

Schools and universities commonly provide outpatient mental health assistance to their students through formal clinics, guidance therapy, or direct collaboration with area community-based providers. Moreover, schools often provide crisis therapy or counseling to students exposed to significant trauma due to violence or bullying in the school or community, or following major devastating events, such as terrorist events or natural disasters. Such therapy or counseling services are commonly provided by local mental health providers.

Incidents of violence in schools spurred the Bush Administration to reconsider whether state and federal laws properly address "the fundamental interests of privacy and individual freedom, safety, and security," and how these laws assist those with mental health needs in getting appropriate care (HHS, DOE, and DOJ 2007, 3). The 2007 "Report to the President" has several recommendations for state and federal actions, including the following:

- Develop guidance that clarifies how information can be shared legally under the **Health Insurance Portability and Accountability Act of 1996 (HIPAA)** and the **Family Educational Rights and Privacy Act of 1974 (FERPA)** and disseminating it to the mental health, education, and law enforcement communities.

609

- Ensure that state and local emergency management teams have clear guidance on the sharing of information as it relates to educational records and FERPA (20 USC § 1232g; 34 CFR Part 99).

- Coordinate best practices in disseminating information about threat assessments for colleges and universities.

Documentation Issues to Consider in Behavioral Healthcare

Behavioral healthcare requires documentation for many types of treatment that may not regularly occur in other settings. These include such issues as seclusion and restraints, suicide watch, minors seeking services, diagnostic interview examination, psychological testing, medication management, psychotherapy sessions, and conservatorship.

Seclusion and Restraints

As mentioned in chapter 5, in most states, only licensed physicians are allowed to issue orders for the use of seclusion or restraints. In some states, however, psychologists, physician assistants, and certified nurse practitioners are also allowed to write such orders under certain conditions. In all cases, health record documentation must support the medical necessity of the services and materials ordered. See **FIGURES 13.3**, **13.4**, and **13.5** for sample forms related to the use of seclusion and restraints. The form used in the behavioral healthcare setting is similar to that used in other healthcare settings.

Orders for physical or pharmaceutical restraint or seclusion must comply with Medicare regulations, state laws, and accreditation standards. In general, orders for restraint or seclusion should be issued only when the procedures are necessary to protect the patient or others from harm. Regulations and standards require specific time limits and continuous observation to prevent injuries to the patient, such as suffocation. Accreditation standards for psychiatric facilities provide more specific guidelines.

Suicide Watch

Patient observation, such as one-to-one staffing or 15-minute checks, should be documented in a patient's health record. (See **FIGURE 13.6** for a sample form.) Studies have found that in some facilities up to 13 percent of psychiatric inpatients require constant observation. Despite observation and monitoring, however, about 75 percent of patients admitted with suicidal thoughts who committed suicide in the hospital denied these thoughts during their last communication with hospital staff (Grant 2007). The cost of constant observation can be significant for a behavioral healthcare facility—as much as 20 percent of the total nursing budget (Grant 2007).

According to the American Psychiatric Association (2006):

The most frequent lawsuits, settlements, and verdicts against psychiatrists are for patients' suicides. …If a malpractice claim is brought against the psychiatrist, documentation of suicide risk assessments assists the court in evaluating the many clinical complexities and ambiguities that exist in the treatment and management of patients at suicide risk.

The failure to document suicide risk assessments and interventions may give the court reason to conclude they were not done. …Thus, it is crucial for the suicide risk assessment to be documented in the medical record.

FIGURE 13.3. Sample restraint order in paper format

Anytown Community

PATIENT LABEL

Patient Behavior/Criteria Present:
- ☐ Climbing out of bed
- ☐ Pulling at dressings, lines, or tubes
- ☐ Attempting to remove dressings, lines, or tubes
- ☐ Unable to follow directions with results that may injure self or others
- ☐ Standing up from chair
- ☐ Other: _____

Patient Behavior Related to:
- ☐ Confusion
- ☐ Delirium
- ☐ Marked agitation
- ☐ Sedation/analgesia
- ☐ Impaired attention and/or concentration
- ☐ Impaired learning ability
- ☐ Other: _____

Type and Number of Restraints:
- ☐ ×1 ☐ ×2 Soft wrist restraint
- ☐ ×1 ☐ ×2 Soft ankle restraint
- ☐ ×1 ☐ ×2 Soft mitten restraint
- ☐ ×4 Leather restraint
- ☐ Vest restraint
- ☐ Chair restraint
- ☐ Other: _____

Time Limitation:
- ☐ Continuous usage
- ☐ At night only
- ☐ When up in chair
- ☐ When family/visitors not at bedside
- ☐ Other: _____

Renewal Order Only

- ☐ Patient examined by physician.
- ☐ Alternatives to use of restraints reviewed by physician/staff.
- ☐ Patient continues to demonstrate behavior leading to use of restraints, as indicated above.

_____
Physician Signature   Date/Time

Telephone/Verbal Order:

Dr. _____ /

_____ ,RN _____
                                                    Date/Time

RESTRAINT ORDER
000011 (11/2002)

Source: AHIMA (2004).

FIGURE 13.4. Sample restraint or seclusion assessment

PRECIPITATING EVENT: Behaviors leading to restraint or seclusion:	Nursing Staff Prompts: *(Check all when completed)*
_____ _____ _____ _____ _____ _____	☐ 1:1 initiated by Charge Nurse ☐ MD evaluation within one (1) hour ☐ Clothing search complete ☐ Denial of Rights Form complete ☐ Order obtained every 4 hours ☐ Add to Treatment Plan *(CRU only)*

Clinical interventions used prior to restraint or seclusion: *(check all that apply)*

☐ **Medication Intervention**   ☐ **De-escalation**   ☐ **Voluntary Time Out**

☐ **Threat Reduction** *(for fear)*
  ☐ Mirror person as far as eye contact
  ☐ Give reassurance of safety
  ☐ No touching without permission
  ☐ Stand with arms at side, palms facing forward
  ☐ Calm, confident vocal tone
  ☐ Slow gestures
  ☐ Use rule of five *(no more than 5 words—each word 5 letters or less)*

☐ **Control** *(for frustration)*
  ☐ Maintain eye contact
  ☐ Assess origin/cause of frustration
  ☐ Stand with palms facing down
  ☐ Speak in confident manner
  ☐ Moderate tone of voice
  ☐ Use rule of five

☐ **Detachment** *(for manipulation)*
  ☐ No direct eye contact
  ☐ Speak in firm voice
  ☐ Turn at an angled position
  ☐ Use rule of five
  ☐ Act in a disengaged manner

☐ **Consequation** *(for intimidation)*
  ☐ Use rule of five
  ☐ Confident posture
  ☐ Maintain direct eye contact
  ☐ Don't threaten or argue
  ☐ Identify consequences

Patient's response to above interventions: _____
_____
(circle one below)
Less restrictive interventions have been attempted unsuccessfully and **seclusion/restraint/ambulatory restraint** is necessary to prevent the following: ☐ Harm to self   ☐ Harm to others

The patient was given the following explanation of reason for seclusion or restraint:_____
_____

Patient grants permission to notify family of seclusion or restraint   ☐ Yes (if yes, document in Progress Notes)
                                                                          ☐ No

☐ Signed consent for involvement of interested party obtained
(If yes, name of person contacted): _____

Release criteria: ☐ Contracts for safety   ☐ Reduced agitation/impulsively
                     ☐ No longer danger to self and/or others

Explain: _____

RN Signature:_____ **Date:**_____ **Time:**_____

County of San Diego
Health and Human Services Agency
Mental Health Services
San Diego County Psychiatric Hospital
RESTRAINT OR SECLUSION ASSESSMENT
HHSA:MHS-225

Patient Identification

Source: County of San Diego (2002a).

FIGURE 13.5. Sample restraint or seclusion flow sheet

TITLE:	RESTRAINT or SECLUSION FLOW SHEET
FORM NUMBER:	HHSA: MHS-226
WHEN	For use of Restraint or Seclusion procedures and ambulatory restraints.
ON WHOM	All patients in seclusion, restraints, or ambulatory restraints.
COMPLETED BY	The flow sheet will be completed by RNs, and LVNs, PTs and/or MHAs.
MODE OF COMPLETION	Handwritten
FORMAT	Restraint or seclusion flow sheet is a preprinted form to include patient's identification, date, shift, time initiated, and initiator RN signature.

The type of Restraint or Seclusion initiated will be checked.

A new form will be used when the first form is completed or when a new date starts.

Signatures and initials of those staff using the form will be placed in the respective boxes.

- **"Describe Patient Behaviors" Section:**
  - ➢ RNs shall document when a patient is placed into seclusion, restraint, or ambulatory restraints and when these measures are renewed, reduced, or discontinued.
  - ➢ Additional pertinent information shall be documented here at least once every hour.
  - ➢ Code numbers from the top of the page shall be used, when applicable.
  - ➢ Additional information may be added to the progress notes.
- **"Every 15 minutes" Section:**
  - ➢ May be completed by RNs, LVNs, PTs, or MHAs.
  - ➢ Add time and initials (end of row).
  - ➢ Check blanks corresponding to each section.
  - ➢ Add code numbers in "brief behavior description" column.
- **"Every 2 hours" Section:**
  - ➢ May be completed by RNs, LVNs, PTs or MHAs.
  - ➢ Add time and initials (end of row).
  - ➢ Check and complete blanks corresponding to each section.
- **"Debriefing" Section:**
  - ➢ Shall be completed by an RN.
  - ➢ Add reason for "no" and additional comments as indicated.
  - ➢ If there are no additional comments, write N/A in the blanks provided.

EXCEPTIONS	None.

FIGURE 13.5. (continued)

Date: _____ Shift: _____ Time Initiated: _____

_____

Initiator RN Signature   *Date*

Check One:	☐ Seclusion	☐ Restraint	☐ Ambulatory Restraints

CODES		Document/check each area every **15 MINUTES** or more frequently as needed.	Document/check each area every TWO (2) HOURS or more frequently as needed.

1. Beating on door/wall	6. Standing still
2. Yelling/screaming	7. Walking/pacing
3. Crying/cursing	8. Thrashing/spitting
4. Laughing/singing	9. Quiet
5. Mumbling	10. Disrobing/sexually inappropriate

11. Other: _____

(RNs, LVNs, PTs, MHAs)

Initials	Signatures

Column headers (vertical):
- Time
- Continual visual & auditory observation
- Patient is breathing without difficulty CIRCULATION CHECKS
- Restraints intact, extremities assessed
- Brief behavior description (USE CODES)
- Offer of foods/fluids
- Offer bathroom/ bedpan
- Range of Motion (10 minutes)
- Pulse & B/P Temperature & Respiration Rate
- **Initials**

Time	Describe Patient Behaviors **(document once every hour)**	RN Initials									

Debriefing within 24 hours after episode ☐ Yes ☐ No If no, give reason_____

Comments:_____

County of San Diego
Health and Human Services Agency
Mental Health Services
San Diego County Psychiatric Hospital

RESTRAINT OR SECLUSION FLOW SHEET

HHSA:MHS-226

Patient Identification

Source: County of San Diego (2002b).

FIGURE 13.6. Inpatient assessment of suicide risk (before and after -discontinuation of suicide precaution)

ASSESSMENT FACTOR	LOW RISK (1 POINT)	MODERATE RISK (2 POINTS)	HIGH RISK (3 POINTS)
Suicidal ideation	No current suicidal thoughts	Intermittent or fleeting suicidal thoughts	Constant suicidal thoughts
Suicide plan	No plan	Has plan without access to planned method	Has carefully thought out plan with actual or potential access to method
Lethality of plan/incident	Low lethality of plan/incident (such as superficial scratching)	Moderate lethality (such as hidden sharps or contraband items)	High lethality of plan/incident (such as hanging, suffocation attempt)
No Harm Contract	Reliably signs No Harm Contract	Signs No Harm Contract but is ambivalent	Unwilling or unable to sign No Harm Contract
Behavioral symptoms: • Anxiety • Hopelessness • Helplessness • Anger/rage • Guilt/shame • Impulsivity • Isolation	None to two symptoms present	Three to four symptoms present	Five to seven symptoms present
Support systems	Several friends, coworkers and relatives available	Few or only one friend	None available
Comments:	Total Score:		
	RN Signature:		
	Date & Time:		
Scoring Directions: 1. Assess each assessment factor. 2. Circle one descriptor for each assessment that best describes the patient. 3. Assign appropriate points (1, 2, or 3) to each factor. 4. Add the points for each assessment factor to arrive at a total score.			
Scoring Key: 6–10 points = Low risk (Zero [0] precautions) 11–14 points = Moderate risk (Alert—continue assessment for another shift) 15 points or above = High risk (Notify physician)	**Patient Label**		

Minors Seeking Services

Some states permit minors to admit themselves into mental health treatment facilities without parental consent; they also permit minors to authorize disclosure of **personal health information (PHI)**. Likewise, if state law permits minors to seek admission for services in a substance abuse program without parental consent, unless the minor lacks the capacity to make a rational choice, only the minor can authorize disclosure of her PHI, including to parents (42 CFR 2, Subpart B, 2.14).

Diagnostic Interview Examination

The first step of the psychiatric evaluation is the assessment, which addresses the onset, duration, and severity of the problem. The provider obtains specific information about the developmental history and family history and reviews and takes into consideration any previous evaluations and testing.

Psychological Testing

Psychologists document the psychological characteristics of patients based on their responses to test questions or stimuli, their behavior during the examination, and previously documented information in the psychological testing report. Test results are explained to the patient. The patient may authorize the psychologist to release the psychological test report.

The American Psychological Association Code of Conduct indicates that the raw test data may be released to the patient or other persons identified in the release. However, the psychologist may refrain from releasing the test data to protect the patient or to keep the information from being misused or misrepresented. Psychologists are responsible for maintaining the integrity and security of test materials. In addition, many states have laws that prevent the test data from being released.

Medication Management

When a patient is prescribed a psychotropic medication, ongoing medical monitoring and evaluation are provided. The prescribing physician does not provide interactive psychiatric treatment at this time, but another clinician may provide such treatment.

Psychotherapy Sessions

A patient's behavioral healthcare record must indicate that he has a psychiatric illness or demonstrates emotional or behavioral symptoms sufficient to intervene with normal functioning. In addition to the date of service, the record must include the time spent in psychotherapy encounters and show that treatment such as behavioral modification, insight and supportive interactions, and discussion of reality were applied to produce therapeutic change. For interactive psychotherapy, the health record also must indicate that the client is unable to interact through normal verbal communication means (for example, art therapy or family therapy). The special confidentiality protections afforded psychotherapy notes under HIPAA (1996) require careful handling. For this reason, organizations must be clear in their understanding of HIPAA's definition of psychotherapy notes.

Psychotherapy notes are also referred to as **process notes**. They capture the therapist's impressions of the client obtained during private, group, joint, or family counseling sessions. The notes contain details considered inappropriate for inclusion in the health record and are used by the provider for future sessions. Psychotherapy notes exclude medication, prescription, and monitoring information; counseling session start and stop times; the modalities and frequencies of treatment furnished; results of clinical tests; and any summary of diagnosis, functional status, treatment plan, symptoms, prognosis, and progress to date.

To qualify as psychotherapy notes, the notes must contain extended direct quotations from both client and therapist. In addition, they must include repeated and systematic references to interpretive insights into the client's intrapsychic dynamics as discussed in the therapy sessions. Finally, the documentation in the notes must weave together the client's unresolved past conflicts or issues with current difficulties. Notes that do not meet these criteria are much better identified as counseling progress notes, which are meant to be useful to the entire treatment team as well as the client.

This distinction is important because psychotherapy notes may not be released unless specifically identified on an authorization form and only with the author's permission.

However, not all therapy documentation requires special handling. The following documentation may be released with a valid authorization:

- Records of the prescription and monitoring of medication

- Counseling session start and stop times

- Modalities and frequency of treatment

- Results of clinical tests

- Any summary of the client's diagnoses, functional status, treatment plan, symptoms, prognosis, and progress to date

In psychiatric settings, clinical observations are typically documented in progress notes. The requirements are similar to those for the acute care record in that they create a chronological report of the patient's condition and response to treatment during her course of treatment, coordination of services provided, and chronological records of vital signs. Behavioral health documentation often includes the 100-point scale **global assessment of functioning (GAF)**, which reflects the clinician's judgment of the individual's overall level of functioning and carrying out activities of daily living.

Conservatorship

When a person is unable to provide for personal needs such as food, shelter, or clothing as the result of a mental disorder, and thereby is gravely disabled and unwilling or incapable of accepting voluntary treatment, he may be recommended for **conservatorship** placement—that is, placed under the care of an appointed guardian. Mental health conservatorship requirements vary from state to state. Acceptable conservatorship documents are created by attorneys and the courts in each state and may differ in format. Conservatorship documents become part of the health record.

Behavioral Health Record Content

The acute psychiatric healthcare record contains a number of assessments and reports pertaining to the patient's treatment.

Psychiatric Assessment

This assessment identifies the client's physical, cognitive, behavioral, emotional, and social status. It also identifies facilitating factors and possible barriers to the patient goals beyond the presenting problems. See **Figure 13.7** for items to be included in the psychiatric assessment.

FIGURE 13.7. Areas to cover in the initial psychiatric assessment

AREA	SOME ELEMENTS
Psychiatric history	Known diagnoses Previous treatments, including drugs and hospitalizations
Medical and family health history	Known disorders Current drugs and treatments
Social history	Education level Marital history Employment history Legal history, including arrests and incarcerations Living arrangements
Developmental history	Family composition and atmosphere during childhood Behavior during schooling Sexual adaptation and experiences
Daily conduct	Use or abuse of alcohol, drugs, and tobacco
Potential for harm to self or others	Suicidal thoughts and plans Intent to harm others

Source: Adapted from *Merck Manual* (2011).

Medical and Psychiatric History

A complete history documents the client's current complaints and symptoms, includes a review of systems, and details her medical, social, and family history.

Physical Examination Report

The physical examination report represents the attending physician's assessment of the patient's current health status. This report should document information on all of the patient's major organ systems or body areas.

Mental Status Exam

The mental status exam is as crucial to psychiatry as the physical exam is to other areas of medicine. Adolf Meyer developed this exam in 1918. He believed that it was important to ask the same questions of every patient so that certain standards could be achieved. The exam describes various mental functions, including appearance, speech, thought process, behavior, affect, orientation, memory, mood, motor skills, intellect, judgment, and insight.

Diagnostic and Therapeutic Orders

Physician's orders are the instructions the physician gives the other healthcare professionals who actually perform diagnostic tests and treatments, administer medications, and provide specific services to a patient. These orders must be legible and must include the date and the physician's signature in a paper-based health record.

Standing orders are orders the medical staff or an individual physician has established as routine care for a specific diagnosis or procedure. Standing orders are commonly used in hospitals, ambulatory surgery facilities, and long-term care facilities. Usually standing orders are preprinted on a single sheet of paper, unless an electronic health record (EHR) is used and the orders are selected from the EHR system. Like other physician's orders, they must be signed, dated, and included in the patient's health record.

Physicians may communicate orders verbally or via telephone when the healthcare organization's policies and procedures or medical staff rules allow. State law and medical staff rules specify which practitioners are allowed to accept and execute verbal and telephone orders. How the orders are to be authenticated and the time period allowed for authentication should also be specified.

Restraint and Seclusion Orders

Specific documentation guidelines and procedures to follow with regard to the use of restraint and seclusion procedures vary by state. However, the guidelines to follow in these matters are those outlined in the Joint Commission's *Comprehensive Accreditation Manual for Behavioral Health Care (CAMBHC)* which is updated annually.

Refer to the "Seclusion and Restraints" section on page 610 for additional discussion regarding seclusion and restraints.

Consultation Reports

Consultation reports document clinical opinions requested from physicians outside the case by the patient's primary or attending physician. They are based on the consulting physicians' examination of the client and a review of the client's health record.

Diagnostic and Therapeutic Procedure Reports

The results of all diagnostic and therapeutic procedures are also included in the patient's health record. Diagnostic procedures consist of laboratory tests performed on blood, urine, and other samples from the patient.

Mandated Reporting

Many states mandate that certain types of reports be completed and forwarded to the appropriate authorities. (Not all are documented in the health record, although a notation may be made in certain circumstances). Examples of mandated reports include, but are not limited to:

- Abuse reports (domestic, child, and elder abuse)

- Tuberculosis

- HIV

- Sexually transmitted diseases

- Legal/police reports, including recommendation to revoke a driver's license

- Duty-to-warn report: Mental health professionals have a duty to warn reasonably identifiable victims when there are known serious threats of violence against them where there is clear evidence of danger to the client or other persons. Most states title these reports differently (for example, in California, the Tarasoff Report [*Tarasoff v. Regents of the University of California* 1976]).

- Possessing, receiving, or purchasing firearms within five years of admission to a behavioral care facility (California Department of Justice 2004)

Treatment/Care Plans

Treatment or care plans are developed based on the patient's needs as identified via the assessments. Plans must specify the patient's goals and objectives, the actions or interventions needed to meet them, and time frames in which to accomplish them. Patients are to be involved in the formulation of their plans and asked for input. They also are asked to agree to the planned course of treatment, care, or services. Each state defines the types of professionals in that state who may act as case managers. Case managers prepare assessments and care plans, which then are included in the client's health record. Care plans are updated when clinically appropriate and when required by organizational policy, state guidelines, and clinical protocols.

Treatment/care plans may be documented via the following:

- Handwritten notes

- EHRs

- Standards of practice

- Decision algorithms

- Clinical protocols or maps

- Individualized preprinted plans of care

Richard Zwolinski (2010) articulates the essential rules for therapy and treatment plans:

1. A mental health treatment plan should be based on a comprehensive and thorough psychosocial evaluation.

2. A mental health treatment plan should be a written plan created by the therapist and patient/client together (except in cases where a severely disabled patient may not be able to contribute).

3. A mental health treatment plan must contain information about a patient's problems, patient's goals, patient's and therapist's objectives, target dates and check-ins, partners in therapy, recommendations, schedule of services, amendments and changes and any other information deemed necessary to successful treatment (though the actual format and names for this information may vary with each therapist).

4. A mental health treatment plan should be referred to during many if not most therapy sessions and both therapist and patient should have access to the plan.

5. A mental health treatment plan is a living, breathing document—it can and should flex and change as treatment progresses.

6. A mental health treatment plan must contain what we can call a "reconstruct clause"; that is, a written clause that states that if goals and objectives are not completed within a certain time-frame, the therapist and patient will revisit the therapist's methods and techniques and the patient's commitment to therapy and decide if they warrant a major change of approach or perhaps even a referral to a new therapist.

7. Any and all courses of therapy or counseling should be based on and utilize a mental health treatment plan.

Outpatient Crisis Plan

Because of the nature of mental illness, clients often develop crisis plans with their therapists. A crisis plan might be viewed in the same way that an advance directive is viewed for individuals in an acute care setting. The crisis plan is the client's direction on what to do and whom to contact should he become mentally incapable of communicating his wishes. The crisis plan does not supersede an advance directive but, rather, complements it.

Progress Notes

In psychiatric settings, clinical observations are typically documented in progress notes. The purpose of such documentation is to create a chronological report of the patient's condition and response to treatment during her course of treatment.

The rules and regulations of the healthcare organization specify which healthcare providers are allowed to enter progress notes into the health record. Typically, these individuals include the patient's attending physician, any consulting physicians who have medical staff privileges, house medical staff, nurses, nutritionists, social workers, and clinical therapists. Depending on the record format the hospital uses, observations may be combined in a single record or separated by discipline.

Progress notes serve to justify further treatment in the facility. In addition, they document the appropriateness and coordination of the services provided. For Medicare purposes, each note must be able to stand alone and justify medical necessity independently.

Nurses keep chronological records of the patient's vital signs (blood pressure, heart rate, respiration rate, and temperature) throughout her hospital stay. Increasingly, vital signs are routinely taken at outpatient care programs. Nurses often keep separate logs showing what medications were ordered and when they were administered.

Diagnostic Information

While the ICD-9-CM is used in reimbursement, behavioral healthcare documentation often reflects the *DSM-IV*. For each disorder included in the *DSM-IV*, a set of diagnostic criteria indicates what symptoms must be present (and for how long) to qualify for a diagnosis and what symptoms must not be present. The *DSM-IV* systematically describes each disorder under the following headings: Diagnostic Features; Subtypes and/or Specifiers; Recording Procedures; Associated Features and Disorders; Specific Culture, Age, and Gender Features; Prevalence; Course; Familial Pattern; and Differential Diagnosis. Diagnoses are categorized into one of five axes:

- Axis I: Clinical Disorders (also includes most V-Codes and conditions that need clinical attention)

- Diagnosis Flow Charts

- Axis II: Personality Disorders and Mental Retardation

- Axis III: General Medical Conditions

- Axis IV: Psychosocial and Environmental Problems

- Axis V: Global Assessment of Functioning Scale

Consent to Treatment

Many healthcare facilities obtain consent to treatment from patients or their legal representatives before providing care or services except in emergency situations. The consent to treatment documents the patient's permission to receive routine services, diagnostic procedures, and medical care. The need to obtain the patient's consent before medical and surgical procedures is based on the legal concept of battery, which is the unlawful touching of a person without his implied or expressed consent.

Individual states may have laws or regulations that define the content of authorizations. When such laws or regulations exist, the treatment program should consult the HIPAA (1996) Privacy Rule to determine how to apply the state requirements.

Implied consent is assumed when a patient voluntarily submits to treatment. The rationale behind implied consent is that one can reasonably assume that the patient understands the nature of the treatment. Expressed consent is a consent that is either spoken or written. Although courts recognize both verbal and written consent, verbal consent is more difficult to prove.

It is primarily the physician's responsibility to ensure that the patient understands the nature of the procedure, alternative treatments, and the procedure's risks, complications, and benefits before it is performed. Medical staff rules or healthcare provider policies usually list the types of services and procedures that require written consent from the patient. Generally, procedures involving the use of anesthetics, the administration of experimental drugs, electroconvulsive therapy, and significant risk of complications require written consent. In addition, some states have passed laws that require written consent forms for certain types of testing procedures (for example, HIV testing).

Advance Directives

An **advance directive** is a written document that names the patient's choice of legal representative for healthcare purposes. The person designated by the patient is then empowered to make healthcare decisions on behalf of the patient in the event the patient is no longer capable of expressing his preferences. **Living wills** and **durable powers of attorney** for healthcare are two examples of advance directives.

Certifications for Holds, Restraints, or Seclusion

When a treating psychiatrist or psychologist finds a patient to be a danger to others or herself or to be gravely disabled as defined by state law, the patient may be held against her will for a certain period, depending on state statute. In some states, the patient can request a judicial review. Patients also may petition the treating physician regarding capacity to consent or refuse antipsychotic medication.

Documentation of Conservatorship

As noted earlier, behavioral health patients may require documentation of conservatorship. This may be recommended when a person is unable to provide for himself. Conservatorship documents become part of the health record.

Refer to page 613 for further discussion of conservatorship.

Discharge Summaries and Client Instructions

The discharge summary is a concise account of the patient's illness, course of treatment, response to treatment, and condition at the time of discharge from the service. The functions of the discharge summary include the following:

- Ensures the continuity of future care by providing information to the patient's attending physician, referring physician, and any consulting physicians

- Provides concise information that can be used to answer information requests from authorized individuals or entities

The discharge summary must be signed by the attending physician. However, there are some exceptions to this rule. For example, some states allow nurses to sign discharge summaries in chemical dependency programs.

The discharge summary also includes instructions for the patient's follow-up care. It is vital that the client or her caregiver be given clear, concise instructions. Ideally, those instructions are communicated both verbally and in writing. The healthcare professional who provides them should sign the health record to indicate that verbal instructions have been issued. In addition, the person receiving the instructions should sign to verify that she understands them. A copy of the written instructions is then filed in the health record.

When someone other than the patient assumes responsibility for the patient's aftercare, the record should indicate that the instructions were given to the party responsible. Documentation of patient education may be accomplished through forms that prompt the person providing instruction to cover important information.

Despite the best efforts of hospital caregivers and physicians, some patients die while hospitalized. In such cases, the attending physician should add a summary statement to the patient's health record documenting the circumstances surrounding the patient's death. The statement can take the form of a final progress note or a separate report, sometimes referred to as the death summary. It should indicate the reason for the client's admission, his diagnosis and course in the hospital, and a description of the events that led to his death.

Information Pertaining to Emergency Care

Emergency care services are primarily delivered in hospital-based emergency departments and freestanding psychiatric hospitals. However, they are also provided in the field by various outreach programs that include psychiatric emergency response teams working in conjunction with the police or emergency medical services. Emergency care documentation is limited to information about the patient's presenting problem and the diagnostic and therapeutic services provided during the episode of care. The services provided in emergency situations focus on diagnosing the problem and stabilizing the patient. Unlike physical illness, in which minor injuries and illnesses may require no further medical treatment, psychiatric emergency patients must be referred to ambulatory care providers for follow-up care. Seriously ill patients are admitted to a hospital for ongoing acute psychiatric care treatment. If the client is determined to be incompetent to provide for her own care, she may be admitted against her will.

Emergency care records must document the instructions or care plan given to the patient as well as the patient's presenting complaint, evaluation, and assessment. Thorough documentation is needed to justify reimbursement, to protect the organization or the patient in future legal proceedings, and to ensure continuity of care.

The following information must be entered into the patient's health record for each emergency care visit:

- Patient's identification (or the reason it could not be obtained)

- Time and means of the patient's arrival at the organization

- Pertinent history of the illness or injury and physical findings, including the patient's vital signs

- Emergency care given to the patient prior to arrival

- Diagnostic and therapeutic orders

- Clinical observations, including the results of treatment

- Reports of procedures, tests, and results

- Diagnostic impression

- Conclusion at the termination of evaluation/treatment, including final disposition, the patient's condition on discharge or transfer, and any instructions given to the patient, the patient's representative, or another healthcare facility for follow-up care

- Documentation of the patient leaving the hospital or emergency department against medical advice, if applicable

Individuals with mental illnesses are encouraged to seek treatment voluntarily, but some individuals may need to be involuntarily admitted for evaluation and treatment. In these cases, a bill of rights for the person who is mentally ill provides a system of due process.

Behavioral Health Accreditation, Regulation, Industry, and Advocacy

Numerous forces in the healthcare environment affect behavioral healthcare and documentation. These forces come from several sources, including accrediting bodies, governmental regulations and recommendations, and changes in the healthcare industry.

Accrediting Bodies

Five widely accepted entities accredit behavioral healthcare organizations: The Joint Commission, the Commission on Accreditation of Rehabilitation Facilities (CARF), the American Osteopathic Association (AOA), the National Committee for Quality Assurance (NCQA), and the Council on Accreditation (COA). These entities issue accreditation and documentation standards that behavioral healthcare organizations may use as benchmarks.

The Joint Commission

The Joint Commission bases its accreditation outcome on the ability of the healthcare organization to demonstrate compliance with specific performance standards. The Joint Commission began accrediting behavioral healthcare facilities in 1971. The accreditation process includes an on-site survey by an interdisciplinary survey team that evaluates on-going compliance with the performance standards specific to the healthcare setting (Joint Commission 2003).

The Joint Commission has specific documentation requirements for behavioral healthcare. Joint Commission Standard IM.6.10 requires behavioral healthcare facilities to maintain complete and accurate medical records for patients assessed, cared for, treated, or served. Medical records must be reviewed on an ongoing basis at the point of care. See **Figure 13.8** for a sample record review (audit) form. This review form details The Joint Commission's documentation requirements for behavioral healthcare organizations.

Behavioral healthcare services currently accredited include mental health care, addiction services, and child welfare and developmentally disabled care in a variety of treatment settings. Depending on the type of state licensure and the funding source, some behavioral healthcare organizations continue to be surveyed under the hospital standards instead of the behavioral health standards.

As in other healthcare settings, Joint Commission accreditation includes an intensive onsite survey process at least once every three years.

In March 2010, The Joint Commission Standards and Survey Procedures Committee approved significant updates and revisions to the current Provision of Care, Treatment, and Services standards for behavioral health care, which went into effective January 1, 2011. Documentation requirements can be found under the following categories:

I. Entry to Care, Treatment, or Services

II. Screening and Assessment

III. Planning Care, Treatment, or Services

IV. Delivery of Care, Treatment, or Services

V. Special Behavioral Procedures

VI. Continuity of Care, Treatment, or Services

Commission on Accreditation of Rehabilitation Facilities

The CARF is similar to The Joint Commission in that it is a not-for-profit organization devoted to ensuring continuous quality improvement in healthcare. However, CARF specifically accredits organizations for quality excellence in rehabilitative and human services. Like The Joint Commission, CARF has developed performance standards that a healthcare organization must meet to pass the survey process (CARF 2011a).

CARF has specific behavioral health standards and surveys a variety of behavioral health settings, including mental health care, substance-abuse care, and other addiction programs. The CARF General Program Standards, Section 2G for behavioral healthcare documentation, state that the individual records must communicate information in

FIGURE 13.8. Sample behavioral healthcare ongoing record review form

	Reviewer Signature						Date						
Date:													
Unit:													
REVIEW QUESTIONS	Enter review date in boxes below												
	Yes							No: Corrected			N/A		
General Information													
Patient identification data on all pages													
All consents completed and signed as required													
Compliance with prohibited abbreviations													
Documentation of "Read back" for telephone order/ critical values (within time frame)													
Times and means of patient arrival													
Documentation if "Left against medical advice"													
Conclusions at termination of treatment, including final disposition, condition, and instructions for follow-up care, treatment, and services (at D/C)													
Initial Screenings & Assessment													
Nursing assessment/documentation complete (no blanks)													
Is there documentation in the computer that the patient was asked about advance directives?													
Is a copy of the advance directive present on the record?													
Is there documentation of the pain scale used to assess the patient's pain?													
Is pain reassessed and pain med effectiveness documented?													
Evidence/documentation that the following screenings/ assessments were performed at point of entry and upon admission according to practice:													
a. Current medication list for reconciliation													
b. Nutritional screening for diet, meals													
c. Universal screening for abuse													
d. Immunizations													
e. Spiritual/educational and cultural needs													
f. Discharge needs													
g. Hx of violence													
h. Fall risk score													
i. Drug/alcohol/tobacco use													

FIGURE 13.8. (continued)

Interdisciplinary care plan:	Yes								No: Corrected			N/A
Is present												
All required elements complete—strength/weakness												
All required signatures present, including patient's												
Reassessment												
Are reassessments documented every shift and when a change occurs in the patient condition?												
Is there documentation of the patient's response to all interventions, including response to medications?												
Documentation of Care												
Is the care plan revised in response to changes in patient condition or in response to changes in the assessments of other disciplines involved in the care?												
Is there documentation of multidisciplinary discharge planning?												
Is there documentation of discharge instructions/ education to patient and/or family?												
Documentation of all elements on graphics present												
Thorough and complete documentation when seclusion/ restraint interventions are utilized												
Physician Care												
Documentation of diagnosis, condition, or indication for—use for each medication ordered												
H&P within 24 hours or documentation of ongoing attempts in progress notes												
Evidence of clinical interpretation of test reports												
Patient and Family Education												
Is there evidence in the record that the education process considers the physical, cognitive, cultural, social, and economic characteristics of the patient?												
Is there evidence that the patient's education is based on the assessed needs, abilities, preferences, and readiness to learn?												
Is there documentation of teaching delivered by appropriate staff or between disciplines?												
Is there documentation that the patient/family has been offered education as appropriate on:												
a. Safe and effective use of medications												
b. Nutrition interventions: modified diet/oral health												
c. Available community resources												
d. Self-care activities/smoking cessation												
e. Discharge instructions												

a manner that is organized, clear, complete, current, and legible. All documents that require signatures must have original or electronic signatures (CARF 2011b).

An individual's record must include the following:

- The date of admission

- Information about the individual's personal representative, conservator, guardian, or representative payee, if any of these have been appointed, including the name, address, and telephone number

- Information about the person to contact in the event of an emergency, including the name, address, and telephone number

- The name of the person currently coordinating the services of the person served

- The location of any other records

- Information about the individual's primary-care physician, including the name, address, and telephone number, when available

- Healthcare reimbursement information, if applicable

- The person's

  - Health history

  - Current medications

  - Preadmission screening, when conducted

  - Documentation of orientation

  - Assessments (see **FIGURES 13.9** and **13.10** for sample psychiatric assessment forms)

  - Individual plan, including reviews

  - Transition plan, when applicable

The discharge summary must include the following elements:

- Date of admission and date of discharge

- Identification of the presenting condition

- Description of the extent to which established goals and objectives were achieved

- Description of the services provided

- The reasons for discharge

- The status of the person served at discharge

- A list of recommendations for services or supports

See Figure 5.14 (p. 222) for a sample discharge form.

FIGURE 13.9. Sample psychiatric assessment form

This is a psychiatric assessment billed as an MMD provided on-site for _____ minutes.

PRESENTING PROBLEM:

      IDENTIFYING DATA/CHIEF COMPLAINT:

      HISTORY OF PRESENT ILLNESS:

CURRENT NEEDS:

      PAST PSYCHIATRIC HISTORY:

DRUG/ALCOHOL HISTORY:

      MEDICAL HISTORY:

      SOCIAL HISTORY:

      CULTURAL & RELIGIOUS ISSUES:

      INSURANCE STATUS:

      VITAL SIGNS:
        Blood pressure: _____ **Temperature:** _____ **Pulse rate:** _____ **Respiratory rate:** _____ **Pain (0-10):** ____

MENTAL STATUS EXAMINATION:

DIAGNOSIS:

      Axis I:
      Axis II:
      Axis III:
      Axis IV:
      Axis V: **GAF Current:**   **Past year:**

CURRENT POTENTIAL FOR HARM:

INTERPRETIVE SUMMARY:

_____
          STAFF PSYCHIATRIST

County of San Diego **Health and Human Services Agency** Mental Health Services SAN DIEGO COUNTY PSYCHIATRIC HOSPITAL PSYCHIATRIC ASSESSMENT	**Patient Name:** **MR#:** **Unit:** **D.O.B.:** **Date**

HHSA:MHS-204

Source: County of San Diego (2002c).

FIGURE 13.10. Sample initial mental health assessment form

Assessment Date:_____

PRESENTING PROBLEM: (Identifying Data/Chief Complaint and History of Present Illness. Summarize client's request for services, **including client's subjective description of the problem.** Include precipitating factors, objective impairing behaviors, including experiences and stigma, if any, and prejudice and client's requests/needs.)

_____
_____
_____
_____
_____
_____
_____
_____
_____
_____
_____
_____
_____

PAST PSYCHIATRIC HISTORY: (Previous mental health treatment—where, when, for how long. Include dates/providers related to any prior psychiatric treatment, history, traumatic and/or significant events; include immigration history, and impact, if any).

_____
_____
_____
_____
_____
_____
_____
_____
_____
_____
_____
_____
_____
_____

FAMILY HISTORY:_____
_____
_____
_____

Any family members with a history of any of the following? (Please, check all that apply)

	Depression	Schizophrenia	Bipolar	Substance Abuse	Suicide	Other	Effective Treatments
Parent							
Sibling							
Children							
Aunt/Uncle							
Grandparent							

County of San Diego
Health and Human Services Agency
Mental Health Services

INITIAL MENTAL HEALTH ASSESSMENT

HHSA:MHS-912 (6/2003)

Client:_____

MR/Client ID #:_____

Program:_____

Page 1 of 5

FIGURE 13.10. (continued)

CULTURE/FAMILY and RECOVERY POTENTIAL:

Birthplace: ( ) San Diego ( ) USA ( ) Other (fill in birthplace and year moved to USA):_____

Language of choice for therapy: ☐English ☐Spanish ☐Vietnamese ☐Other (fill in language)_____

Ethnicity: ☐ Latino/Hispanic ☐ African American ☐ Asian/Pacific Islander (fill in):_____

☐ White ☐ American Indian ☐ Other (fill in):_____

Culture-specific symptomatology/explanations for behavior (may reference Appendix I of DSM-IV-TR):_____
_____
_____

Family/Community Support System: (Live alone? Describe it, including alternative relationship support, if any. Who is supportive? Community groups, e.g., AA/NA)
_____
_____

Socioeconomic Factors: (educational achievement, occupation, income source, and level)
_____
_____

Religious/Spiritual Issues: (Is R/S important in your life? If yes, is it a source of strength in your recovery process? Describe how/who: persons, practices.)
_____
_____
_____

ASSETS/STRENGTHS: (What abilities or skills do you have that you would choose to develop during your recovery? What new ones might you choose to develop?)
_____
_____
_____

MEDICAL HISTORY: (Indicate any significant medical history related to client's current mental health condition, including dates/providers related to prior treatment, as well as client's adjustment to co-occurring disabilities.)
_____
_____
_____
_____

Current Medication(s)	*Dose*	Frequency	Taken as Prescribed?
			☐YES ☐NO
			☐YES ☐NO
			☐YES ☐NO
			☐YES ☐NO

ALLERGIES AND ADVERSE MEDICATION REACTIONS:

☐ NKA(s)

☐ Other (s)_____

HEALING AND HEALTH: (Alternative healing practices/beliefs. Apart from mental health professionals, who—or what—helps you deal with disability/illness? Describe.)
_____
_____
_____

County of San Diego Health and Human Services Agency Mental Health Services	Client:_____
	MR/Client ID #:_____
INITIAL MENTAL HEALTH ASSESSMENT	Program:_____
HHSA:MHS-912 (6/2003)	Page 2 of 5

FIGURE 13.10. (continued)

NAME OF CURRENT PRIMARY CARE PHYSICIAN:
May we consult? ☐Yes ☐No   **Date Last Seen:** _____   **Release of Information Form:** ☐Yes ☐No

_____

Name   Address   Phone number (including area code)

CLIENT'S HOSPITAL OF CHOICE:

_____

Name   Address   Phone number (including area code)

SUBSTANCE USE INFORMATION: Indicate if no history of use ☐   History unknown ☐

Type:	Date of Last Use	Amount of Last Use	Frequency and Amount of Use	Length of Time Using	Age of First Use
_____	_____	_____	_____	_____	_____
_____	_____	_____	_____	_____	_____
_____	_____	_____	_____	_____	_____
_____	_____	_____	_____	_____	_____
_____	_____	_____	_____	_____	_____
_____	_____	_____	_____	_____	_____

MENTAL STATUS EXAM:

Level of Consciousness:	☐ Alert	☐ Lethargic	☐ Stuporous		
Orientation:	☐ Person	☐ Place	Time ☐ Day ☐ Month ☐ Year	☐ Current Situation	☐ None
Appearance:	☐ Clean	☐ Well-Nourished	☐ Malodorous	☐ Disheveled	☐ Malnourished	☐ Reddened Eyes
Speech:	☐ Normal	☐ Slurred	☐ Loud	☐ Pressured	☐ Slow	☐ Mute
Thought Process:	☐ Coherent	☐ Tangential	☐ Circumstantial	☐ Incoherent	☐ Loose Association	
Behavior:	☐ Cooperative	☐ Evasive	☐ Uncooperative	☐ Threatening	☐ Agitated	☐ Combative
Affect:	☐ Appropriate	☐ Blunted	☐ Flat	☐ Restricted	☐ Labile	☐ Other
Intellect:	☐ Normal	☐ Below Normal	☐ Paucity of Knowledge	☐ Vocabulary Poor	☐ Poor Abstraction	☐ Uncooperative
Mood:	☐ Euthymic	☐ Elevated	☐ Euphoric	☐ Depressed	☐ Anxious	☐ Irritable
Memory:	☐ Normal	☐ Poor Recent	☐ Poor Remote	☐ Inability to Concentrate	☐ Confabulation	☐ Amnesia
Judgment:	☐ Normal	☐ Poor	☐ Unrealistic	☐ Unmotivated	☐ Uncertain	
Motor:	☐ Normal	☐ Decreased	☐ Agitated	☐ Tremors	☐ Tics	☐ Repetitive Motions
Insight:	☐ Normal	☐ Adequate	☐ Marginal	☐ Poor		

Note: A narrative mental status exam may be done on a progress note, in lieu of above.

County of San Diego
Health and Human Services Agency
Mental Health Services

INITIAL MENTAL HEALTH ASSESSMENT

HHSA:MHS-912 (6/2003)

Client:_____

MR/Client ID #:_____

Program:_____

Page 3 of 5

FIGURE 13.10. (continued)

| Visual Hallucinations: | ☐No | ☐Yes | Specify:_____ |

Visual Hallucinations: ☐No ☐Yes Specify:_____

Auditory Hallucinations: ☐No ☐Yes Specify:_____

Delusions: ☐No ☐Yes Specify:_____

Other Information (optional):_____

<u>**POTENTIAL FOR HARM:**</u> (Include risk factors, e.g., chronic illness, recent loss of job, age)

Current SI: ☐ No ☐ Yes Specify plan (method, vague, passive, imminent):_____

_____

_____

Access to means: ☐ No ☐ Yes Specify:_____

Previous Attempts: ☐ No ☐ Yes Specify:_____

_____

_____

Client Contract for Safety: ☐ No ☐ Yes Specify in Progress Notes:_____

Current III: ☐ No ☐ Yes Specify Plan (vague, intent, with/without means):_____

_____

_____

_____

Identified Victim: ☐ No ☐ Yes Name and Contact Information:_____

_____

☐ No ☐ Yes Tarasoff warning: _____

Client No Harm Contract: ☐ No ☐ Yes Specify in Progress Notes:_____

History of Violence: ☐ No ☐ Yes Specify Type (past, current):_____

_____

History of Domestic Violence: _____

History of Abuse: ☐ No ☐ Yes Specify Type (past, current):_____

_____

_____

Abuse Reported: ☐ No ☐ Yes

Probation Officer Contact Info:

_____

Name   Address   Phone (including Area Code)

<u>**CONVICTION OF FELONY AND JAIL TIME:**</u> ☐ No ☐ Yes

<u>What was the conviction for? Length of jail time?</u>

_____

_____

DSM IV DIAGNOSIS: Impairment/Disability Use DSM-IV-TR Codes. Indicate (P) – Primary and (S) – Secondary	**Enter P in front of primary**	**DIAGNOSTIC CODE**
AXIS I		
AXIS I		
AXIS I		
AXIS II		
AXIS III Relevant Medical Conditions:		
AXIS IV Psychosocial and Environmental Problems:		
AXIS V Current GAF: **Highest in Past Year:**		

County of San Diego
Health and Human Services Agency
Mental Health Services

INITIAL MENTAL HEALTH ASSESSMENT

HHSA:MHS-912 (6/2003)

Client:_____

MR/Client ID #:_____

Program:_____

Page 4 of 5

FIGURE 13.10. (continued)

INTERPRETIVE SUMMARY: (Justification for diagnosis. Summarize and integrate all information gathered from other sources to render clinical judgments regarding intensity, length of treatment, and recommendations for services. Clearly state those emotional or behavioral symptoms that interfere with normal functioning. Include evaluation of client's ability and willingness to solve the client's presenting problem.)

_____
_____
_____
_____
_____
_____
_____
_____
_____
_____
_____
_____
_____

_____

Medical Necessity Met: ☐ Yes ☐ No   NOA Issued: ☐ Yes ☐ No (Medi-Cal Clients only)

REHABILITATION/RECOVERY/RECOMMENDATIONS: (List in-house clinical services as well as names of agencies/clinicians currently being received or recommended.)

1. ☐ Assisted Living Services	7. ☐ Employment Services	13. ☐ RAP Plan
2. ☐ Community Services	8. ☐ Group Therapy	14. ☐ Recovery Programs/Socialization Services
3. ☐ Case Management Services	9. ☐ Housing Services	15. ☐ Substance Abuse
4. ☐ Crisis Residential/Hospitalization	10. ☐ Individual Therapy	16. ☐ Support Group
5. ☐ Day Rehabilitation	11. ☐ Medical Treatment	17. ☐ Other
6. ☐ Education/Support	12. ☐ Medication Management	

Number and explain below:

_____ ☐ Current: _____

_____ ☐ Proposed Referral: _____

_____ ☐ Current: _____

_____ ☐ Proposed Referral: _____

_____ ☐ Current: _____

_____ ☐ Proposed Referral: _____

_____ ☐ Current: _____

_____ ☐ Proposed Referral: _____

_____ ☐ Current: _____

_____ ☐ Proposed Referral: _____

Completed by: _____   _____   _____   _____
             Signature   Title   Date   Time Spent

Cosignature: _____   _____   _____
(if required)   Signature   Title   Date

County of San Diego Health and Human Services Agency Mental Health Services **INITIAL MENTAL HEALTH ASSESSMENT** HHSA:MHS-912 (6/2003)	**Client:** _____ **MR/Client ID #:** _____ **Program:** _____ Page 5 of 5

Source: County of San Diego (2003).

Other items to include are correspondence pertinent to the person served, authorization for release of information, and documentation of internal or external referrals.

Entries should be made to the records of the persons served within the time frame specified by the organization's policy. If duplicate information or reports from the main record of a person served exist, or if working files are maintained, such materials are not substituted for the main record; are considered secondary documents, with the main record of the person served receiving first priority; and are maintained in such a manner as to protect confidentiality. See chapter 5 for additional discussion of documentation policies and procedures. In the behavioral healthcare setting, policies and procedures will mirror those used in acute care, except for those situations noted in this chapter.

American Osteopathic Association

The AOA accredits mental health, substance abuse, and several other types of organizations under the Healthcare Facilities Accreditation Program (HFAP). It was developed in 1943 and implemented in 1945 for annual hospital surveys (AOA 2007).

Eligibility requirements specify that behavioral healthcare organizations do the following (AOA 2007):

- Meet state licensing requirements

- Have bylaws that specify acceptance of the HFAP certification process

- Have operated for at least three months prior to application

- Meet basic service requirements as well as requirements based on the type of organization seeking accreditation

National Committee for Quality Assurance

The NCQA was established in 1990 and began its accreditation program for **managed behavioral healthcare organizations (MBHOs)** in 1997. NCQA has been a central figure in driving improvement throughout the healthcare system, helping to elevate the issue of healthcare quality to the top of the national agenda (NCQA 2011).

Its accreditation model is based on the specific organization type or services provided. For example, if providing medical care under a **managed care organization (MCO)** and behavioral health services, standards for both the MCO and MBHO are used in the accreditation survey. Eligibility requirements are specific to the type of accreditation or certification being sought.

NCQA accreditation includes a rigorous review against standards for improving behavioral healthcare access and services and the process of credentialing practitioners (NCQA 2011). For MBHOs this includes the following:

- Quality management and improvement

- Utilization management

- Credentialing and recredentialing

- Members' rights and responsibilities

- Preventive health

The NCQA's accreditation of MBHOs rewards organizations that focus on quality (NCQA 2007). The NCQA has developed a report card for MBHOs to inform the public of how well they meet quality-of-care standards as developed by NCQA. These reports help to drive the healthcare system to a higher level of performance.

The NCQA MBHO accreditation program is designed to:

- Foster accountability among MBHOs for the quality of care and services that members receive

- Provide employers, public purchasers, plans, and consumers with meaningful information regarding MBHOs

- Strengthen MBHO systems for population-based continuous quality improvement programs

- Encourage effectiveness in the provision of behavioral healthcare by addressing the need for prevention, early intervention, and coordination of behavioral healthcare with medical care

The NCQA's focus is to provide information that enables consumers to make informed healthcare decisions and choices.

Council on Accreditation

The COA was founded in 1977 by the Child Welfare League of America and Family Service America. Currently, 98 programs or services can be accredited under COA. Those related to behavioral health include the following:

- Mental health services

- Psychosocial and psychiatric rehabilitation services

- Case management services

- Counseling services

- Treatment/therapeutic foster care

- Day treatment services

COA accredits human service and behavioral healthcare organizations using a community-based social services model. The healthcare organization, in general, is accredited, as are specific individual programs. Organizations seeking COA accreditation can be public or private, can be not-for-profit or for-profit, and must provide at least one service for which COA has developed standards. All required licensures or certifications must be obtained, and the organization must be able to demonstrate its independence for review as a legal entity.

An organization is evaluated against best-practice standards, which are developed using a consensus model with input from a wide range of service providers, funders, experts, policy makers, and consumers.

Accreditation is based on quality documentation. Required behavioral healthcare documentation elements include the following (COA 2008).

Screening assessments:

- Identifying information, including name, date of birth, and Social Security number (if available)

- Current residence

- Emergency health needs

- Emergency contacts (if any)

- Safety, imminent danger, or risk of future harm, as applicable

- Legal status

Comprehensive basic assessments:

- Information gathered for a screening/intake assessment

- A preliminary evaluation of the request or need for service

- The person's and/or family's strengths and resources

- Family relationships and formal and informal support systems

- The person's past or current use of services from this organization or other organizations

- Independent living skills, activities of daily living assessment, as applicable

- A screening for family violence, abuse or neglect, or exploitation

- Mental health status and developmental screening, as applicable

- Trauma screening

- Alcohol and other drug use screening

- Educational and vocational information

- Financial status, including financial assistance and insurance coverage

- Housing status, history, and a description of living conditions

- Other information necessary to provide services

Comprehensive psychosocial assessments:

- Information gathered for the screening/intake assessment and basic assessment

- Psychiatric issues

- A mental status exam

- Alcohol and other drug use assessment

- Assessment of nonsubstance addictive behaviors

Government Regulation

Some of the more influential government agencies affecting delivery of behavioral healthcare are Centers for Medicare and Medicaid Services (CMS), the HIPAA Privacy Rule, and the Substance Abuse and Mental Health Services Administration (SAMHSA).

Centers for Medicare and Medicaid Services

The CMS is a division of the US Department of Health and Human Services (HHS). CMS plays an integral role in the quality of care provided to those individuals who use the behavioral healthcare system. It monitors expenses related to behavioral healthcare and provides mental health benefits to eligible recipients through its Medicare program (CMS 2010a). Additionally, CMS oversees the quality improvement organizations (QIOs), which monitor medical necessity, quality of care, and the appropriateness of reimbursed services in behavioral healthcare settings.

Behavioral healthcare organizations that participate in the Medicare program must comply with federal standards issued by the CMS called the Conditions of Participation (COP) (CMS 2006). Standard 482.61 addresses special health record requirements for inpatient psychiatric hospitals and states: "the medical records maintained by a psychiatric hospital must permit determination of the degree and intensity of the treatment provided to individuals who are furnished services in the institution." In other words, the documentation must support the amount and level of services provided. A facility's documentation policies must be developed in alignment with these requirements to be in compliance.

Documentation standards specified in the COP for psychiatric hospitals include the following:

- **Development of assessment/diagnostic data:** Health records must stress the psychiatric components of the record, including history of findings and treatment provided for the psychiatric condition for which the patient is hospitalized.

- **Psychiatric evaluation:** Each patient must receive a psychiatric evaluation within 60 hours of admission. It must include a medical history noting the mental status of the patient, the onset of illness and circumstances leading to admission, attitudes and behavior, and intellectual and memory functioning.

- **Treatment plan:** Each patient must have an individual comprehensive treatment plan based on an inventory of the patient's strengths and disabilities. The treatment must be documented in such a way as to ensure that all active therapeutic efforts are included.

- **Recording progress:** Progress notes must be recorded by the doctor responsible for the care of the patient, the nurse, the social worker, and, when appropriate, others significantly involved in active treatment. The frequency of progress notes is determined by the condition of the patient, but they must be recorded at least weekly for the first two months and at least once a month thereafter. Progress notes must contain recommendations for revisions in the treatment plan as indicated and precise assessment of the patient's progress in accordance with the original or revised treatment plan.

- **Discharge planning and discharge summary:** The health record must have a discharge summary that includes a summary of the patient's hospitalization, recommendations from appropriate services concerning follow-up or aftercare, and a brief summary of the patient's condition on discharge.

Quality Improvement Organizations

Formerly known as peer review organizations, QIOs are entities operating under the funding of CMS (2010b). Their primary function is to assess and improve the quality of healthcare provided to consumers. Often advocating for healthcare consumers, QIOs perform retrospective record reviews, conduct national and local quality improvement studies, and investigate consumer complaints regarding the quality of care provided in a number of settings. The record reviews influence healthcare organizations to comply with governmental documentation standards.

Although QIOs do not specifically review mental health facilities, care provided to individuals with mental illness is monitored in other settings in which behavioral healthcare is sought, such as rehabilitation facilities and emergency departments. QIOs also protect the integrity of the Medicare funds by ensuring that services are provided only when medically appropriate or necessary. QIOs are dedicated to protecting the rights of individuals receiving behavioral healthcare services.

HIPAA Privacy Rule

Behavioral healthcare organizations are considered **covered entities (CEs)** under HIPAA. However, other federal laws may carry additional privacy considerations. Substance-abuse programs must meet the HIPAA guidelines and the more stringent *Code of Federal Regulations*, 42 CFR 2. Some behavioral health organizations also provide **early childhood intervention (ECI)** services. ECI services are currently exempt from HIPAA; the privacy of these records is covered by FERPA (20 USC §1232g, 34 CFR 99), a federal law that protects the privacy of student education records.

Although HIPAA and FERPA do not necessarily influence the format of mental healthcare documentation, both of these laws restrict the release of mental health information about a person who may be a threat to himself or others.

The federal law governing the confidentiality of records of alcohol and drug abuse clients requires that the client authorize disclosure of PHI to any other entity that is not specifically permitted by these regulations. However, 42 CFR 2 does not permit authorized disclosures that would be self-incriminating, except when clients have been referred for services by the courts (42 CFR 2, §2.33 and §2.35). **FIGURE 13.11** describes the circumstances in which information may be disclosed without authorization as long as the Privacy Rule and state law permit the disclosure. The health information manager would do well to read the full text in 42 CFR 2 (HHS 2002).

Federal regulations that cover the confidentiality of PHI on alcohol and drug abuse patients apply to recipients of the information. Recipients are prohibited from redisclosing information they have received under authorization (42 CFR 2, §2.12[d]). This is in contrast to the Privacy Rule (HHS 2002b), which requires the CE to inform patients that

FIGURE 13.11. Disclosure and alcohol and drug abuse treatment programs

Alcohol and drug treatment programs that are regulated under 42 CFR, Part 2 may only disclose protected health information *without* authorization in the following circumstances:

- Communication within and between a program and with an entity having direct administrative control over the program and its personnel who need the information in connection with their duties that arise out of the provision of services provided (Subpart B, §2.12[c][3])

- Communication between a program and a business associate/qualified service organization (§2.12[c][4])

- Limited information to law enforcement and the courts when a client has committed a crime on program property or against program staff (§2.12[c][5]

- Limited information to report suspected child abuse and neglect (§2.12[c][6]

- For medical emergency to medical personnel (Subpart D, §2.51)

- For research activities (Subpart D, §2.52)

- For program audit and evaluation activities (§2.53)

- Upon a court order following the special 42 CFR, Part 2, "good cause" hearing (Subpart E, §2.61 and §2.63) (Note: Other than for purposes of criminal investigation or prosecution, anyone having a legally recognized interest in a disclosure may apply for a hearing [§2.64].)

- Situations in which certain entities apply for the good cause hearing to criminally investigate or prosecute a client (§2.65) or the program (§2.66)

their information is no longer protected after it has been disclosed. Because it is more protective, 42 CFR 2 supersedes the Privacy Rule.

One of the most difficult situations related to privacy of clients in a substance-abuse program occurs when state law generally permits—or even requires—disclosure in response to a subpoena or court order. To maintain privacy, a patient would need to enlist an attorney to respond to a court order. With the exception of a court order following a "good cause" hearing to which all parties have been notified to appear, including the provider, 42 CFR 2, §2.31, requires an authorization for the provider to respond to the subpoena, warrant, or court order that meets the requirements of the regulations (HHS 2002b).

Substance Abuse and Mental Health Services Administration

The **Substance Abuse and Mental Health Services Administration (SAMHSA)** is a federal agency of HHS established in 1992 to target substance abuse and mental health services to the people most in need. SAMHSA has proved that prevention works, treatment is effective, and people recover from mental and substance use disorders. Through SAMHSA's mission, to reduce the impact of substance abuse and mental illness on America's communities, eight strategic initiatives have been identified (SAMHSA 2011b):

1. **Prevention of Substance Abuse and Mental Illness**: Creating communities where individuals, families, schools, faith-based organizations, and workplaces take action to promote emotional health and reduce the likelihood of mental illness, substance abuse (including tobacco), and suicide.

2. **Trauma and Justice**: Reducing the pervasive, harmful, and costly health impact of violence and trauma by integrating trauma-informed approaches throughout health, behavioral health, and related systems and addressing the behavioral health needs of people involved in or at risk of involvement in the criminal and juvenile justice systems.

3. **Military Families**: Supporting America's service men and women—active duty, National Guard, reserve, and veteran—together with their families and communities—by leading efforts to ensure that needed behavioral health services are accessible and that outcomes are positive.

4. **Recovery Support**: Partnering with people in recovery from mental and substance use disorders to guide the behavioral health system and promote individual-, program-, and system-level approaches that foster health and resilience; increase permanent housing, employment, education, and other necessary supports; and reduce barriers to social inclusion.

5. **Health Reform**: Broadening health coverage to increase access to appropriate high-quality care and to reduce disparities that currently exist between the availability of services for substance abuse, mental disorders, and other medical conditions such as HIV/AIDS.

6. **Health Information Technology**: Ensuring that the behavioral health system, including states, community providers, and peer and prevention specialists, fully participates with the general healthcare delivery system in the adoption of health information technology and interoperable EHRs.

7. **Data, Outcomes, and Quality**: Realizing an integrated data strategy and a national framework for quality improvement in behavioral health care that will inform policy, measure program impact, and lead to improved quality of services and outcomes for individuals, families, and communities.

8. **Public Awareness and Support**: Increasing the understanding of mental and substance use disorders to achieve the full potential of prevention, help people recognize mental and substance use disorders and seek assistance with the same urgency as any other health condition, and make recovery the expectation.

SAMHSA supports the use of EHRs, as they allow behavioral health professionals to engage their patients without waiting for the exchange of paper records between departments and organizations and thereby facilitate the flow of critical information and improve patient treatment. In addition, with appropriate privacy and security safeguards, SAMHSA advocates for health information exchange between states and territories.

Healthcare Industry Forces

Healthcare industry forces focus on patient care and cost controls. These include managed care, integrated delivery systems, performance improvement, outcomes assessment and management, and growth of outpatient and partial treatment settings. All of these focus areas influence a facility's documentation requirements and will vary from organization to organization.

Managed Care

As with other service types in the healthcare delivery system, behavioral healthcare must take measures to control the cost of services. Managed care entities have added behavioral health benefits to their plans and routinely monitor compliance with contractual agreements. In many circumstances, however, benefits provided for behavioral health services are less than those provided for traditional medical treatment. For this reason, many employers have established EAPs to provide employees with access to brief and limited counseling or therapy services during times of need. This service is often fully paid for by the employer.

The NCQA **Standards and Guidelines for the Accreditation of Managed Behavioral Health Organizations** outlines standards and features in-depth explanations and examples of how to meet the standards, accreditation scoring guidelines and points, and accreditation outcomes and reporting categories. From the 2010 NCQA MBHO accreditation requirements, the standards for treatment record documentation (QI 12) include the following:

- Does the organization establish and distribute treatment record policies that address confidentiality, documentation standards, record keeping, and availability?

- Does the organization have methods to improve treatment record keeping where appropriate?

Integrated Delivery Systems

Providers and organizations commonly offer a variety of healthcare services. For example, one organization may provide acute care services, home healthcare services, and behavioral healthcare services under the same organizational name. As with any other healthcare provider, reliable and timely access to health information in such an **integrated delivery system (IDS)** is critical to the successful delivery of high-quality care. Yet, this is one of the most significant challenges in this type of healthcare system.

It is not uncommon for individual disciplines to establish and maintain separate and distinct records of care (commonly referred to as clinical records) in the IDS. Thus, the provider must have a well-maintained information management system or other reliable client indexing system that allows for the identification of shared clients. This permits optimal communication among providers in each discipline within the network or IDS arrangement and ensures continuity of care for the client.

Performance Improvement

Performance improvement activities are an important aspect of any industry in the healthcare delivery system. Behavioral healthcare facilities accredited by The Joint Commission or CARF demonstrate an excellence in high-quality service provision by maintaining compliance with hundreds of quality standards developed by the accreditation bodies. Accrediting bodies such as The Joint Commission and CARF closely monitor organizational policies and procedures related to PI activities (CARF 2011a).

The NCQA 2011 accreditation requirements for quality improvement include the following:

- Quality improvement program structure

- Program operations

- Health services contracting

- Availability of practitioners and providers

- Accessibility of services

- Member satisfaction

- Clinical practice guidelines

- Continuity and coordination between behavioral health and managed care

- Clinical measurement activities

- Effectiveness of the quality improvement program

- Standards for treatment record documentation

- Delegation of quality improvement

The Joint Commission accreditation requirements for performance improvement include the following:

- The hospital collects data to monitor its performance (PI.01.01.01).

- The hospital compiles and analyzes data (PI.02.01.01).

- The hospital improves performance on an ongoing basis (PI.03.01.01).

- The hospital uses data from clinical/service screening indicators and human resource screening indicators to assess and continuously improve staffing effectiveness. Note: This standard is not in effect at this time (PI.04.01.01).

Outcomes Assessment and Management

Outcomes assessment is an effective tool used to monitor the success of a plan from beginning to end. In behavioral health, it is a way to determine whether care and services were prescribed appropriately and provided to assist the client in achieving the expected or desired outcome.

Although behavioral healthcare experts report that individuals suffering from behavioral health conditions may never be "cured" in the traditional sense of the word, it is widely accepted that many of these individuals can achieve a fairly independent lifestyle when diagnosed and treated properly.

Growth of Outpatient and Partial Treatment Settings

As the cost of inpatient services rises, many individuals are seeking behavioral health services through outpatient or partial-treatment settings. These options provide the client with a stable healthcare provider at a significantly lower expense. However, not all insurers or payers cover outpatient or partial treatment.

Organizations and Advocacy Groups

In addition to the accrediting organizations, several other organizations support, fund, and influence some behavioral healthcare services. While these organizations may not have specific documentation requirements, they are included here because of their influence in the industry.

National Alliance on Mental Illness

The National Alliance on Mental Illness (NAMI) is a nonprofit organization dedicated to providing advocacy and support to individuals affected by mental illness (such as schizophrenia, bipolar disorder, major depressive disorders). NAMI not only assists individuals with the mental illness but also works with their families. NAMI is "dedicated to improving the lives of individuals and families affected by mental illness" (NAMI 2011).

Mental Health America

Mental Health America (MHA) (formerly National Mental Health Association) is a nonprofit organization created to assist the more than 54 million Americans with mental disorders. Through its public advocacy, education, and research programs, MHA hopes to elevate public knowledge of mental health issues, encourage reform, and promote the effective use of qualified prevention and recovery programs (MHA 2011).

MHA's mission is to promote mental health, prevent mental and substance use conditions, and achieve victory over mental illnesses and addictions through advocacy, education, research, and service. This is accomplished by providing information, advocacy, and access to quality behavioral health services for all Americans.

MHA has over 300 affiliates in 41 states and the District of Columbia throughout the nation that provide

- direct access to a broad range of self-help and professional recovery support for people facing mental health challenges,

- housing and supported employment for adults with severe mental illnesses or referrals to services, and

- easy access to comprehensive mental health screenings, which enable individuals to identify a need for help.

The Health Information Management Professional's Role in Behavioral Healthcare

The health information management (HIM) professional is a vital part of any behavioral healthcare organization. From the onset of care, the HIM professional is able to provide best-practice guidance and expertise on documentation issues, compliance issues, and general record maintenance issues.

FIGURE 13.12 lists several questions to assist in improving behavioral healthcare documentation.

Successful HIM practices throughout the continuum of behavioral care contribute to the safety and quality of care provided to clients, effective outcomes monitoring, and positive customer satisfaction. As the keepers of information and data, HIM professionals play an integral, indispensable, and powerful role.

To provide accurate and timely assistance, it is critical that the HIM professional understands the complexity of the behavioral healthcare system, its rules and regulations, and its unique position in the healthcare delivery system. Protecting the confidentiality,

FIGURE 13.12. Questions for improving behavioral healthcare documentation

- Is there documentation of medical necessity: in other words, does documentation indicate why services are necessary?
- Does the diagnosis warrant the particular treatment being offered?
- Are correct diagnostic codes being used?
- Does the patient have the cognitive or communication skills necessary to benefit from treatment?
- Could services be provided by someone other than a mental health professional?
- Is there documentation of symptoms, goals, and client's capacity to participate in treatment?
- Do progress notes relate to the interventions prescribed on the treatment plan?
- Do progress notes document all services being prescribed on the treatment plan?
- Does documentation justify the duration or frequency of services?
- Does documentation justify any extension of services?
- Are services being provided by a qualified professional?
- Is documentation timely, legible, and signed?
- Is billing timely and accurate?
- Are services provided within the standard payer definitions and do these align with correct CPT codes?

Source: Martins and Nicholson 2008, 242.

privacy, and security of mental health and substance abuse records, as well as all related PHI, has become very complicated. Health information managers, who also may be privacy officers, have significant responsibilities regarding implementation of the various laws regulating use and disclosure of PHI. For this reason, it is imperative that they be familiar with federal and state laws and keep abreast of new legislation.

Because of their daily oversight of PHI use and disclosure in behavioral healthcare organizations, HIM professionals also are well qualified—and should therefore come forward—to take part in the revision or development of laws and standards of practice related to the privacy, confidentiality, and security of behavioral healthcare PHI. Their contribution is valuable and necessary (and perhaps sometimes overlooked) within the overall healthcare industry and beyond.

Health information managers working in substance-abuse programs must ensure that the organization's workforce understands that with the exception of a court order following a "good cause" hearing, communication of PHI without an authorization is prohibited, and even when a judge finds reason for PHI disclosure, information is restricted to that which is essential to fulfill the purpose of the order. Without authorization, as stated in 42 CFR 2, §2.13, 2.31, 2.61ff, disclosure in response to a subpoena, court order, or warrant is prohibited. This rule preempts less protective state laws.

EHRs in Behavioral Healthcare

Behavioral healthcare has been slow to embrace EHR technology. Although behavioral health programs in larger hospitals may have migrated from paper to electronic documentation, many behavioral health providers (private practices, solo practitioners, and community-based agencies) continue to use paper-based health record systems. The reasons range from cost of software, to lack of information technology staff and resources, to a concern for complete privacy and security of client information.

On April 15, 2010, Congressman Patrick J. Kennedy (D-RI) and Congressman Tim Murphy (R-PA) introduced the Health Information Technology Extension for Behavioral Health Services Act of 2010. This legislation would extend the incentives for the "meaningful use" of EHRs established through the American Recovery and Reinvestment Act of 2009 by ensuring the eligibility of many behavioral and mental health professionals, psychiatric hospitals, behavioral and mental health treatment facilities, and substance abuse treatment facilities.

The American Recovery and Reinvestment Act provided $20 billion in incentives and grants to healthcare providers and hospitals to establish interoperable EHR systems throughout the nation. These benefits extend to most physicians, chiropractors, dentists, optometrists, podiatrists, and hospitals. However, an important sector of the healthcare community is excluded: clinical psychologists, clinical social workers, psychiatric hospitals, substance use treatment facilities, and mental health treatment facilities.

"Health information technology is a critical component of health reform. Proper use of health information technology will address some of the challenges that hospitals, practitioners and facilities encounter when delivering mental and behavioral health services. Furthermore, this bill will ensure that mental and behavioral health providers are included in the nation's plan to achieve widespread adoption of health information technology," said Congressman Alcee L. Hastings (D-FL) (as quoted in Kennedy 2010). Behavioral healthcare organizations will benefit from the implementation of EHRs. The immediate availability of documentation to trusted providers will assist in emergent client needs and well as ongoing care. Medical and treatment errors can be reduced from the use of decision support software. Reimbursement for services can be expedited with completed clinical record documentation required before billing occurs.

Summary

The need for HIM professionals working in the behavioral healthcare setting to have a thorough knowledge and understanding of laws, rules, regulations, standards, and best practices is crucial to the operation of the organization. Many federal and state laws focus specifically on behavioral healthcare.

The variety of behavioral healthcare settings requires documentation for many types of treatment that may not regularly occur in other settings. These include such issues as seclusion and restraints, suicide watch, and minors seeking services. The content of the record also varies to include psychiatric assessment and psychological testing reports pertaining to the patient's treatment. Add to this the numerous accrediting bodies that have an impact on behavioral healthcare and documentation. As with other healthcare settings, measures must be taken to control the costs and services of behavioral health. Healthcare industry forces in behavioral healthcare influence a facility's documentation requirements which have to be monitored for compliance.

References

American Osteopathic Association (AOA). 2007. *Accreditation of Colleges of Osteopathic Medicine: COM Accreditation Standards and Procedures.* Chicago, IL: American Osteopathic Association.

American Psychiatric Association (APA). 2006. Practice Guideline for the Assessment and Treatment of Patients with Suicidal Behaviors. http://www.psychiatryonline.com/pracGuide/pracGuideTopic_14.aspx.

American Psychiatric Association (APA). 2000. *Diagnostic and Statistical Manual of Mental Disorders DSM-IV-TR*, 4th ed. Arlington, VA: American Psychiatric Association.

American Recovery and Reinvestment Act (ARRA). 2009. CMS Information Related to the Economic Recovery Act of 2009, Health Information Technology. http://www.cms.gov/Recovery/11_HealthIT.asp.

American Residential Treatment Association. 2011. http://www.artausa.org/

American Psychological Association. 2010. Ethical Principles of Psychologists and Code of Conduct. http://www.apa.org/ethics/code/index.aspx

California Department of Justice. 2004. Assembly Bill (AB) 157 - Revised Mental Health Reporting Requirements. CCR AB 1587 (Chapter 578, Statutes of 1999). http://www.dmh.ca.gov/DMHDocs/docs/notices99/99-17.pdf.

Centers for Medicare and Medicaid Services (CMS). 2010a. Medicare and Your Mental Health Benefits. http://www.medicare.gov/publications/pubs/pdf/10184.pdf.

Centers for Medicare and Medicaid Services (CMS). 2010b. Quality Improvement Organizations Overview. http://www.cms.gov/QualityImprovementOrgs.

Centers for Medicare and Medicaid Services. 2006. Conditions of Participation for Hospitals; Final Rule. 42 CFR Part 482. *Federal Register* 71(227): 68672–68695.

Commission on Accreditation of Rehabilitation Facilities (CARF). 2011a. Behavioral Health. http://www.carf.org/Programs/BH.

Commission on Accreditation of Rehabilitation Facilities (CARF). 2011b. What Does CARF Accredit? http://www.carf.org/Accreditation.

Council on Accreditation (COA). 2008. *COA Accreditation and Standards*. http:// www.coastandards.org/standards.php.

County of San Diego 2003. *Initial Mental Health Assessment*. San Diego: Health and Human Services Agency.

County of San Diego. 2002a. *Restraint or Seclusion Assessment*. San Diego: Health and Human Services Agency.

County of San Diego. 2002b. *Restraint or Seclusion Flow Sheet*. San Diego: Health and Human Services Agency.

County of San Diego. 2002c. *Psychiatric Assessment*. San Diego: Health and Human Services Agency.

Family Educational Rights and Privacy Act (FERPA). 20 U.S.C. § 1232g; 34 CFR Part 99. 1974.

Grant, J. E. 2007. Failing the 15-minute Suicide Watch: Guidelines to Monitor Patients. *Current Psychiatry* 6 (6): 41–43.

Health Insurance Portability and Accountability Act (HIPAA) of 1996. Public Law 104-191. http://www.gpoaccess.gov/cfr/index.html.

The Joint Commission. 2003. Facts about the Joint Commission on Accreditation of Healthcare Organizations. http://www.jointcommission.com.

The Joint Commission. 2010. *Behavioral Health Care Accreditation Program, 2011 Chapter: Care, Treatment, and Services*. Oakbrook Terrace, IL: The Joint Commission.

Kennedy, P. 2010 (April 15). Press release: Kennedy, Tim Murphy introduce health information technology extension for Behavioral Health Services Act Of 2010. http://www.votesmart.org/public-statement/499095/kennedy-tim-murphy-introduce-health-information-technology-extension-for-behavioral-health-services-act-of-2010.

Kessler, R.C., Berglund, P., Demler, O, Jin, R., Merikangas, K.R., and E. E. Walters. 2005. Lifetime Prevalence and Age-of-Onset Distributions of DSM-IV Disorders in the National Comorbidity Survey Replication. *Archives of General Psychiatry* 62:593–602.

Martins, L., and R. Nicholson. 2008. Compliance Considerations in Behavioral Health Facilities. In *Health Information Management Compliance: Guidelines for Preventing Fraud and Abuse*, edited by S. Bowman. Chicago: AHIMA.

Mental Health America (MHA). 2011. Mental Illness and the Family: Is Hospitalization Necessary. http://www.nmha.org/go/information/get-info/mi-and-the-family/is-hospitalization-necessary.

Merck Manual. 2011. Areas to Cover in the Initial Psychiatric Assessment. http://www.merckmanuals.com/professional/psychiatric_disorders/approach_to_the_patient_with_mental_symptoms/routine_psychiatric_assessment.html#v1024529.

National Alliance on Mental Illness (NAMI). 2011. About NAMI. http://www.nami.org/Content/NavigationMenu/Inform_Yourself/About_NAMI/About_NAMI.htm.

National Committee on Quality Assurance (NCQA). 2011. 2011 MBHO Accreditation Requirements. http://www.ncqa.org/tabid/94/Default.aspx.

National Committee on Quality Assurance (NCQA). 2007. MBHO Standards and Guidelines. http://www.ncqa.org/tabid/378/Default.aspx.

National Council for Community Behavioral Healthcare (NCBBH). 2011. About Us: History. http://www.thenationalcouncil.org/cs/history.

National Institute of Mental Health (NIMH). 2010a. Prevalence of Serious Mental Illness Among U.S. Adults by Age, Sex, and Race. http://www.nimh.nih.gov/statistics/pdf/NSDUH-SMI-Adults.pdf.

National Institute of Mental Health (NIMH). 2010b. "The Numbers Count: Mental Disorders in America." http://www.nimh.nih.gov.

National Mental Health Association (NMHA). 2004. "About NMHA." http://www.nmha.org.

Substance Abuse and Mental Health Services Administration. 2011a. "The Confidentiality of Alcohol and Drug Abuse Patient Records Regulation and the HIPAA Privacy Rule: Implications for Alcohol and Substance Abuse Programs." http://ncadistore.samhsa.gov/catalog/productDetails.aspx?ProductID=16873.

Substance Abuse and Mental Health Services Administration. 2011b. SAMHSA's Eight Strategic Initiatives. http://www.samhsa.gov/about/strategy.aspx.

Substance Abuse and Mental Health Services Administration. 2010. Mental Health Programs, Homelessness. http://mentalhealth.samhsa.gov/cmhs/Homelessness.

Tarasoff v. Regents of the University of California, 17 Cal. 3d 425, 551 P.2d 334, 131 Cal. Rptr. 14 (1976). http://www.publichealthlaw.net/Reader/docs/Tarasoff.pdf.

US Department of Health and Human Services (HHS). 2002a. Confidentiality of Alcohol and Drug Abuse Patient Records; Final Rule. 42 CFR Part 2.63 *Federal Register*. http://www.access.gpo.gov/nara/cfr/waisidx_02/42cfr2_02.html.

US Department of Health and Human Services (HHS). 2002b. The Privacy Rule. http://www.hhs.gov/ocr/privacy/hipaa/administrative/privacyrule/index.html.

US Department of Health and Human Services (HHS), Department of Education (DOE), Department of Justice (DOJ). 2007. Report to the President on Issues Raised by the Virginia Tech Tragedy. http://www.hhs. gov/vtreport.pdf.

US Department of Health and Human Services (HHS), Office of the Surgeon General. 2001. Mental Health: Culture, Race, Ethnicity." Supplement to "Mental Health: Report of the Surgeon General. http://www .surgeongeneral.gov/library/mentalhealth/cre/sma-01-3613.pdf.

Zwolinski, R. 2010. Richard's Seven Rudiments of the Mental Health Treatment Plan. http://blogs. psychcentral.com/therapy-soup/2010/04/richards-seven-rudiments-of-the-mental-health-treatment-plan.

Chapter 14

Exploring Other Healthcare Settings

Cheryl Gregg Fahrenholz, RHIA, CCS-P

Objectives

- Describe the regulatory and legal standards that apply to all healthcare providers
- Explain services provided by, specific regulations for, professional associations for, and health record requirements for the following healthcare providers:

Solo practitioners

- Chiropractors
- Dental practitioners
- Licensed complementary/alternative care providers
- Midlevel practitioners
- Nurse midwives
- Optometrists
- Physicians
- Podiatrists
- Psychologists/mental health workers

Ambulatory care practices

- Ambulatory surgery centers
- Cancer treatment centers
- Convenient care centers/retail medical clinics
- Diagnostic imaging centers
- Diagnostic sleep centers
- Diagnostic/therapeutic centers
- Endoscopy centers
- Medical/dental centers
- Mobile health units
- Outpatient rehabilitation centers

- Public health clinics
- Renal dialysis centers
- Rehabilitation centers
- Telehealth/nonsurgical centers
- Telehealth/surgical centers
- Urgent care centers

Governmental providers

- Correctional facilities
- Indian health services
- Military hospitals
- Veterans Administration health system

Other practitioners and providers

- Blood banks
- Coordinated school programs
- Critical access hospitals
- University-based health services
- Veterinarians

Key Terms

Accreditation Association for Ambulatory Health Care (AAAHC)

American Board of Medical Specialties (ABMS)

Cancer treatment center

Certification Commission for Health Information Technology (CCHIT)

Commission on Cancer (CoC)

Convenient care center

Current Dental Terminology (CDT)

Electronic medication administration record (eMAR)

Family Educational Rights and Privacy Act of 1974 (FERPA)

National Center for Complementary and Alternative Medicine (NCCAM)

National Conference on Correctional Health Care (NCCHC)

Nurse practitioner (NP)

Outpatient rehabilitation center (ORC)

Physician assistant (PA)

Resource and Patient Management System (RPMS)

Retail medical clinic

Telemedicine

Urgent care center

Veterans Health Administration (VHA)

Introduction

Health records are maintained in many settings other than those described in the first 13 chapters of this book. This chapter presents a brief overview of these other healthcare settings. The type of care each provides is described, and the health record practices of each are explored. In addition, documentation requirements from accrediting bodies, licensure, or government regulations are examined. Professional association and advocacy groups associated with the setting are also described. Finally, the chapter provides a review of any healthcare settings where the electronic health record (EHR) is currently in use or is emerging. Because the chapter only provides an overview of each alternative setting, additional references and resources are provided at the end of the chapter.

The types of healthcare settings are divided into four groups. First, outpatient settings where care is provided by a solo practitioner are explored. These settings include the practices of physicians, podiatrists, psychologists, chiropractors, nurse midwives, dental professionals, optometrists, and licensed complementary or alternative care providers (including acupuncturists, massage therapists, and naturopathic physicians).

The second type is outpatient/ambulatory, where some combination of physicians, ancillary clinicians, and nursing staff provide care. These settings include renal dialysis centers, public health clinics, mental health clinics, integrative medicine clinics, and rehabilitation centers. Rehabilitation centers can actually provide inpatient or outpatient care or both—so both are explored for this setting.

The third type of setting includes hospitals and clinics managed by the government to provide care to veterans or members of the armed services and their dependents, as well as to prisoners. These settings include military hospitals and clinics, Veterans Administration hospitals, and correctional facilities. Finally, the fourth type includes blood banks and veterinary practices.

Regulations Common to All Healthcare Providers

Certain regulations and laws apply to all healthcare providers—at least those settings providing services to humans. Veterinary services are also explored in this chapter, but because they do not provide healthcare services to humans, they are not bound by the laws and regulations addressed here. Specific laws and regulations for veterinarians are addressed in the section on veterinary care.

Federal law, specifically the Health Insurance Portability and Accountability Act (HIPAA), applies to all healthcare practitioners, regardless of the type of healthcare provided or the location of the care, Specifically, HIPAA protects the privacy and security of all patients' protected health information, which is defined as any information that includes patient identifiers and clinical information of any type. Patients have the right to, and therefore all healthcare providers have the responsibility to ensure that patients can do the following:

1. Obtain and inspect a copy of their health records

2. Request a correction of inaccurate health information

3. Find out where their health information has been shared for purposes other than care, payment, or healthcare administrative purposes

4. Request special restrictions on the use or disclosure of their health information

5. Request that the provider share their health information with them in a particular way

6. See a provider's policy on confidentiality

In addition to HIPAA, healthcare providers who treat Medicaid or Medicare patients must adhere to the US Department of Health and Human Services (HHS) Office of the Inspector General healthcare compliance regulations. Medicare Conditions of Participation (COP) apply to any healthcare provider who treats Medicare patients. Federal and state regulations apply to any healthcare provider who treats Medicaid patients. And every provider is bound by his state's department of health rules and statutes. Every healthcare provider must, at a minimum, be licensed in the state where she practices. In the sections that follow, we discuss for each healthcare provider, where they exist, health record regulations, accrediting body requirements, and licensing issues.

Outpatient Private Practitioners or Solo Practitioners

In this section, we look at private practitioners or healthcare practitioners who may practice as solo practitioners. For health information management (HIM) professionals, the opportunity to work with these providers will be more likely when they practice in groups. For example, a large physician practice of 10 or more physicians is more likely to employ an HIM professional. However, every healthcare provider, even solo practitioners, has HIM needs. Often, individual practitioners may employ an HIM professional as a contractor for specific needs or look to HIM professionals to provide educational and training services through their professional associations.

Physicians

The most common location for a physician–patient encounter in the United States is the physician office. Each year, patients make about 1 billion visits to physician offices, or an average of three visits per person per year. This accounts for 27 percent of all spending in healthcare (Cherry, Woodwell, and Rechtsteiner 2007). According to the American Medical Association, about one-third of the 662,000 practicing physicians are in solo practice. About 25 percent are in groups of 2 to 4 physicians, 15 percent are in groups of 5 to 9 physicians, 17 percent are in groups of 10 to 49, and 5 percent are in groups with more than 50 physicians (Kane 2001). The most frequent reasons to visit physician offices in 2007 were hypertension, arthritis, hyperlipidemia, diabetes preventive care, immunizations, and annual exams. Physician office appointments include visits to primary care practitioners, specialists, and surgeons. In 2007, 52 percent of all physician office visits were to primary care physicians. The number of visits increases each year.

In addition to the regulations common to all healthcare providers, the American Recovery and Reinvestment Act of 2009 (ARRA) and Health Information Technology for Economic and Clinical Health (HITECH) Act meaningful use requirements apply to physician practices. The criteria for physicians are slightly different from those for hospitals and healthcare systems. However, physicians are required to comply with the EHR criteria by 2015. Physicians can choose to participate in Medicaid or Medicare incentives. To qualify as a Medicaid-eligible provider for meaningful use, the physician must be non–hospital based, do more than 30 percent Medicaid encounters, and assign her incentives to the organization (that is, physician group practice), where the EHR is employed in a meaningful way. In a 2009 survey, 42 percent of physicians reported using a partial or complete EHR in their office practices (Higgins 2010). **Figure 14.1** illustrates physician EHR usage.

FIGURE 14.1. Physicians using EHRs

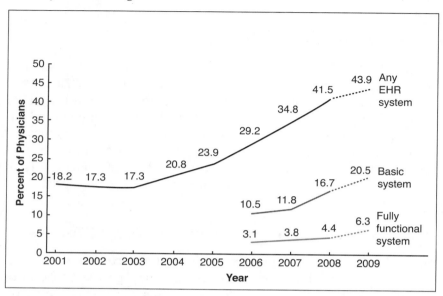

Source: CDC 2010.

Physicians must be licensed by the state(s) where they practice and are subject to inspection by the state department of health. Physicians are also subject to regulation by any private insurance companies from which they accept payment for services. Many physicians seek additional certification through the **American Board of Medical Specialties (ABMS)**. The ABMS provides board certification for more than 145 specialties and subspecialties (ABMS 2011). (See **TABLE 14.1**).

Most physicians belong to the professional association of their specialty. For example, a family practice physician is likely to belong to the American Academy of Family Practitioners. This association acts as both professional association and board-certifying entity for family practice physicians. Other associations' physicians may belong to include the American Medical Association and state or local medical societies.

TABLE 14.1. ABMS-recognized physician specialty and subspecialty certificates

GENERAL CERTIFICATE(S)	SUBSPECIALTY CERTIFICATES
American Board of Allergy and Immunology	
Allergy and immunology	No subspecialties
American Board of Anesthesiology	
Anesthesiology	Critical care medicine Hospice and palliative medicine Pain medicine Pediatric anesthesiology[1] Sleep medicine[2]
American Board of Colon and Rectal Surgery	
Colon and rectal surgery	No subspecialties
American Board of Dermatology	
Dermatology	Dermatopathology Pediatric dermatology

TABLE 14.1. (continued)

GENERAL CERTIFICATE(S)	SUBSPECIALTY CERTIFICATES
American Board of Emergency Medicine	
Emergency medicine	Emergency medical services[3] Hospice and palliative medicine Medical toxicology Pediatric emergency medicine Sports medicine Undersea and hyperbaric medicine
American Board of Family Medicine	
Family medicine	Adolescent medicine Geriatric medicine Hospice and palliative medicine Sleep medicine Sports medicine
American Board of Internal Medicine	
Internal medicine	Adolescent medicine Advanced heart failure and transplant Cardiology Cardiovascular disease Clinical cardiac electrophysiology Critical care medicine Endocrinology, diabetes, and metabolism Gastroenterology Geriatric medicine Hematology Hospice and palliative medicine Infectious disease Interventional cardiology Medical oncology Nephrology Pulmonary disease Rheumatology Sleep medicine Sports medicine Transplant hepatology
American Board of Medical Genetics	
Clinical biochemical genetics* Clinical cytogenetics* Clinical genetics (MD)* Clinical molecular genetics*	Medical biochemical genetics Molecular genetic pathology
American Board of Neurological Surgery	
Neurological surgery	No subspecialties
American Board of Nuclear Medicine	
Nuclear medicine	No subspecialties
American Board of Obstetrics and Gynecology	
Obstetrics and gynecology	Critical care medicine Female pelvic medicine and reconstructive surgery[1] Gynecologic oncology Hospice and palliative medicine Maternal and fetal medicine Reproductive endocrinology/infertility

TABLE 14.1. (continued)

GENERAL CERTIFICATE(S)	SUBSPECIALTY CERTIFICATES
American Board of Ophthalmology	
Ophthalmology	No subspecialties
American Board of Orthopaedic Surgery	
Orthopaedic surgery	Orthopaedic sports medicine Surgery of the hand
American Board of Otolaryngology	
Otolaryngology	Neurotology Pediatric otolaryngology Plastic surgery within the head and neck Sleep medicine
American Board of Pathology	
Anatomic pathology and clinical pathology* Pathology–anatomic* Pathology–clinical*	Blood banking/transfusion medicine Cytopathology Dermatopathology Neuropathology Pathology–chemical Pathology–forensic Pathology–hematology Pathology–medical microbiology Pathology–molecular genetic Pathology–pediatric
American Board of Pediatrics	
Pediatrics	Adolescent medicine Child abuse pediatrics Developmental-behavioral pediatrics Hospice and palliative medicine Medical toxicology Neonatal-perinatal medicine Neurodevelopmental disabilities Pediatric cardiology Pediatric critical care medicine Pediatric emergency medicine Pediatric endocrinology Pediatric gastroenterology Pediatric hematology-oncology Pediatric infectious diseases Pediatric nephrology Pediatric pulmonology Pediatric rheumatology Pediatric transplant hepatology Sleep medicine Sports medicine
American Board of Physical Medicine and Rehabilitation	
Physical medicine and rehabilitation	Hospice and palliative medicine Neuromuscular medicine Pain medicine Pediatric rehabilitation medicine Spinal cord injury medicine Sports medicine

TABLE 14.1. (continued)

GENERAL CERTIFICATE(S)	SUBSPECIALTY CERTIFICATES
American Board of Plastic Surgery	
Plastic surgery	Plastic surgery within the head and neck Surgery of the hand
American Board of Preventive Medicine	
Aerospace medicine* Occupational medicine* Public health and general preventive medicine*	Medical toxicology Undersea and hyperbaric medicine
American Board of Psychiatry and Neurology	
Psychiatry* Neurology* Neurology with special qualification in child neurology*	Addiction psychiatry Child and adolescent psychiatry Clinical neurophysiology Epilepsy[4] Forensic psychiatry Geriatric psychiatry Hospice and palliative medicine Neurodevelopmental disabilities Neuromuscular medicine Pain medicine Psychosomatic medicine Sleep medicine Vascular neurology
American Board of Radiology	
Diagnostic radiology* Radiation oncology* Medical physics*	Hospice and palliative medicine Neuroradiology Nuclear radiology Pediatric radiology Vascular and interventional radiology
American Board of Surgery	
Surgery* Vascular surgery*	Complex general surgical oncology[1] Hospice and palliative medicine Pediatric surgery Surgery of the hand Surgical critical care
American Board of Thoracic Surgery	
Thoracic surgery	Congenital cardiac surgery
American Board of Urology	
Urology	Female pelvic medicine and reconstructive surgery[1] Pediatric urology

*Specific disciplines within the specialty where certification is offered.
[1]Approved 2011; first issue to be determined.
[2]Approved 2011; first issue November 2011.
[3]Approved 2010; first issue to be determined.
[4]Approved 2010; first issue 2013.

Source: ABMS 2011.

Most states closely regulate the content of patient records. Therefore, HIM professionals must be familiar with state law. To illustrate the level of complexity and detail that may apply to regulations for patient health records in physicians' offices, see **FIGURE 14.2**. In response to a simple question about the length of record retention in physician offices in the state of

FIGURE 14.2. Record retention

How long must a physician's office maintain a patient's medical records?
There is no general law requiring a physician to maintain medical records for a specific period of time. However, there are situations or government health plans that require a provider/physician to maintain their records for a certain period of time. Several laws specify a three-year retention period: Welfare and Institutions Code section 14124.1 (which relates to Medi-Cal patients), Health and Safety Code section 1797.98(e) (for services reimbursed by Emergency Medical Services Fund), and Health and Safety Code section 11191 (when a physician prescribes, dispenses or administers a Schedule II controlled substance). The Knox-Keene Act requires that HMO medical records be maintained a minimum of two years to ensure that compliance with the act can be validated by the Department of Corporations. In Workers' Compensation Cases, qualified medical evaluators must maintain medical-legal reports for five years. Health and Safety Code section 123145 indicates that providers who are licensed under section 1205 as a medical clinic shall preserve the records for seven years. However, there is no general statute which relates to all other types of medical records.

Source: State of California 2010.

California, the Medical Board of California cites seven different statutes. In addition, each state has specific requirements governing health record retention when a physician practice closes. HIM professionals should review the applicable state regulations.

Podiatrists

Podiatric medicine focuses on diagnosing and treating foot, ankle, and lower extremity disorders. In the early 1900s, although there were orthopedic surgeons to treat musculoskeletal disorders, there was no medical profession dedicated to foot and ankle care and treatment. Dr. Scholl, commonly known for Dr. Scholl's footwear and foot care products, is the father of podiatric medicine. He started his career in a shoe store, where he became so concerned with customers' painful foot conditions that he enrolled in medical school. He earned his MD degree at Illinois Medical College and made it his lifelong mission to improve people's health, comfort, and well-being through their feet. In 1912, he founded the second college of podiatric medicine in the United States. Today, podiatrists must attend four years of medical school through one of the eight podiatric medical schools in the United Stated to receive a doctor of podiatric medicine (DPM) degree. Then they must complete a two- or three-year residency program and meet state licensing requirements. There are approximately 12,200 podiatrists in the United States today.

Podiatrists are subject to the same regulations as physicians, including the ARRA and HITECH Act meaningful use of the EHR requirements. The American Podiatric Medical Association (APMA) is the professional and certification board for podiatrists. The APMA established specialty boards in podiatric medicine to certify advanced qualifications in podiatric orthopedics, podiatric surgery, and primary podiatric medicine. Certification is considered an earned credential for those podiatric physicians who have achieved certain levels of skill and ability based on the completion of specific advanced training and clinical experience and examination.

HIM professionals should be familiar with the state laws and hospital-specific regulations regarding podiatrists. For example, if a podiatrist is able to admit patients to the hospital setting in a particular state, Medicare COP still require that certain reports, such as the history and physical and the discharge summary, be signed by an doctor of medicine or a doctor of osteopathy.

Midlevel Practitioners

The term *midlevel practitioner* means an individual practitioner, other than a physician, dentist, veterinarian, or podiatrist, who is licensed, registered, or otherwise permitted by the United States or the jurisdiction in which he practices, to dispense a controlled substance in the course of professional practice. Examples of midlevel practitioners include, but are not limited to, nurse practitioners, nurse midwives, nurse anesthetists, clinical nurse specialists, and physician assistants (DOJ 2010).

Nurse practitioners (NPs) are advanced practice nurses who, as a discipline, have been providing healthcare services similar to those of a doctor since 1965. Most NPs have master's degrees, and many have doctorate degrees. There are about 140,000 NPs nationwide. NPs diagnose and treat a wide range of health problems. They have a unique approach and stress both *care* and *cure*. Besides clinical care, NPs focus on health promotion, disease prevention, health education, and counseling (AANP 2010). Although in some states NPs are permitted to provide patient care independently in an office setting, NPs in hospital settings work under the direct supervision of a physician. HIM professionals should be familiar with state laws and hospital regulations regarding the documentation and billing requirements specific to the NP.

Physician assistants (PAs) practice in all 50 states. Of the 75,000 PAs in practice in 2008, more than 43 percent worked in group practices or solo physician offices, and more than one third were found in hospitals (AAPA 2010). State medical and PA practice acts and regulations generally allow physicians broad delegatory authority, which permits flexible, customized team practice. However, the Centers for Medicare and Medicaid Services (CMS) requires direct physician supervision. HIM professionals should be familiar with both state laws and hospital regulations regarding the documentation and billing requirements specific to the PA.

Psychologists/Mental Health Professionals

Mental health professionals may practice independently, in a group with several other mental health professionals, or for a healthcare organization. Nonphysician mental health professionals are discussed in this section.

Psychologists, therapists, and mental health counselors are licensed by the state where they practice. Every state has different requirements for education, training, and certification. **Figure 14.3** shows the Massachusetts law that addresses record-keeping requirements for psychologists. HIM professionals must be familiar with the laws in their state that address health information and health record keeping for all healthcare providers whose health records they are responsible for maintaining. In addition, HIM professionals should be familiar with the hospital-specific regulations regarding documentation by behavioral health professionals in the health record. And, because mental health records have additional confidentiality protections under HIPAA, HIM professionals should be familiar with and follow these regulations (addressed in chapter 2). The American Psychological Association (APA) is the largest professional association for psychologists, with over 150,000 members worldwide. The National Association of Social Workers (NASW), which also claims 150,000 members, is the professional association for social workers.

Psychologists

Some psychologists have a master's degree (MA or MS) in psychology while others have a doctoral degree (PhD, PsyD, or EdD) in clinical, educational, counseling, or research

FIGURE 14.3. Massachusetts law on record-keeping requirements for psychologists

Commonwealth of Massachusetts
Division of Medical Assistance
Provider Manual Series
Psychologist Manual

411.413: Recordkeeping Requirements

(A) Payment for any service listed in 130 CMR 411.000 is conditioned upon its full and complete documentation in the member's medical record. The psychologist must maintain a record (chart or folder) of all psychology services provided to a member for a period of at least six years following the date of service. The record must be identified by the name of the member and the date or dates of testing. The record must contain the following information:

    (1) the referral source;

    (2) the reason for the referral;

    (3) for a personality evaluation or an assessment of organic mental disorders, a brief description of behavioral observations, and any other personal information elicited during testing;

    (4) the protocol of responses to the tests used;

    (5) a summary of scores; and

    (6) a comprehensive written report describing the psychological evaluation and interpretation of responses.

(B) Release of information in the record is limited to the following:

    (1) those instances required by federal or state statute or regulation in accordance with the confidentiality provisions of the profession; and

    (2) qualified personnel or consultants of the Department or the US Department of Health and Human Services for the purpose of monitoring the provision of services in accordance with 130 CMR 411.000.

Source: Commonwealth of Massachusetts 2003, iv.

psychology. Most states license psychologists to practice psychology. They can provide psychological testing or evaluations, treat emotional and behavioral problems and mental disorders, and provide psychotherapy.

Social Workers

Social workers have a bachelor's degree (BA, BS, or BSW), a master's degree (MA, MS, MSW, or MSSW), or a doctoral degree (DSW or PhD). In most states, social workers take an examination to be licensed to practice social work (LCSW or LICSW), and the type of license depends on their level of education and practice experience. Social workers provide various services, including assessment and treatment of psychiatric illnesses, case management, hospital discharge planning, and psychotherapy. Most organizations allow social workers to document discharge planning in the progress notes, but behavioral health information requires separate documentation.

Psychiatric/Mental Health Nurses

Psychiatric/mental health nurses may have various degrees ranging from associate's, to bachelor's (BSN), to master's (MSN or APRN), to doctoral (DNSc, PhD). Depending on their level of education and licensing, they provide a broad range of psychiatric and medical services, including the assessment and treatment of psychiatric illnesses, case management, and psychotherapy. In some states, some psychiatric nurses may prescribe and monitor medication.

Licensed Professional Counselors

Licensed professional counselors have a master's degree (MA) in psychology, counseling, or a similar discipline, and typically have two years of postgraduate experience. They may provide services that include diagnosis and counseling (individual, family/group, or both). They have a license issued in their state and may be certified by the National Academy of Certified Clinical Mental Health Counselors (NAMI 2010).

Dentists

Dentists are an integral part of every patient's healthcare team. Modern dental hygiene has influenced many other medical advances. Dentists may be the first to spot certain diseases, such as throat and mouth cancers. All dentists attend dental school for four years after earning their bachelor's degree. Depending on their specialty, dentists earn either a DMD (doctor of dental medicine) or DDS (doctor of dental surgery) degree. Then, they may spend anywhere from one to five additional years in residency. All dentists are licensed by the state where they practice. Board certification is available for general dentistry and dental specialties through their respective boards. Dentists restore, replace, and extract teeth. They also correct misaligned teeth and provide oral health instruction.

After dental school, dentists spend one to two years in residency. Endodontists focus their treatment on the dental nerves and pulp and perform surgeries such as root canal. Oral and maxillofacial surgeons focus on injuries and defects of the neck, head, and jaw. They treat conditions such as temporomandibular joint disorder and oral cancer. Oral surgeons spend four years in surgical residency after dental school. Orthodontists address problems related to irregular dental development and missing teeth, problems needing braces to correct. They spend three years in residency after dental school. Periodontists treat gum disease and problems related to the supporting bones. They also spend three years in residency after dental school.

Like physicians, DMDs and DDSs can be members of a hospital's medical staff. Specific documentation and oversight requirements may apply to DMDs or DDSs. HIM professionals should be familiar with hospital-specific regulations regarding documentation by these disciplines. These practitioners are also subject to the HITECH Act and meaningful use of the EHR criteria. As a result of digital imaging and communications in medicine technology and the dental professions' reliance on X-ray technology in everyday treatment, dentists are some of the first healthcare providers to use EHRs. Dentists also have their own coding and classification system, **Current Dental Terminology (CDT)**. CDT was created by the American Dental Association to categorize and bill dental services in a uniform manner. CDT is designated by the federal government under HIPAA as the national terminology for reporting dental services. Specific record-keeping requirements for dentists are governed by the state department of health where the dentist practices.

Optometrists

The American Optometric Association (AOA) represents approximately 36,000 doctors of optometry (ODs). Optometrists serve patients in nearly 6,500 communities across the country. In 3,500 of those communities, optometrists are the only eye doctors. DOs provide two thirds of all primary eye care in the United States. The AOA's Code of Ethics states that optometrists must "ensure confidentiality and privacy of patients' protected health and other personal information." ODs attend four years of optometry school after completing their undergraduate education. ODs are licensed by the state where they practice and must conform to all of the laws of that state.

Licensed Complementary and Alternative Medicine Providers

Many types of licensed complementary and alternative medicine (CAM) are practiced in the United States. In the 1990s, the National Institutes of Health recognized the increasing role CAM was playing and formed the **National Center for Complementary and Alternative Medicine (NCCAM)** to serve as a resource for these types of practices. Because much of CAM is not currently regulated, patients must be cautious. The Academic Consortium for Complementary and Alternative Health Care (ACCAHC) was formed to help patients and CAM practitioners. The ACCAHC recommends that patients only seek treatment from licensed practitioners. Licensed CAM practitioners are joining hospitals and healthcare systems to provide "integrative medicine"—that is, alternative medicine within the context of traditional medicine. For example, many cancer centers employ acupuncturists because certain acupuncture treatments have been proven to alleviate the side effects of chemotherapy treatment. The five types of licensed CAM practitioners are discussed in this section.

Acupuncture and Oriental Medicine Practitioners

Acupuncture is an ancient healing technique that involves the insertion of very thin needles into points on the body to move energy (or *chi*), thereby improving symptoms. Most acupuncturists are also licensed to practice herbal medicine. Acupuncture has been proven, through clinical trials, to be effective for treating certain types of ailments, such as arthritis, back pain, the side effects of chemotherapy, migraine headaches, and nausea and vomiting associated with pregnancy. Acupuncture and Oriental medicine practitioners (AOM) practitioners require an additional three to four years of education beyond the undergraduate level. They must also pass a national certification exam. AOM practitioners are licensed in 46 states and must abide by the state requirements for licensure, record keeping, and practice. There are approximately 17,000 AOM practitioners in the United States who have graduated from from 54 Oriental medicine schools. Their professional association is the Association of Acupuncture and Oriental Medicine. Often, CAM professionals are more closely regulated than traditional healthcare practitioners. **Figure 14.4** shows the level of detail required for record keeping and, in particular, addresses the use of the EHR by acupuncturists.

Chiropractors

A complementary and alternative healthcare profession, chiropractic medicine focuses on diagnosing and treating mechanical disorders of the spine and musculoskeletal system. The treatments are designed to affect the nervous system and improve overall health. There are 19 chiropractic medical schools in the United States, all four-year programs, each requiring a minimum of 90 undergraduate credit hours for entry. Chiropractors must also pass a national certification exam. The American Chiropractic Association is their national association, representing approximately 15,000 chiropractors. Chiropractors are licensed in the state where they practice and must abide by the laws of that state. **Figure 14.5** shows the Kentucky state law regarding record keeping for chiropractors. Compare figure 14.5 with figure 14.4 for acupuncture and notice the different record-keeping requirements for the two professions and the different ways a state may approach the guidelines and laws. HIM professionals may work directly for CAM professionals, or they may work for a hospital where CAM professionals are employed. In either case, HIM professionals must be familiar with the state laws for each of the different types of CAM professionals.

FIGURE 14.4. New Jersey laws regarding electronic record keeping for licensed acupuncturists

NJ Statute 13:35-9.11 [Acupuncturist] **Preparation of patient records; computerized records; access to or release of information; confidentiality,** **transfer or disposal of records**

Treatment records shall be maintained for a period of seven years from the date of the most recent entry.

1. To the extent applicable, professional treatment records shall reflect: i. The dates of all treatments; ii. The patient complaint; iii. The history; iv. Progress notes; and v. Any orders for tests or consultations and the results thereof.

2. Corrections and/or additions may be made to an existing record, provided that each change is clearly identified as such, dated and initialed by the certificate holder;

3. A patient record *which is prepared and maintained on a personal or other computer shall be prepared and maintained as follows:*

    i. The patient record shall contain at least two forms of identification, for example, name and record number or any other specific identifying information;

    ii. The entry made by the acupuncturist shall be made contemporaneously with the treatment and shall contain the date of service, date of entry, and full printed name of the treatment provider. The acupuncturist shall finalize or "sign" the entry by means of a confidential personal code ("CPC") and include date of the "signing";

    iii. The acupuncturist may dictate a dated entry for later transcription. The transcription shall be dated and identified as "preliminary" until reviewed, finalized and dated by the acupuncturist as provided in (b)3ii above;

    iv. The computer system shall contain an internal permanently activated date and time recordation for all entries, and shall automatically prepare a back-up copy of the file;

    v. The computer system shall be designed in such manner that after "signing" by means of the CPC, the existing entry cannot be changed in any manner. Notwithstanding the permanent status of a prior entry, a new entry may be made at any time and may indicate correction to a prior entry;

    vi. Where more than one acupuncturist is authorized to make entries into the computer file of any professional treatment record, the acupuncturist responsible for the acupuncture practice shall assure that each such person obtains a CPC and uses the file program in the same manner;

    vii. A copy of each day's entry, identified as preliminary or final as applicable, shall be made available to a physician responsible for the patient's care, to a representative of the Board of Acupuncture Examiners, the Attorney General or the Division of Consumer Affairs no later than 10 days after notice, or to a patient within 30 days of the request, or promptly in the event of emergency.

    viii. An acupuncturist wishing to continue a system of computerized patient records, which system does not meet the requirements of (b)3i through vii above, shall promptly initiate arrangements for modification of the system which shall be completed by October 18, 2000. In the interim, the acupuncturist shall assure that, on the date of the first treatment of each patient treated subsequent to October 18, 1999, the computer entry for that first visit shall be accompanied by a hard copy printout of the entire computer-recorded treatment record. The printout shall be dated and initialed by the attending acupuncturist. Thereafter, a hard copy shall be prepared for each subsequent visit, continuing to the date of the changeover of computer program, with each page initialed by the treating acupuncturist.

Source: State of New Jersey 2005.

Naturopathic Doctors

Naturopathy is a school of medical philosophy and practice that focuses on improving health and treating disease chiefly by assisting the body's intrinsic ability to recuperate from illness and injury. According to the Association of Accredited Naturopathic Medical Colleges (www.aanmc.org), naturopathic doctors (NDs) practice according to six principles, among which is the healing power of nature. Some of the top conditions that NDs treat are fatigue, menstruation/hormonal issues, allergies, depression/insomnia, fibromyalgia, and thyroid disorders. Licensed NDs must complete four years of naturopathic medical

FIGURE 14.5. Kentucky laws regarding record keeping of chiropractors

201 KAR 21:100 Minimum standards for record keeping/itemized statements

Section 1. Office Visits—Recordkeeping.
 	
1. The patient's records shall include the history, exams, re-exams, diagnosis, update diagnosis, standing orders or plan of care (updated as needed or at re-exam), and appropriate diagnostic and imaging studies. This information shall be legibly recorded in the patient's records and properly identified.
 	
2. Legible documentation, whether electronically generated, computer generated, typewritten or hand written, shall record each visit, and shall include the following:
 	
  a. Date of the visit;
 	
  b. Patient symptoms, comment and interval history, if any;
 	
  c. Procedures performed, if any;
 	
  d. Additional pertinent comments, instructions, or orders; and
 	
  e. The doctor's name.

Source: State of Kentucky 2006.

school at one of six accredited schools after their undergraduate education is completed. They must also pass a national certification exam. The 14 states that license NDs to practice medicine are

1. Alaska
2. Arizona
3. California
4. Connecticut
5. Hawaii
6. Idaho
7. Kansas
8. Maine
9. Montana
10. New Hampshire
11. Oregon
12. Utah
13. Vermont
14. Washington

Licensed Massage Therapists

Licensed massage therapists (LMTs) are becoming more integral to healthcare, especially in academic medical centers. LMTs are regulated by the state where they practice. They must complete anywhere from 500 to 1,000 hours of professional training from an accredited institution and pass a national certification exam before they can be licensed. LMTs are governed by the record-keeping laws of their states.

Direct-Entry Midwives

Direct-entry midwifery refers to an educational path that does not require prior nursing training to enter the profession. (Direct-entry midwives are different from NP midwives. NPs are addressed in the earlier section on midlevel practitioners.) Certified professional midwives (CPMs) are direct-entry midwives who are nationally certified and licensed in the states where they practice. In response to numerous state initiatives that call for the legalization of midwifery practice and the increased utilization of midwives as maternity care providers, midwives across the United States have come together to define and establish standards for international certification. The North American Registry of Midwives, the Midwives' Alliance of North America, and the Midwifery Education and Accreditation Council have joined together to create the internationally accepted CPM credential to preserve the unique, woman-centered forms of practice that are common to midwives attending out-of-hospital births.

Outpatient Ambulatory Integrated Clinical Settings

Integrated clinical settings discussed in this section include several types of ambulatory care, outpatient rehabilitation centers, renal dialysis centers, public health clinics, cancer treatment centers, and mobile health units.

Ambulatory Care

The percentage of healthcare that is provided in an ambulatory setting has grown significantly in the past 15 years. Today, almost half of all healthcare expenses are derived from care provided in an outpatient setting. The number of ambulatory visits is much greater than the number of inpatient visits: 1.1 billion ambulatory visits to approximately 35 million inpatient visits. Until recently, much of the focus has been on HIM in the hospital setting, so health information professionals have a great opportunity to bring improvement to ambulatory areas. The list of different types of ambulatory settings is quite extensive, so we will focus on those that can be accredited by The Joint Commission.

Although Joint Commission accreditation is voluntary, most healthcare organizations look to The Joint Commission as the standard-setting institution. Many will seek the accreditation because they believe it helps position them as a higher-quality alternative than a competitor who is not accredited. Many of the ambulatory care providers that can seek accreditation through The Joint Commission are listed in the following sections. For a complete list, see The Joint Commission's "Facts about Ambulatory Care Accreditation" (Joint Commission 2011). In each case, ambulatory centers must seek licensure from and abide by the laws of the state where they are located. This includes record-keeping laws that the HIM professionals employed there must know and apply.

Many ambulatory care centers are owned by or affiliated with a local hospital. In such cases, HIM may be centralized. Ambulatory care centers that are freestanding must employ their own credentialed HIM professionals.

FIGURE 14.6. Types of organizations accredited by AAAHC

- Ambulatory healthcare clinics
- Ambulatory surgery centers
- Birthing centers
- College and university health centers
- Community health centers
- Dental group practices
- Diagnostic imaging centers
- Endoscopy centers
- Federally qualified community health centers
- Health maintenance organizations (HMOs)
- Independent physician associations
- Indian health centers
- Lithotripsy centers
- Managed care organizations

- Medical home organizations
- Military healthcare facilities
- Multispecialty group practices
- Occupational health centers
- Office-based anesthesia organizations
- Office-based surgery centers and practices
- Oral and maxillofacial surgeons' offices
- Pain management centers
- Podiatry practices
- Radiation oncology centers
- Single-specialty group practices
- Surgical recovery centers
- Urgent or immediate care centers
- Women's health centers

The **Accreditation Association for Ambulatory Health Care (AAAHC)** defines standards for many types of ambulatory settings (AAAHC 2010). See **Figure 14.6** for a complete list of these settings.

Ambulatory Surgical Centers

CMS defines an ambulatory surgical center (ASC) as "any distinct entity that operates exclusively for the purpose of providing surgical services to patients not requiring hospitalization." ASCs can be freestanding or based within a hospital. The plan for their patients is to admit and discharge them on the same day. However, some ASC patients who experience complications may require admission to a hospital. The attraction of a freestanding ASC is usually convenience, personalized attention, and posh accommodations. The most common procedures performed at an ASC are hernia repair; skin repair or excision; ear tube insertion or removal; eye surgery, such as cataract removal or retina repair; plastic or cosmetic surgery; repair of muscles, tendons, ligaments, and joints; carpal tunnel release; tonsillectomy; cardiac catheterization; colonoscopy; other gastric endoscopies; gallbladder removal; and hysterectomies.

The Ambulatory Surgery Center Association is the membership and advocacy organization for ASCs. It provides member benefits and services and lobbies for legislative, regulatory, and other challenges at the federal and state levels. **Figure 14.7** contains the health record requirements for ASCs under the Medicare COP.

Convenient Care

Convenient care centers are also referred to as **retail medical clinics**. They are relatively new to the healthcare industry in the United States and have begun to spring up in the past five years. Many national drugstore chains, such as CVS, Walgreens, and RiteAid, have convenient care centers staffed by physicians, PAs, NPs, and nurses located within the store, facilitating the prescription-filling process. Patients can generally be seen for

FIGURE 14.7. Conditions of participation for ASCs

416.47—ASCs: Condition for coverage medical records
The ASC must maintain complete, comprehensive, and accurate medical records to ensure adequate patient care.

a. Standard: Organization. The ASC must develop and maintain a system for the proper collection, storage, and use of patient records.

b. Standard: Form and content of record. The ASC must maintain a medical record for each patient. Every record must be accurate, legible, and promptly completed. Medical records must include at least the following:

   1. Patient identification.

   2. Significant medical history and results of physical examination.

   3. Pre-operative diagnostic studies (entered before surgery), if performed.

   4. Findings and techniques of the operation, including a pathologist's report on all tissues removed during surgery, except those exempted by the governing body.

   5. Any allergies and abnormal drug reactions.

   6. Entries related to anesthesia administration.

   7. Documentation of properly executed informed patient consent.

   8. Discharge diagnosis.

Source: 42 CFR Parts 410, 416, and 419.

minor complaints, flu shots, or physical exam for administrative purposes. Convenient care centers must be licensed by the state where they are located and must comply with all the state department of health's regulations regarding healthcare providers. These organizations may employ a health information professional to oversee the HIM needs of several different locations.

Diagnostic Imaging Centers

Diagnostic imaging centers can provide convenience for patients and often have a much shorter waiting time than a hospital imaging department. The Joint Commission provides voluntary accreditation for diagnostic imaging centers that offer up to the full range of imaging services, including computed tomography (CT) scanning, magnetic resonance imaging (MRI), cardiac imaging, ultrasound, mammography, digital X-ray, fetal ultrasound, molecular imaging, nuclear imaging, and woman's imaging. The American College of Radiology also offers voluntary accreditation for imaging centers. Their accreditation includes MRI, radiation oncology, mammography, CT scan, positive emission tomography scan, stereotactic breast biopsy, and ultrasound. Imaging centers must be licensed by the state where they are located and must comply with all the state department of health's regulations regarding healthcare providers. Depending on the size of the organization, they may employ one or more HIM professionals. Imaging centers likely need HIM expertise for coding as well as information management, because coding and billing for radiology procedures can be complex.

Diagnostic Sleep Centers

To accommodate the many Americans who experience chronic sleep disorders, sleep centers have been established throughout the country over the past 10 years. Sleep disorders have been correlated with obesity, hypertension, heart disease, impotence, depression, and attention deficit/hyperactivity disorder in some patients. Because the diagnosis of these conditions is growing, so is the need for sleep disturbance analysis. Ten years ago, a group of physicians with specialty training in neurology, sleep medicine, pulmonary medicine, oral surgery, and otolaryngology decided to create the sleep center concept, directed by a multispecialty approach that would offer patients innovative as well as classic options for the treatment of snoring and obstructive sleep apnea. Diagnostic sleep centers (DSCs) therefore do standard testing in addition to snore localization studies. While most DSCs are in freestanding locations or within hospitals, some have begun to offer patients the option of sleeping in a hotel or at home and having the DSC transport its mobile labs to the location. DSCs must be licensed by the state where they are located and must comply with all the state department of health's regulations regarding healthcare providers. HIM expertise is needed for information management (including release of information), coding, and billing purposes.

Diagnostic/Therapeutic Centers

These centers combine the diagnostic activities of imaging (and others) with treatment so the patient can receive the entire spectrum of services in one location. Services that may be offered by a diagnostic/treatment center include imaging and other diagnostic testing, laboratory testing, cardiac diagnostics and therapeutics, neurophysiology (such as electroencephalograms, electromyograms, and electronystagmograms), and cancer treatment. These organizations are licensed by the states where they are located and must comply with all state department of health's regulations for healthcare providers. Depending on the size of the organization, HIM professionals may be employed for coding and billing expertise as well as health information management functions.

Endoscopy Centers

Endoscopy centers generally provide gastroenterology endoscopies and are staffed by gastroenterologists. The appeal to patients is the ease of service and expertise/focus on this specific health concern. These organizations are licensed by the states where they are located and must comply with all state department of health regulations for healthcare providers. HIM professionals may be employed for coding, billing, and HIM functions.

Medical/Dental Centers

The Joint Commission provides accreditation for these types of ambulatory centers. Since we have discussed physicians and dentists as solo practitioners, the details about these types of practices can be reviewed in the relevant earlier sections.

Telehealth/Nonsurgical

Telemedicine is the use of medical information transmitted from one site to another via electronic communications to improve a patient's health status. Closely associated with telemedicine is the term "telehealth," which is often used to encompass a broader definition of remote healthcare that does not always involve clinical services. Videoconferencing; transmission of still images; e-health, including patient portals; remote monitoring of vital signs; continuing medical education; and nursing call centers are all considered part of telemedicine and telehealth (ATA 2010).

Telemedicine dates back to the 1960s with NASA's efforts to provide healthcare services to astronauts. Since that time, several pilot projects introduced the concept of telemedicine to patients in rural areas without access to specialists. Today, telemedicine is provided in every state and may encompass services to patients in rural areas, patients in correctional facilities and nursing homes, and homebound patients; remote monitoring for intensive care units and emergency departments; cardiac telemetry; and fetal monitoring. Although telemedicine can be provided by physicians at any location, it is most often delivered from academic medical centers or large healthcare systems with access to many specialists. Teleradiology is the most common type of telemedicine. Physicians in any specialty can use telemedicine, but dermatologists, ophthalmologists, and pathologists have found significant added value through telemedicine. Overall, telemedicine services can be categorized as one of the following:

1. Direct clinical, preventive, diagnostic, and therapeutic services

2. Consultative and follow-up services

3. Remote monitoring, including the remote reading and interpretation of results of patient's procedures

4. Rehabilitative services

The American Telemedicine Association (ATA) is the professional and educational accreditation body. Reimbursement for telemedicine services is quite complex and changing as payers continue to reconsider payment policies. Because of the nature of telemedicine, there are specific health information needs. For example, order and informed consents must be modified to take into consideration the nature of the visit. The patient must consent not only to the format of the telemedicine visit but also to being recorded during the visit. **FIGURE 14.8** contains a list of data elements that the ATA recommends referring physicians provide on their requests for telemedicine services. On a consultation, the report must contain the location of the physician and the location of the patient.

Patients must consent to a telemedicine consultation just as they would to any face-to-face encounter with a physician. If the transmitted images will be recorded as part of the diagnostic or therapeutic process, the consent form should include discussion of the capture and use of the images. A facility's policy should address information ownership and how images or recordings will be maintained. Images and recordings should be considered part of the patient's medical record and should be kept for the same time period state law requires medical records to be kept. A note should be made in the patient's record indicating the availability and location of these recordings.

Telemedicine uses store forward technology, which means that images, data, and other recordings are transmitted from the patient's (remote) site to the provider's site during the tele-appointment. These electronic data need to be preserved and made available for the provider to review before each appointment. In addition to the electronic recordings of the visit, a traditional patient record must also be kept. HIM professionals may also be employed to assist with the coding and billing for telemedicine services.

Telehealth/Surgical

Considered a subset of telemedicine, telesurgery has the same logistical and management issues. The nature of the service, however, makes telesurgery unique. Until the past few years, telesurgery was used primarily by the military. A surgeon using a robotic surgery system in a hospital typically sits across the room from a patient. Looking through a three-dimensional monitor, the surgeon uses a joystick to control the robot, which is armed with surgical tools and a camera. Robotic surgeries are useful for minimally invasive procedures and have been used to repair blockages between the kidney and the

FIGURE 14.8. Telemedicine referral: Clinical information

Clinical Data Recommended to Be Documented for a Telemedicine Referral
• Reason for consultation (pull-down choices: diagnosis, second opinion, recommendation for treatment, other [type in option])
• Patient's chief complaint (rash, growth, acne, nail, hair, other [type in option])
• Location(s) (free text or graphic image for point and click)
• Duration (free text or pull-down options to include "since birth")
• Chronicity (pull-down menu: intermittent, persistent, other [free text])
• Associated signs and symptoms (pull-down menu: pruritus, tenderness, burning, other [type in option])
• Palliative factors (free text)
• Exacerbating factors (free text)
• Number of Images (integers)
• PMHx (defaults to noncontributory unless information is typed in as free text)
• PSHx (defaults to noncontributory unless information is typed in as free text)
• Fam Hx (defaults to noncontributory unless information is typed in as free text)
• ROS (defaults to noncontributory unless information is typed in as free text)
• Medications (defaults to none unless information is typed in as free text)
• Allergies (defaults to NKDA unless information is typed in as free text)
• Biopsy results/laboratory data (free text)
• Provisional (your) diagnosis (free text)
• Specific questions (free text)

Source: ATA 2009.

ureter or to remove the prostate. In the civilian world, telesurgery is still being performed with the surgeon in the same room as the patient, or the next room. It is only a matter of time, however, before long-distance surgeries are available to people in rural areas or other locations where access to the best expertise may not have been possible before.

Urgent Care Centers

Urgent care centers provide walk-in, extended-hour access for acute illness and injury care that is beyond the scope or availability of the typical primary care practice. According to the Urgent Care Association of America (UCAOA), there are more than 8,500 urgent care centers in the United States. The UCAOA certifies urgent care centers, which have a broader and deeper scope of services than retail clinics/convenient care centers but are not equivalent to emergency departments. Urgent care ideally helps reserve the nation's emergency department resources for more serious, life-threatening conditions. Most urgent care centers use some form of an EHR. Clinical documentation, coding, billing, and HIPAA concerns may be present along with HIM needs. Depending on the size of the center, they may employ one or many HIM professionals. Urgent care centers are licensed in the state where they are located and must comply with all state laws.

Mobile Health Units

Mobile health units are typically large vans or vehicles that bring screening services and health education to communities and rural areas in which residents do not have easy access to health services. For example, the services offered by the Medical University of South Carolina's Hollings Health Center's 40-foot mobile unit van include (MUSC 2011)

- Mammograms

- Digital rectal exams and prostate-specific antigen tests

- Visual inspection for skin cancer

- Pelvic exams and Pap smears

- Oral exams of the mouth and neck

Outpatient Rehabilitation Center

The **outpatient rehabilitation center (ORC)** provides an integrated, multidisciplinary program. It brings together specialized rehabilitation personnel to upgrade the physical functions of disabled individuals. The center's staff must include a physician and provide services of physical therapists, occupational therapists, and speech therapists. Generally, patients receive physical therapy care in an outpatient setting for a minor injury or following discharge from an inpatient rehabilitation hospital. ORCs usually treat patients following injury, fracture, heart attack, or stroke. Some ORCs also offer addiction and substance abuse treatment. The Commission on Accreditation of Rehabilitation Facilities (CARF) accredits ORCs. CARF accredits the following types of service programs:

- Aging services

- Behavioral health

- Child and youth services

- Durable medical equipment providers

- Medical rehabilitation

- Opiod rehabilitation

- Vision rehabilitation

In addition, healthcare providers can be accredited by CARF for specific rehabilitation programs, including those for pediatric specialty, amputation, brain injury, spinal cord, stroke, and pain relief. Each program has its own health information requirements. In addition to CARF-specific requirements, the HIM professional must be aware of federal and state-specific health record requirements for these types of services. **FIGURE 14.9** contains the health record requirements for rehabilitation centers under the Medicare COP. Note that the sections highlighted are those that are specific to the type of care provided in a rehabilitation facility.

Renal Dialysis Centers

Renal dialysis centers are facilities where individuals with kidney disease or those awaiting a kidney transplant receive assistance from equipment that performs the necessary kidney functions. Individuals receiving renal dialysis are either waiting for a suitable donor kidney or cannot receive a kidney donation at this time. Renal dialysis on a

FIGURE 14.9. COP for rehabilitation facilities

§485.60 Condition of Participation: Clinical records. The facility must maintain clinical records on all patients in accordance with accepted professional standards and practice. The clinical records must be completely, promptly, and accurately documented, readily accessible, and systematically organized to facilitate retrieval and compilation of information.

a. **Standard: Content.** Each clinical record must contain sufficient information to identify the patient clearly and to justify the diagnosis and treatment. Entries in the clinical record must be made as frequently as is necessary to insure effective treatment, and must be signed by personnel providing services. All entries made by assistant level personnel must be countersigned by the corresponding professional. Documentation on each patient must be consolidated into one clinical record that must contain—

1. The initial assessment and subsequent reassessments of the patient's needs;

2. Current plan of treatment;

3. Identification data and consent or authorization forms;

4. Pertinent medical history, past and present;

5. A report of pertinent physical examinations if any;

6. Progress notes or other documentation that reflect patient reaction to treatment, tests, or injury, or the need to change the established plan of treatment; and

7. Upon discharge, a discharge summary including patient status relative to goal achievement, prognosis, and future treatment considerations.

b. **Standard: Protection of clinical record information.** The facility must safeguard clinical record information against loss, destruction, or unauthorized use. The facility must have procedures that govern the use and removal of records and the conditions for release of information. The facility must obtain the patient's written consent before releasing information not required to be released by law.

c. **Standard: Retention and preservation.** The facility must retain clinical record information for 5 years after patient discharge and must make provision for the maintenance of such records in the event that it is no longer able to treat patients.

frequent or daily basis is provided for effective kidney functioning. Under a doctor's supervision, these units are staffed by registered nurses and certified technicians and operate on an outpatient basis. They are often located within a hospital or as an outpatient facility. Some large corporations operate outpatient renal dialysis centers throughout the nation. Both Davita and Fresenius specialize in end-stage renal disease care. Davita employs more than 34,000 staff in more than 2,200 facilities, and Fresenius employs more than 30,000 staff in 1,700 facilities nationwide.

Because all dialysis patients are covered by Medicare, CMS has a special interest in obtaining and providing data about the quality of care provided at renal dialysis centers. The following three specific quality measures are collected and posted on the CMS website for dialysis patients:

- **Anemia**—number of patients at a facility whose anemia (low red blood cell count) was not controlled (hemoglobin less than 10.0 g/dL or hemoglobin greater than 12.0 g/dL)

- **Hemodialysis adequacy**—number of patients at a facility who had enough waste removed from their blood during dialysis treatments (urea reduction ratio of 65 or greater)

- **Patient survival**—if the patients treated at a facility generally live longer than, as long as, or not as long as expected.

Because of these criteria and the importance of each center, documentation must be as accurate as possible. Physicians and other clinicians in the centers are likely to need education, review, and feedback from the HIM professionals employed in these facilities.

Public Health Clinics

Most public health clinics provide services similar to those in a physician's office. They are usually sponsored and managed by a government entity, community, or religious organization. Clinics typically focus on primary care, but they may also provide obstetrical, gynecological, dental, mental health, and substance abuse services. The federal government provides nationwide free-clinic care through the Health Resources and Services Administration (HRSA). Federally funded clinics can be located on the HRSA website (ask.hrsa. gov/pc).The federal government's definition of a clinic requires that the facility meet the following test of physician participation: three or more physicians practicing medicine together provide the clinic's medical services, and at least one physician is present during all clinic hours to perform medical services. Residents often provide many of the services at clinics. The most common services clinics provide are immunizations, prenatal and post-neonatal care, and contraception. The most common conditions clinics treat are allergic reactions, asthma (mild to moderate wheezing), broken bones, minor burns, minor cuts, dehydration, diarrhea, earaches and infections, low fevers, rashes and bumps, sprains, and sore throats. Public health clinics must meet both federal requirements (if they are federally funded) and state laws for the states in which they are located. Health record activities and responsibilities are similar to those in a physician's office or ambulatory care center.

Cancer Treatment Centers

Cancer treatment centers specialize in providing comprehensive cancer treatment, including radiation and chemotherapy. Many also offer patient education and family counseling services.

Established by the American College of Surgeons in 1922, the multidisciplinary **Commission on Cancer (CoC)** sets standards for quality multidisciplinary cancer care. The CoC Approvals Program encourages hospitals, treatment centers, and other facilities to improve their quality of patient care through various cancer-related programs. These programs are concerned with prevention, early diagnosis, pretreatment evaluation, staging, and optimal treatment, as well as rehabilitation, surveillance for recurrent disease, support services, and end-of-life care.

The availability of a full range of medical services and a multidisciplinary team approach to patient care at approved cancer treatment centers has resulted in approximately 80 percent of all newly diagnosed cancer patients being treated in CoC-approved cancer programs.

Recognizing that cancer is a complex group of diseases, the CoC Cancer Program Standards promote consultation among surgeons, medical and radiation oncologists, diagnostic radiologists, pathologists, and other cancer specialists (CoC 2009). This multidisciplinary cooperation results in improved patient care.

The following five elements contribute to the success of a CoC-approved cancer program (CoC 2009):

1. The clinical services provide state-of-the-art pretreatment evaluation, staging, treatment, and clinical follow-up for cancer patients seen at the facility for primary, secondary, tertiary, or quaternary care.

2. The cancer committee leads the program through setting goals, monitoring activities, evaluating patient outcomes, and improving care.

3. The cancer conferences provide a forum for patient consultation and contribute to physician education.

4. The quality improvement program is the mechanism for evaluating and improving patient outcomes.

5. The cancer registry and database form the basis for monitoring the quality of care.

Records regarding chemotherapy and radiotherapy treatment must be retained for a patient's lifetime. Premature destruction of such documentation may result in a preventable death or inappropriate subsequent treatment.

Government Healthcare Settings

The government healthcare settings discussed in this section are the Veterans Health Administration, other military healthcare systems, correctional facilities, and Indian Health Services. The government provides funding for a variety of providers who fit the criteria as federally qualified health centers (FQHCs). According to HHS (2011), "FQHCs are 'safety net' providers such as community health centers, public housing centers, outpatient health programs funded by the Indian Health Service, and programs serving migrants and the homeless. The main purpose of the FQHC Program is to enhance the provision of primary care services in underserved urban and rural communities." FQHCs are not a type of provider, so they are not covered in detail in this book.

Veterans Health Administration

The **Veterans Health Administration (VHA)** runs the largest integrated healthcare system in the country, with 153 hospitals and more than 1,000 clinics and nursing homes employing 14,800 doctors and 61,000 nurses serving 5.3 million veterans. See chapter 5 for an in-depth discussion of the VHA EHR. In addition to the inpatient and outpatient VHA facilities discussed in chapter 5, the VHA also has a personal health record (PHR) for all veterans called My Healthe Vet.

My HealtheVet offers veterans, active-duty soldiers, and their dependents and caregivers Internet access to VHA healthcare information and services. Launched nationwide in 2003, My HealtheVet is a free, online PHR that empowers veterans to become informed partners in their healthcare. Veterans can access trusted, secure, and current health and benefits information and record and store important health and military history information at their convenience. With My HealtheVet, one can access

- Nine healthy living centers

- Disease and conditions centers

- Mental health information

- Trusted health and medical information

- Info on VHA benefits and services

- Local VHA events and activities

- Personal health journals

- Vitals tracking and graphing

- Military health history

- Activity and food journals

The VHA includes provides more than 1.2 million dental treatment visits each year; employs more than 800 dentists, 900 dental assistants, 185 dental hygienists, and 300 dental technicians; and operates command centers to coordinate services. There are many opportunities for HIM professionals at VHA settings. Some are in traditional HIM roles, such as HIM director or privacy officer. The VHA hospitals began requiring ICD-9-CM coding for all diagnoses and procedures in the 1990s and now reimburses for inpatient care using a prospective payment system similar to the diagnosis-related group (DRG system). In addition, the VHA is constantly involved in developing new information technology, which provides HIM professionals with additional opportunities to use their expertise in a technology role.

The VHA maintains the most comprehensive and integrated EHR system in the world, known as VistA. VistA is used as a case study in this book, and its contents and format are addressed in detail in chapter 6.

Other Military Healthcare Systems

The Military Health System (MHS) is a global medical network within the Department of Defense that provides care to all US military personnel worldwide. Equipped with 59 hospitals and 364 health clinics, MHS delivers care to 9.6 million service members, veterans, and family members. The US Army, Navy, and Air Force all have their own healthcare systems. Other branches of the armed forces use healthcare from one of these branches or from the private sector. The Army manages 25 hospitals and 17 clinics, the Navy manages 17 hospitals and 46 clinics, and the Air Force manages 5 hospitals and 62 clinics. All care is tracked and managed using ICD-9-CM and CPT codes in military hospitals, just as in civilian hospitals. Payments are calculated using a DRG system for inpatient stays. In addition to documentation and coding responsibilities, HIM staff at other military facilities have responsibilities similar to those in acute care hospitals and outpatient clinics.

The MHS is integrating its EHR to the VistA EHR. These two large EHR integration efforts have also provided some private-sector opportunities to begin integration through the National Health Information Network, providing additional employment and career development opportunities for HIM professionals.

Correctional Facilities

As of 2008, approximately 2.4 million people were incarcerated in the United States. These individuals are in federal and state correctional facilities, local jails, military jails, and juvenile correctional facilities. Approximately 500 facilities are accredited by **National Conference on Correctional Healthcare (NCCHC)**. **Table 14.2** provides the number of incarcerated individuals by correctional facility type.

Most states use telemedicine to some degree in their correctional facilities. States like Arizona and California estimate that they save millions of dollars per year by providing telemedicine services (where appropriate) to inmates instead of transporting them to

TABLE 14.2 Incarcerated individuals in the United States

USA AND TERRITORIES INCARCERATED POPULATION	NUMBER OF INMATES IN 2008
Total	2,424,279
Federal and state prisons	1,518,559
Territorial prisons	13,576
Local jails	785,556
Immigration and Customs Enforcement facilities	9,957
Military facilities	1,651
Jails in Indian country	2,135
Juvenile facilities	92,845

Source: US Bureau of Justice Statistics 2009.

hospitals for care. Correctional facilities need to be aware of the special considerations for healthcare and HIM surrounding telehealth services. These considerations are addressed in the earlier section on telehealth.

Every correctional facility is governed by the laws of the state where it is located. States have specific laws that address medical care and health records of inmates. At a minimum, HIM professionals providing services to correctional facilities need to be aware of state laws. For those facilities that are accredited by the NCCHC, HIM professionals should be aware of its requirements. NCCHC accreditation promotes and documents an efficient, well-managed system of healthcare delivery in correctional facilities. Standards must be met in the following areas:

- Facility governance and administration
- Maintaining a safe and healthy environment
- Personnel and training
- Healthcare services support
- Inmate care and treatment
- Health promotion and disease prevention
- Special inmate needs and services
- Health records

As an example of state requirements, **Figure 14.10** contains the Massachusetts state law regarding health records for inmates in Massachusetts prisons.

Indian Health Service

The Indian Health Service (IHS), an agency within HHS, provides federal health services to American Indians and Alaska Natives. The provision of health services to members of federally recognized tribes grew out of the relationship between the federal government and Indian tribes, established in 1787. The IHS is the principal federal healthcare provider and health advocate for Indian people The IHS provides a comprehensive health service

FIGURE 14.10. Massachusetts health record requirements in correctional facilities

Commonwealth of Massachusetts
MINIMUM STANDARDS GOVERNING MEDICAL RECORDS AND THE CONDUCT OF PHYSICAL EXAMINATIONS IN CORRECTIONAL FACILITIES

205.500: Medical Record to be Maintained: Each inmate shall have an individual medical record which shall be kept separate from any other administrative records.

205.501: Record to be Accurate: An accurate and complete medical record shall be maintained for each inmate from the time of admission to the time of discharge.

205.502: Responsibility of Physician: The completion of the medical record shall be the responsibility of the attending physician. Orders for treatment and all reports shall be legibly entered into the medical record, either in ink or in type, and signed by the physician submitting such orders or reports.

205.503: Record to be Transferred with Inmates: At any time an inmate is transferred to another correctional or health care facility, a copy of the medical record or a summary sheet (*See* 105 CMR 205.600 Appendix A) shall accompany the inmate. Any portion of the record, which is not reasonably completed at the time of the transfer, shall be completed and a copy delivered to such facility within 72 hours of said transfer. The medical record and/or summary sheet which accompany the inmate shall be sealed and given into the custody of the transportation officer responsible for the transfer of the inmate and shall be delivered to the person responsible for the maintenance of the medical records at the receiving facility.

205.504: Confidentiality: The medical staff shall maintain and use medical records in a manner which ensures the confidentiality of the information contained therein. Only those persons who need access to the record in order to provide medical services to the inmate or fulfill statutory obligations, and those persons specifically authorized by the inmate to see the record, shall have access to the records and information in them. The Department of Public Health staff shall have access to the records and information in them for the purpose of determining compliance.

205.505: Inspection of Records: Medical records may be inspected by the inmate to whom they relate, by his/her attorney or by any other person upon written authorization from the inmate. The inmate's signature on the written authorization shall be witnessed by a correctional facility's staff person. Copies of such records shall be furnished within 72 hours of request. Fees for such copies shall not exceed the fees required for copying public documents.

205.600: Contents of Medical Record: Every medical record used in a correctional facility shall consist of, but need not be limited to, the following:

A. Admissions Health Screening Report

B. Health History

C. Physical Examination or Physical Examination

D. Problem List

E. Progress Note

F. Medication Log Sheet

G. Order Sheet

205.601: Additional Requirements of Medical Record: In addition to those forms required by 105 CMR 205.600, the medical record shall also include any and all appropriate discharge summaries, referral reports and laboratory and diagnostic results.

205.602: All Visits to be Recorded: All contacts for the purpose of receiving medical care that the inmate has with a health care staff person shall be recorded in the appropriate place in the medical record.

205.603: Identification and Filing: The correctional facility shall maintain a system of identification and filing to insure rapid access to each patient's medical record, regardless of the physical form or method of storage of records.

205.604: Storage Space: The correctional facility shall provide adequate equipment and space for the storage of active and inactive medical records. The records shall be maintained so as to be safe from fire and water damage and from unauthorized use. Pursuant to M.G.L. c. 111, § 70 the medical records shall be retained for a period of 30 years from the last entry therein.

Source: Adapted from Commonwealth of Massachusetts 1996.

delivery system for approximately 1.9 million American Indians and Alaska Natives who belong to 564 federally recognized tribes in 35 states. Services are provided at 33 IHS hospitals, 59 health centers, and 50 health stations. The IHS employs approximately 2,700 nurses, 900 physicians, 400 engineers, 500 pharmacists, and 300 dentists, as well as other health professionals totaling more than 15,000 (IHS 2010).

The **Resource and Patient Management System (RPMS)** is the IHS enterprise health information system. The RPMS consists of more than 60 software applications and is used at approximately 400 IHS, tribal, and urban locations. The RPMS is certified by the **Certification Commission for Health Information Technology (CCHIT)**, a recognized certification body for EHRs. Aggregate data are used to report on clinical performance measures to Congress. The IHS also maintains a centralized database of patient encounters and administrative data for statistical purposes, performance measurement for accreditation, and public health and epidemiological studies. The IHS telecommunications infrastructure connects IHS, tribal, and urban facilities and links to the HHS telecommunications network. The IHS participates in HHS enterprise-wide initiatives to improve information technology (IT) infrastructure and works with the Department of Veterans Affairs and other federal partners to develop software and share technology resources. These collaborations are reflected in the IHS IT architecture and five-year plan (IHS 2010). Health record and data collection and analysis activities are an important component of IHS opportunities for HIM professionals.

Other Healthcare Settings

Other healthcare settings provide a variety of services and include blood banks, healthcare services for students, veterinary practices, and critical access hospitals.

Blood Banks

A blood bank is a place where blood is collected from donors, typed, separated into components, stored, and prepared for transfusion to recipients. A blood bank may be a free-standing facility or part of a larger laboratory in a hospital. Typically, each donated unit of blood (whole blood) is separated into multiple components, such as red blood cells, plasma, and platelets. An increasingly common blood bank procedure is apheresis, or the process of removing a specific component of the blood, such as platelets, and returning the remaining components, such as red blood cells and plasma, to the donor. This process allows more of one particular part of the blood to be collected than could be separated from a unit of whole blood. Apheresis is also performed to collect plasma (the liquid part of the blood) and granulocytes (white blood cells) (MedicineNet.com 2010). The American Red Cross is the organization responsible for most blood drives. America's Blood Centers is a nonprofit organization that operates 600 blood banks in the United States.

Blood banks are licensed and regulated by the US Food and Drug Administration. As of 2004, each time a patient receives blood products, the product and the patient's bracelet must be scanned using **electronic medication administration record (eMAR)** technology. As a result, the labeling of blood products by blood banks during the collection process is highly regulated. See **FIGURE 14.11** for a sample of the bar code for the blood product and the patient receiving the product. Information obtained from individuals who are donating is generally stored electronically. Each time patients donate blood, they must answer health history questions to ensure that they are still eligible to donate. HIM professionals can be involved in information management and quality control activities in blood banks. The American Association of Blood Banks is a professional and accrediting association for the industry.

FIGURE 14.11. Sample bar code form for blood banks

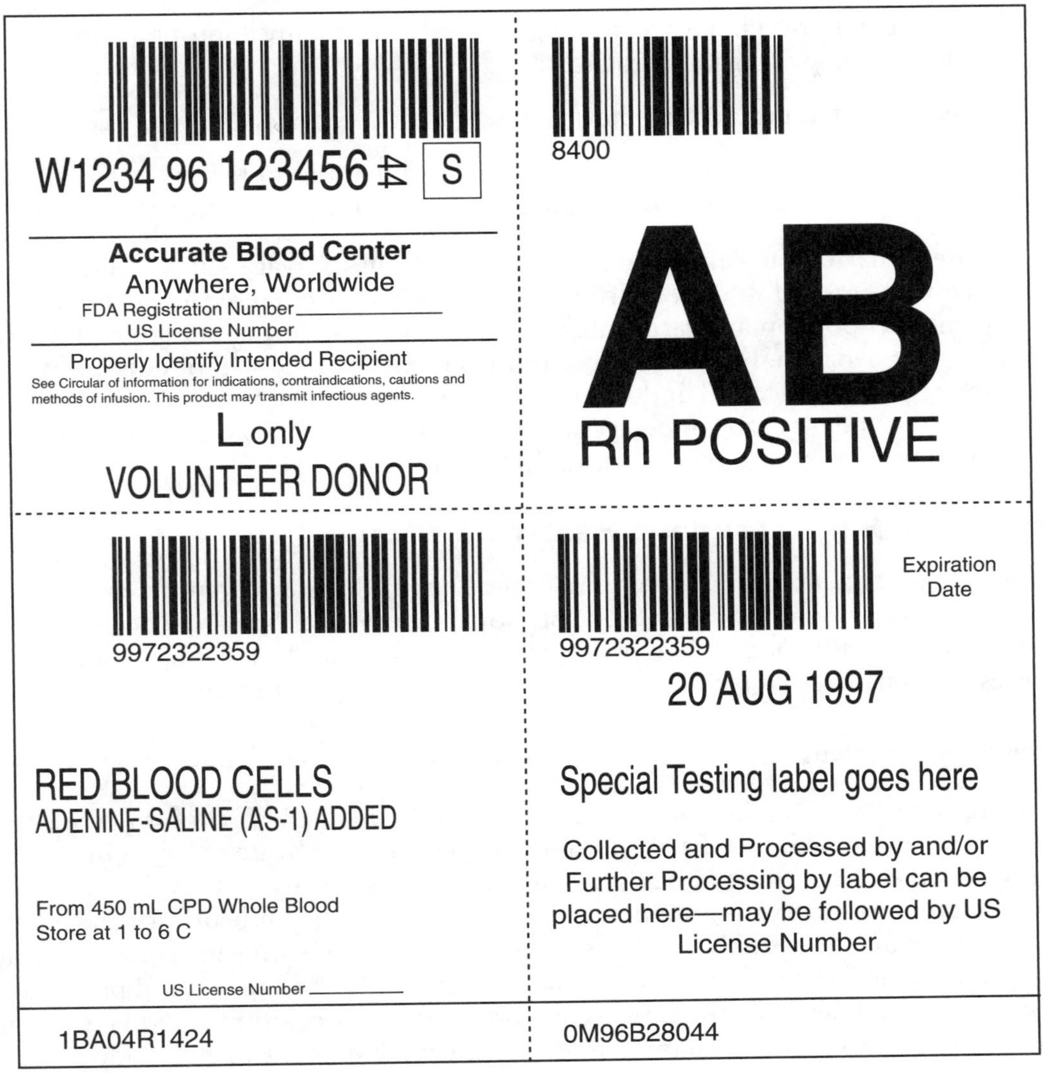

W1234 96 123456 ⊥⊥ [S]

Accurate Blood Center
Anywhere, Worldwide
FDA Registration Number_____
US License Number
Properly Identify Intended Recipient
See Circular of information for indications, contraindications, cautions and
methods of infusion. This product may transmit infectious agents.
L only
VOLUNTEER DONOR

8400

AB
Rh POSITIVE

9972322359

9972322359
20 AUG 1997

Expiration
Date

RED BLOOD CELLS
ADENINE-SALINE (AS-1) ADDED

Special Testing label goes here

Collected and Processed by and/or
Further Processing by label can be
placed here—may be followed by US
License Number

From 450 mL CPD Whole Blood
Store at 1 to 6 C

US License Number_____

1BA04R1424

0M96B28044

Source: FDA 2010.

Coordinated School Health Programs

According to the website for the American Association for School Health, all the strategies, activities, and services that are offered by, in, or in association with schools and designed to promote students' physical, emotional, and social development make up a school's health program.

When a school works with students, their families, and their community to provide these strategies, activities, and services in a coordinated, planned way, the term *coordinated school health program* applies. Ideally, a coordinated school health program includes the following:

- A healthful environment
- Nursing and other health services that students need to stay in school
- Nutritious and appealing school meals

- Opportunities for physical activity that include physical education

- Health education that covers a range of developmentally appropriate topics taught by knowledgeable teachers

- Programs that promote the health of school faculty and staff

- Counseling, psychological, and social services that promote healthy social and emotional development and remove barriers to students' learning

Congress enacted the **Family Educational Rights and Privacy Act (FERPA) of 1974** to protect the privacy of student educational records. Educational records maintained by the student's school contain vaccination histories, information about sports physicals, counseling for behavioral problems, and records of visits to the school nurse. Privacy of education records is protected under FERPA. An institution must have written permission from the adult student or the underage student's parent or legal guardian before releasing any information from a student's educational record.

University-Based Student Health Services

University student centers provide primary healthcare; disease prevention services; and counseling for personal, academic, and vocational concerns to their students. Promotion of a healthy lifestyle is one of their main goals. FERPA laws and regulations apply to state colleges, universities, and technical schools that receive federal funding.

Veterinary Practices

There are 80,000 veterinarians and 28 four-year veterinary medical schools in the United States. Veterinary practices differ significantly from other healthcare practices in that they do not provide care to human beings. While it is still necessary to provide quality care and maintain health records for animals, they do not have the same privacy and security rights as humans. As result, the processes are not nearly as stringent. However, health information practices for veterinary practices are governed by state law and professional association guidelines. The American Veterinary Medical Association (AVMA) is the professional association for veterinary professionals. The AVMA code of ethics addresses the maintenance and content of health records, stating the following (AVMA 2010):

- Veterinary medical records are an integral part of veterinary care. The records must comply with the standards established by state and federal law.

- Medical records are the property of the practice and the practice owner. The original records must be retained by the practice for the period required by statute.

- Ethically, the information within veterinary medical records is considered privileged and confidential. It must not be released except by court order or consent of the patient's owner.

- Veterinarians are obligated to provide copies or summaries of medical records when requested by the client. Veterinarians should secure a written release to document that request.

- Without the express permission of the practice owner, it is unethical for a veterinarian to remove, copy, or use the medical records or any part of any record.

FIGURE 14.12. Veterinary health record requirements in California State law

California Code of Regulations, Title 16, Section 2032.3 states:

Every veterinarian performing any act requiring a license pursuant to the provisions of Chapter 11, Division 2, of the code, upon any animal or group of animals shall prepare a legible, written or computer generated record concerning the animal or animals which shall contain the following information available:

1. Name or initials of the veterinarian responsible for entries.

2. Name, address and phone number of the client.

3. Name or identity of the animal, herd or flock.

4. Except for herds or flocks, age, sex, breed, species, and color of the animal.

5. Dates (beginning and ending) of custody of the animal, if applicable.

6. A history or pertinent information as it pertains to each animal, herd, or flock's medical status.

7. Data, including that obtained by instrumentation, from the physical examination.

8. Treatment and intended treatment plan, including medications, dosages and frequency of use.

9. Records for surgical procedures shall include a description of the procedure, the name of the surgeon, the type of sedative/anesthetic agents used, their route of administration, and their strength if available in more than one strength.

10. Diagnosis or tentative diagnosis at the beginning of custody of animal.

11. If relevant, a prognosis of the animal's condition.

12. All medications and treatments prescribed and dispensed, including strength, dosage, quantity, and frequency.

13. Daily progress, if relevant, and disposition of the case.

Source: California Department of Consumer Affairs, Veterinary Medical Board 2010.

Veterinarians and their practices are licensed by the state where they are located, and they must abide by the applicable laws. Most states address health record-keeping practices of veterinarians. **FIGURE 14.12** is the California state law that describes the responsibilities of veterinarians in regards to the health records of the animals they treat.

Critical Access Hospitals

Critical access hospitals (CAHs) must be located in a rural area and meet one of the following criteria:

- More than 35 miles from another hospital

- 15 miles from another hospital in mountainous terrain or areas with only secondary roads

A CAH is a hospital that is certified to receive cost-based reimbursement from Medicare. The reimbursement that CAHs receive is intended to improve their financial performance and thereby reduce hospital closures. CAHs are certified under a different set of Medicare COP that are more flexible than those for acute care hospitals. There are 1,305 certified CAHs located throughout the United States (RAC 2010). Staffing requirements for CAHs are different from those for acute care hospitals, as follow (RAC 2010):

- **Medical staff**: A CAH must have at least one physician, but he or she is not required to be on site. Midlevel practitioners can be an active, independent part of the CAH medical staff and provide direct service to patients. CAHs are required to provide oversight by a physician, but the oversight provisions are very liberal. This can be especially useful in communities that have had difficulty recruiting physicians.

- **Nursing staff**: General acute care hospitals are required to have a registered nurse (RN) on-site 24 hours a day, seven days a week. CAHs have more flexibility regarding staffing levels for nurses. The federal requirements allow for the hospital to close (and so have no RN on staff) if the facility is empty. State requirements vary. Some states may offer flexibility by allowing a licensed practical nurse to cover a shift in place of an RN when there are no acute patients, for example. Contact your state survey agency for details.

However, CAHs must continue to meet their state licensure requirements if they are stricter than the COP. The COP for CAH Health Records are provided in **Figure 14.13**.

HIM professionals should be familiar with both the Medicare COP and the state-specific regulations for health records in a CAH. EHR and health information exchange (HIE) provide opportunities for CAHs to improve the quality of care while decreasing costs. In addition, the increased use of technology for HIE provides additional career opportunities for HIM professionals.

FIGURE 14.13. Medicare COP for CAHs: Clinical records

---

a. Standard: Records system.

1. The CAH maintains a clinical records system in accordance with written policies and procedures.

2. The records are legible, complete, accurately documented, readily accessible, and systematically organized.

3. A designated member of the professional staff is responsible for maintaining the records and for ensuring that they are completely and accurately documented, readily accessible, and systematically organized.

4. For each patient receiving health care services, the CAH maintains a record that includes, as applicable.

   i. Identification and social data, evidence of properly executed informed consent forms, pertinent medical history, assessment of the health status and health care needs of the patient, and a brief summary of the episode, disposition, and instructions to the patient;

   ii. Reports of physical examinations, diagnostic and laboratory test results, including clinical laboratory services, and consultative findings;

   iii. All orders of doctors of medicine or osteopathy or other practitioners, reports of treatments and medications, nursing notes and documentation of complications, and other pertinent information necessary to monitor the patient's progress, such as temperature graphics, progress notes describing the patient's response to treatment; and

   iv. Dated signatures of the doctor of medicine or osteopathy or other health care professional.

b. Standard: Protection of record information--(1) The CAH maintains the confidentiality of record information and provides safeguards against loss, destruction, or unauthorized use.

2. Written policies and procedures govern the use and removal of records from the CAH and the conditions for the release of information.

3. The patient's written consent is required for release of information not required by law.

c. Standard: Retention of records. The records are retained for at least 6 years from date of last entry, and longer if required by State statute, or if the records may be needed in any pending proceeding.

Source: 42 CFR 485.638 2004.

A Note on Health Plans and Insurers

While original health record documentation is not created by health plans or health insurers, these organizations are users of the information they contain. And, in fact, there is a close relationship between health insurers and the HIM department in most healthcare organizations as health insurers seek to legitimately obtain documentation to help make coverage determinations. Health plans are interested not only in individual patient health information for coverage purposes but also in aggregate data for analysis. Health plans use aggregate data in planning, strategy, quality, and pricing. Health plans/health insurers provide an additional career opportunity for the HIM professional. The HIM professional's expertise in coding, data analysis, and EHRs can be used in the health plan setting.

America's Health Insurance Plans (AHIP) is the national association that represents nearly 1,300 member companies providing health insurance coverage to more than 200 million Americans (AHIP 2010). *US News & World Report* rates the top health plans each year. In 2010, the top 10 plans were all health maintenance organizations (HMOs) and included such plans as Harvard Pilgrim and Geisinger HMO (*US News & World Report* 2010). These plans are rated based on patient satisfaction and quality indicators. The largest health plans include United Health Group, Well Point, Aetna, Humana, and Cigna (*Fortune* 2010). United Health Group, the largest commercial insurer, had 2009 revenues of $87 billion and employs over 80,000 people (UHG 2010). Other insurers that provide career opportunities for HIM professionals include Medicare and Medicaid.

Summary

Healthcare is provided to patients in a myriad of settings other than the traditional hospital and healthcare systems described in earlier chapters. These settings can be generally grouped into solo (or group) practices, ambulatory care practices, government providers, and other providers, such as blood banks and critical access hospitals. Each type of setting has its own professional association and accrediting organization. In addition, each must maintain health records for the care provided. Most of these healthcare settings are beginning to pursue the transformation of health information from a paper-based or hybrid format into an electronic format. In each case, the HIM professional must become familiar with the specific federal, state, and regulatory requirements for health information in each setting. In addition, each setting presents new and growing career opportunities for the HIM professional.

References

42 CFR Parts 410, 416, and 419. 2008. Medicare Program: Changes to the Hospital Outpatient Prospective Payment System and CY 2009 Payment Rates; Changes to the Ambulatory Surgical Center Payment System and CY 2009 Payment Rates; Hospital Conditions of Participation: Requirements for Approval and Re-Approval of Transplant Centers To Perform Organ Transplants—Clarification of Provider and Supplier Termination Policy Medicare and Medicaid Programs: Changes to the Ambulatory Surgical Center Conditions for Coverage; Final Rule. http://edocket.access.gpo.gov/2008/pdf/E8-26212.pdf.

42 CFR Parts 410, 411, 414 et al. 2009. Medicare Program; Payment Policies Under the Physician Fee Schedule and Other Revisions to Part B for CY 2010; Final Rule; Medicare Program; Solicitation of Independent Accrediting Organizations To Participate in the Advanced Diagnostic Imaging Supplier Accreditation Program; Notice. http://edocket.access.gpo.gov/2009/E9-26502.htm.

42 CFR 485.638. 2004. Centers for Medicare and Medicaid Services. Conditions of Participation: Specialized Providers. http://edocket.access.gpo.gov/cfr_2004/octqtr/42cfr485.638.htm.

Accreditation Association for Ambulatory Health Care (AAAHC). 2010. Types of Organizations Accredited. http://www.aaahc.org/eweb/dynamicpage.aspx?webcode=types_accredited.

American Academy of Nurse Practitioners (AANP). 2010. About NPs. http://www.aanp.org/AANPCMS2/AboutAANP/About+NPs.htm.

American Academy of Physician Assistants (AAPA). 2010. Our Practice Areas. http://www.aapa.org/about-pas/our-practice-areas.

American Board of Medical Specialties (ABMS). 2011. Specialties and Subspecialties. http://www.abms.org/Who_We_Help/Physicians/specialties.aspx.

American College of Nurse-Midwives (ACNM). 2005. Standards for the Practice of Midwifery. http://www.midwife.org.

American Optometric Association. 2007. Code of Ethics. http://www.aoa.org/documents/Code-of-Ethics_Adopted-June-2007.pdf.

American Telemedicine Association (ATA). 2010. About Telemedicine. http://www.americantelemed.org/i4a/pages/index.cfm?pageID=3308.

American Telemedicine Association (ATA). 2009. Practice Guidelines for Videoconferencing-based Telemedicine. http://www.atmeda.org/files/public/standards/PracticeGuidelinesforVideoconferencing-Based%20TelementalHealth.pdf.

American Veterinary Medicine Association (AVMA). 2010. AVMA Policy. http://www.avma.org/issues/policy/ethics.asp.

America's Health Insurance Plans (AHIP). 2010. About AHIP. http://www.ahip.org/content/default.aspx?bc=31.

California Department of Consumer Affairs, Veterinary Medical Board. 2010. About Us. http://www.vmb.ca.gov/about_us/cc_medrk.shtml.

Centers for Disease Control and Prevention. 2010. Electronic Medical Record/Electronic Health Record Use by Office-based Physicians: United States 2008 and Preliminary 2009. http://www.cdc.gov/nchs/data/hestat/emr_ehr/emr_ehr.pdf.

Cherry, D.S., D.A. Woodwell, and E.A. Rechtsteiner. 2007. National Ambulatory Medical Care Survey: Advance Data from Vital and Health Statistics 387: 1–40. http://www.cdc.gov/nchs/data/ad/ad387.pdf.

Commission on Cancer. 2009. About Accreditation. http://www.facs.org/cancer/coc/whatis.html.

Commonwealth of Massachusetts. 2003. *Commonwealth of Massachusetts Division of Medical Assistance Provider Manual Series, Psychologist Manual.* Transmittal letter PSY-20. http://www.mass.gov/Eeohhs2/docs/masshealth/regs_provider/regs_psychologist.pdf.

Commonwealth of Massachusetts. 1996. 105 CMR: Department of Public Health. http://www.mass.gov/Eeohhs2/docs/dph/regs/105cmr205.pdf.

Department of Justice (DOJ). 2010. 21 CFR Sec 1300.01 (b28). http://www.deadiversion.usdoj.gov/drugreg/practioners/mlp_by_state.pdf.

Fortune. 2010. Annual Ranking of America's Largest Companies. http://money.cnn.com/magazines/fortune/fortune500/2009/industries/223/index.html.

Higgins, G. 2010. Adoption of the EHR in Physician Office Settings. http://healthsystemcio.com/2010/02/01/adoption-of-the-ehr-in-physician-office-settings.

Indian Health Service (IHS). 2010. Indian Health Service Introduction. http://www.ihs.gov/PublicInfo/ PublicAffairs/Welcome_Info/IHSintro.asp.

The Joint Commission. 2011. Facts about Ambulatory Care Accreditation. http://www.jointcommission. org/assets/1/18/Ambulatorycare_1_11.pdf.

Kane, C. 2004 (February). Practice Arrangements of Patient Care Physicians, 2001. In *Physician Marketplace Report*, 1–9. Chicago: American Medical Association.

Medical University of South Carolina (MUSC). 2011. Hollings Cancer Center: Outreach: Mobile Health Unit. http://www.muschealth.com/cancer/outreach/mobile.htm.

MedicineNet.com. 2010. Definition of Blood Bank. http://www.medterms.com/script/main/art. asp?articlekey=13184.

National Alliance on Mental Illness (NAMI). 2010. Mental Health Professionals: Who They Are and How to Find One. http://www.nami.org/Content/ContentGroups/Helpline1/Mental_Health_Professionals_Who_ They_Are_and_How_to_Find_One.htm.

National Hospital Ambulatory Medical Care Survey: 2007 Outpatient Department Summary (2009):1 -48. http://www.cdc.gov/nchs/data/nhsr/nhsr028.pdf.

Rural Assistance Center (RAC). 2010. CAH Frequently Asked Questions. http://www.raconline.org/info_ guides/hospitals/cahfaq.php#whatis.

State of California. 2010. Medical Board of California: General Office Practices/Protocols—Frequently Asked Questions. http://www.medbd.ca.gov/consumer/complaint_info_questions_practice.html#8.

State of Kentucky. 2006. 201 KAR 21:100. Minimum Standards for Recordkeeping/Itemized Statements. http://www.lrc.state.ky.us/kar/201/021/100.htm.

State of New Jersey. 2005. Chapter 35: Board of Medical Examiners. http://www.state.nj.us/oag/ca/laws/ acuregs.pdf.

United Health Group (UHG). 2010. Why Work Here. http://careers.unitedhealthgroup.com/ Why-Work-Here.aspx.

US Bureau of Justice Statistics. 2009. Prisoners in 2008. http://bjs.ojp.usdoj.gov/index. cfm?ty=pbdetail&iid=1763.

US Department of Health and Human Services (HHS). 2011. Federally Qualified Health Center: Rural Health Fact Sheet Series. https://www.cms.gov/MLNProducts/downloads/fqhcfactsheet.pdf.

US Food and Drug Administration (FDA). 2010. Bar Code Requirements for Blood Banks. http://www.fda. gov/BiologicsBloodVaccines/NewsEvents/WorkshopsMeetingsConferences/ucm113326.htm.

US News & World Report. 2010. Best Health Insurance Plans. http://health.usnews.com/directories/ health-plans/index_html/plan_cat+commercial.

Glossary

Accountable Care Organization (ACO): An organization of healthcare providers accountable for the quality, cost, and overall care of Medicare beneficiaries who are assigned and enrolled in the traditional fee-for-service program

Accreditation: 1. A voluntary process of institutional or organizational review in which a quasi-independent body created for this purpose periodically evaluates the quality of the entity's work against preestablished written criteria 2. A determination by an accrediting body that an eligible organization, network, program, group, or individual complies with applicable standards 3. The act of granting approval to a healthcare organization based on whether the organization has met a set of voluntary standards developed by an accreditation agency

Accreditation Association for Ambulatory Health Care (AAAHC): A professional organization that offers accreditation programs for ambulatory and outpatient organizations such as single-specialty and multispecialty group practices, ambulatory surgery centers, college/university health services, and community health centers

Accreditation Commission for Health Care (ACHC): An organization that provides quality standards and accreditation programs for home health and other healthcare organizations

Accreditation organization: A professional organization that establishes the standards against which healthcare organizations are measured and conducts periodic assessments of the performance of individual healthcare organizations

Activities of daily living (ADL): The basic activities of self-care, including grooming, bathing, ambulating, toileting, and eating

Acute care: Medical care of a limited duration that is provided in an inpatient hospital setting to diagnose and/or treat an injury or a short-term illness

Administrative information: Information used for administrative and healthcare operations purposes, such as billing and quality oversight

Adult foster care: Care provided for individuals or small groups of adults who need help functioning or who cannot live safely on their own

Advanced decision support: Automated clinical practice guidelines that are built in to electronic health record systems and designed to support clinical decision making

Advance directive: A legal, written document that describes the patient's preferences regarding future healthcare or stipulates the person who is authorized to make medical decisions in the event the patient is incapable of communicating his or her preferences

Agency for Healthcare Research and Quality (AHRQ): The branch of the US Public Health Service that supports general health research and distributes research findings and treatment guidelines with the goal of improving the quality, appropriateness, and effectiveness of healthcare services

Aggregate data: Data extracted from individual health records and combined to form de-identified information about groups of patients that can be compared and analyzed

Allied health professional: A credentialed healthcare worker who is not a physician, nurse, psychologist, or pharmacist (for example, a physical therapist, dietitian, social worker, or occupational therapist)

Ambulatory care: Preventive or corrective healthcare services provided on a nonresident basis in a provider's office, clinic setting, or hospital outpatient setting

American Association for Accreditation of Ambulatory Surgery Facilities (AAAASF): An organization that provides an accreditation program to ensure the quality and safety of medical and surgical care provided in ambulatory surgery facilities

American Board of Medical Specialties (ABMS): A board that provides certification for physicians in more than 145 specialties and subspecialties

American College of Radiology (ACR): Diagnostic medical imaging accrediting body that has accredited nearly 16,000 facilities in the United States

American College of Surgeons (ACS): The scientific and educational association of surgeons formed to improve the quality of surgical care by setting high standards for surgical education and practice

American National Standards Institute (ANSI): An organization that governs standards in many aspects of public and private business; developer of the Health Information Technology Standards Panel

American Osteopathic Association (AOA): The professional association of osteopathic physicians, surgeons, and graduates of approved colleges of osteopathic medicine that inspects and accredits osteopathic colleges and hospitals

American Recovery and Reinvestment Act of 2009 (ARRA): An economic stimulus package enacted by the 111th United States Congress in February 2009; signed into law by President Obama on February 17th, 2009; an unprecedented effort to jumpstart the economy, create/save millions of jobs, and put a down payment on addressing long-neglected challenges; an extraordinary response to a crisis unlike any since the Great Depression; includes measures to modernize our nation's infrastructure, enhance energy independence, expand educational opportunities, preserve and improve affordable health care, provide tax relief, and protect those in greatest need; *Also called* **Recovery Act; Stimulus**

American Society for Testing and Materials (ASTM): A national organization whose purpose is to establish standards on materials, products, systems, and services

Analysis: Review of health record for proper documentation and adherence to regulatory and accreditation standards

Ancillary services: 1. Tests and procedures ordered by a physician to provide information for use in patient diagnosis or treatment 2. Professional healthcare services such as radiology, laboratory, or physical therapy

Application: In AHIMA's data quality management model, the purpose for which data are collected

Assisted living: A type of freestanding long-term care facility where residents receive necessary medical services but retain a degree of independence

Attending physician: The physician primarily responsible for the care and treatment of a patient

Authentication: 1. The process of identifying the source of health record entries by attaching a handwritten signature, the author's initials, or an electronic signature 2. Proof of authorship that ensures, as much as possible, that log-ins and messages from a user originate from an authorized source

Autopsy report: Written documentation of the findings from a postmortem pathological examination

Bar code medication administration (BCMA): An electronic system of administering medication that makes use of specific bar code identifiers for each medication

Behavioral healthcare: A broad array of psychiatric services provided in acute, long-term, and ambulatory care settings; includes treatment of mental disorders, chemical dependency, mental retardation, and developmental disabilities, as well as cognitive rehabilitation services

Biomedical research: The process of systematically investigating subjects related to the functioning of the human body

Board and care home: A small, private long-term care facility, usually with 20 or fewer residents; also referred to as a residential care facility or group home

Board certified: A designation given to a physician or other health professional who has passed an exam from a medical specialty board and is thereby certified to provide care within that specialty

Cancer treatment center: A center that specializes in providing comprehensive cancer treatment, including radiation and chemotherapy. Many also offer patient education and family counseling services

Cardiology report: A report written by a cardiologist interpreting the results of cardiac diagnostic tests

Care plan: The specific goals in the treatment of an individual patient, amended as the patient's condition requires, and the assessment of the outcomes of care; serves as the primary source for ongoing documentation of the resident's care, condition, and needs

CARF: *See* **Commission on Accreditation of Rehabilitation Facilities**

Case management: 1. The ongoing, concurrent review performed by clinical professionals to ensure the necessity and effectiveness of the clinical services being provided to a patient 2. A process that integrates and coordinates patient care over time and across multiple sites and providers, especially in complex and high-cost cases, with goals of continuity of care, cost-effectiveness, quality, and appropriate utilization 3. The process of developing a specific care plan for a patient that serves as a communication tool to improve quality of care and reduce cost

Case-mix analysis: A method of analyzing health records by grouping patients according to a predefined set of characteristics; used to determine Medicare reimbursements

Case-mix index (CMI): The average relative weight of all cases treated at a given facility or by a given physician, which reflects the resource intensity or clinical severity of a specific group in relation to the other groups in the classification system; calculated by dividing the sum of the weights of diagnosis-related groups for patients discharged during a given period by the total number of patients discharged

Census: The number of inpatients present in a healthcare facility at any given time

Centers for Disease Control and Prevention (CDC): A group of federal agencies that oversee health promotion and disease control and prevention activities in the United States

Centers for Medicare and Medicaid Services (CMS): The division of the Department of Health and Human Services that is responsible for developing healthcare policy in the United States and for administering the Medicare program and the federal portion of the Medicaid program and maintaining the procedure portion of the International Classification of Diseases, ninth revision, Clinical Modification (ICD-9-CM); called the Health Care Financing Administration (HCFA) prior to 2001

Certificate of destruction: A document that constitutes proof that a health record was destroyed and that includes the method of destruction, the signature of the person responsible for destruction, and inclusive dates for destruction

Certification: 1. The process by which a duly authorized body evaluates and recognizes an individual, institution, or educational program as meeting predetermined requirements 2. An evaluation performed to establish the extent to which a particular computer system, network design, or application implementation meets a prespecified set of requirements

Certification Commission for Healthcare Information Technology (CCHIT): An independent, voluntary, private-sector initiative organized as a limited liability corporation that has been awarded a contract by the US Department of Health and Human Services (HHS) to develop, create prototypes for, and evaluate the certification criteria and inspection process for electronic health record products (EHRs)

Civilian Health and Medical Program of the Uniformed Services (CHAMPUS): A federal program providing supplementary civilian-sector hospital and medical services beyond that which is available in military treatment facilities to military dependents, retirees and their dependents, and certain others

Clinical data repository (CDR): A central database that focuses on clinical information

Clinical decision support (CDS) system: A special subcategory of clinical information systems that is designed to help healthcare providers make knowledge-based clinical decisions

Clinical documentation: Any manual or electronic notation (or recording) made by a physician or other healthcare clinician related to a patient's medical condition or treatment

Clinical documentation specialist: A specialist who performs documentation reviews as part of a clinical documentation improvement program

Clinical information: Health record documentation that describes the patient's condition and course of treatment

Clinical Laboratory Improvement Amendments (CLIA): Passed in 1988, the amendments established quality standards for all laboratory testing to ensure the accuracy, reliability, and timeliness of patient test results regardless of where the test is

Clinical pathway: A tool designed to coordinate multidisciplinary care planning for specific diagnoses and treatments

Clinical practice guidelines: A detailed, step-by-step guide used by healthcare practitioners to make knowledge-based decisions related to patient care and issued by an authoritative organization such as a medical society or government agency; *See* **clinical protocol**

Clinical privileges: The authorization granted by a healthcare organization's governing board to a member of the medical staff that enables the physician to provide patient services in the organization within specific practice limits

Clinical protocol: Specific instructions for performing clinical procedures established by authoritative bodies, such as medical staff committees, and intended to be applied literally and universally; *See* **clinical practice guidelines**

Clinical trial: 1. A controlled research study involving human subjects that is designed to evaluate prospectively the safety and effectiveness of new drugs, tests, devices, or interventions 2. Experimental study in which an intervention or treatment is given to one group in a clinical setting and the outcomes compared with a control group that did not have the intervention or treatment or that had a different intervention or treatment

Closing practice policy: Policy that directs an organization to send informational letters to patients of physicians who are closing their practices at a facility

CMS quality measures: Information publicly reported by hospitals to the Centers for Medicare and Medicaid Services (CMS); introduced by the United States Department of Health and Human Services in 2001 to help measure or quantify healthcare processes, outcomes, patient perceptions, and organizational structure and systems

Code of Federal Regulations (CFR): The official collection of legislative and regulatory guidelines mandated by final rules published in the *Federal Register*

Collection: 1. The part of the billing process in which payment for services performed is obtained 2. In AHIMA's data quality management model, it is the process by which data elements are accumulated

College of American Pathologists (CAP): A medical specialty organization of board-certified pathologists that owns and holds the copyright to SNOMED CT®

Commission on Accreditation of Rehabilitation Facilities (CARF): A private, not-for-profit organization that develops customer-focused standards for behavioral healthcare and medical rehabilitation programs and accredits such programs on the basis of its standards

Commission on Cancer (CoC): Established by the American College of Surgeons in 1922, this entity sets standards for quality multidisciplinary cancer care. These programs are concerned with prevention, early diagnosis, pretreatment evaluation, staging, and optimal treatment, as well as rehabilitation, surveillance for recurrent disease, support services, and end-of-life care

Community Health Accreditation Program (CHAP): A group that surveys and accredits home healthcare and hospice organizations

Comorbidity: 1. A medical condition that coexists with the primary cause for hospitalization and affects the patient's treatment and length of stay 2. Pre-existing condition that, because of its presence with a specific diagnosis, causes an increase in length of stay by at least one day in approximately 75 percent of the cases (as in complication and comorbidity [CC])

Compliance guidance: The information provided by the Office of the Inspector General of the Department of Health and Human Services to help healthcare organizations develop internal controls that promote adherence to applicable federal and state guidelines

Complication and/or comorbidity (CC): Illness or injury that coexists with the condition for which the patient is primarily seeking healthcare

Complication: 1. A medical condition that arises during an inpatient hospitalization (for example, a postoperative wound infection) 2. Condition that arises during the hospital stay that prolongs the length of stay at least one day in approximately 75 percent of the cases (as in complication and comorbidity [CC])

Comprehensive assessment: Patient-specific medical assessment that accurately reflects the patient's current health status and includes information that may be used to demonstrate the patient's progress toward desired outcomes

Computer output to laser disk/enterprise report management (COLD/ERM) technology: Technology that electronically stores documents and distributes them with fax, e-mail, web, and traditional hard-copy print processes

Computer-based patient record: An electronic record of health-related information on an individual that conforms to nationally recognized interoperability standards and that can be created, managed, and consulted by authorized clinicians and staff across more than one healthcare organization; *Also called* **electronic health record**

Computerized physician order entry (CPOE): Electronic prescribing system that allows physicians to write prescriptions and transmit them electronically. These systems usually contain error prevention software that provides the user with prompts that warn against the possibility of drug interaction, allergy, or overdose and other relevant information

Concurrent query: A question posed to the documenting physician during the patient's hospital stay; used to obtain additional, clarifying documentation to improve both the quality of documentation in the patient's record and the treatment of the patient

Conditions of Participation: The administrative and operational guidelines and regulations under which facilities are allowed to take part in the Medicare and Medicaid programs; published by the Centers for Medicare and Medicaid Services, a federal agency under the Department of Health and Human Services; *Also called* **Conditions for Coverage**

Confidentiality: A legal and ethical concept that establishes the healthcare provider's responsibility for protecting health records and other personal and private information from unauthorized use or disclosure

Consent to treatment: Legal permission given by a patient or a patient's legal representative to a healthcare provider that allows the provider to administer care and/or treatment or to perform surgery and/or other medical procedures

Conservatorship: The placement of a patient under the care of an appointed guardian; can be recommended when a person is unable to provide for basic personal needs as the result of a mental disorder and is unwilling or incapable of accepting voluntary treatment

Consolidated Health Informatics (CHI) initiative: The effort to achieve CHI through federal agencies spearheaded by the Office of National Coordinator for Health Information Technology

Consultation report: Health record documentation that describes the findings and recommendations of consulting physicians

Continuing care retirement community: An organization established to provide housing and services, including healthcare, to people of retirement age

Continuous quality improvement (CQI): 1. A management philosophy that emphasizes the importance of knowing and meeting customer expectations, reducing variation within processes, and relying on data to build knowledge for process improvement 2. A component of total quality management (TQM) that emphasizes ongoing performance assessment and improvement planning

Continuum of care: The range of healthcare services provided to patients, from routine ambulatory care to intensive acute care; the emphasis is on treating individual patients at the level of care required by their course of treatment with the assurance of communication between caregivers

Convenient care centers: Clinics, often associated with national drugstore chains, at which patients are generally seen for minor complaints, flu shots, or physical exams; *Also known as* **retail medical clinics**

Core measure/core measure set: Standardized performance measures developed to improve the safety and quality of healthcare (for example, core measures are used in the Joint Commission's ORYX initiative)

Corporate negligence: The failure of an organization to exercise the degree of care considered reasonable under the circumstances that resulted in an unintended injury to another party

Court order: An official direction issued by a court judge and requiring or forbidding specific parties to perform specific actions

Covered entity (CE): Any healthcare provider or contractor that transmits individually identifiable health information in electronic form

Credentialing: The process of reviewing and validating the qualifications (degrees, licenses, and other credentials) of physicians and other licensed independent practitioners, for granting medical staff membership to provide patient care services

Critical access hospitals (CAHs): 1. Hospitals that are excluded from the outpatient prospective payment system because they are paid under a reasonable cost-based system as required under section 1834(g) of the Social Security Act 2. Small facilities that give limited outpatient and inpatient hospital services to people in rural areas

Current Dental Terminology (CDT): A medical code set of dental procedures, maintained and copyrighted by the American Dental Association (ADA), referred to as the Uniform Code on Dental Procedures and Nomenclatures until 1990

Data: The dates, numbers, images, symbols, letters, and words that represent basic facts and observations about people, processes, measurements, and conditions

Data collection: The process by which data are gathered

Data dictionary: A descriptive list of the names, definitions, and attributes of data elements to be collected in an information system or database whose purpose is to standardize definitions and ensure consistent use

Data exchange standards: Protocols that help ensure that data transmitted from one system to another remain comparable

Data set: A list of recommended data elements with uniform definitions that are relevant for a particular use

Database: An organized collection of data, text, references, or pictures in a standardized format, typically stored in a computer system for multiple applications

Database management system (DBMS): Computer software that enables the user to create, modify, delete, and view the data in a database

Day treatment: A program that provides individuals with mental health treatment that is more intense than the services provided on an outpatient basis; day treatment services are typically provided eight hours a day, Monday through Friday, during the workday

Deemed status: An official designation indicating that a healthcare facility is in compliance with the Medicare Conditions of Participation; to qualify for deemed status, facilities must be accredited by the Joint Commission or AOA

Deficiency systems: Paper- or computer-based processes designed to track and report elements of documentation missing from the health records of discharged patients

Demographic information: Information used to identify an individual, such as name, address, gender, age, and other information linked to a specific person

Department of Health and Human Services (HHS): The cabinet-level federal agency that oversees all the health- and human-services–related activities of the federal government and administers federal regulations

Derived data: Data that consist of factual details aggregated or summarized from a group of health records that provide no means to identify specific patients; it is not considered part of the legal health record though it has the same level of confidentiality

Destruction of records: The act of breaking down the components of a health record into pieces that can no longer be recognized as parts of the original record

Diagnosis-related groups (DRGs): A unit of case-mix classification adopted by the federal government and some other payers as a prospective payment mechanism for hospital inpatients in which diseases are placed into groups because related diseases and treatments tend to consume similar amounts of healthcare resources and incur similar amounts of cost; in the Medicare and Medicaid programs, one of more than 500 diagnostic classifications in which cases demonstrate similar resource consumption and length-of-stay patterns. Under the prospective payment system (PPS), hospitals are paid a set fee for treating patients in a single DRG category, regardless of the actual cost of care for the individual

Diagnostic and Statistical Manual of Mental Disorders, Fourth Revision (DSM-IV): A nomenclature developed by the American Psychiatric Association to standardize the diagnostic process for patients with psychiatric disorders, which includes codes that correspond to ICD-9-CM codes; most recent version is fourth edition (text revision), or DSM-IV-TR, published in 2000

Diagnostic codes: Numeric or alphanumeric characters used to classify and report diseases, conditions, and injuries

Digital information: Data or information represented in an encoded, computer-readable format

Discharge summary: A summary of the resident's stay at a healthcare facility that is used along with the postdischarge plan of care to provide continuity of care upon discharge from the facility

Disease index: A list of diseases and conditions of patients sequenced according to the code numbers of the classification system in use

Do-not-resuscitate (DNR): An order written by the treating physician stating that in the event the patient suffers cardiac or pulmonary arrest, cardiopulmonary resuscitation should not be attempted

Dumping: The illegal practice of transferring uninsured and indigent patients who need emergency services from one hospital to another (usually public) hospital solely to avoid the cost of providing uncompensated services. EMTALA, passed in 1986 and implemented in 1990, contains provisions intended to curtail this practice

Durable power of attorney (DPOA): A power of attorney that remains in effect even after the principal is incapacitated; some are drafted so that they only take effect when the principal becomes incapacitated

e-Discovery: Refers to Amendments to Federal Rules of Civil Procedure and Uniform Rules Relating to Discovery of Electronically Stored Information; wherein audit trails, the source code of the program, metadata, and any other electronic information that is not typically considered the legal health record is subject to motion for compulsory discovery

Electronic document management system (EDMS): A storage solution based on digital scanning technology in which source documents are scanned to create digital images of the documents that can be stored electronically on optical disks

Electronic health record (EHR): An electronic record of health-related information on an individual that conforms to nationally recognized interoperability standards and that can be created, managed, and consulted by authorized clinicians and staff across more than one healthcare organization

Electronic medication administration record (EMAR): A system designed to prevent medication errors by checking a patient's medication information against his or her barcoded wristband

Elements of performance (EP): The Joint Commission's specific performance expectations and/or structures or processes that must be in place for an organization to provide safe, high-quality care, treatment, and services

Emergency and trauma care: The medical-surgical care provided to individuals whose injuries or illnesses require urgent care to address conditions that could be life threatening or disabling if not treated immediately

Emergency Medical Treatment and Active Labor Act (EMTALA): A 1986 law enacted as part of the Consolidated Omnibus Reconciliation Act largely to combat "patient dumping"—the transferring, discharging, or refusal to treat indigent emergency department patients because of their inability to pay

Employee Assistance Programs (EAPs): Outpatient programs designed to provide employees with immediate access to psychological counseling on a limited basis; may be provided on site or through local providers

Encoder: Specialty software used to facilitate the assignment of diagnostic and procedural codes according to the rules of the coding system

Encounter note: The record of clinical observations of a patient in the hospital, recorded in chronological order by every physician and clinician who sees or treats the patient in an ambulatory setting; *Also known as* **visit note**.

Enterprise master patient index (EMPI): An index that provides access to multiple repositories of information from overlapping patient populations that are maintained in separate systems and databases

Evidence-based documentation: A system of high-quality clinical documentation in which physicians and clinicians follow a set of criteria that requires all entries in the patient record to be legible, reliable, precise, complete, consistent, clear, and timely

Evidence-based medicine: Healthcare services based on clinical methods that have been thoroughly tested through controlled, peer-reviewed biomedical studies

Expressed consent: The spoken or written permission granted by a patient to a healthcare provider that allows the provider to perform medical or surgical services

Face sheet: Usually the first page of the health record, which contains patient identification, demographics, date of admission, insurance coverage or payment source, referral information, hospital stay dates, physician information, and discharge information, as well as the name of the responsible party, emergency and additional contacts, and the resident's diagnoses

Facility-specific index: Databases established by healthcare facilities to meet their individual, specific needs for customer care or other reporting requirements. These indexes make it possible to retrieve health records in a variety of ways including by disease, physician, operation, or other data element. Prior to computerization in healthcare, these indexes were kept on cards. Today, most are compiled from databases routinely developed by the facility

Facility-specific registry: A healthcare database consisting of data extracted from individual records; used for research and improvement in customer care

Failed/missed appointment policy: Policy that tracks appointments that are canceled or missed. A failed/missed appointment policy should state the required documentation of information concerning the missed appointment

Federal Register: The daily publication of the US Government Printing Office that reports all changes in regulations and federally mandated standards, including HCPCS and ICD-9-CM codes

Federal Rules of Civil Procedure (FRCP): Rules established by the US Supreme Court setting the "rules of the road" and procedures for federal court cases. FRCP were amended in 2006 to include electronic records and continue to be very important as benchmarks in how these records can be used in courts, not only federal, but state and other courts as well. Record custodianship is widely discussed within the FRCP

Financial data: The data collected for the purpose of managing the assets and expenses of a business (for example, a healthcare organization, a product line); in healthcare, data derived from the charge generation documentation associated with the activities of care and then aggregated by specific customer grouping for financial analysis

Flow chart: A graphic tool that uses standard symbols to visually display detailed information, including time and distance, of the sequential flow of work of an individual or a product as it progresses through a process

Food and Drug Administration (FDA): The federal agency responsible for controlling the sale and use of pharmaceuticals, biological products, medical devices, food, cosmetics, and products that emit radiation, including the licensing of medications for human use

Functional independence measure (FIM): Measure used to evaluate the level of independence of patients in long-term acute-care (LTCH) settings where the focus of care is on extensive rehabilitation of the patient. FIM includes 18 items that are scored on a scale of 1 to 7, with 1 being the most dependent and 7 being the most independent. Total scores range between 18 and 126. FIM scores can be used as outcome measures by LTCHs

Functionality standards: Standards that define the components that an electronic health record needs to support the functions for which it is designed; HL7 standards are an example

General consent to treatment: A consent signed upon admission to the facility that allows the clinical staff to provide care and treatment for the resident and that usually includes the resident's agreement to pay for the services provided by the facility, to assign insurance benefits to the facility, and to allow the facility to obtain or release health records for payment purposes; *Also called* **general consent**

Global Assessment of Functioning (GAF) Scale: A 100-point tool rating overall psychological, social, and occupational functioning of individuals, excluding physical and environmental impairment

Hand-off communication: Communication of patient information between caregivers. The Joint Commission standard 2E recommends that each healthcare organization implement a standardized approach to "hand-off" communications, including an opportunity to ask and respond to questions

Healthcare Facilities Accreditation Program (HFAP): An accreditation program managed by the American Osteopathic Association that offers services to a number of healthcare facilities and services, including laboratories, ambulatory care clinics, ambulatory surgery centers, behavioral health and substance abuse treatment facilities, physical rehabilitation facilities, acute care hospitals, critical access hospitals, and hospitals providing postdoctoral training for osteopathic physicians

Healthcare information standards: Guidelines developed to standardize data throughout the healthcare industry (for example, developing uniform terminologies and vocabularies)

Healthcare Integrity and Protection Data Bank (HIPDB): A database maintained by the federal government to provide information on fraud-and-abuse findings against US healthcare providers

Health Care and Education Reconciliation Act of 2010 (P.L. 111-152) (HCERA): A federal law enacted by Congress through reconciliation in order to make changes to the Patient Protection and Affordable Care Act. HCERA was signed into law by President Barack Obama on March 30, 2010; *Also called HR 4872*

Health Care Quality Improvement Act: A regulation enacted in 1986 to monitor the quality of care provided and the medical necessity of services

Health data repository: A database that will provide immediate nationwide access to local data in the event of a primary system failure or system unavailability. It is an effort to improve data accessibility and increase disaster preparedness

Health informatics standards: A set of standards that describe accepted methods for collecting, maintaining, and/or transferring healthcare data among computer systems

Health information exchange (HIE): The exchange of health information electronically between providers and others with the same level of interoperability, such as labs and pharmacies

Health information exchange organization (HIEO): An organization that supports, oversees, or governs the exchange of health-related information among organizations according to nationally recognized standards

Health information management (HIM) professionals: Individuals who have received professional training at the associate or baccalaureate degree level in the management of health data and information flow throughout healthcare delivery systems; formerly known as **medical record technicians** or **medical record administrators**

Health Information Technology for Economic and Clinical Health (HITECH) Act: Legislation created to stimulate the adoption of EHR and supporting technology in the United States. Signed into law on February 17, 2009, as part of ARRA.

Health Insurance Portability and Accountability Act of 1996 (HIPAA): The federal legislation enacted to provide continuity of health coverage, control fraud and abuse in healthcare, reduce healthcare costs, and guarantee the security and privacy of health information; limits exclusion for pre-existing medical conditions, prohibits discrimination against employees and dependents based on health status, guarantees availability of health insurance to small employers, and guarantees renewability of insurance to all employees regardless of size; requires covered entities (most healthcare providers and organizations) to transmit healthcare claims in a specific format and to develop, implement, and comply with the standards of the Privacy Rule and the Security Rule; and mandates that covered entities apply for and utilize national identifiers in HIPAA transactions; *Also called* the Kassebaum-Kennedy Law; **Public Law 104-191**

Health Level 7 (HL7): An international organization of healthcare professionals dedicated to creating standards for the exchange, management, and integration of electronic information

Health record: 1. Information relating to the physical or mental health or condition of an individual, as made by or on behalf of a health professional in connection with the care ascribed that individual 2. A medical record, health record, or medical chart that is a systematic documentation of a patient's medical history and care

Health record analysis: A concurrent or ongoing review of health record content performed by caregivers or HIM professionals while the patient is still receiving inpatient services to ensure the quality of the services being provided and the completeness of the documentation being maintained; *Also called* **health record review**

Health services research: Research conducted on the subject of healthcare delivery that examines organizational structures and systems as well as the effectiveness and efficiency of healthcare services

History: Part of a patient's medical record; a summary of the patient's illness provided by the patient and documented by the attending physician

HITECH Act: See Health Information Technology for Economic and Clinical Health (HITECH)

Home Assessment Validation and Entry (HAVEN): A type of data-entry software used to collect Outcome and Assessment Information Set (OASIS) data and then transmit them to state databases; imports and exports data in standard OASIS record format, maintains agency/patient/employee information, enforces data integrity through rigorous edit checks, and provides comprehensive online help. HAVEN is used in the home health prospective payment system (HHPPS)

Home care: *See* **home health**

Home health (HH): An umbrella term that refers to the medical and nonmedical services provided to patients and their families in their places of residence; *also called* **home care**

Home health agency (HHA): A program or organization that provides a blend of home-based medical and social services to homebound patients and their families for the purpose of promoting, maintaining, or restoring health or of minimizing the effects of illness, injury, or disability; these services include skilled nursing care, physical therapy, occupational therapy, speech therapy, and personal care by home health aides

Home healthcare: The medical and/or personal care provided to individuals and families in their places of residence with the goal of promoting, maintaining, or restoring health or minimizing the effects of disabilities and illnesses, including terminal illnesses

Home health resource group (HHRG): A classification system for the home health prospective payment system (HHPPS) derived from the data elements in the Outcome and Assessment Information Set (OASIS) with 80 home health episode rates established to support the prospective reimbursement of covered home care and rehabilitation services provided to Medicare beneficiaries during 60-day episodes of care; a six-character alphanumeric code is used to represent a severity level in three domains

Hospice care: The medical care provided to persons with life expectancies of six months or less who elect to forgo standard treatment of their illness and to receive only palliative care

Hospitalist: Physicians employed by teaching hospitals to play the role that admitting physicians fulfill in hospitals that are not affiliated with medical training programs

Hybrid health record: A combination of paper and electronic records; a health record that includes both paper and electronic elements

Identifier standards: Recommended methods for assigning unique identifiers to individuals (patients and clinical providers), corporate providers, and healthcare vendors and suppliers

Imaging reports: Radiologists' written interpretations of imaging procedures such as X-ray examinations, CT scans, MRI and positron-emission tomography; imaging reports generally include patient and image identification data, the physician's order for the test, the name and date of the test performed, the type and amount of radiopharmaceutical administered, and the radiologist's interpretation of the images

Implied consent: The type of permission that is inferred when a patient voluntarily submits to treatment

Incidence: The number of new cases of a specific disease

Incident: An occurrence in a medical facility that is inconsistent with accepted standards of care

Incident report: A quality or performance management tool used to collect data and information about potentially compensable events (events that may result in death or serious injury)

Index: An organized (usually alphabetical) list of specific data that serves to guide, indicate, or otherwise facilitate reference to the data

Individual-based system tracer activity: An on-site survey process used by The Joint Commission to explore a specific system or process across the organization, evaluating the integration of related processes, coordination, and communication among disciplines and departments; *See also* **tracer methodology**

Individual tracer activity: An on-site survey process used by The Joint Commission to evaluate the care experience of a specific patient while he is in the hospital; analyzes a hospital's system of providing care, treatment, and services used; *See also* **tracer methodology**

Information: Data that have been deliberately selected, processed, and organized to be useful

Informed consent: 1. A legal term referring to a patient's right to make his or her own treatment decisions based on the knowledge of the treatment to be administered or the procedure to be performed 2. An individual's voluntary agreement to participate in research or to undergo a diagnostic, therapeutic, or preventive medical procedure

Inpatient: A patient who is provided with room, board, and continuous general nursing services in an area of an acute care facility where patients generally stay at least overnight

Inpatient facility: Facility that provides patients with around-the-clock care; may be a dedicated portion of a hospital or may stand alone

Institute of Medicine (IOM): A branch of the National Academy of Sciences whose goal is to advance and distribute scientific knowledge with the mission of improving human health

Integrated delivery system (IDS): A system that combines the financial and clinical aspects of healthcare and uses a group of healthcare providers, selected on the basis of quality and cost management criteria, to furnish comprehensive health services across the continuum of care

Integrated healthcare network: A group of healthcare organizations that collectively provides a full range of coordinated healthcare services ranging from simple preventative care to complex surgical care

Integrated health records: A system of health record organization in which all the paper forms are arranged in strict chronological order and mixed with forms created by different departments

International Classification of Diseases, tenth revision, Clinical Modification (ICD-10-CM®): The coding classification system that will replace ICD-9-CM, Volumes 1 and 2, on October 1, 2013. ICD-10-CM is the United States' clinical modification of the World Health Organization's ICD-10. ICD-10-CM has a total of 21 chapters and contains significantly more codes than ICD-9-CM, providing the ability to code with a greater level of specificity

International Classification of Diseases, tenth revision, Procedure Coding System (ICD-10-PCS): The coding classification system that will replace ICD-9-CM, Volume 3, on October 1, 2013. ICD-10-PCS has 16 sections and contains significantly more procedure codes than ICD-9-CM, providing the ability to code procedures with a greater level of specificity

Interval note: Health record documentation that describes the patient's course between two closely related hospitalizations directed toward the treatment of the same complaint when a patient has been discharged and readmitted within 30 days

Intraoperative anesthesia record: Health record documentation that describes the entire surgical process from the time the operation began until the patient left the operating room

The Joint Commission: A private, voluntary, not-for-profit organization that evaluates and accredits hospitals and other healthcare organizations on the basis of predefined performance standards; formerly known as the Joint Commission on Accreditation of Healthcare Organizations or JCAHO

Joint Commission on Accreditation of Healthcare Organizations (JCAHO): Name used for Joint Commission on Accreditation of Hospitals when it began to accredit more nonhospital healthcare settings in 1987; now known as **The Joint Commission**

Joint Commission on Accreditation of Hospitals (JCAH): Private, voluntary, not-for-profit organization formed in 1952 to accredit hospitals on the basis of predefined performance standards; now known as **The Joint Commission.**

Labor and delivery record: Health record documentation that takes the place of an operative report for patients who give birth in the obstetrics department of an acute care hospital

Laboratory report: The analysis of a laboratory procedure, generated automatically by electronic testing equipment or written by a medical technologist or other specialist; reports include patient and laboratory identification, the name and date of the test performed, the signature of the laboratory technologist or scientist who performed the test, and the results of the test

Legal health record (LHR): Documents and data elements that a healthcare provider may include in response to legally permissible requests for patient information

Liability: 1. A legal obligation or responsibility that may have financial repercussions if not fulfilled 2. An amount owed by an individual or organization to another individual or organization

Licensure: The legal authority or formal permission from authorities to carry on certain activities that by law or regulation require such permission (applicable to institutions as well as individuals)

Living will: A directive that allows an individual to describe in writing the type of healthcare that he or she would or would not wish to receive

Longitudinal health record: A permanent, coordinated patient record of significant information listed in chronological order and maintained across time, ideally from birth to death

Long-term acute care: The medical care provided to individuals who are clinically complex and have multiple acute and chronic conditions requiring an average length of stay greater than 25 days in long-term care hospitals certified as acute care hospitals

Long-term care: Healthcare services provided in a nonacute care setting to chronically ill, aged, disabled, or mentally handicapped individuals

Long-term care hospital (LTCH): According to the Centers for Medicare and Medicaid Services (CMS), a hospital with an average length of stay for Medicare patients that is 25 days or longer, or a hospital excluded from the inpatient prospective payment system and that has an average length of stay for all patients that is 20 days or longer

Loss prevention: A risk management strategy that includes developing and revising policies and procedures that are both facility-wide and department specific

Loss reduction: A component of a risk management program that encompasses techniques used to manage events or claims that already have taken place

Major diagnostic category (MDC): Under diagnosis-related groups (DRGs), one of 25 categories based on single or multiple organ systems into which all diseases and disorders relating to that system are classified

Managed behavioral healthcare organization (MBHO): A type of healthcare organization that delivers and manages all aspects of behavioral healthcare or the payment for care by limiting providers of care, discounting payment to providers of care, and/or limiting access to care

Managed care organization (MCO): A type of healthcare organization that delivers medical care and manages all aspects of the care or the payment for care by limiting providers of care, discounting payment to providers of care, and/or limiting access to care; *also called* coordinated care organization

Master patient index (MPI): A patient-identifying directory referencing all patients related to an organization and which also serves as a link to the patient record or information, facilitates patient identification, and assists in maintaining a longitudinal patient record from birth to death

Meaningful use criteria: The requirements healthcare providers must meet to receive federal incentive payments for implementing different phases of an EHR between 2011 and 2015

Medicaid: An entitlement program that oversees medical assistance for individuals and families with low incomes and limited resources; jointly funded between state and federal governments and legislated by the Social Security Act

Medical necessity: 1. The likelihood that a proposed healthcare service will have a reasonable beneficial effect on the patient's physical condition and quality of life at a specific point in his or her illness or lifetime 2. Healthcare services and supplies that are proven or acknowledged to be effective in the diagnosis, treatment, cure, or relief of a health condition, illness, injury, disease, or its symptoms and to be consistent with the community's accepted standard of care. Under medical necessity, only those services, procedures, and patient care warranted by the patient's condition are provided 3. The concept that procedures are only eligible for reimbursement as a covered benefit when they are performed for a specific diagnosis or specified frequency; *Also called* **need-to-know principle**

Medical record delinquency rate: Rate of delinquent payments for health services calculated by dividing the monthly average number of discharges by the monthly average number of delinquent records at a hospital

Medical specialties: A group of clinical specialties that concentrates on the provision of nonsurgical care by physicians who have received advanced training in internal medicine, pediatrics, cardiology, endocrinology, psychiatry, oncology, nephrology, neurology, pulmonology, gastroenterology, dermatology, radiology, and nuclear medicine, among many other concentrations

Medical staff bylaws: Standards governing the practice of medical staff members; typically voted upon by the organized medical staff and the medical staff executive committee and approved by the facility's board; governs the business conduct, rights, and responsibilities of the medical staff; medical staff members must abide by these bylaws in order to continue practice in the healthcare facility

Medically complex patients: Patients who require specialized care, including intensive therapies and nursing care, for a longer period than a short-term community hospital has the capacity to provide

Medicare: A federally funded health program established in 1965 to assist with the medical care costs of Americans 65 years of age and older as well as other individuals entitled to Social Security benefits owing to their disabilities

Medicare quality indicators: Criteria determined by Medicare that, if present in a patient's record, are likely to result in better outcomes than if they are not present; examples include smoking cessation counseling and aspirin given to patients within minutes of their admission to the emergency department

Medicare severity diagnosis-related groups (MS-DRGs): The US government's 2007 revision of the DRG system, the MS-DRG system better accounts for severity of illness and resource consumption; *See also* **diagnosis-related group (DRG)**

Medication administration records (MARs): The records used to document the date and time each dose and type of medication is administered to a patient

Medication list: An ongoing record of the medications a patient has received in the past and is taking currently; includes names of medications, dosages, amounts dispensed, dispensing instructions, prescription dates, discontinued dates, and the problem for which the medication was prescribed

MedPAR data: Data from the Medicare Provider Analysis and Review (MEDPAR) database system, a database containing information and files submitted by fiscal intermediaries that is used by the Office of the Inspector General to identify suspicious billing and charge practices

Mental Health America (MHA): A nonprofit organization created to assist the more than 54 million Americans with mental disorders; provides information, advocacy, and access to quality behavioral health services for all Americans

Mental Health Parity Act (MHPA): A regulation enacted in 1996 to monitor the quality of care provided and the medical necessity of services

Messaging standards: Standards that support the uniform format and sequence of data during transmission from one healthcare entity to another; *Also called* **communication standards; transmission standards**

Minimum Data Set (MDS 3.0): A core set of screening, clinical, and functional status elements, including common definitions and coding categories, which forms the foundation of a comprehensive assessment for all residents of nursing homes certified to participate in Medicare or Medicaid

Morbidity: The state of being diseased (including illness, injury, or deviation from normal health); the number of sick persons or cases of disease in relation to a specific population

Mortality: 1. The incidence of death in a specific population 2. The loss of subjects during the course of a clinical research study; *Also called* **attrition**

National Alliance for Health Information Technology (NAHIT): A partnership of government and private sector leaders from various healthcare organizations that worked toward using technology to achieve improvements in patient safety, quality of care, and operating performance; founded in 2002; ceased operations in 2009

National Center for Complementary and Alternative Medicine (NCCAM): A resource for licensed complementary and alternative medicine practices, formed by the National Institutes of Health in the 1990s

National Centers for Health Statistics (NCHS): The federal agency responsible for collecting and disseminating information on health services utilization and the health status of the population in the United States; developed the clinical modification to the

International Classification of Diseases, Ninth Revision (ICD-9) and is responsible for updating the diagnosis portion of the ICD-9-CM

National Committee for Quality Assurance (NCQA): A private not-for-profit accreditation organization whose mission is to evaluate and report on the quality of managed care organizations in the United States

National Committee on Vital and Health Statistics (NCVHS): A public policy advisory board that recommends policy to the National Center for Health Statistics and other health-related federal programs

National Conference on Correctional Health Care (NCCHC): Organization that accredits approximately 500 federal and state correctional facilities, local jails, military jails, and juvenile correctional facilities

National Council for Prescription Drug Programs (NCPDP): A not-for-profit ANSI-accredited standards development organization founded in 1977 that develops standards for exchanging prescription and payment information

National health information infrastructure (NHII): An initiative set forth to improve the effectiveness, efficiency, and overall quality of health and healthcare in the United States; a comprehensive knowledge-based network of interoperable systems of clinical, public health, and personal health information that would improve decision-making by making health information available when and where it is needed; the set of technologies, standards, applications, systems, values, and laws that support all facets of individual health, healthcare, and public health

National Practitioner Data Bank (NPDB): A data bank established by the federal government through the 1986 Health Care Quality Improvement Act that contains information on professional review actions taken against physicians and other licensed healthcare practitioners that healthcare organizations are required to verify as part of the credentialing process

National Quality Forum: A private, not-for-profit membership organization created to develop and implement a nationwide strategy to improve the measurement and reporting of healthcare quality

National Resource Center for Health Information Technology: Organization that provides technical assistance for health information technology projects

National Vital Statistics System (NVSS): The oldest and most successful example of intergovernmental data sharing in public health, and the shared relationships, standards, and procedures that form the mechanism by which NCHS collects and disseminates the nation's official vital statistics. These data are provided through contracts between NCHS and vital registration systems operated in the various jurisdictions and legally responsible for the registration of vital events—births, deaths, marriages, divorces, and fetal deaths

Nationwide Health Information Network (NHIN): A set of standards, services, and policies that enable secure health information exchange over the Internet. The network provides a foundation for the exchange of health information across diverse entities, within communities, and across the country, helping to achieve the goals of the HITECH Act

Neurology report: Report describing the neurological status of patients

Notice of privacy practices: A statement (mandated by the HIPAA Privacy Rule) issued by a healthcare organization that informs individuals of the uses and disclosures of patient-identifiable health information that may be made by the organization, as well as the individual's rights and the organization's legal duties with respect to that information

Notifiable disease: A disease that must be reported to a government agency so that regular, frequent, and timely information on individual cases can be used to prevent and control future cases of the disease

Nurse practitioner (NP): A registered nurse (RN) with advanced training authorized to provide basic primary healthcare, diagnosing and treating common acute illnesses and injuries, including prescribing medications

Nursing assessment: The assessment performed by a nurse to obtain clinical and personal information about a patient shortly after he or she has been admitted to a nursing unit

Nursing facility: A comprehensive term for long-term care facilities that provide nursing care and related services on a 24-hour basis for residents requiring medical, nursing, or rehabilitative care

Nutritional assessment: The assessment performed by a registered dietitian to obtain information about a patient's diet history, weight and height, appetite and food preferences, and food sensitivities and allergies

OASIS: *See* **Outcomes and Assessment Information Set**

Office for Civil Rights (OCR): Department in HHS responsible for enforcing civil rights laws that prohibit discrimination on the basis of race, color, national origin, disability, age, sex, and religion by healthcare and human services entities over which OCR has jurisdiction, such as state and local social and health services agencies, and hospitals, clinics, nursing homes, or other entities receiving federal financial assistance from HHS. This office also has the authority to ensure and enforce the HIPAA Privacy and Security Rules; OCR is responsible for investigating all alleged violations of the Privacy and Security Rules

Office of the Inspector General (OIG): Mandated by Public Law 95-452 (as amended) to protect the integrity of Department of Health and Human Services (HHS) programs, as well as the health and welfare of the beneficiaries of those programs. The OIG has a responsibility to report both to the Secretary and to the Congress program and management problems and recommendations to correct them. The OIG's duties are carried out through a nationwide network of audits, investigations, inspections, and other mission-related functions performed by OIG components

Office of the National Coordinator for Health Information Technology (ONC): The principal federal entity charged with coordination of nationwide efforts to implement and use the most advanced health information technology and the electronic exchange of health information. The position of National Coordinator was created in 2004, through an Executive Order, and legislatively mandated in the Health Information Technology for Economic and Clinical Health Act (HITECH Act) of 2009

Omnibus Budget Reconciliation Act (OBRA) of 1987: Federal legislation passed in 1987 that required the Health Care Financing Administration (now renamed the Centers for Medicare and Medicaid Services) to develop an assessment instrument (called the resident assessment instrument) to standardize the collection of patient data from skilled nursing facilities

Ongoing records review: *See* **open-record review**

Open-record review: A review of the health records of patients currently in the hospital or under active treatment; part of the Joint Commission survey process

Operation index: A list of the operations and surgical procedures performed in a healthcare facility, which is sequenced according to the code numbers of the classification system in use

Operative report: A formal document that describes the events surrounding a surgical procedure or operation and identifies the principal participants in the surgery

ORYX: The Joint Commission's initiative that supports the integration of outcomes data and other performance measurement data into the accreditation process; often referred to as ORYX

Outcomes and Assessment Information Set (OASIS): A standard core assessment data tool developed to measure the outcomes of adult patients receiving home health services under the Medicare and Medicaid programs

Outcome: 1. The end result of healthcare treatment, which may be positive and appropriate or negative and diminishing 2. The performance (or nonperformance) of one or more processes, services, or activities by healthcare providers

Outcomes assessment: An evaluation that measures the actual outcomes of patient care and service against predetermined criteria (expected outcomes), based on the premise that care is delivered in order to bring about certain results; *Also called* **outcomes analysis**

Outpatient: A patient who receives ambulatory care services in a hospital-based clinic or department

Outpatient facility: A care facility that provides clients with access to a stable treatment provider on an outpatient basis; such care may occur in a formal office setting or in the patient's residence

Outpatient rehabilitation center (ORC): Facility that brings together specialized rehabilitation personnel to upgrade the physical functions of disabled individuals; staff must include a physician and provide services of physical therapists, occupational therapists, and speech therapists

Outstanding record policy: Policy that details the length of time for which a medical record can be kept in the clinic or physician's office

Partial stay: A program that provides individuals with mental health treatment that is more intense than the services provided on an outpatient basis; typically a four-hour-a-day, Monday through Friday program in which treatment may be provided in the morning, afternoon, or early evening

Pathology report: A type of health record or documentation that describes the results of a microscopic and macroscopic evaluation of a specimen removed or expelled during a surgical procedure

Patient assessment instrument (PAI): A standardized tool used to evaluate the patient's condition after admission to, and at discharge from, the healthcare facility

Patient-Centered Medical Home (PCMH): A program to provide comprehensive primary care that partners physicians with the patient and their family to allow better access to healthcare and improved outcomes

Patient outcome measures: The determined change in a patient's condition, calculated on a completed episode of care that begins with admission to a home health agency (or a resumption of care following an inpatient facility stay) and ends with discharge or transfer to an inpatient facility

Patient Protection and Affordable Care Act (PPACA): A federal statute that was signed into law on March 23, 2010. Along with the Health Care and Education Reconciliation Act of 2010 (signed into law on March 30, 2010), the Act is the product of the healthcare reform agenda of the Democratic 111th Congress and the Obama administration

Patient Self-Determination Act (PSDA): The federal legislation that requires healthcare facilities to provide written information on the patient's right to issue advance directives and to accept or refuse medical treatment

Patient-specific/identifiable data: 1. Data in the health record that relate to a particular patient identified by name 2. Personal information that can be linked to a specific patient, such as age, gender, date of birth, and address-specific data

Patient's rights: Rights conferred to Medicare patients by the Medicare Conditions of Participation, such as the right to receive accurate information, the right to choose healthcare providers, and the right to access emergency services.

Peer Review Act: A regulation enacted in 1982 to monitor the quality of care provided and the medical necessity of services

Performance improvement (PI): The continuous study and adaptation of a healthcare organization's functions and processes to increase the likelihood of achieving desired outcomes

Performance measurement: The process of comparing the outcomes of an organization, work unit, or employee against preestablished performance plans and standards

Periodic performance review (PPR): An organizational self-assessment conducted at the halfway point between triennial on-site accreditation surveys conducted by the Joint Commission

Personal health record (PHR): An electronic or paper health record maintained and updated by an individual for himself or herself; a tool that individuals can use to collect, track, and share past and current information about their health or the health of someone in their care

Physician assistant (PA): A healthcare professional licensed to practice medicine with physician supervision

Physician index: A list of patients and their physicians usually arranged according to the physician code numbers assigned by the healthcare facility

Physician's orders: A physician's written or verbal instructions to the other caregivers involved in a patient's care

Picture archiving and communication system (PACS): An integrated computer system that obtains, stores, retrieves, and displays digital images (in healthcare, radiological images)

Plan of care (POC): A term referring to Medicare home health services for homebound beneficiaries that must be delivered under a plan established by a physician

Policy: 1. Governing principle that describes how a department or an organization is supposed to handle a specific situation or execute a specific process 2. Binding contract issued by a healthcare insurance company to an individual or group in which the company promises to pay for healthcare to treat illness or injury; such contracts may also be referred to as **health plan agreements** and **evidence of coverage**

Population-based registry: A type of registry that includes information from more than one facility in a specific geopolitical area, such as a state or region

Population-based statistics: Statistics based on a defined population rather than on a sample drawn from the same population

Postoperative anesthesia record: Health record documentation that contains information on any unusual events or complications that occurred during surgery as well as information on the patient's condition at the conclusion of surgery and after recovery from anesthesia

Precise clinical documentation: Accurate, exact, and strictly defined documentation; one of the seven criteria for high-quality clinical documentation

Preoperative anesthesia evaluation: An assessment performed by an anesthesiologist to collect information on a patient's medical history and current physical and emotional condition that will become the basis of the anesthesia plan for the surgery to be performed

Prevalence rate: The proportion of people in a population who have a particular disease at a specific point in time or over a specified period of time

Primary care: The continuous and comprehensive care provided at first contact with the healthcare provider in an ambulatory care setting

Primary data: *See* **Patient-specific/identifiable data**

Primary data source (in healthcare): A record developed by healthcare professionals in the process of providing patient care

Principal diagnosis: The disease or condition that was present on admission, was the principal reason for admission, and received treatment or evaluation during the hospital stay or visit *or* the reason established after study to be chiefly responsible for occasioning the admission of the patient to the hospital for care

Principal procedure: The procedure performed for the definitive treatment of a condition (as opposed to a procedure performed for diagnostic or exploratory purposes) or for care of a complication

Priority focus area (PFA): One of 14 areas that the Joint Commission considers vital in the successful operation of a hospital; includes processes, systems, and structures that have a substantial effect on patient care services

Priority focus process (PFP): A process used by the Joint Commission to collect, analyze, and create information about a specific organization being accredited in order to customize the accreditation process

Privacy: The quality or state of being hidden from, or undisturbed by, the observation or activities of other persons, or freedom from unauthorized intrusion; in healthcare-related contexts, the right of a patient to control disclosure of protected health information

Privileged communication: The protection afforded to the recipients of professional services that prohibits medical practitioners, lawyers, and other professionals from disclosing the confidential information that they learn in their capacity as professional service providers

Problem list: A list of illnesses, injuries, and other factors that affect the health of an individual patient, usually identifying the time of occurrence or identification and resolution

Problem-oriented health record: Patient record in which clinical problems are defined and documented individually; *Also called* **problem-oriented medical record**

Procedural codes: The numeric or alphanumeric characters used to classify and report the medical procedures and services performed for patients

Procedure: 1. A document that describes the steps involved in performing a specific function 2. An action of a medical professional for treatment or diagnosis of a medical condition 3. The steps taken to implement a policy

Process notes: Psychotherapy notes that capture the therapist's impressions of the client, obtained during private, group, joint, or family counseling sessions; contain extended direct quotations from both client and therapist and include repeated references to insights discussed in the therapy sessions

Professional certification organizations: Private societies and membership organizations that establish professional qualification requirements and clinical practice standards for specific areas of medicine, nursing, and allied health professions

Progress notes: The documentation of a patient's care, treatment, and therapeutic response, which is entered into the health record by each of the clinical professionals involved in a patient's care, including nurses, physicians, therapists, and social workers

Prohibited abbreviations: Acronyms, abbreviations, and symbols that cannot be used in health records because they are prone to misinterpretation

Prospective Payment Act: A regulation enacted in 1982 to monitor the quality of care provided and the medical necessity of services

Prospective payment system (PPS): A type of reimbursement system that is based on preset payment levels rather than actual charges billed after the service has been provided; specifically, one of several Medicare reimbursement systems based on predetermined payment rates or periods and linked to the anticipated intensity of services delivered as well as the beneficiary's condition

Protected health information (PHI): Individually identifiable health information, transmitted electronically or maintained in any other form, that is created or received by a healthcare provider or any other entity subject to HIPAA requirements

Protocol: In healthcare, a detailed plan of care for a specific medical condition based on investigative studies; in medical research, a rule or procedure to be followed in a clinical trial; in a computer network, a rule or procedure used to address and ensure delivery of data

Public health: An area of healthcare that deals with the health of populations in geopolitical areas, such as states and counties

Qualitative analysis: A review of the health record to ensure that standards are met and to determine the adequacy of entries documenting the quality of care

Quality: The degree or grade of excellence of goods or services, including, in healthcare, meeting expectations for outcomes of care

Quality improvement organization (QIO): An organization that performs medical peer review of Medicare and Medicaid claims, including review of validity of hospital diagnosis and procedure coding information; completeness, adequacy, and quality of care; and appropriateness of prospective payments for outlier cases and nonemergent use of the emergency room. Until 2002, called peer review organization

Quality indicator: A standard against which actual care may be measured to identify a level of performance for that standard

Recovery audit contractor (RAC): A governmental program whose goal is to identify improper payments made on claims of healthcare services provided to Medicare beneficiaries. Improper payments may be overpayments or underpayments

Recovery room record: A type of health record documentation used by nurses to document the patient's reaction to anesthesia and condition after surgery; *Also called* recovery room report

Redisclosure: The release, transfer, provision of access to, or divulging in any other manner of patient health information that was generated by an external source to others outside of the organization and its workforce members

Regional health information organization (RHIO): A health information organization that brings together healthcare stakeholders within a defined geographic area and governs health information exchange among them for the purpose of improving health and care in the community

Regional home health intermediaries (RHHI): Private companies that contract with Medicare to pay home health bills and check on the quality of home healthcare

Registry: A collection of care information related to a specific disease, condition, or procedure that makes health record information available for analysis and comparison

Regulation: A rule established by an administrative agency of government. The difference between a statute and a regulation is regulations must be followed by any healthcare organization participating in the related program. Administrative agencies are responsible for implementing and managing the programs instituted by state and federal statutes

Rehabilitation care: The process of restoring the disabled insured to maximum physical, mental, and vocational independence and productivity (commensurate with their limitations) through the identification and development of residual capabilities, job modifications, or retraining

Reimbursement: Compensation or repayment for healthcare services

Release and disclosure: The processes that make health record information available to legitimate users

Release of information (ROI): The process of disclosing patient-identifiable information from the health record to another party

Request for anticipated payment (RAP): The first of two Centers for Medicare and Medicaid Services forms used at the opening of a prospective payment system episode to ask for one of two split-percentage payments; not a claim according to Medicare statutes

Research: An inquiry process aimed at discovering new information about a subject or revising old information. Investigation or experimentation aimed at the discovery and interpretation of facts, revision of accepted theories or laws in the light of new facts, or practical application of such new or revised theories or laws; the collecting of information about a particular subject

Resident assessment instrument (RAI): A uniform assessment instrument developed by the Centers for Medicare and Medicaid Services to standardize the collection of skilled nursing facility patient data; includes the Minimum Data Set 2.0, triggers, and resident assessment protocols; *See* **Minimum Data Set**

Resident assessment protocol (RAP): A summary of a long-term care resident's medical condition and care requirements

Residential program: A behavioral healthcare setting that offers daily professional treatment and provides a home-like environment for residents to build self-esteem, develop relationships, and improve life skills

Resource and Patient Management System (RPMS): The Indian Health Service's enterprise health information system; consists of more than 60 software applications and is used at approximately 400 IHS, tribal, and urban locations

Retail medical clinics: Clinics, often associated with national drugstore chains, at which patients are generally seen for minor complaints, flu shots, or physical exams; *Also referred to as* **convenient care clinics**

Retention: 1. Mechanisms for storing records, providing for timely retrieval, and establishing the length of times that various types of records will be retained by the healthcare organization 2. The ability to keep valuable employees from seeking employment elsewhere

Retrospective query: A question posed to the documenting or attending physician after the patient has been discharged to obtain additional, clarifying documentation to improve the specificity and completeness of the data used to assign diagnosis and procedure codes in the patient's health record

RHHI Outcomes and Assessment Information Set Verification (ROVER) protocol: An automated accuracy software application used to review home health claims submitted by home health agencies that are paid under the HHA prospective payment system; uses health records to verify that the information on an HHA-completed OASIS reflects the patient's condition and the services actually delivered during a particular episode

Risk-adjusted outcome: Measure of the change in a patient's condition during an episode of care by a home health agency, adjusted to compensate for differences in the patient population served by different home health agencies

Risk evaluation: The final step in the risk management process, which involves evaluating each piece of the process in order to determine whether objectives are being met

Risk prevention: One component of a successful risk management program

Secondary care: A general term for healthcare services provided by a specialist at the request of the primary care physician

Secondary data: Compiled information on groups of people or patients that does not identify any particular patient; *Also referred to as* **aggregate data**

Secondary data source: Data derived from the primary patient record, such as an index or a database

Secondary diagnosis: A statement of those conditions coexisting during a hospital episode that affect the treatment received or the length of stay

Sentinel event: According to the Joint Commission, an unexpected occurrence involving death or serious physical or psychological injury, or the risk thereof. Serious injury specifically includes loss of limb or function. The phrase "or risk thereof" includes any process variation for which a recurrence would carry a significant chance of serious adverse outcome. Such events are called "sentinel" because they signal the need for immediate investigation and response

Seven criteria for high-quality clinical documentation: Requirement for all entries in the patient record to be legible, reliable, precise, complete, consistent, clear, and timely

Severity of illness (SI or SOI): A type of supportive documentation reflecting objective clinical indicators of a patient illness (essentially the patient is sick enough to be at an identified level of care) and referring to the extent of physiologic decompensation or organ system loss of function

Shadow chart policy: Policy requiring that all original information and medical reports be kept in the medical record located in the HIM department; discourages physicians from keeping copies of records or reports in a shadow chart in their offices

Skilled-nursing care: The professional nursing care and related medical, therapeutic, psychosocial, and personal services provided in a residential setting to individuals recovering from injuries or illnesses or the residual effects of injuries or illnesses after the acute phase of the condition has resolved

Skilled nursing facility (SNF): A long-term care facility with an organized professional staff and permanent facilities (including inpatient beds) that provides continuous nursing and other health-related, psychosocial, and personal services to patients who are not in an acute phase of illness but who primarily require continued care on an inpatient basis

Source-oriented health record: A health record in which information is arranged according to the patient care department that provided the care

Source-system data: The data from which interpretations, summaries, and notes are derived; examples include radiological film or scans, laboratory values, pathology slides, video and audio recordings, and EKG tracings

Standards and Guidelines for the Accreditation of Managed Behavioral Health Organizations (MBHOs): Determined by the National Committee for Quality Assurance; outlines standards and features in-depth explanations and examples of how to meet the standards, accreditation scoring guidelines and points, and accreditation outcomes and reporting categories

Standing order: An order the medical staff or an individual physician has established as routine care for a specific diagnosis or procedure

State Operations Manual: Manual regulating the care provided in skilled nursing facilities

Statute: A piece of legislation written and approved by a state or federal legislature and then signed into law by the state's governor or the president

Statute of limitations: A specific time frame allowed by a statute or law for bringing litigation

Structure and content standards: Common data elements and definitions of the data elements to be included in an electronic patient record

Subacute care: A type of step-down care provided after a patient is released from an acute care hospital (including nursing homes and other facilities that provide medical care, but not surgical or emergency care)

Subpoena: A command to appear at a certain time and place to give testimony on a certain matter; *Also called* **subpoena ad testificandum**

Subpoena duces tecum: A written order commanding a person to appear, give testimony, and bring all documents, papers, books, and records described in the subpoena. The devices are used to obtain documents during pretrial discovery and to obtain testimony during trial

Substance Abuse and Mental Health Services Administration (SAMHSA): A division of the Department of Health and Human Services which in 2004 published a document explaining the relationship between HIPAA and the Alcohol and Drug Abuse Regulations regarding confidentiality and release of information

Summary list: *See* **problem list**

Surgical specialties: A group of clinical specialties that concentrates on the provision of surgical services by physicians who have received advanced training in obstetrics and gynecology, ophthalmology, orthopedics, cardiovascular surgery, otorhinolaryngology, trauma surgery, neurosurgery, thoracic surgery, urology, plastic and reconstructive surgery, anesthesiology, and pathology

Systematized Nomenclature of Medicine–Clinical Terms® (SNOMED CT®): A concept-based terminology consisting of more than 110,000 concepts with linkages to more than 180,000 terms with unique computer-readable codes

Tax Equity and Fiscal Responsibility Act of 1982 (TEFRA): The federal legislation that modified Medicare's retrospective reimbursement system for inpatient hospital stays by requiring implementation of diagnosis-related groups and the acute care prospective payment system

Technical standards: Rules for how EHR data must be transmitted from one computer system to another

Telemedicine: A telecommunications system that links healthcare organizations and patients from diverse geographic locations and transmits text and images for (medical) consultation and treatment; *Also called* **telehealth**

Telephone encounter: Advice or patient follow-up communicated via telephone

Tertiary care: Care centered on the provision of highly specialized and technologically advanced diagnostic and therapeutic services in inpatient and outpatient hospital settings

Third-party payer: An insurance company (for example, Blue Cross/Blue Shield) or healthcare program (for example, Medicare) that pays or reimburses healthcare providers (second party) and/or patients (first party) for the delivery of medical services

Tracer methodology: A process the Joint Commission surveyors use during the on-site survey to analyze an organization's systems, with particular attention to identified priority focus areas, by following individual patients through the organization's healthcare process in the sequence experienced by the patients; an evaluation that follows (traces) the hospital experiences of specific patients to assess the quality of patient care; part of the new Joint Commission survey processes

Transcriptionist: A specially trained typist who understands medical terminology and translates physicians' verbal dictation into written reports

Transfer record: A review of the patient's acute stay along with current status, discharge and transfer orders, and any additional instructions that accompanies the patient when he or she is transferred to another facility; *Also called a* referral form

Transfusion record: Health record documentation that includes information on the type and amount of blood products a patient received, the source of the blood products, and the patient's reaction to them

Unannounced survey: An on-site assessment conducted by The Joint Commission as part of a hospital's accreditation process

Uniform Ambulatory Care Data Set (UACDS): A data set developed by the National Committee on Vital and Health Statistics consisting of a minimum set of patient- or client-specific data elements to be collected in ambulatory care settings

Uniform Hospital Discharge Data Set (UHDDS): A core set of data elements adopted by the US Department of Health, Education, and Welfare in 1974 that are collected by hospitals on all discharges and all discharge abstract systems

Unique identifier: A type of information that refers to only one individual or organization

Urgent care center: A clinical setting that provides walk-in, extended-hour access for acute illness and injury care that is beyond the scope or availability of the typical primary care practice

Utilization management (UM): 1. A collection of systems and processes to ensure that facilities and resources, both human and nonhuman, are used maximally and are consistent with patient care needs 2. A program that evaluates the healthcare facility's efficiency in providing necessary care to patients in the most effective manner

Utilization review (UR): The process of determining whether the medical care provided to a specific patient is necessary according to preestablished objective screening criteria at time frames specified in the organization's utilization management plan

Veterans Health Information Systems and Technology Architecture (VistA): The EHR of the Veterans Administration Healthcare System; consists of an integrated system of software applications that directly supports patient care at Veterans Health Administration healthcare facilities

Veterans Health Administration (VHA): The component of the US Department of Veterans Affairs that implements the medical assistance program of the VA

Visit notes: The records of clinical observations of a patient in the hospital, recorded in chronological order by every physician and clinician who sees or treats the patient in an ambulatory setting; *Also referred to as* **encounter notes**

Vital statistics: Data related to births, deaths, marriages, and fetal deaths

Vocabulary standards: A list or collection of clinical words or phrases with their meanings; also, the set of words used by an individual or group within a particular subject field

Warehousing: The acquisition of all the business data and information from potentially multiple, cross-platform sources, such as legacy databases, departmental databases, and online transaction-based databases, and then the warehouse storage of all the data in one consistent format used to analyze data for decision-making purposes

Working documents: Administrative information that should not be considered part of the legal health record and should not be produced in response to a court order, subpoena, or request for the health record

World Health Organization (WHO): The United Nations specialized agency created to ensure the attainment by all peoples of the highest possible levels of health; responsible for a number of international classifications, including the International Statistical Classification of Diseases & Related Health Problems (ICD-10) and the International Classification of Functioning, Disability & Health (ICF)

Index

Page numbers followed by *t* indicate tables, charts, graphs, or reproductions of standard forms.

A

AAAASF. *See* American Association for Accreditation of Ambulatory Surgery Facilities

AAAHC. *See* Accreditation Association for Ambulatory Health Care

Abbreviations, 133, 325–326

ABMS (American Board of Medical Specialties), 654*t*–657*t*

Academic Consortium for Complementary and Alternative Health Care (ACCAHC), 662

Academic medical centers, 145

Access
consumer's right to, 103
federal laws, 48–49
issues for HIM professionals, 29
Joint Commission standards, 355
during transition from paper to EHRs, 362–366

Access control, 145

Accidents, in long-term care settings, 548

Accountable care organization (ACO), 74

Account numbers, 189

Accreditation, 432–477
acute care hospital requirements, 461–471
ambulatory care, 483–497, 665
AOA standards, 470–471
behavioral healthcare, 624–637, 642–643
CMS quality measures, 447–450
CMS regulations, 442–447
defined, 84, 461, 483
federal healthcare statutes, 436–441
federal patient safety legislation, 441–442
federal requirements for special health record protection, 454–457
federal/state general requirements, 434–436
healthcare corporate compliance, 451–454
home care/hospice, 553, 584, 590
internal hospital policies/procedures, 471–476
Joint Commission standards, 84, 462–470, 476
long-term care hospitals, 515–516
Medicaid eligibility/administration, 459–461
ORC, 671
origins of, 4
protection of EHRs, 355
skilled-nursing facilities, 545–546
state requirements, 457–461

Accreditation Association for Ambulatory Health Care (AAAHC), 12, 490–491, 666*t*

Accreditation Commission for Healthcare (ACHC), 495

Accreditation Manual for Ambulatory Care Organizations (Joint Commission), 485

Accreditation Manual for Ambulatory Surgical Centers (Joint Commission), 504

Accreditation organizations, 78. *See also specific organizations and programs, e.g.:* The Joint Commission

ACHC (Accreditation Commission for Healthcare), 495

Acknowledgments (term), 190

ACO (accountable care organization), 74

ACP (American College of Physicians), 11

ACR (American College of Radiology), 493–494, 667

Acronyms, 325–326

ACS (American College of Surgeons), 3

Active deployment (MPIs), 167–168, 179

T

W

Z